AF703933

Neurophysiology in Clinical Practice

Neurophysiology in Clinical Practice

Neurophysiology in Clinical Practice

Editor: Rosalyn Pryor

AMERICAN
MEDICAL PUBLISHERS
www.americanmedicalpublishers.com

AMERICAN
MEDICAL PUBLISHERS
www.americanmedicalpublishers.com

Cataloging-in-Publication Data

Neurophysiology in clinical practice / edited by Rosalyn Pryor.
p. cm.
Includes bibliographical references and index.
ISBN 979-8-88740-316-8
1. Neurophysiology. 2. Neurobiology. 3. Brain--Diseases. I. Pryor, Rosalyn.
QP355.2 .N48 2023
612.8--dc23

© American Medical Publishers, 2023

American Medical Publishers,
41 Flatbush Avenue,
1st Floor, New York,
NY 11217, USA

ISBN 979-8-88740-316-8 (Hardback)

This book contains information obtained from authentic and highly regarded sources. Copyright for all individual chapters remain with the respective authors as indicated. All chapters are published with permission under the Creative Commons Attribution License or equivalent. A wide variety of references are listed. Permission and sources are indicated; for detailed attributions, please refer to the permissions page and list of contributors. Reasonable efforts have been made to publish reliable data and information, but the authors, editors and publisher cannot assume any responsibility for the validity of all materials or the consequences of their use.

Trademark Notice: Registered trademark of products or corporate names are used only for explanation and identification without intent to infringe.

Contents

Contents

Preface

The branch of medical science which deals with the study of the function of the nervous system as well as its measurement and evaluation is known as neurophysiology. It lies at the intersection of neuroscience and physiology. It involves analysis of the functional properties of neurons, glia, and networks. Clinical neurophysiology focuses on the study of the central and peripheral nervous systems through the recording of bioelectrical activity. Some of the areas of study within this field are epilepsy, developmental clinical neurophysiology, psychophysiology and psychopathology, and motor control and movement disorders. This book is a valuable compilation of topics, ranging from the basic to the most complex advancements in the field of neurophysiology. Also included herein is a detailed explanation of the various concepts and clinical applications of this area of study. Students, researchers, and medical experts associated with neurology will benefit alike from this book.

The information shared in this book is based on empirical researches made by veterans in this field of study. The elaborative information provided in this book will help the readers further their scope of knowledge leading to advancements in this field.

Finally, I would like to thank my fellow researchers who gave constructive feedback and my family members who supported me at every step of my research.

Editor

1

Mapping and Analysis of the Connectome of Sympathetic Premotor Neurons in the Rostral Ventrolateral Medulla of the Rat Using a Volumetric Brain Atlas

*Bowen Dempsey[1], Sheng Le[1], Anita Turner[1], Phil Bokiniec[1], Radhika Ramadas[1], Jan G. Bjaalie[2], Clement Menuet[3], Rachael Neve[4], Andrew M. Allen[3], Ann K. Goodchild[1] and Simon McMullan[1]**

[1] Faculty of Medicine and Health Sciences, Neurobiology of Vital Systems, Macquarie University, Sydney, NSW, Australia, [2] Department of Anatomy, Institute of Basic Medical Sciences, University of Oslo, Oslo, Norway, [3] Department of Physiology, University of Melbourne, Melbourne, VIC, Australia, [4] Viral Core Facility, McGovern Institute for Brain Research, Massachusetts Institute of Technology, Cambridge, MA, USA

***Correspondence:**
Simon McMullan
simon.mcmullan@mq.edu.au

Spinally projecting neurons in the rostral ventrolateral medulla (RVLM) play a critical role in the generation of vasomotor sympathetic tone and are thought to receive convergent input from neurons at every level of the neuraxis; the factors that determine their ongoing activity remain unresolved. In this study we use a genetically restricted viral tracing strategy to definitively map their spatially diffuse connectome. We infected bulbospinal RVLM neurons with a recombinant rabies variant that drives reporter expression in monosynaptically connected input neurons and mapped their distribution using an MRI-based volumetric atlas and a novel image alignment and visualization tool that efficiently translates the positions of neurons captured in conventional photomicrographs to Cartesian coordinates. We identified prominent inputs from well-established neurohumoral and viscero-sympathetic sensory actuators, medullary autonomic and respiratory subnuclei, and supramedullary autonomic nuclei. The majority of inputs lay within the brainstem (88–94%), and included putative respiratory neurons in the pre-Bötzinger Complex and post-inspiratory complex that are therefore likely to underlie respiratory-sympathetic coupling. We also discovered a substantial and previously unrecognized input from the region immediately ventral to nucleus prepositus hypoglossi. In contrast, RVLM sympathetic premotor neurons were only sparsely innervated by suprapontine structures including the paraventricular nucleus, lateral hypothalamus, periaqueductal gray, and superior colliculus, and we found almost no evidence of direct inputs from the cortex or amygdala. Our approach can be used to quantify, standardize and share complete neuroanatomical datasets, and therefore provides researchers with a platform for presentation, analysis and independent reanalysis of connectomic data.

Keywords: connectome, RVLM, sympathetic, rabies, volumetric, segmentation, respiratory-sympathetic, mesoscale

INTRODUCTION

The nascent field of *connectomics* applies rapidly developing ultrastructural, trans-synaptic tracing, and whole brain imaging technologies to identify neural circuits at micro-, meso-, and macroscopic resolutions. The central tenet of the connectomic approach is that insights regarding both the functional properties of specific neural circuits and general brain organizational principles may be gained by definitively resolving network architecture (Carandini, 2012; Denk et al., 2012; Mitra, 2014).

Ultrastructural approaches such as serial block-face electron microscopy can comprehensively identify local synaptic connectivity, but are limited by the enormous time and costs associated with data acquisition and analysis, and are therefore best suited to the examination of small regions of brain in high detail (discussed by Lichtman and Denk, 2011; Wanner et al., 2015). Investigators interested in mapping more diffuse circuits have instead monitored the trans-synaptic spread of replication-competent neurotropic viruses such as rabies (Ugolini, 1995; Kelly and Strick, 2000; Dum et al., 2016) and alpha herpes variants (Strack et al., 1989; Rinaman and Schwartz, 2004; McGovern et al., 2012; reviewed by Nassi et al., 2015; Wojaczynski et al., 2015).

In recent years glycoprotein-deleted EnvA-pseudotyped rabies [SADΔG(EnvA)] has emerged as a flagship tool for tracing connectomes in experimental animals (Wickersham et al., 2007b; Callaway and Luo, 2015). The key insights made by Callaway and colleagues in developing this system are that the ability of SADΔG(EnvA) to enter populations of target neurons and retrogradely spread to monosynaptically connected partners can be controlled by selective expression of the EnvA receptor, TVA, and the rabies glycoprotein respectively. Here we apply this approach to resolve the afferent connectome of putative sympathetic premotor neurons in the rostral ventrolateral medulla (RVLM) of the Sprague Dawley rat.

This population, approximately half of which are adrenergic C1 neurons (Stornetta, 2009), is a major source of the glutamatergic drive that maintains sympathetic vasomotor tone and therefore determines arterial blood pressure (Guyenet, 2006). The factors that determine the ongoing activity of these neurons have for several decades remained an unresolved core issue in the field of autonomic neuroscience (Coote, 2007; Guyenet et al., 2013): electrophysiological recordings from anesthetized animals suggest that RVLM sympathetic premotor neurons are a point of convergence for inputs from visceral and somatic reflex pathways (Brown and Guyenet, 1984; McMullan et al., 2008), from the central respiratory pattern generator (McAllen, 1987; Miyawaki et al., 1995; Verberne et al., 1999; Moraes et al., 2013), hypothalamus (Yang and Coote, 1998; Allen, 2002; Horiuchi et al., 2004; Korim et al., 2014), and higher centers including the prefrontal cortex and amygdala (Gelsema et al., 1989; Verberne, 1996), and that ongoing synaptic drive supports their activity (Lipski et al., 1996). However, the relative contributions of inputs from these regions, and in particular the level of input derived from local medullary neurons, has remained elusive.

Our strategy was first to use a recombinant herpes vector with a retrograde transduction profile, HSV-hCMV-YTB, to drive the expression of TVA, rabies glycoprotein, and a fluorescent reporter (YFP) in neurons that project to the interomediolateral cell column of the spinal cord (IML), a major site of termination of sympathetic premotor neurons. We then focally microinjected SADΔG(EnvA)-mCherry into the RVLM, selectively restricting its access to TVA-expressing bulbospinal neurons. This enabled us to map brain-wide sources of synaptic input to bulbospinal RVLM neurons using an image alignment tool based on the Waxholm volumetric atlas of the rat brain (Papp et al., 2014; Kjonigsen et al., 2015).

MATERIALS AND METHODS

Experiments were approved by Macquarie University Animal Ethics Committee and conformed to the Australian Code of Practice for the Care and Use of Animals for Scientific Purposes.

Vector Preparation

SADΔG Production

Rabies glycoprotein-transcomplemented SADΔG-mCherry (Wickersham et al., 2007a) and SADΔG(EnvA)-mCherry was produced and titrated as described by Osakada and Callaway (2013); the titers used for injections were 2×10^9 and 6.8×10^7 IU/ml respectively. SADΔG(EnvA)-mCherry purity was determined by infection of naïve HEK cells and determined to contain approximately 5.3×10^3 unpseudotyped virions per ml. Injection of SADΔG(EnvA)-mCherry in the absence of YTB expression resulted in no labeling in two control experiments.

Retrograde HSV Vectors

A recombinant herpes simplex type1 (HSV) vector with a retrograde tropism was used to drive expression of rabies glycoprotein, TVA, and YFP (HSV-hCMV-YTB). The gene cassette was derived from the pCAG-YTB plasmid (Addgene 26721) and cloned into recombinant HSV amplicons under the control of the human cytomegalovirus promoter. HSV-hCMV-YTB was supplied at 3×10^8 IU/ml and diluted 1:4 with 0.9% saline containing blue fluorescent polystyrene spheres immediately prior to injection to mark the injection site (1:10,000, Thermo Scientific, Australia, 09980508). Control vectors that drive the expression of reporter proteins (HSV-hCMV-GFP, HSV-hCMV-mCherry) were used in initial experiments to determine the time course of protein translation and segment the anatomical boundary of the RVLM. Control vectors were used undiluted and animals sacrificed after 4–5 days.

Vector Injections

Spinal Cord Injections of Retrograde Herpes Vectors

Adult male Sprague Dawley rats (165–500 g) were anesthetized with intraperitoneal ketamine (75 mg/kg; Parnell Laboratories, Australia) mixed with medetomidine (0.75 mg/kg; Pfizer Animal Health, Australia) and treated with prophylactic antibiotics (100 mg/kg Cephazolin sodium, i.m.; Mayne Pharma, Australia) and analgesia (2.5–10 mg/kg Carprofen, s.c.; Norbrook Pharmaceuticals, Australia). Two 500 nl injections of HSV-hCMV-YTB were made over 5–10 min at coordinates corresponding to the left T2 IML as previously described (Turner et al., 2013). Injections were separated by 1 mm rostrocaudally and the pipette was left in position after injections for approximately 5 min before its slow retraction. At the end of surgery anesthesia was reversed with atipamazole (1 mg/kg s.c., Pfizer Animal Health, Australia) and rats were observed until ambulatory and then returned to their home cages. Rats were monitored closely for the remainder of the experiment with additional analgesia as required. For experiments in which HSV-hCMV-GFP/mCherry control vectors were used the same general surgical approach was employed, but vector injections were made bilaterally at the T2 and/or T10 spinal cord.

Brainstem Microinjections

One to five days after injection of HSV-hCMV-YTB rats were prepared for surgery as described above and positioned in a stereotaxic frame in the skull flat position. The left facial nucleus, an anatomical landmark directly rostral to the RVLM, was mapped using a micropipette containing SADΔG(EnvA)-mCherry by recording antidromic field potentials evoked by stimulation of the facial nerve (Turner et al., 2013). Fifty to seventy five nl of SADΔG(EnvA)-mCherry was microinjected 100–300 μm caudal to the facial nucleus at a depth equivalent to the ventral surface of the facial nucleus. The pipette was left in position for ~5 min prior to its withdrawal. Rats were treated as described above and allowed to recover for up to 7 days.

In initial experiments we observed histological signs of injury in HSV-hCMV-YTB-transduced neurons that were independent of rabies infection. Neurons developed a blebby appearance with retracted dendrites and spheroidal somata about 7 days after spinal injections, suggesting latent toxicity of the HSV vector. This effect was largely mitigated by dilution of HSV-hCMV-YTB.

We also found that longer intervals between HSV and rabies injections were associated with more off-target infection of bulbospinal (TVA-expressing) neurons outside of the RVLM (especially the paraventricular nucleus, midline raphe, rostral ventromedial medulla and C3 regions). Such neurons were easily identified by their dual expression of mCherry and YFP: contaminated experiments were excluded from analysis. Optimal results were obtained when SADΔG(EnvA)-mCherry was injected 24 h after HSV-hCMV-YTB and animals kept for a further 6 days.

Histology

Animals were euthanized with sodium pentobarbital (>150 mg/kg, Lethabarb, Virbac, Australia) and immediately transcardially perfused with 300 ml ice cold heparinized saline followed by 300 ml 4% paraformaldehyde. The brain and thoracic spinal cord were then removed and post-fixed overnight. With the assistance of a brain matrix, brains were cut coronally 2 mm caudal to the olfactory bulb and mounted frontal pole down on a vibratome plate so that the ventral surface of the brain was approximately perpendicular to the plate. The entire brain was sectioned at 50 μm in the coronal plane using a Leica VT1200S vibrating microtome and collected in 4 bins in 0.01 M Tris-phosphate buffered saline (TPBS). Pot 1 was mounted directly onto glass slides to maintain section order. Brainstem sections from a second pot were processed for YFP and TH immunoreactivity so that starter neurons could be identified. The other pots were transferred to cryoprotectant solution (500 μM polyvinylpyrrolidone, 76.7 mM Na_2HPO_4, 26.6 mM NaH_2PO_4, 876 mM sucrose, 5 mM ethylene glycol) for storage at − 20°C.

Immunohistochemistry and *In situ* Hybridization

Sections were permeabilized in TPBS containing 0.2% Triton-100 for 3 × 15 min and blocked for nonspecific binding in TPBS containing 2% bovine serum albumin and 0.2% Triton-100 for 1 h at room temperature. Primary antibodies (see **Table 1**) were added to the blocking buffer and sections were incubated for 48 h at 4°C. Sections were washed in TPBS 3 × 30 min and incubated in secondary antibodies for 12 h at 4°C. Processed sections were washed again in TPBS 3 × 30 min before being mounted on glass slides with Dako fluorescence mounting medium and cover slipped. ISH was conducted to examine double labeling of rabies-infected input neurons with GAD67 mRNA, a marker of GABAergic neurons, and GLYT2 mRNA, a marker of glycinergic neurons. ISH probes and processing were identical to those described by Bowman et al. (2013) and Le et al. (2016) respectively.

Imaging

For whole-brain mapping of rabies-infected neurons every 4th histological section lying between the cervical spinal cord and the most rostral section containing labeled neurons was imaged under epifluorescence (Zeiss AxioImager Z2 microscope, 10x/0.30 NA M27 objective lens running ZEN 2011). Images were obtained from sections that were immediately mounted during cutting, preserving order, except for sections from the RVLM region; these data were obtained from alternative sections that were processed for YFP and TH immunoreactivity. Neurons that contained both YFP and mCherry were classified as starter neurons and were further sub-classified as TH-immunoreactive (C1) or TH-negative (non-C1). Input neurons and C1/non-C1 starter neurons were manually annotated on each image using Zen software; the pixel coordinates of annotated neurons were then extracted from file metadata using the ImageJ/FIJI package (NIH, Bethesda, Maryland, USA) and tabulated.

Epifluorescence imaging at 10x permitted efficient imaging of whole-brain datasets at the expense of sensitivity, biasing against lightly labeled or small neurons. This was particularly problematic for detection of lightly-labeled TH-immunoreactive starter neurons; confocal reimaging (20x objective, Leica TCS SP5X) of three sections containing starter neurons previously imaged and analyzed as described above indicated that approximately a third of the C1 starter neurons detected under confocal had been identified as non-C1 under epifluorescence (19/27 vs. 13/27). This problem did not apply to detection of rabies-infected neurons, which were unambiguously labeled.

Image Alignment and Anchoring

Image alignment and anchoring was achieved using a beta version of the AligNII tool embedded in Navigator-3 (N3), a web-based data management system currently under development of the University of Oslo Neuroinformatics group (see Figure 5

TABLE 1 | Antibody Table.

Type	Antigen	Species	Tag	Conc.	Clonality	Manufacturer	Cat No./RRID
1°	TH	Mouse	N/A	1:1000	Mono	Sigma	T1299/AB_477560
1°	NK1R	Rabbit	N/A	1:1000	Poly	Sigma	S8305/AB_261562
1°	Vasopressin	Rabbit	N/A	1:1000	Poly	Millipore	AB1565/AB_11212336
1°	Choline Acetyltransferase (ChAT)	Goat	n/a	1:800	Poly	Chemicon, Millipore	AB144P/AB_2079751
1°	GFP	Rabbit	N/A	1:500	Poly	Life Technologies	A6455/AB_2313717
2°	Rabbit IgG (H+L chain)	Donkey	Alexa Fluor® 488	1:500	Poly	Life Technologies	A21206/AB_141708
2°	Rabbit IgG (H+L chain)	Donkey	Alexa Fluor® 647	1:500	Poly	Life Technologies	A31573/AB_10561706
2°	Mouse IgG (H+L chain)	Donkey	Alexa Fluor® 647	1:500	Poly	Life Technologies	A31571/AB_162542
2°	Sheep IgG (H+L chain)	Donkey	Alexa Fluor® 647	1:500	Poly	Jackson Immunoresearch	713-605-003/AB_2340750

in Papp et al., 2016). An overview of the image alignment workflow is provided in **Figure 1**: microscope images were contrast-optimized for differentiation of gray and white matter and uploaded to N3 where the section images were overlaid onto virtual sections of the Waxholm atlas template, a whole brain MRI dataset obtained from a male Sprague Dawley rat (Papp et al., 2014). The cut angle of the MRI dataset was manually adjusted to match the histological section, allowing the user to align histological sections cut at any plane to the reference dataset and therefore compensating for deviations from standard cutting planes or tissue distortion. Once each image was optimally aligned to its MRI equivalent the image was considered "anchored"; geometric vectors corresponding to the rostrocaudal level of the image origin, deviation from the vertical and horizontal planes, scaling and rotation were calculated by the anchoring tool in the N3 platform and exported as metadata. With this information the position of any point in a histological image could be converted to 3-dimensional Waxholm coordinates in Microsoft Excel. Waxholm coordinates are by convention presented in the xyz format (lateral, rostrocaudal, dorsoventral) with a voxel resolution of 39 μm. The interested reader is directed toward CutNii, a freely downloadable explorer and custom-angle slicer for the Waxholm dataset (Csucs and Bjaalie, 2015), which is similar to the N3 tool used for image alignment (although it does not allow overlay or anchoring of histological images).

Volumetric Brain Modeling

The raw MRI data and corresponding segmentation model of the Waxholm Sprague Dawley rat were downloaded from the International Neuroinformatics Coordinating Facility Software Center (Papp et al., 2015) and imported into Imaris volumetric imaging software (Version 8.1, Bitplane AG, Switzerland) following conversion to the Biorad format in ImageJ. Each segmented area was individually rendered using the Imaris "contour surface" function, resulting in a surface-rendered model that incorporates regions demarcated in Waxholm space. Tabulated Waxholm coordinates of Input, non-C1 starter, and C1 starter neurons were then imported using a Python script (*"CreateSpotsFromFile,"* http://open.bitplane.com/tabid/235/Default.aspx?id=70), resulting in a 3d model of the Waxholm brain populated with points corresponding to identified neurons. Another script was then used to automatically quantify the number of input neurons that lay within each segmented region (*"Spots split into surface objects,"* http://open.bitplane.com/tabid/235/Default.aspx?id=19). The Imaris-rendered Waxholm brain (containing the RVLM connectomic dataset) is available as a supplementary download and can be used freely by other researchers (http://datadryad.org/resource/doi:10.5061/dryad.q5t5s). The dataset can also be viewed with the free Imaris SceneViewer program (www.bitplane.com). The voxel coordinates of starter and input neurons are included in tabulated format in **Data Sheet 1**.

Segmentation of the Facial Nucleus, RVLM, Bötzinger and Pre-Bötzinger Complex in Waxholm Space

The Waxholm segmentation model does not differentiate brainstem subnuclei, so we used the locations of bulbospinal TH-immunoreactive RVLM neurons as the basis for segmentation of the RVLM. Data were obtained from six rats in which neurons projecting to the T2 and/or T10 spinal segments were retrogradely labeled by HSV-hCMV-GFP or -mCherry control vectors. Vector injections and histology were conducted as described above and 273 TH-positive bulbospinal RVLM neurons were annotated and anchored in Waxholm space. The lateral coordinates of all neurons were represented as being on *both* sides of the brainstem for segmentation; two-dimensional contour maps indicating the density of labeling were then generated for each dorsoventral level using the Plotly visualization tool (https://plot.ly, 10 voxel resolution). Contours enclosing pixels that contained >2 neurons/10 pixel radius in the horizontal plane were converted to an image stack, imported into the virtual Waxholm rat brain using Imaris, and surface rendered to define the boundaries of the RVLM (**Video 1**).

The extent of the facial nucleus was annotated directly from the Waxholm MRI dataset in Imaris; the Bötzinger and pre-Bötzinger Complex were defined as longitudinal cylinders, 500 μm in diameter that ran center-aligned and immediately ventral to nucleus ambiguus. The Bötzinger region was defined as starting at the caudal pole of the facial nucleus and running 600 μm caudal; the pre-Bötzinger Complex was defined as

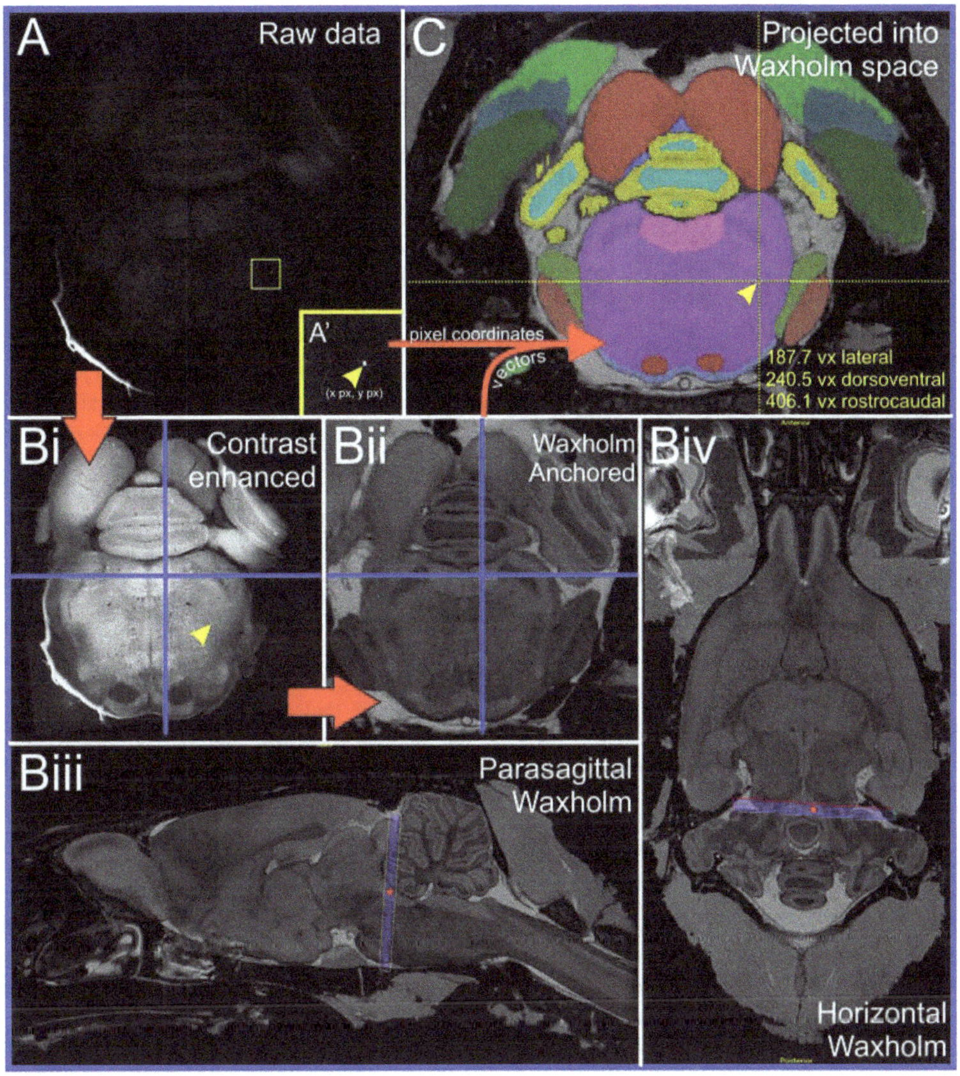

FIGURE 1 | Anchoring workflow. (A) Original coronal epifluorescence image showing the location of a single rabies-labeled input neuron (yellow box, inset in **A'**). Following manual annotation, the pixel coordinates of the neuron were exported to a spreadsheet and the image contrast adjusted for optimal visualization of anatomical landmarks **(Bi)**. The image was then aligned to a corresponding section plane through the Waxholm atlas template **(Bii)** using a beta version of an image alignment/anchoring tool embedded in the Navigator-3 system. The anchoring tool allowed accurate positioning of the image plane in the MRI-derived atlas template. The orientation of the plane of the image is close to coronal, as shown in the blue frames in **(Biii)** and **(Biv)**. The parasagittal plane through the atlas template shown in **(Biii)** corresponds to the vertical blue line in **(Bi)** and **(Bii)**, whereas the horizontal plane in **(Biv)** corresponds to the horizontal blue lines in **(Bi)** and **(Bii)**. The red dots in **(Biii)** and **(Biv)** represent the intersections with the horizontal and parasagittal planes, respectively. Anchoring vectors generated by Navigator-3 were then used to translate the pixel co-ordinates of annotated neurons into xyz Waxholm coordinates and integrated into the Waxholm segmentation model **(C)**.

running between 700 and 1200 μm caudal to the facial nucleus (Le et al., 2016).

Cluster Analysis

K-means analysis was used to partition groups of input neurons based on their 3d distribution. The algorithm determines clusters by assigning data points to a closest mean (centroid), assigned initially at random and iteratively refined as data points are sequentially accumulated within a cluster. Analysis was performed and density plots generated in "R project" (R Foundation for Statistical Computing, Vienna, Austria, 2005, http://www.r-project.org). The voxel coordinates of input neurons segregated by cluster are provided in **Data Sheet 2**.

RESULTS

Retrograde Transduction of Spinally Projecting Neurons and Segmentation of the RVLM in Waxholm-Space

Microinjection of HSV vectors at the thoracic spinal cord drove reporter expression in bulbospinal neurons within

12 h, with maximal expression apparent by 2-4 days. Reporter-labeled neurons spanned the RVLM, rostral ventromedial medulla (RVMM), and midline raphe region, and were identified in other sympathetic premotor nuclei such as the C3, paraventricular, A5, and locus coeruleus (**Supplementary Image 1**).

The distribution of TH-immunoreactive neurons labeled by HSV control vectors was plotted in Waxholm co-ordinates (**Figure 1**) and was used to define the anatomical boundaries of the RVLM (**Supplementary Image 1**). The geometric epicenter was located at Waxholm coordinates 198 lateral, 313 rostrocaudal, 182 dorsoventral (**Supplementary Images 1D–F**), corresponding to a position 1.78 mm lateral to the midline, 117 μm rostral to the caudal pole of the facial nucleus, and 339 μm dorsal to the ventral surface of the medulla immediately beneath the epicenter. The segmentation defined a dorsoventrally flattened ovoid (**Supplementary Images 1G–I**) in which the long axis runs medial in more rostral sections and spans Waxholm coordinates 176–218 lateral (2.6–1 mm lateral to midline), 287–327 rostrocaudal (900 μm caudal to 663 μm rostral to caudal pole of the facial nucleus) and 174–198 dorsoventral (within 897 μm from the ventral surface of the brainstem). This region contained 86% of TH-positive bulbospinal neurons used to generate the segmentation ($n = 236$) and corresponds well with the pressor region that encompasses the rostral RVLM and perifacial zone (Goodchild and Moon, 2009).

Monosynaptic Tracing Was Predominantly Restricted to Putative RVLM Sympathetic Premotor Neurons

Data from 4 animals were selected for detailed connectomic analysis. As illustrated in **Supplementary Image 2**, unilateral injection of HSV-hCMV-YTB directed at the second thoracic (T2) IML resulted in retrograde transduction of bulbospinal neurons in the ventrolateral medulla, the majority of which were ipsilateral to the injection site (82% (71–88) [mean (range), $n =$ 4 rats]). Subsequent injection of SADΔG(EnvA)-mCherry in the RVLM resulted in the primary infection of bulbospinal RVLM neurons. As shown in **Figure 2**, bulbospinal "starter" neurons were identified by their co-expression of YFP and mCherry and many were immunoreactive for TH (**Figure 2B'**).

Neurons were counted on every fourth section: on average 38 starter neurons were identified per animal (range: 19–67), of which 40% (30–45) were confirmed as TH-positive C1 neurons under epifluorescence (which underrepresents the proportion of C1 starter neurons by up to 50%: see Methods–Imaging). Seventy eight percent (74–87%) of starter neurons lay within the Waxholm RVLM boundary defined above (**Figure 2C**). Ectopic starter neurons that fell outside the RVLM were observed around the lateral and dorsal perimeter of the facial nucleus and adjacent sympathetic premotor nuclei which included the rostral ventromedial medulla (RVMM), caudal raphe and contralateral RVLM. **Video 1** shows the Waxholm MRI dataset overlaid with the distribution of C1 and non-C1 starter neurons from 4 rats subjected to detailed analysis, along with the boundary of the RVLM region.

Inputs to Putative RVLM Sympathetic Premotor Neurons Predominantly Arise from Medullary Nuclei

Monosynaptic input neurons were identified throughout the brain as mCherry, non-YFP neurons. 1298 input neurons were identified in total [325 (220–561) per animal], corresponding to an input: starter ratio of 9.8 (4.4–13.4). The overall distribution of input neurons is shown in **Figures 3A,B**: although the absolute number of input neurons and efficiency of trans-synaptic spread was variable, the overall pattern of inputs was consistent between animals: input neurons were encountered from the most caudal point quantified, the cervical medullary junction, to the hypothalamus at the level of the optic chiasm, with a pronounced [77% (75–80)] ipsilateral bias. Nodal edge-length analysis (the shortest distance between each neuron and the epicenter of the RVLM) indicates that most input neurons lie in close proximity to the RVLM, with 50% of inputs residing within 2.5 mm (2.3–2.7) with a progressively diminishing proportion of inputs identified at increasing distances: only 10% of monosynaptic input neurons lie more than 5 mm from the RVLM (**Figure 3C**). Input neurons were also distributed throughout the thoracic and cervical spinal cord, although these data were not quantified.

A script that automatically counts the number of neurons within each region of the Waxholm atlas was used to quantify the regional distribution of input neurons. These data are graphically represented in **Figure 4** and tabulated in **Table S1**: the overwhelming majority of inputs resided within the Waxholm-defined boundary of the brainstem 92% (88–94), with inputs arising from the forebrain and midbrain accounting for 3% each and the remainder originating in the cervical spinal cord and cerebellum. Sub-nuclei of the brainstem are not well represented in the current iteration of the Waxholm atlas; of those regions thus far defined the highest source of input was the RVLM itself, which contained 14% of input neurons.

K-means analysis was used to objectively group input neurons based on their spatial distribution. We empirically determined that 12 was an appropriate number of clusters (k) by which to partition the dataset by plotting the percentage of variance explained by clusters generated for k-values 1–20 and identifying a point at which the increase in explained variance was marginal for further increases in k, denoted by an "elbow" in the curve (**Figure 3Dii**, inset). The 12 clusters identified accounted for 89.3% of variance in the dataset (**Figure 3**); a detailed overview of identified clusters and their correspondence to the literature is presented in **Table S2.** Eight of 12 input clusters were located within the medulla, the largest of which (Cluster 2) encompassed the ipsilateral RVLM (including occasional trans-synaptically labeled C1 neurons: **Figure 2B**), Bötzinger region (**Figure 5D**), nucleus ambiguus (**Figure 5G**), and choline acetyltransferase (ChAT)-immunoreactive cells in a region of the ventral lateral tegmental field (**Figure 6A**) that may represent the rat analog of the post-inspiratory complex (PiCo: Anderson et al., 2016). In a sample of 21 input neurons identified as lying within the Bötzinger region using previously published criteria (Le et al., 2016), none contained glycine

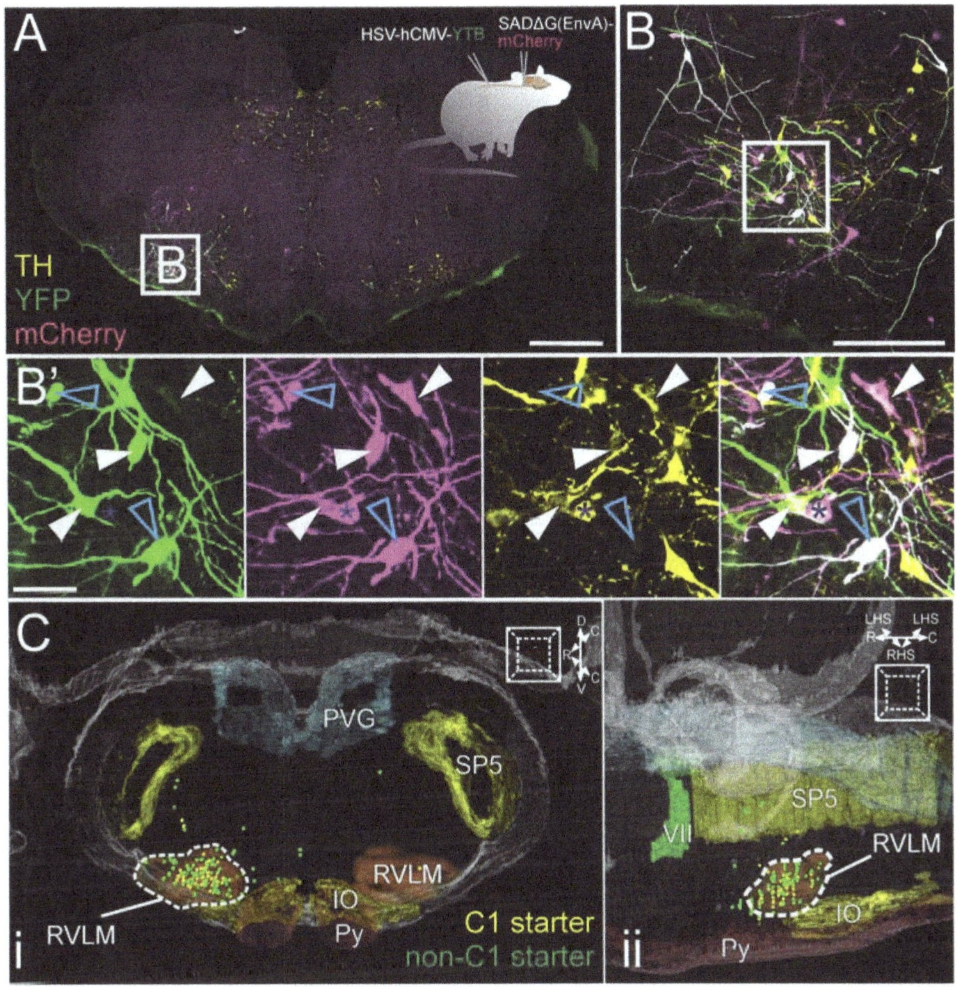

FIGURE 2 | Experimental strategy (inset in A): HSV-hCMV-YTB was injected at the T2 IML, retrogradely driving the expression of TVA, rabies glycoprotein, and YFP in spinally projecting neurons. SADΔG(EnvA)-mCherry was subsequently injected into the RVLM, exclusively infecting neurons that express TVA, and seeding trans-synaptic infection of monosynaptically connected input neurons. **(A)** Coronal brainstem section at the level of the rostral ventrolateral medulla (RVLM) processed for immunoreactivity to TH and YFP; starter neurons are defined by the expression of both YFP and mCherry. **(B)** Confocal detail with magnified **(B')** examples of C1 (solid arrowheads) and non-C1 (cyan arrowheads) starter neurons (individual channels and merged image). Blue asterisk indicates a C1 input neuron. **(C)** Distribution of C1 (yellow) and non-C1 (green) starter neurons from four experiments plotted in Waxholm space, shown from coronal **(Ci)** and parasagittal **(Cii)** perspectives. Anatomical landmarks are Waxholm-segmented boundaries of the inferior olive (IO), spinal trigeminal nucleus (SP5), RVLM, pyramidal tract (Py), facial nerve (VII), and periventricular gray (PVG). Scale bars 1000 μm **(A)**, 250 μm **(B)**, and 100 μm **(B')**.

transporter 2 mRNA, a marker for respiratory function in this region (**Figure 6B**, Schreihofer et al., 1999). Adjacent clusters enveloped the dorsal LTF (Cluster 3) and pre-Bötzinger Complex (Cluster 4, **Figure 5E**), including neurokinin-1 receptor (NK1R) immunoreactive neurons (**Figure 6C**), a putative marker for respiratory function in this region (Gray et al., 2001). Cluster 4 also spanned the rostral ventral respiratory group and caudal ventrolateral medulla (CVLM: **Figure 5A**), including confirmed GABAergic CVLM neurons (**Figure 6D**). Input clusters also included the rostral ventromedial medulla and caudal Raphe nuclei (Cluster 7) and a distinct input from the region immediately ventral to the nucleus prepositus hypoglossi (Cluster 9, **Figure 5B**). Other brainstem clusters spanned the intermediate and commissural nucleus of the solitary tract (NTS: **Figure 5C**, Cluster 6), the caudal pressor area and caudal ventral respiratory group (Cluster 10), and the ventral aspect of the contralateral medulla (Cluster 5). A flythrough of the entire dataset, projected onto the MRI Waxholm dataset and segregated by color into its component clusters, is presented in **Video 2**.

Supramedullary Nuclei Constitute a Minor Source of Input to RVLM Sympathetic Premotor Neurons

Supramedullary inputs included diffuse pontine clusters that encompassed the ipsilateral (Cluster 1) and contralateral (Cluster 11) A5 adrenergic cell group, subcoeruleus, Kölliker-Fuse, and medial and lateral parabrachial nuclei. The single midbrain

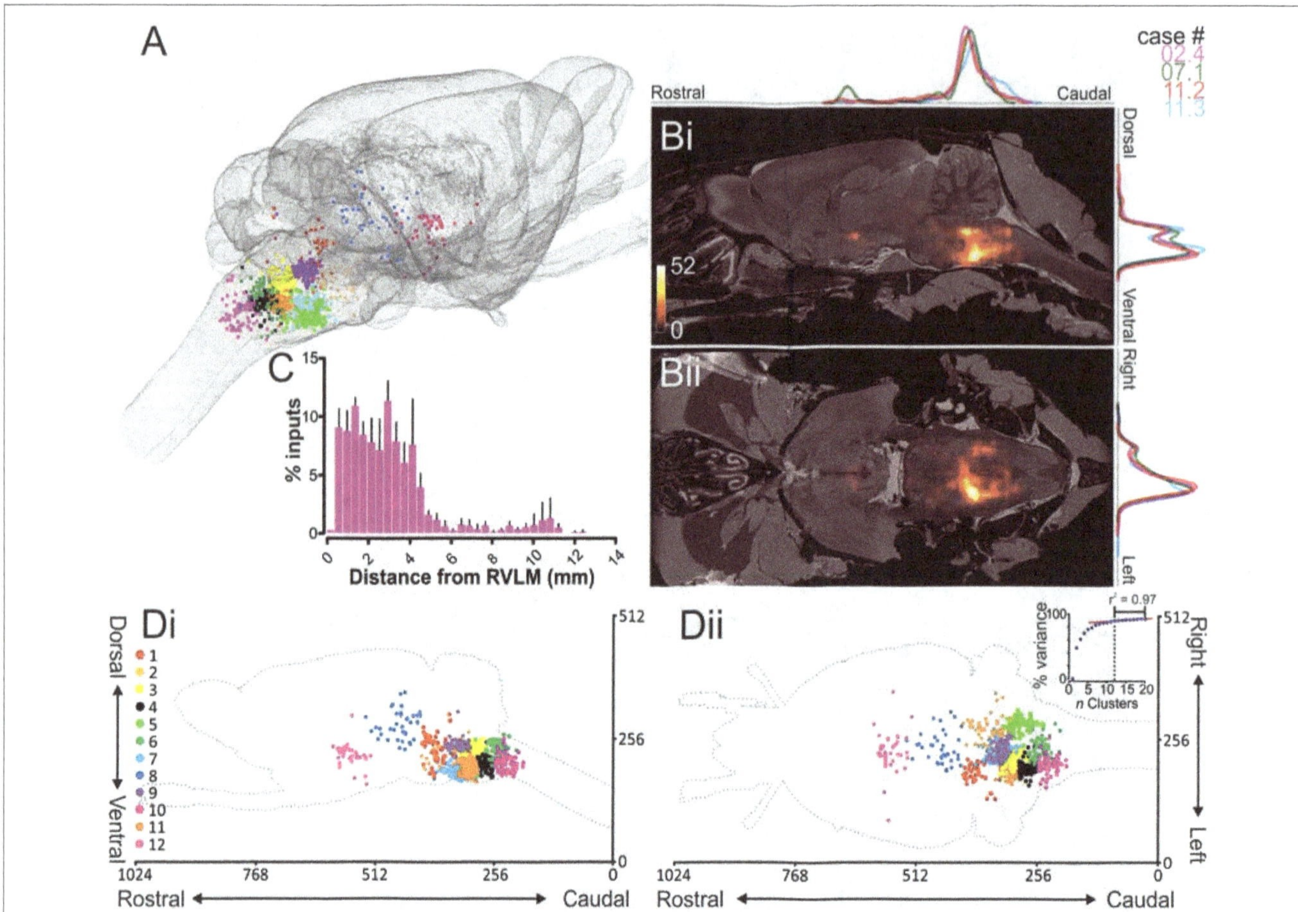

FIGURE 3 | Distribution of monosynaptic input neurons. (A) Input neurons to putative sympathetic premotor neurons in the rostral ventrolateral medulla (RVLM) segregated into 12 distinct clusters and plotted in the Waxholm volumetric rat atlas. **(B)** Heat maps showing input neuron density overlaid on the Waxholm MRI dataset in the parasagittal **(i)** and horizontal **(ii)** planes. Scale indicates number of neurons per 10 voxels. Normalized plots of input densities for individual experiments are plotted alongside heat maps. **(C)** Absolute distance of input neurons from RVLM epicenter ($n = 4$ rats). **(D)** Cluster plots presented in the sagittal **(i)** and horizontal **(ii)** planes. Inset in **(Dii)** shows the proportion of total variance accounted for by incremental increases in cluster number; the turning point of the curve, after which slope becomes linear, occurs at 12 clusters.

cluster (Cluster 8) incorporated the lateral and ventrolateral periaqueductal gray (PAG) and colliculi, and a hypothalamic cluster (Cluster 12) composed from neurons residing within the paraventricular hypothalamic nucleus, including confirmed vasopressinergic neurons (**Figures 5F, 6E**) and neurons in the lateral and perifornical hypothalamic areas.

DISCUSSION

The objective of the current study was to definitively and quantitatively map the afferent connectome of putative RVLM sympathetic premotor neurons, a regulatory axis through which convergent sensory and limbic inputs are thought to summate to produce baseline sympathetic nerve activity. We identified prominent inputs from well-established neurohumoral and viscero-sympathetic actuators such as the area postrema and NTS, and inputs that spanned medullary autonomic (A5, RVLM, ventromedial medulla, CVLM, LTF) and respiratory nuclei (Bötzinger, pre-Bötzinger Complex, PiCo, rostral ventral respiratory group), as well as supramedullary autonomic nuclei (paraventricular nucleus, ventrolateral PAG, lateral hypothalamus) (Dampney, 1994b; Guyenet, 2006; Card et al., 2011; Stornetta et al., 2016). However, the most striking feature of the connectome is its diffuse distribution, which contrasts with the nodal ball-and-stick schemes sometimes used to conceptualize it (Dampney, 1994a; Pilowsky and Goodchild, 2002; Guyenet, 2006), and its strong weighting toward local inputs, with around 14% of input neurons residing within the RVLM region and 30% of inputs lying within 1 mm of the RVLM epicenter. In contrast, the dataset includes a relatively low number of inputs from the forebrain (3%) and midbrain (3%), and a virtual absence of inputs from locus coeruleus, the amygdala, cortex and subfornical organ and median preoptic nucleus, despite compelling prior evidence for both functional and neuroanatomical connectivity (Dampney et al., 1987; Cassell and Gray, 1989; Gelsema et al., 1989; Verberne, 1996; Saha, 2005; Card et al., 2011; Bou Farah

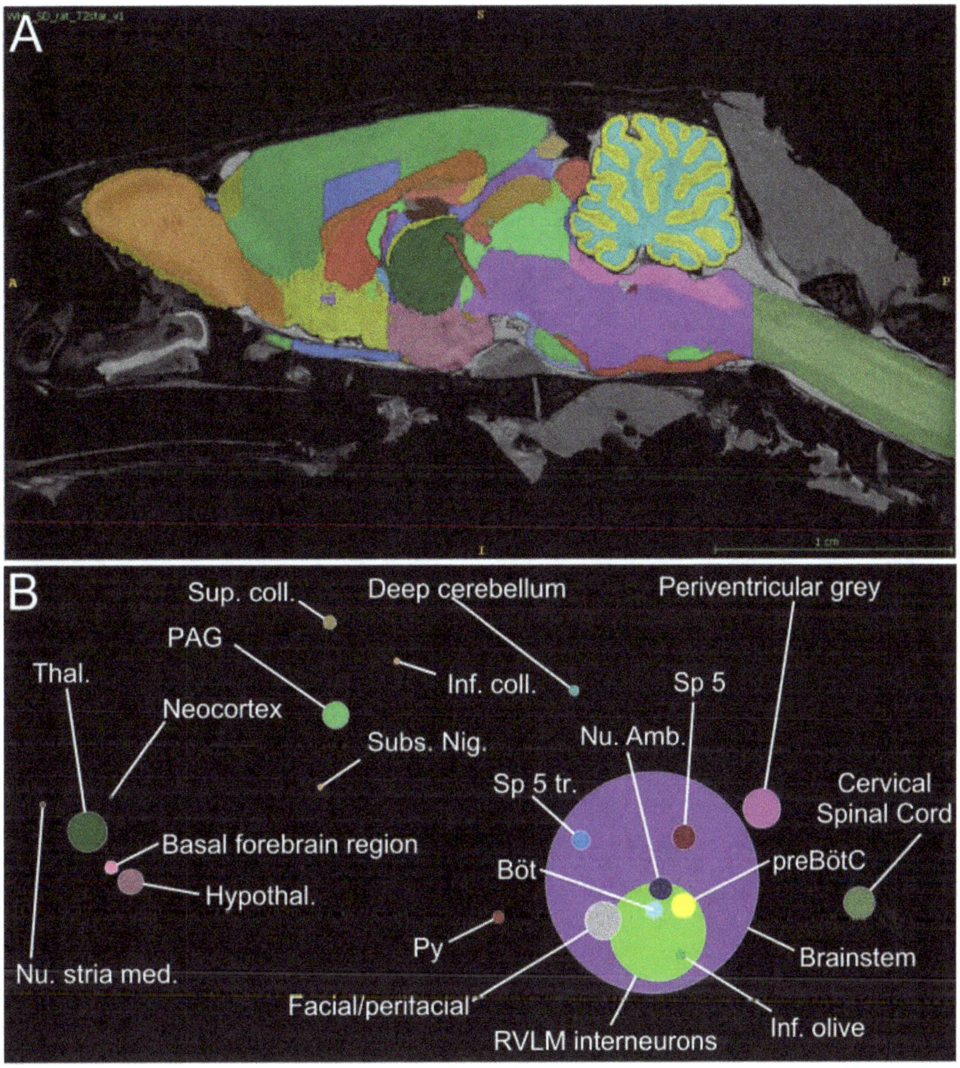

FIGURE 4 | RVLM input neurons organized by Waxholm segment. (A) Parasagittal view through the Waxholm volumetric atlas for reference; different colors indicate different brain segments. **(B)** Proportions of input neurons per Waxholm segment (summed from 4 experiments) colored and positioned according to their corresponding Waxholm regions. The diameter of each circle corresponds to the number of inputs therein. See **Table S2** for source data and abbreviations.

et al., 2016). This pattern of connectivity is consistent with qualitative data from in a similar study that targeted TH-synthesizing RVLM neurons in the mouse (Stornetta et al., 2016) and supports the argument that RVLM sympathetic premotor neurons play little, if any, role in the generation of sympathoexcitatory responses to acute psychological stress or conditioned fear (Dayas et al., 2001; Carrive and Gorissen, 2008; Furlong et al., 2014; Dampney, 2015), although it does not rule out the possibility that input from cortical and limbic structures could be indirect, perhaps involving disynaptic relays through the abundant monosynaptically connected RVLM interneurons identified in this study. Alternatively, as the current study focused exclusively on inputs received by sympathetic premotor neurons that project to the T2 thoracic spinal cord, it could be that higher centers provide a more (numerically) significant input to RVLM neurons that project to other spinal segments.

The minor input received from supramedullary centers is unlikely to represent a limitation of SADΔG(EnvA), as distance is not thought to impair its labeling efficiency (Callaway and Luo, 2015; Schwarz et al., 2015). Furthermore, inputs from the amygdala and cortex were observed in control experiments using rabies glycoprotein-transcomplemented SADΔG-mCherry and retrograde herpes vectors, and have been reported in studies that used classical chemical tracers (Bowman et al., 2013; Bou Farah et al., 2016), confirming that these structures innervate the RVLM region; apparently just not those neurons targeted in the current study. Taken at face value, these data suggest that inputs from numerous local brainstem structures predominate in their capacity to influence sympathetic nerve activity compared

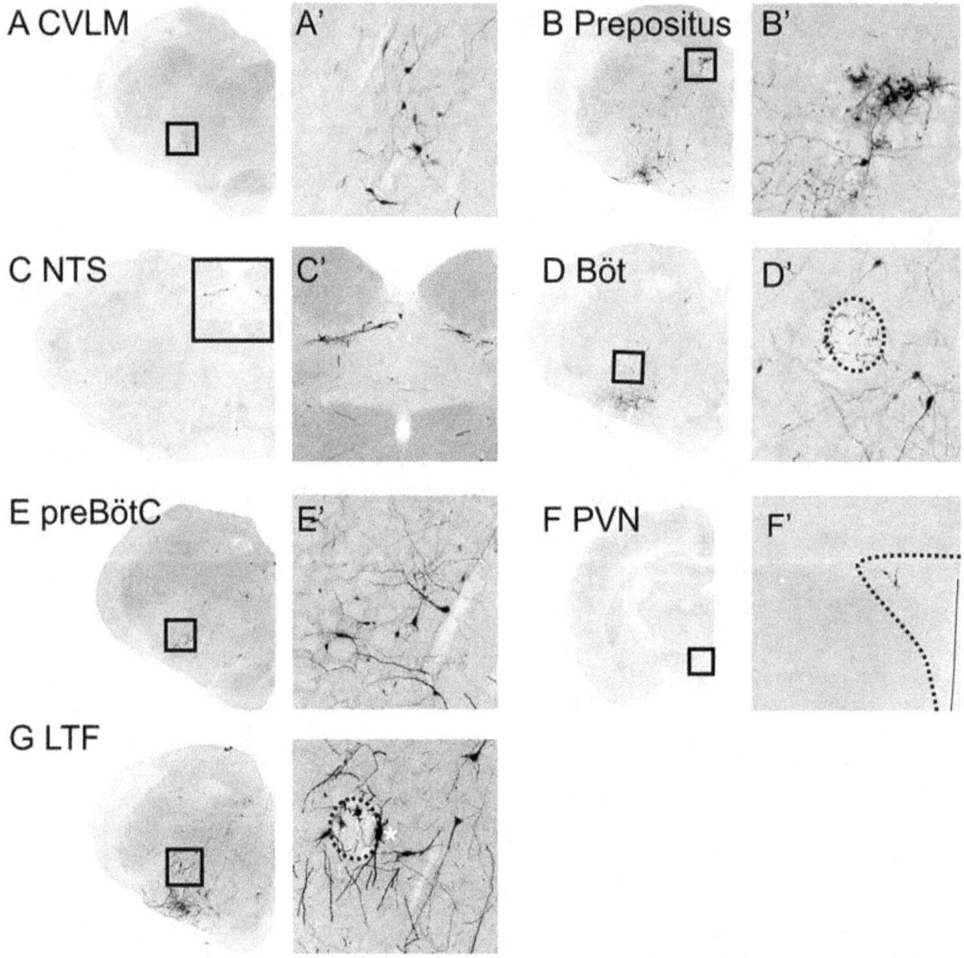

FIGURE 5 | Medullary inputs to RVLM sympathetic premotor neurons. Inverted epifluorescence micrographs with high power insets **(A'–F')** of boxed regions illustrating monosynaptic inputs from the caudal ventrolateral medulla (CVLM: **A**), nucleus prepositus **(B)**, nucleus of the solitary tract (NTS: **C**), Bötzinger (Böt: **D**), pre-Bötzinger Complex (preBötC: **E**), paraventricular nucleus of the hypothalamus (PVN: **F**) and lateral tegmental field (LTF: **G**). Nucleus ambiguus is indicated by the hatched ovals in **(D,G)**. *in Panel **(G)** indicates a TH-positive starter neuron.

to more distant regions, with the caveat that identification of monosynaptically connected neurons does not necessarily denote activity of those inputs: rabies spread is a function of synaptic strength, not synaptic activity (Ugolini, 1995; Brennand et al., 2011).

RVLM sympathetic premotor neurons include both C1 and non-C1 neurons, which differ in their functional and neurochemical phenotypes (Schreihofer and Guyenet, 1997; Stornetta et al., 2001) and may play differing roles in the generation of baseline sympathetic nerve activity and the elaboration of sympathetic reflexes (Schreihofer and Guyenet, 2000; Schreihofer et al., 2000; Madden et al., 2006; Burke et al., 2011). We used a herpes vector with a retrograde tropism to transduce putative sympathetic premotor neurons based on their axonal trajectory, allowing us to target both C1 and non-C1 bulbospinal neurons. One potential limitation of this approach is that SADΔG(EnvA)-mCherry injected into the RVLM could have theoretically infected TVA-expressing spinally-projecting neurons from other brain regions, either as a result of trans-synaptic spread (to spinally projecting neurons that provide collateral input to RVLM sympathetic premotor neurons) or by direct infection of axons that traverse the RVLM. Evidence of such "ectopic" starter neurons was apparent in pilot experiments, but was largely eliminated by limiting the interval between herpes and rabies injections to 24 h and by diluting the herpes vector. We speculate that TVA is differentially expressed on the somata but not the axons of herpes-transduced neurons at 24 h, accounting for the selective accessibility of RVLM neurons at this time-point, and conclude that bulbospinal RVLM neurons do not receive collateral input from other spinally projecting neurons because we did not see any evidence of ectopically infected spinally projecting neurons in other brain regions.

A notable deviation from the standard autonomic circuit model is the discovery of a conspicuous input from the region of the prepositus hypoglossi, a brainstem nucleus conventionally

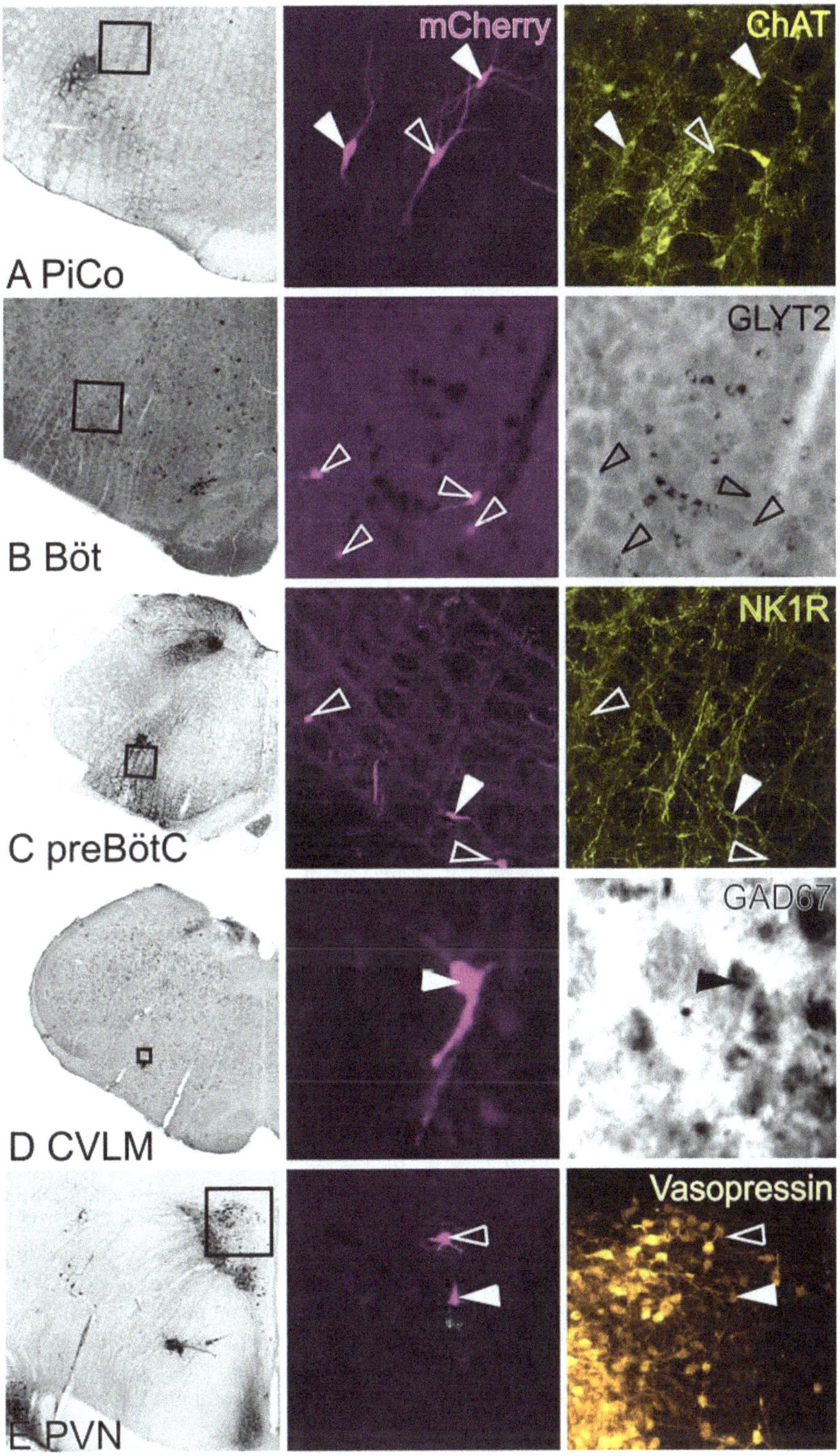

FIGURE 6 | Neurochemical phenotypes of input neurons. Left hand panels are low power images of *in situ* hybridization/immunohistochemistry indicating region shown in high power images. Middle panel shows rabies-labeled input neurons, right panels show *in situ* hybridization/immunofluorescence. Closed arrowheads indicate double-labeled neurons; open arrowheads indicate the positions of rabies labeled input neurons. **(A)** ChAT-immunoreactive input neurons in the region of the lateral reticular formation that corresponds to the mouse PiCo. **(B)** Bötzinger input neurons were abundant but none were identified as GlyT2-positive. **(C)** NK1R-positive and -negative pre-Bötzinger Complex inputs. **(D)** GAD67-positive input neurons in the CVLM. **(E)** Vasopressin-positive and -negative PVN inputs. PiCo: post-inspiratory complex, Böt: Bötzinger, preBötC: pre-Bötzinger Complex, CVLM: caudal ventrolateral medulla, PVN: paraventricular nucleus.

associated with vestibulo-occulomotor integration (McCrea, 1988) but also previously shown to drive pressor responses to glutamate microinjection (Talman and Robertson, 1991). Rabies-labeled prepositus neurons reside along the axonal trajectory of RVLM bulbospinal neurons (Lipski et al., 1995; Stornetta et al., 2016) but are not labeled by traditional retrograde tracers injected at the RVLM pressor region (Dampney, 1994b) (or retrograde rabies/herpes vectors—data not shown): we speculate that trans-synaptic infection of this population may have been via axoaxonic contacts or via the distal dendrites of starter neurons. Future functional studies will be required to elucidate the functional significance of this input.

Our dataset provides unequivocal evidence of monosynaptic inputs from respiratory subnuclei, providing clues to the neuroanatomical substrate responsible for respiratory-sympathetic coupling, the entrainment of sympathetic nerve activity to the phasic bursting of the central respiratory rhythm generator. Although direct interaction between respiratory and cardiovascular neurons in the brainstem has long been suspected (reviewed by Pilowsky et al., 1996; Taylor et al., 1999; Zoccal et al., 2014), technical difficulties have until now precluded unambiguous examination of this hypothesis. We found no evidence that input neurons in the Bötzinger region were glycinergic, (a functional marker of Bötzinger respiratory neurons: Schreihofer et al., 1999; Ezure et al., 2003), undermining the hypothesis that Bötzinger neurons are a source of inhibitory input to sympathetic premotor neurons (Sun et al., 1997). This is consistent with the observation that blockade of RVLM glycinergic transmission does not alter respiratory-sympathetic coupling (Guyenet et al., 1990), and suggests that the close appositions identified by Sun et al. (1997) may not represent functional synapses, an acknowledged limitation of light microscopy for reliable identification of synaptic contacts (Murphy et al., 1995; Descarries and Mechawar, 2000).

On the other hand, we identified pre-Bötzinger Complex input neurons that were immunoreactive for NK1R, a putative marker of glutamatergic inspiratory neurons in this region (Gray et al., 2001; Guyenet and Wang, 2001; Stornetta et al., 2003), providing a plausible structural basis for the inspiratory-locked sympathoexcitation evident in some sympathetic outflows (reviewed by Häbler et al., 1994; Pilowsky et al., 1996) and RVLM sympathetic premotor neurons (McAllen, 1987; Moraes et al., 2013). We also identified inputs from ChAT-immunoreactive neurons in the region of the LTF that may correspond to the PiCo, a group of glutamatergic cholinergic neurons recently reported to underlie the generation of postinspiratory activity in the mouse (Anderson et al., 2016). Although functional studies of the PiCo are yet to be replicated in the rat, we tentatively hypothesize that excitatory input from its analog could underlie the prominent post-inspiratory activity seen in rat lumbar and splanchnic sympathetic nerve activities (Haselton and Guyenet, 1989; Burke et al., 2010; Korim et al., 2012).

Few input neurons were found in the medullary retrotrapezoid/parafacial region that lies close to the ventral brainstem surface immediately adjacent to the RVLM. As this population is not thought to directly contribute to respiratory-sympathetic coupling (Moraes et al., 2012) their neurochemical phenotype was not studied in detail: such inputs that were identified did not conform to the small fusiform morphology or reticular distribution typical of RTN CO_2-sensing neurons (Stornetta et al., 2006).

Like other mesoscale connectomes, the RVLM connectome is diffuse and highly non-uniform in its distribution. This level of complexity makes it difficult to conceptualize as a whole, and makes identification of its major subdivisions susceptible to operator bias. Principle component analysis (cluster analysis) provides a simple and unbiased way to do this but suffers some potential drawbacks. First, selection of the appropriate number of clusters (the value of k) is inexact; it can be estimated by examining the degree of variance accounted for by iterative increases in k and identifying the "elbow" after which the relationship between k and variance becomes linear (Thorndike, 1953: in the current study $k = 12$). However, as this value is a function of the variance of the dataset, one would expect k to increase if more experimental data were added—in other words, if one analyzed 10,000 input neurons instead of 1,000, the sensitivity of the analysis would be higher and it would resolve clusters not currently detectable. Second, cluster analysis was performed on the pooled connectomic dataset, rather than on each individual experiment. Although the overall normalized distribution of inputs was reproducible between experiments, this means that experiments in which a large number of input neurons were detected influence cluster detection more than those in which fewer inputs were detected. Taken together, cluster analysis of connectomic datasets should be seen as a useful platform for breaking complicated datasets down into a readily digestible overview, rather than a definitive structural analysis tool.

Overall, the spatial distribution of the RVLM connectome adheres to two key organizational principles evident when examining interregional connectivity profiles [i.e., at the macroscopic resolution: reviewed by Bullmore and Sporns (2012)]. The first is reciprocity, that is, regions innervated by the collateral branches of putative sympathetic premotor neurons such as the NTS, RVLM, CVLM/A1, raphe and PAG (Card et al., 2006; McMullan and Pilowsky, 2012; Stornetta et al., 2016) all in turn provide afferent input to RVLM sympathetic premotor neurons. The second is spatial embedding: RVLM sympathetic premotor neurons are more likely to receive input from nearby neurons than distant ones. The spatial embedding evident in the rat RVLM connectome is in striking accordance with the nodal edge-length distribution of the mouse mesoscale connectome, the most detailed whole brain connectivity atlas currently available (Oh et al., 2014), and in particular the spatial distribution of reciprocally connected nodes (Henriksen et al., 2016) (see **Supplementary Image 3** for direct comparison). This supports the proposition, reviewed by Bullmore and Sporns (2012), that highly conserved general principles likely govern circuit topography irrespective of species, brain region, cell type or scale, and provides for the first time cell-type specific connectomic data that can be used to test general brain connectivity models.

Cell-specific connectome tracing provides unique insights into the organization of circuits that control populations of neurons selected based on their genetic, functional, or projection profiles (Yonehara et al., 2013; Pollak Dorocic et al., 2014; Pollock et al., 2014; Wertz et al., 2015). However, one of the challenges to this approach lies in the analysis and presentation of the data. A common strategy is to align histological images with corresponding plates from a stereotaxic atlas, count the number of neurons that reside within each segmented region, and then tabulate the output (Pollak Dorocic et al., 2014; Schwarz et al., 2015). Although superficially straightforward, we found that the reliability of this approach depends greatly on the expertise of the operator and can be compromised by even small misalignments in cutting plane. We calculate that each degree in deviation in the lateral plane results in an offset of ~280 μm rostrocaudal at the widest point of the rat brain, (which is further exaggerated by any deviation in the dorsoventral plane). Perfect histological cutting planes are virtually impossible to achieve, and so data presented in this way are intrinsically error-prone. The longevity of data presented as #cells/region are further undermined by the evolving taxonomy of the brain, variation in segmentation and nomenclature used by different reference atlases, and the ongoing discovery of new cell groups. An alternative approach is to present imaging data in its entirety, either as an online repository of still (Pollak Dorocic et al., 2014) or video images (Stanek et al., 2014). This allows other investigators to access the raw data, but independent analysis is hampered by the enormous volume of imaging data and the time commitment required to reanalyze it.

Our approach sidesteps both of these limitations: alignment of a 3d reference atlas to the histological image (rather than the other way around) eliminates potential errors caused by imperfect cutting angle or tissue distortion. Second, the compact size (current study <100 kb) and standardization of the positional metadata make it amenable to sharing and independent reanalysis, and eliminates the need for other investigators to directly interact with cumbersome raw imaging data (current study >300 Gb). Routine publication of such metadata would enable researchers to present complex neuroanatomical datasets in a standardized and transparent format that improves utility and reproducibility.

The promise of the connectomic approach is reflected by its widespread adoption and the continued refinement of connectome-tracing viral vectors (Osakada et al., 2011; McGovern et al., 2015; Kim et al., 2016; Reardon et al., 2016; Zingg et al., 2017), but tools that compile and quantify connectomic datasets remain primitive. The approach described here allows the quantification, standardization, and sharing of complete neuroanatomical datasets, and therefore provides a platform by which researchers may independently visualize, analyze, and compare each other's data. Bioinformatics at a single-cell resolution may allow researchers to move beyond the ball-and-stick diagrams often used to conceptualize the organization of spatially diffuse real-world neuronal networks (Rockland, 2015) and realize the full potential of novel connectomic technologies.

AUTHOR CONTRIBUTIONS

Conceptualization: SM, AG, and AA; Methodology: BD, RN, and SM; Software: JB; Formal analysis: SL, BD, AT, and SM; Investigation: BD, AT, SL, CM, and SM; Resources: RR, PB, RN, and JB; Data curation: SL, BD, and SM; Writing—Original Draft: BD, AG, and SM; Writing—Review and Editing: All authors; Visualization: BD and SM; Supervision: SM; Project Administration: SM; Funding Acquisition: SM, AA, and AG.

ACKNOWLEDGMENTS

The authors thank Sid Henriksen, Mark Wronkiewicz, and Rich Pang for their assistance in the preparation of the manuscript, Elsa Mardones for providing laboratory access and equipment, and Gergely Csucs, Dmitri Darine, and Maja Puchades for providing technical assistance and advice on the use of the tool for image anchoring. pSADΔG-mCherry genome plasmid (Addgene 32636), pcDNA-SADB19N (Addgene 32630), pcDNA-SADB19P (Addgene 32631), pcDNA-SADB19L (Addgene 32632), and pcDNA-SADB19G (Addgene 32633) plasmids and B7GG, EnvA-BHK and TVA-HEK cell lines were kindly provided by Professor Ed Callaway. This work was supported by grants from the Australian Research Council Discovery Scheme (DP120100920), the Australian National Health & Medical Research Council (APP1030301), The Human Brain Project through the European Union Seventh Framework Program (604102), the Norwegian Node of the International Neuroinformatics Coordinating Facility (INCF) and Macquarie University. BD thanks the Adam J Berry Memorial Fund, Australian Academy of Sciences, and NIH for their support.

SUPPLEMENTARY MATERIAL

Supplementary Image 1 | Segmentation of the RVLM in Waxholm space. **(A)** Experimental strategy: HSV vectors encoding GFP or mCherry were microinjected into the T2 or T10 spinal cord and **(B)** retrogradely transduced RVLM neurons (boxed area) were classified as C1 or non-C1; **(C)** shows examples of C1 neurons labeled from the T10 segment (open cyan arrowhead) and from both the T2 and T10 segments (closed white arrowhead). **(D)** Waxholm coordinates of 273 bulbospinal C1 neurons were plotted as 2d heat maps at each horizontal plane (detail in **D'**): the epicenter is indicated by crosshairs in the corresponding horizontal **(D)**, coronal **(E)**, and parasagittal **(F)** sections through the Waxholm MRI dataset. **(G–I)** Coordinates of individual bulbospinal C1 neurons (green spheres) and segmentation that enclosed 86% of neurons (green surface) plotted in 3d model of the Waxholm brain. Regional landmarks are the facial nerve (VII: red) and inferior olive (IO: orange).

Supplementary Image 2 | Retrograde transduction of spinally projecting neurons by HSV-hCMV-YTB. Coronal section at the level of the RVLM showing YFP expression in spinally projecting neurons 7 days after vector injection. Reporter expression was predominantly ipsilateral to the injection side; most transduced neurons were found in the RVLM, RVMM, and ventral raphe nuclei.

Supplementary Image 3 | Spatial distribution of rat rostral ventrolateral medulla (RVLM) input neurons identified in the current study (magenta,

plotted as distance from RVLM epicenter) compared to normalized nodal edge length distributions of reciprocal (blue) and non-reciprocal (black) nodes contained within the Allen Mouse Brain Connectivity Atlas. Mouse connectivity data adapted with permission from Henriksen et al. (2016).

Video 1 | Positions of C1 (yellow) and non-C1 (green) starter neurons in Waxholm space. Data shown first plotted on the Waxholm MRI volume, then in the Waxholm segmentation model, and finally (with monosynaptically connected input neurons, magenta), in the whole brain model.

Video 2 | Virtual flythrough showing the positions of monosynaptically connected input neurons colored according to cluster and projected onto the Waxholm MRI dataset. The video starts at the caudal end of the Waxholm MRI dataset, presented in the coronal plane, and flies in the rostral direction. The audio channel denotes the number of input neurons per section.

Table S1 | RVLM input neurons sorted according to Waxholm-defined region.

Table S2 | Key to cluster analysis and relevant literature. Abbreviations: A1, A1 noradrenergic group; BötC, Bötzinger Complex; C3, C3 adrenergic group; CPA, caudal pressor area; KF, Kolliker-Fuse; LHA, lateral hypothalamic area; MCPA, medullocervical pressor area; MPB/LPB, medial & lateral parabrachial nucleus; mRaphe, midline Raphe; NTS, nucleus of the solitary tract; Pe, perifornical hypothalamus; PiCo, postinspiratory complex; Pr, nucleus prepositus; preBötC, pre-Bötzinger Complex; PVN, paraventricular nucleus; Ramb, nucleus retroambiguus; RVLM, rostral ventrolateral medulla; RVMM, rostral ventromedial medulla; rVRG/cVRG, rostral & caudal ventral respiratory group; SC, superior colliculus; SubLC, sub-coeruleus; VL/LPAG, ventrolateral & lateral periaqueductal gray; vLTF/dLTF, ventral & dorsal lateral tegmental field; ZI, zona incerta.

Data Sheet 1 | Waxholm co-ordinates of entire dataset, segregated by experiment number and cell type (C1 or non-C1 starter neurons and input neurons).

Data Sheet 2 | Waxholm co-ordinates and Kmeans analysis of input neurons, segregated by cluster number.

REFERENCES

Allen, A. M. (2002). Inhibition of the hypothalamic paraventricular nucleus in spontaneously hypertensive rats dramatically reduces sympathetic vasomotor tone. *Hypertension* 39, 275–280. doi: 10.1161/hy0202.104272

Anderson, T. M., Garcia, A. J., Baertsch, N. A., Pollak, J., Bloom, J. C., Wei, A. D., et al. (2016). A novel excitatory network for the control of breathing. *Nature* 536, 76–80. doi: 10.1038/nature18944

Bou Farah, L., Bowman, B. R., Bokiniec, P., Karim, S., Le, S., Goodchild, A. K., et al. (2016). Somatostatin in the rat rostral ventrolateral medulla: origins and mechanism of action. *J. Comp. Neurol.* 524, 323–342. doi: 10.1002/cne.23846

Bowman, B. R., Kumar, N. N., Hassan, S. F., McMullan, S., and Goodchild, A. K. (2013). Brain sources of inhibitory input to the rat rostral ventrolateral medulla. *J. Comp. Neurol.* 521, 213–232. doi: 10.1002/cne.23175

Brennand, K. J., Simone, A., Jou, J., Gelboin-Burkhart, C., Tran, N., Sangar, S., et al. (2011). Modelling schizophrenia using human induced pluripotent stem cells. *Nature* 473, 221–225. doi: 10.1038/nature09915

Brown, D. L., and Guyenet, P. G. (1984). Cardiovascular neurons of brain stem with projections to spinal cord. *Am. J. Physiol.* 247, R1009–R1016.

Bullmore, E., and Sporns, O. (2012). The economy of brain network organization. *Nat. Rev. Neurosci.* 13, 336–349. doi: 10.1038/nrn3214

Burke, P. G., Abbott, S. B., McMullan, S., Goodchild, A. K., and Pilowsky, P. M. (2010). Somatostatin selectively ablates post-inspiratory activity after injection into the Botzinger complex. *Neuroscience* 167, 528–539. doi: 10.1016/j.neuroscience.2010.01.065

Burke, P. G., Neale, J., Korim, W. S., McMullan, S., and Goodchild, A. K. (2011). Patterning of somatosympathetic reflexes reveals nonuniform organization of presympathetic drive from C1 and non-C1 RVLM neurons. *Am. J. Physiol. Regul. Integr. Comp. Physiol.* 301:R1112. doi: 10.1152/ajpregu.00131.2011

Callaway, E. M., and Luo, L. (2015). Monosynaptic circuit tracing with glycoprotein-deleted rabies viruses. *J. Neurosci.* 35, 8979–8985. doi: 10.1523/JNEUROSCI.0409-15.2015

Carandini, M. (2012). From circuits to behavior: a bridge too far? *Nat. Neurosci.* 15, 507–509. doi: 10.1038/nn.3043

Card, J. P., Kobiler, O., McCambridge, J., Ebdlahad, S., Shan, Z., Raizada, M. K., et al. (2011). Microdissection of neural networks by conditional reporter expression from a Brainbow herpesvirus. *Proc. Natl. Acad. Sci. U.S.A.* 108, 3377–3382. doi: 10.1073/pnas.1015033108

Card, J. P., Sved, J. C., Craig, B., Raizada, M., Vazquez, J., and Sved, A. F. (2006). Efferent projections of rat rostroventrolateral medulla C1 catecholamine neurons: implications for the central control of cardiovascular regulation. *J. Comp. Neurol.* 499, 840–859. doi: 10.1002/cne.21140

Carrive, P., and Gorissen, M. (2008). Premotor sympathetic neurons of conditioned fear in the rat. *Eur. J. Neurosci.* 28, 428–446. doi: 10.1111/j.1460-9568.2008.06351.x

Cassell, M. D., and Gray, T. S. (1989). The amygdala directly innervates adrenergic (C1) neurons in the ventrolateral medulla in the rat. *Neurosci. Lett.* 97, 163–168. doi: 10.1016/0304-3940(89)90157-2

Coote, J. H. (2007). Landmarks in understanding the central nervous control of the cardiovascular system. *Exp. Physiol.* 92, 3–18. doi: 10.1113/expphysiol.2006.035378

Csucs, G., and Bjaalie, J. G. (2015). *CutNII for Waxholm Space Atlas of the Sprague Dawley Rat Brain.* INCF Software Center. Available online at: https://www.nitrc.org/frs/shownotes.php?release_id=3396

Dampney, R. A. (1994a). Functional organization of central pathways regulating the cardiovascular system. *Physiol. Rev.* 74, 323–364.

Dampney, R. A. (1994b). The subretrofacial vasomotor nucleus: anatomical, chemical and pharmacological properties and role in cardiovascular regulation. *Prog. Neurobiol.* 42, 197–227. doi: 10.1016/0301-0082(94)90064-7

Dampney, R. A. (2015). Central mechanisms regulating coordinated cardiovascular and respiratory function during stress and arousal. *Am. J. Physiol. Regul. Integr. Comp. Physiol.* 309, R429–R443. doi: 10.1152/ajpregu.00051.2015

Dampney, R. A., Czachurski, J., Dembowsky, K., Goodchild, A. K., and Seller, H. (1987). Afferent connections and spinal projections of the pressor region in the rostral ventrolateral medulla of the cat. *J. Auton. Nerv. Syst.* 20, 73–86. doi: 10.1016/0165-1838(87)90083-X

Dayas, C. V., Buller, K. M., Crane, J. W., Xu, Y., and Day, T. A. (2001). Stressor categorization: acute physical and psychological stressors elicit distinctive recruitment patterns in the amygdala and in medullary noradrenergic cell groups. *Eur. J. Neurosci.* 14, 1143–1152. doi: 10.1046/j.0953-816x.2001.01733.x

Denk, W., Briggman, K. L., and Helmstaedter, M. (2012). Structural neurobiology: missing link to a mechanistic understanding of neural computation. *Nat. Rev. Neurosci.* 13, 351–358. doi: 10.1038/nrn3169

Descarries, L., and Mechawar, N. (2000). Ultrastructural evidence for diffuse transmission by monoamine and acetylcholine neurons of the central nervous system. *Prog. Brain Res.* 125, 27–47. doi: 10.1016/S0079-6123(00)25005-X

Dum, R. P., Levinthal, D. J., and Strick, P. L. (2016). Motor, cognitive, and affective areas of the cerebral cortex influence the adrenal medulla. *Proc. Natl. Acad. Sci. U.S.A.* 113, 9922–9927. doi: 10.1073/pnas.1605044113

Ezure, K., Tanaka, I., and Kondo, M. (2003). Glycine is used as a transmitter by decrementing expiratory neurons of the ventrolateral medulla in the rat. *J. Neurosci.* 23, 8941–8948.

Furlong, T. M., McDowall, L. M., Horiuchi, J., Polson, J. W., and Dampney, R. A. (2014). The effect of air puff stress on c-Fos expression in rat hypothalamus and brainstem: central circuitry mediating sympathoexcitation and baroreflex resetting. *Eur. J. Neurosci.* 39, 1429–1438. doi: 10.1111/ejn.12521

Gelsema, A. J., Agarwal, S. K., and Calaresu, F. R. (1989). Cardiovascular responses and changes in neural activity in the rostral ventrolateral medulla elicited by electrical stimulation of the amygdala of the rat. *J. Auton. Nerv. Syst.* 27, 91–100. doi: 10.1016/0165-1838(89)90091-X

Goodchild, A. K., and Moon, E. A. (2009). Maps of cardiovascular and respiratory regions of rat ventral medulla: focus on the caudal medulla. *J. Chem. Neuroanat.* 38, 209–221. doi: 10.1016/j.jchemneu.2009.06.002

Gray, P. A., Janczewski, W. A., Mellen, N., McCrimmon, D. R., and Feldman, J. L. (2001). Normal breathing requires preBotzinger complex neurokinin-1 receptor-expressing neurons. *Nat. Neurosci.* 4, 927–930. doi: 10.1038/nn0901-927

Guyenet, P. G. (2006). The sympathetic control of blood pressure. *Nat. Rev. Neurosci.* 7, 335–346. doi: 10.1038/nrn1902

Guyenet, P. G., Darnall, R. A., and Riley, T. A. (1990). Rostral ventrolateral medulla and sympathorespiratory integration in rats. *Am. J. Physiol.* 259, R1063–R1074.

Guyenet, P. G., Stornetta, R. L., Bochorishvili, G., Depuy, S. D., Burke, P. G., and Abbott, S. B. (2013). C1 neurons: the body's EMTs. *Am. J. Physiol. Regul. Integr. Comp. Physiol.* 305, R187–R204. doi: 10.1152/ajpregu.00054.2013

Guyenet, P. G., and Wang, H. (2001). Pre-Botzinger neurons with preinspiratory discharges "*in vivo*" express NK1 receptors in the rat. *J. Neurophysiol.* 86, 438–446.

Häbler, H. J., Janig, W., and Michaelis, M. (1994). Respiratory modulation in the activity of sympathetic neurones. *Prog. Neurobiol.* 43, 567–606. doi: 10.1016/0301-0082(94)90053-1

Haselton, J. R., and Guyenet, P. G. (1989). Central respiratory modulation of medullary sympathoexcitatory neurons in rat. *Am. J. Physiol.* 256, R739–R750.

Henriksen, S., Pang, R., and Wronkiewicz, M. (2016). A simple generative model of the mouse mesoscale connectome. *eLife* 5:e12366. doi: 10.7554/eLife.12366

Horiuchi, J., McAllen, R. M., Allen, A. M., Killinger, S., Fontes, M. A., and Dampney, R. A. (2004). Descending vasomotor pathways from the dorsomedial hypothalamic nucleus: role of medullary raphe and RVLM. *Am. J. Physiol. Regul. Integr. Comp. Physiol.* 287, R824–R832. doi: 10.1152/ajpregu.00221.2004

Kelly, R. M., and Strick, P. L. (2000). Rabies as a transneuronal tracer of circuits in the central nervous system. *J. Neurosci. Methods* 103, 63–71. doi: 10.1016/S0165-0270(00)00296-X

Kim, E. J., Jacobs, M. W., Ito-Cole, T., and Callaway, E. M. (2016). Improved monosynaptic neural circuit tracing using engineered rabies virus glycoproteins. *Cell Rep.* 15, 692–699. doi: 10.1016/j.celrep.2016.03.067

Kjonigsen, L. J., Lillehaug, S., Bjaalie, J. G., Witter, M. P., and Leergaard, T. B. (2015). Waxholm Space atlas of the rat brain hippocampal region: three-dimensional delineations based on magnetic resonance and diffusion tensor imaging. *Neuroimage* 108, 441–449. doi: 10.1016/j.neuroimage.2014.12.080

Korim, W. S., Bou Farah, L., McMullan, S., and Verberne, A. J. (2014). Orexinergic activation of medullary premotor neurons modulates the adrenal sympathoexcitation to hypothalamic glucoprivation. *Diabetes* 63, 1895–1906. doi: 10.2337/db13-1073

Korim, W. S., Egwuenu, E., Fong, A. Y., McMullan, S., Cravo, S. L., and Pilowsky, P. M. (2012). Noxious somatic stimuli diminish respiratory-sympathetic coupling by selective resetting of the respiratory rhythm in anaesthetized rats. *Exp. Physiol.* 97, 1093–1104. doi: 10.1113/expphysiol.2012.066365

Le, S., Turner, A. J., Parker, L. M., Burke, P. G., Kumar, N. N., Goodchild, A. K., et al. (2016). Somatostatin 2a receptors are not expressed on functionally identified respiratory neurons in the ventral respiratory column of the rat. *J. Comp. Neurol.* 524, 1384–1398. doi: 10.1002/cne.23912

Lichtman, J. W., and Denk, W. (2011). The big and the small: challenges of imaging the brain's circuits. *Science* 334, 618–623. doi: 10.1126/science.1209168

Lipski, J., Kanjhan, R., Kruszewska, B., and Rong, W. (1996). Properties of presympathetic neurones in the rostral ventrolateral medulla in the rat: an intracellular study "*in vivo*". *J. Physiol.* 490, 729–744. doi: 10.1113/jphysiol.1996.sp021181

Lipski, J., Kanjhan, R., Kruszewska, B., and Smith, M. (1995). Barosensitive neurons in the rostral ventrolateral medulla of the rat *in vivo*: morphological properties and relationship to C1 adrenergic neurons. *Neuroscience* 69, 601–618. doi: 10.1016/0306-4522(95)92652-Z

Madden, C. J., Stocker, S. D., and Sved, A. F. (2006). Attenuation of homeostatic responses to hypotension and glucoprivation after destruction of catecholaminergic rostral ventrolateral medulla (RVLM) neurons. *Am. J. Physiol. Regul. Integr. Comp. Physiol.* 291, R751–R759. doi: 10.1152/ajpregu.00800.2005

McAllen, R. M. (1987). Central respiratory modulation of subretrofacial bulbospinal neurones in the cat. *J. Physiol.* 388, 533–545. doi: 10.1113/jphysiol.1987.sp016630

McCrea, R. A. (1988). Neuroanatomy of the oculomotor system. The nucleus prepositus. *Rev. Oculomot. Res.* 2, 203–223.

McGovern, A. E., Davis-Poynter, N., Rakoczy, J., Phipps, S., Simmons, D. G., and Mazzone, S. B. (2012). Anterograde neuronal circuit tracing using a genetically modified herpes simplex virus expressing EGFP. *J. Neurosci. Methods* 209, 158–167. doi: 10.1016/j.jneumeth.2012.05.035

McGovern, A. E., Driessen, A. K., Simmons, D. G., Powell, J., Davis-Poynter, N., Farrell, M. J., et al. (2015). Distinct brainstem and forebrain circuits receiving tracheal sensory neuron inputs revealed using a novel conditional anterograde transsynaptic viral tracing system. *J. Neurosci.* 35, 7041–7055. doi: 10.1523/JNEUROSCI.5128-14.2015

McMullan, S., Pathmanandavel, K., Pilowsky, P. M., and Goodchild, A. K. (2008). Somatic nerve stimulation evokes qualitatively different somatosympathetic responses in the cervical and splanchnic sympathetic nerves in the rat. *Brain Res.* 1217, 139–147. doi: 10.1016/j.brainres.2008.04.034

McMullan, S., and Pilowsky, P. M. (2012). Sympathetic premotor neurones project to and are influenced by neurones in the contralateral rostral ventrolateral medulla of the rat *in vivo*. *Brain Res.* 1439, 34–43. doi: 10.1016/j.brainres.2011.12.058

Mitra, P. P. (2014). The circuit architecture of whole brains at the mesoscopic scale. *Neuron* 83, 1273–1283. doi: 10.1016/j.neuron.2014.08.055

Miyawaki, T., Pilowsky, P., Sun, Q. J., Minson, J., Suzuki, S., Arnolda, L., et al. (1995). Central inspiration increases barosensitivity of neurons in rat rostral ventrolateral medulla. *Am. J. Physiol.* 268, R909–R918.

Moraes, D. J. A., Dias, M. B., Cavalcanti-Kwiatkoski, R., Machado, B. H., and Zoccal, D. B. (2012). Contribution of the retrotrapezoid nucleus/parafacial respiratory region to the expiratory-sympathetic coupling in response to peripheral chemoreflex in rats. *J. Neurophysiol.* 108, 882–890. doi: 10.1152/jn.00193.2012

Moraes, D. J., Da Silva, M. P., Bonagamba, L. G., Mecawi, A. S., Zoccal, D. B., Antunes-Rodrigues, J., et al. (2013). Electrophysiological properties of rostral ventrolateral medulla presympathetic neurons modulated by the respiratory network in rats. *J. Neurosci.* 33, 19223–19237. doi: 10.1523/JNEUROSCI.3041-13.2013

Murphy, S. M., Pilowsky, P. M., Sun, Q. J., and Llewellyn-Smith, I. J. (1995). Thyrotropin-releasing hormone-immunoreactive varicosities synapse on rat phrenic motoneurons. *J. Comp. Neurol.* 359, 310–322. doi: 10.1002/cne.903590209

Nassi, J. J., Cepko, C. L., Born, R. T., and Beier, K. T. (2015). Neuroanatomy goes viral! *Front. Neuroanat.* 9:80. doi: 10.3389/fnana.2015.00080

Oh, S. W., Harris, J. A., Ng, L., Winslow, B., Cain, N., Mihalas, S., et al. (2014). A mesoscale connectome of the mouse brain. *Nature* 508, 207–214. doi: 10.1038/nature13186

Osakada, F., and Callaway, E. M. (2013). Design and generation of recombinant rabies virus vectors. *Nat. Protoc.* 8, 1583–1601. doi: 10.1038/nprot.2013.094

Osakada, F., Mori, T., Cetin, A. H., Marshel, J. H., Virgen, B., and Callaway, E. M. (2011). New rabies virus variants for monitoring and manipulating activity and gene expression in defined neural circuits. *Neuron* 71, 617–631. doi: 10.1016/j.neuron.2011.07.005

Papp, E. A., Csucs, G., and Bjaalie, J. G. (2015). "Sprague Dawley Atlas v2 bundle", in *Waxholm Space Atlas of the Sprague Dawley Rat Brain* (INCF Software Center: The International Neuroinformatics Coordinating Facility). Available online at: https://www.nitrc.org/projects/whs-sd-atlas/

Papp, E. A., Leergaard, T. B., Calabrese, E., Johnson, G. A., and Bjaalie, J. G. (2014). Waxholm Space atlas of the Sprague Dawley rat brain. *Neuroimage* 97, 374–386. doi: 10.1016/j.neuroimage.2014.04.001

Papp, E. A., Leergaard, T. B., Csucs, G., and Bjaalie, J. G. (2016). Brain-wide mapping of axonal connections: workflow for automated detection and spatial analysis of labeling in microscopic sections. *Front. Neuroinform.* 10:11. doi: 10.3389/fninf.2016.00011

Pilowsky, P., Arnolda, L., Chalmers, J., Llewellyn-Smith, I., Minson, J., Miyawaki, T., et al. (1996). Respiratory inputs to central cardiovascular neurons. *Ann. N.Y. Acad. Sci.* 783, 64–70. doi: 10.1111/j.1749-6632.1996.tb26707.x

Pilowsky, P. M., and Goodchild, A. K. (2002). Baroreceptor reflex pathways and neurotransmitters: 10 years on. *J. Hypertens.* 20, 1675–1688. doi: 10.1097/00004872-200209000-00002

Pollak Dorocic, I., Fürth, D., Xuan, Y., Johansson, Y., Pozzi, L., Silberberg, G., et al. (2014). A whole-brain atlas of inputs to serotonergic neurons of the dorsal and median raphe nuclei. *Neuron* 83, 663–678. doi: 10.1016/j.neuron.2014.07.002

Pollock, J. D., Wu, D. Y., and Satterlee, J. S. (2014). Molecular neuroanatomy: a generation of progress. *Trends Neurosci.* 37, 106–123. doi: 10.1016/j.tins.2013.11.001

Reardon, T. R., Murray, A. J., Turi, G. F., Wirblich, C., Croce, K. R., Schnell, M. J., et al. (2016). Rabies virus CVS-N2c(ΔG) strain enhances retrograde synaptic transfer and neuronal viability. *Neuron* 89, 711–724. doi: 10.1016/j.neuron.2016.01.004

Rinaman, L., and Schwartz, G. (2004). Anterograde transneuronal viral tracing of central viscerosensory pathways in rats. *J. Neurosci.* 24, 2782–2786. doi: 10.1523/JNEUROSCI.5329-03.2004

Rockland, K. S. (2015). About connections. *Front. Neuroanat.* 9:61. doi: 10.3389/fnana.2015.00061

Saha, S. (2005). Role of the central nucleus of the amygdala in the control of blood pressure: descending pathways to medullary cardiovascular nuclei. *Clin. Exp. Pharmacol. Physiol.* 32, 450–456. doi: 10.1111/j.1440-1681.2005.04210.x

Schreihofer, A. M., and Guyenet, P. G. (1997). Identification of C1 presympathetic neurons in rat rostral ventrolateral medulla by juxtacellular labeling *in vivo*. *J. Comp. Neurol.* 387, 524–536. doi: 10.1002/(SICI)1096-9861(19971103)387:4<524::AID-CNE4>3.0.CO;2-4

Schreihofer, A. M., and Guyenet, P. G. (2000). Sympathetic reflexes after depletion of bulbospinal catecholaminergic neurons with anti-DbetaH-saporin. *Am. J. Physiol. Regul. Integr. Comp. Physiol.* 279, R729–R742.

Schreihofer, A. M., Stornetta, R. L., and Guyenet, P. G. (1999). Evidence for glycinergic respiratory neurons: botzinger neurons express mRNA for glycinergic transporter 2. *J. Comp. Neurol.* 407, 583–597. doi: 10.1002/(SICI)1096-9861(19990517)407:4<583::AID-CNE8>3.0.CO;2-E

Schreihofer, A. M., Stornetta, R. L., and Guyenet, P. G. (2000). Regulation of sympathetic tone and arterial pressure by rostral ventrolateral medulla after depletion of C1 cells in rat. *J. Physiol.* 529(Pt 1), 221–236. doi: 10.1111/j.1469-7793.2000.00221.x

Schwarz, L. A., Miyamichi, K., Gao, X. J., Beier, K. T., Weissbourd, B., Deloach, K. E., et al. (2015). Viral-genetic tracing of the input-output organization of a central noradrenaline circuit. *Nature* 524, 88–92. doi: 10.1038/nature14600

Stanek, E., IV, Cheng, S., Takatoh, J., Han, B.-X., and Wang, F. (2014). Monosynaptic premotor circuit tracing reveals neural substrates for oro-motor coordination. *Elife.* 3:e02511 doi: 10.7554/elife.02511

Stornetta, R. L. (2009). Neurochemistry of bulbospinal presympathetic neurons of the medulla oblongata. *J. Chem. Neuroanat.* 38, 222–230. doi: 10.1016/j.jchemneu.2009.07.005

Stornetta, R. L., Inglis, M. A., Viar, K. E., and Guyenet, P. G. (2016). Afferent and efferent connections of C1 cells with spinal cord or hypothalamic projections in mice. *Brain Struct. Funct.* 221, 4027–4044. doi: 10.1007/s00429-015-1143-3

Stornetta, R. L., Moreira, T. S., Takakura, A. C., Kang, B. J., Chang, D. A., West, G. H., et al. (2006). Expression of Phox2b by brainstem neurons involved in chemosensory integration in the adult rat. *J. Neurosci.* 26, 10305–10314. doi: 10.1523/JNEUROSCI.2917-06.2006

Stornetta, R. L., Rosin, D. L., Wang, H., Sevigny, C. P., Weston, M. C., and Guyenet, P. G. (2003). A group of glutamatergic interneurons expressing high levels of both neurokinin-1 receptors and somatostatin identifies the region of the pre-Botzinger complex. *J. Comp. Neurol.* 455, 499–512. doi: 10.1002/cne.10504

Stornetta, R. L., Schreihofer, A. M., Pelaez, N. M., Sevigny, C. P., and Guyenet, P. G. (2001). Preproenkephalin mRNA is expressed by C1 and non-C1 barosensitive bulbospinal neurons in the rostral ventrolateral medulla of the rat. *J. Comp. Neurol.* 435, 111–126. doi: 10.1002/cne.1196

Strack, A. M., Sawyer, W. B., Platt, K. B., and Loewy, A. D. (1989). CNS cell groups regulating the sympathetic outflow to adrenal gland as revealed by transneuronal cell body labeling with pseudorabies virus. *Brain Res.* 491, 274–296. doi: 10.1016/0006-8993(89)90063-2

Sun, Q. J., Minson, J., Llewellyn-Smith, I. J., Arnolda, L., Chalmers, J., and Pilowsky, P. (1997). Botzinger neurons project towards bulbospinal neurons in the rostral ventrolateral medulla of the rat. *J. Comp. Neurol.* 388, 23–31. doi: 10.1002/(SICI)1096-9861(19971110)388:1<23::AID-CNE2>3.0.CO;2-Q

Talman, W. T., and Robertson, S. C. (1991). Nucleus prepositus hypoglossi. A medullary pressor region. *Hypertension* 17, 1173–1176. doi: 10.1161/01.HYP.17.6.1173

Taylor, E. W., Jordan, D., and Coote, J. H. (1999). Central control of the cardiovascular and respiratory systems and their interactions in vertebrates. *Physiol. Rev.* 79, 855–916.

Thorndike, R. L. (1953). Who belongs in the family? *Psychometrika* 18, 267–276. doi: 10.1007/BF02289263

Turner, A., Kumar, N., Farnham, M., Lung, M., Pilowsky, P., and McMullan, S. (2013). Rostroventrolateral medulla neurons with commissural projections provide input to sympathetic premotor neurons: anatomical and functional evidence. *Eur. J. Neurosci.* 38, 2504–2515. doi: 10.1111/ejn.12232

Ugolini, G. (1995). Specificity of rabies virus as a transneuronal tracer of motor networks: transfer from hypoglossal motoneurons to connected second-order and higher order central nervous system cell groups. *J. Comp. Neurol.* 356, 457–480. doi: 10.1002/cne.903560312

Verberne, A. J. (1996). Medullary sympathoexcitatory neurons are inhibited by activation of the medial prefrontal cortex in the rat. *Am. J. Physiol.* 270, R713–R719.

Verberne, A. J., Stornetta, R. L., and Guyenet, P. G. (1999). Properties of C1 and other ventrolateral medullary neurones with hypothalamic projections in the rat. *J. Physiol.* 517(Pt 2), 477–494. doi: 10.1111/j.1469-7793.1999.0477t.x

Wanner, A. A., Kirschmann, M. A., and Genoud, C. (2015). Challenges of microtome-based serial block-face scanning electron microscopy in neuroscience. *J. Microsc.* 259, 137–142. doi: 10.1111/jmi.12244

Wertz, A., Trenholm, S., Yonehara, K., Hillier, D., Raics, Z., Leinweber, M., et al. (2015). PRESYNAPTIC NETWORKS. Single-cell-initiated monosynaptic tracing reveals layer-specific cortical network modules. *Science* 349, 70–74. doi: 10.1126/science.aab1687

Wickersham, I. R., Finke, S., Conzelmann, K. K., and Callaway, E. M. (2007a). Retrograde neuronal tracing with a deletion-mutant rabies virus. *Nat. Methods* 4, 47–49. doi: 10.1038/nmeth999

Wickersham, I. R., Lyon, D. C., Barnard, R. J., Mori, T., Finke, S., Conzelmann, K. K., et al. (2007b). Monosynaptic restriction of transsynaptic tracing from single, genetically targeted neurons. *Neuron* 53, 639–647. doi: 10.1016/j.neuron.2007.01.033

Wojaczynski, G. J., Engel, E. A., Steren, K. E., Enquist, L. W., and Patrick Card, J. (2015). The neuroinvasive profiles of H129 (herpes simplex virus type 1) recombinants with putative anterograde-only transneuronal spread properties. *Brain Struct. Funct.* 220, 1395–1420. doi: 10.1007/s00429-014-0733-9

Yang, Z., and Coote, J. H. (1998). Influence of the hypothalamic paraventricular nucleus on cardiovascular neurones in the rostral ventrolateral medulla of the rat. *J. Physiol.* 513(Pt 2), 521–530. doi: 10.1111/j.1469-7793.1998.521bb.x

Yonehara, K., Farrow, K., Ghanem, A., Hillier, D., Balint, K., Teixeira, M., et al. (2013). The first stage of cardinal direction selectivity is localized to the dendrites of retinal ganglion cells. *Neuron* 79, 1078–1085. doi: 10.1016/j.neuron.2013.08.005

Zingg, B., Chou, X.-l., Zhang, Z.-g., Mesik, L., Liang, F., Tao, H. W., et al. (2017). AAV-mediated anterograde transsynaptic tagging: mapping corticocollicular input-defined neural pathways for defense behaviors. *Neuron* 93, 33–47. doi: 10.1016/j.neuron.2016.11.045

Zoccal, D. B., Furuya, W. I., Bassi, M., Colombari, D. S. A., and Colombari, E. (2014). The nucleus of the solitary tract and the coordination of respiratory and sympathetic activities. *Front. Physiol.* 5:238. doi: 10.3389/fphys.2014.00238

2

Hypotensive Response to Angiotensin II Type 2 Receptor Stimulation in the Rostral Ventrolateral Medulla Requires Functional GABA-A Receptors

Laura Légat [1, 2, 3], Sofie Brouwers [1, 2, 3], Ilse J. Smolders [1] and Alain G. Dupont [1, 2, 3]*

[1] Laboratory of Pharmaceutical Chemistry, Drug Analysis and Drug Information (FASC), Research Group Experimental Pharmacology (FFAR), Center for Neurosciences (C4N), Vrije Universiteit Brussel, Brussels, Belgium, [2] Cardiovascular Center, Universitair Ziekenhuis Brussel, Brussels, Belgium, [3] Department of Clinical Pharmacology and Clinical Pharmacy, Universitair Ziekenhuis Brussel, Brussels, Belgium

Correspondence:
Laura Légat
laura.legat@vub.be

Objectives: Angiotensin II, glutamate and gamma-aminobutyric acid (GABA) interact within the rostral ventrolateral medulla (RVLM) and the paraventricular nucleus (PVN) modulating the central regulation of blood pressure and sympathetic tone. Our aim was to assess the effects of local angiotensin II type 2 receptor stimulation within the RVLM and the PVN on neurotransmitter concentrations and mean arterial pressure (MAP).

Methods: *In vivo* microdialysis was used for measurement of extracellular glutamate and GABA levels and for local infusion of the angiotensin II type 2 receptor agonist Compound 21 in the RVLM and the PVN of conscious normotensive Wistar rats. The MAP response to local Compound 21 was monitored with a pressure transducer under anaesthesia. Angiotensin II type 2 receptor selectivity was assessed using the angiotensin II type 2 receptor antagonist PD123319; the GABA-A receptor antagonist bicuculline was used to assess the involvement of GABA-A receptors.

Results: Infusion of Compound 21 (0.05 μg/μl/h) in the RVLM significantly increased GABA levels and lowered blood pressure. These effects were abolished by co-infusion with PD123319. No changes in neurotransmitter levels or effects on blood pressure were seen with PD123319 infusion alone. Co-infusion of bicuculline abolished the Compound 21 evoked decrease in MAP. Infusion of Compound 21 within the PVN did not change extracellular neurotransmitter levels nor MAP.

Conclusion: Selective stimulation of angiotensin II type 2 receptor within the RVLM by local Compound 21 infusion reduces blood pressure and increases local GABA levels in normotensive rats. This hypotensive response requires functional GABA-A receptors, suggesting that GABAergic neurons are involved in the sympatho-inhibitory action underlying this hypotensive response.

Keywords: renin-angiotensin-system, angiotensin II type 2 receptor, compound 21, mean arterial pressure, gamma-aminobutyric acid, rostral ventrolateral medulla

INTRODUCTION

Angiotensin II (Ang II) is the most important effector within the renin-angiotensin-aldosterone system (RAAS), mediating its actions through the angiotensin II type 1 receptors (AT1R), and angiotensin II type 2 receptors (AT2R). Activation of the AT1R mediates most known effects of Ang II, such as vasoconstriction, renal sodium retention, promotion of inflammatory responses, vascular smooth muscle cell proliferation and hypertrophy. The AT2R counteracts these AT1R effects and mediates vasodilation, apoptosis, natriuresis and anti-inflammatory, anti-proliferative and anti-fibrotic responses (de Gasparo et al., 2000; Padia and Carey, 2013). It has been demonstrated that activation of the AT2R, part of the "protective arm" of the RAAS, leads to therapeutic protective effects against myocardial and brain injury (Namsolleck et al., 2014). Despite the fact that AT2R stimulation causes vasodilation *ex* and *in vivo,* due to the dominating AT1R mediated vasoconstrictor tone, peripheral AT2R stimulation *in vivo* does not cause lowering in blood pressure (Steckelings et al., 2012).

The brain RAAS plays a major role in the regulation of blood pressure and sympathetic tone and that brain Ang II induces tonic sympatho-excitatory effects resulting in blood pressure increases through stimulation of central AT1R (Guyenet, 2006; Dupont and Brouwers, 2010). However, the possible role of the central AT2R herein are incompletely understood although recent data support the involvement of central AT2Rs in the regulation of blood pressure and sympathetic tone (Gao and Zucker, 2011; Li et al., 2012). Intracerebroventricular (icv) injection of Ang II in AT2R-knockout mice was reported to result in a larger increase in blood pressure compared to wild type mice, suggesting a counter-regulatory protective role of brain AT2R in the regulation of blood pressure (Siragy et al., 1999; Li et al., 2003).

The development of the first orally active, selective, non-peptide agonist of the AT2R, Compound 21 (C21) offers the possibility to selectively and specifically investigate AT2R mediated effects (Wan et al., 2004; Steckelings et al., 2011). C21 was reported to induce cardio-, cerebro-, and nephroprotective as well as anti-inflammatory effects in different animal models. Although we, as others, could not demonstrate a putative hypotensive response after peripheral administration of a range of different doses of C21, with or without concomitant AT1R blockade (Yang et al., 2011; Brouwers et al., 2013, 2015), we did observe significant blood pressure decreases after chronic icv infusion of C21 (Yang et al., 2011; Brouwers et al., 2015). Specific and selective stimulation of brain AT2R with C21 evoked a sustained hypotensive response not only in normotensive but also in spontaneously hypertensive rats *in vivo.* In addition, we observed that this hypotensive response was associated with sympatho-inhibition and increased spontaneous baroreflex sensitivity (Steckelings et al., 2012; Brouwers et al., 2015).

The central regulation of blood pressure involves different parts of the brain. However, the most important site within the brainstem, involved in the short- and longterm central regulation of the blood pressure is the rostral ventrolateral medulla (RVLM) region, the so-called "pressor area," which is responsible for the sympathetic drive. The RVLM receives inputs from multiple integrative areas in the hypothalamus and the medulla and is the main region from which the sympathetic outflow from the brain originates (Guyenet, 2006; Dupont and Brouwers, 2010). The neurons in the paraventricular nucleus (PVN) of the hypothalamus have projections to the RVLM and are also known to significantly affect sympathetic output indirectly through modulation of the neurons within the RVLM region (Guyenet, 2006; Dupont and Brouwers, 2010). Therefore, the RVLM and the PVN are generally considered the two most appropriate sites to study the central regulation of sympathetic activity. Neuronal excitability in the RVLM and the PVN are mainly modulated by the "classical" excitatory and inhibitory neurotransmitters, glutamate and gamma-aminobutyric acid (GABA), respectively (Miyawaki et al., 1996; Butcher and Cechetto, 1998; Tasker et al., 1998; Li et al., 2006; Hatam and Ganjkhani, 2012).

Brain Ang II, acting through AT1R, increases the sympathetic outflow through stimulation of glutamatergic neurons in the RVLM (Dupont and Brouwers, 2010). The presence of AT2R in the RVLM opposing the effect of neuronal stimulation through the AT1R has also been demonstrated (Gao et al., 2008a). Current evidence suggests that AT2R in the RVLM may mediate a sympatho-inhibitory effect (Gao et al., 2008a,b). Brain angiotensin peptides, glutamate and GABA appear to interact within the RVLM and the PVN to regulate sympathetic tone and blood pressure (Li et al., 2006; Dupont and Brouwers, 2010).

In the present study we aimed to further investigate the possible role of AT2R located within the RVLM-PVN axis and their interaction with glutamate and GABA in the central regulation of blood pressure. We therefore assessed blood pressure changes and possible effects on local glutamate and GABA concentrations in response to local unilateral administration of C21 within the RVLM and the PVN through microdialysis.

MATERIALS AND METHODS

Animals

All experiments were carried out on normotensive male albino Wistar rats (Charles River Laboratories, France) weighing between 250 and 300 g. Animals were kept in the animal house of the Vrije Universiteit Brussel minimum 1 week before surgery at constant temperature (24°C) and relative humidity (50%) with 12 h light-dark cycle and had *ad libitum* food and water. All protocols used and described for animal experiments on rats ($n = 4$–9 per experimental group) were carried out according to the National and European guidelines for animal experimental research and were approved by the Ethical Committee for Animal Experiments of the Faculty of Medicine and Pharmacy of the VUB. All possible steps were taken to avoid animals' suffering at each stage of the experiment.

Drugs

S-(+)-1-[(4-(Dimethylamino)-3-methylphenyl)methyl]-5-(diphenylacetyl)-4,5,6,7-tetrahydro-1H-imidazo[4,5-c]pyridine-6-carboxylic acid di(trifluoroacetate) salt hydrate (PD123319) and bicuculline were purchased form Sigma-Aldrich Co. (St.

Louis, USA). Compound 21 (C21) was provided by Vicore Pharma AB (Göteborg, Sweden). Doses of C21, PD133319 and bicuculline were selected based on previous studies (Smolders et al., 1995a; Brouwers et al., 2015).

Experimental Protocol

Normotensive Wistar rats were first subjected to brain surgery, as described in "*surgical procedures*" for implantation of a guide cannula. The following day, samples were collected through *in vivo* microdialysis on freely moving rats allowing us to measure neurotransmitters at many time points in each animal. All dialysis samples were analyzed by high performance liquid chromatography for measurement of glutamate and GABA levels. On day three, the same rats as used for microdialysis experiments were anaesthetized in order to cannulate the right carotid artery for continuous monitoring of mean arterial pressure (MAP) with a pressure transducer and the pharmacological experiments were repeated.

Post-mortem evaluation was done after each experiment in order to exclude animals with inaccurately implanted probes.

Surgical Procedures

Animals were anaesthetized prior to surgery with a ketamine/diazepam mixture (90/4.5 mg/kg) intraperitoneally and received ketoprofen (4 mg/kg) subcutaneously. A stainless steel cannula (CMA12, Solna, Sweden) was stereotaxically implanted into the left RVLM (AP: −2.2, L: −12.3, V: 7) or left PVN (AP: −0.5, L: −1.8, V: 7), according to the atlas of Paxinos and Watson (1998) and fixed with dental cement.

In vivo Microdialysis

After overnight recovery, rats were single housed in experimental cages and the microdialysis probe (CMA12/1 mm membrane length, Solna, Zweden) was inserted into the guide-cannula. For collection of basal brain dialysates, the microdialysis probe was continuously perfused at a flow rate of 2 μl/min with modified Ringer's solution (147 mM NaCl, 2.3 mM $CaCl_2$, 4 mM KCl). Samples were collected with a temporal resolution of 20 min and split into two aliquots of 15 μl. The experiment proceeded through perfusion with modified Ringer's solution for 120 min. Consecutively, one of the treatments at a rate of 2 μl/min: [C21 (0.05 μg/μl/h), PD123319 (0.05 μg/μl/h) or C21 (0.05 μg/μl/h) + PD123319 (0.05 μg/μl/h)] were dissolved in modified Ringer's solution and perfused through the microdialysis probe for 120 min and finally modified Ringer's solution for 120 min. Samples were stored at −20°C and thawed prior to analysis.

Determination of Glutamate and GABA Dialysate Levels via Liquid Chromatography

Two distinct chromatographic systems were used in the present study to determine glutamate and GABA dialysate levels following there derivatization with o-phtalaldehyde and β-mercapto-ethanol or tert-butylthiol respectively. Glutamate concentrations were determined using reversed-phase narrowbore liquid chromatography with gradient elution and fluorescence detection as described previously (Smolders et al., 1995b), while GABA was analyzed by reversed-phase microbore liquid chromatography with isocratic elution and electrochemical detection as described in detail in Van Hemelrijck et al. (2005).

Mean Arterial Pressure (MAP) Measurements

Animals were anaesthetized prior to surgery by 4% sevoflurane gas, and during surgery anaesthesia was maintained by 2.5% sevoflurane administration. The right jugular vein was catheterized for fluid maintenance (saline 0.9%), and the right carotid artery was cannulated for continuous monitoring of MAP with a pressure transducer (HP Hewlett Packard, Boebingen, Germany). The experimental protocol started after a 30 min equilibration period following surgery in order to record baseline values before the administration of the pharmacological compounds. The experiment proceeded through perfusion of modified Ringer's solution for 30 min. Consecutively, one of the treatments at a rate of 2 μl/min: [C21 (0.05 μg/μl/h), PD123319 (0.05 μg/μl/h), bicuculline (100 μM), C21 (0.05 μg/μl/h) + PD123319 (0.05 μg/μl/h) or C21 (0.05 μg/μl/h) + bicuculline (100 μM)] were dissolved in modified Ringer's solution and perfused through the microdialysis probe for 120 min, and finally modified Ringer's solution for 30 min.

Post-mortem Evaluation

At the end of every experiment, rats were killed by an overdose of Nembutal. In order to fix the brain, perfusing was performed by 4% paraformaldehyde solution and removed brains were preserved on formol. After slicing brain tissue, probe localization and tissue damage were histologically verified and evaluated post-mortem by a neutral red staining in order to exclude animals with inaccurately implanted probes.

Statistical Analysis

Data are expressed as mean ± standard error of the mean (SEM), all calculations and graphs were obtained using Graphpad Prism 4.03 (Graphpad Software Inc., San Diego, CA, USA). The mean values of the basal microdialysis samples obtained before drug administration were considered as the 100% baseline value for each animal. All neurotransmitter (glutamate and GABA) results were expressed as percentages of this baseline value ± SEM. All MAP measurements are shown as the MAP by SEM. For determination of intragroup differences of the treatment an one-way ANOVA for repeated measures followed by *post-hoc* Dunnett's multiple comparison test was used. Subsequently, for the microdialysis results, an area under the curve (AUC) analysis was performed to determine if there was an overall difference in neurotransmitter (glutamate and GABA) concentrations between different compounds. AUC values, expressed in arbitrary units, were compared by a Kruskal Wallis test with Dunn's multiple comparison *post-hoc* test. A value of $p < 0.05$ was considered to be statistically significant.

RESULTS

AT2R-Mediated Changes in Neurotransmitter Concentrations in the RVLM

The baseline values for glutamate and GABA in the microdialysis samples of the RVLM were 432 ± 219 nM for glutamate and 10 ± 5 nM for GABA in the group receiving 0.01 μg/μl/h C21 (data not shown), and 44±12 nM for glutamate (**Figure 1A**) ($n = 4$) and 3 ± 1 nM for GABA (**Figure 1B**) ($n = 6$) in the group receiving 0.05 μg/μl/h C21. No changes from baseline levels were seen for glutamate or GABA levels during infusion of C21 (0.01 μg/μl/h) within the RVLM (data not shown). Infusion of the higher dose of C21 (0.05 μg/μl/h) within RVLM significantly increased GABA levels ($p < 0.05$; **Figure 1B**) but tended to decrease glutamate levels (**Figure 1A**), with a subsequent return to baseline levels for both transmitters after switching the infusion again to Ringer's solution alone.

In the group receiving 0.05 μg/μl/h PD123319 alone, average baseline dialysate concentrations of the RVLM were 354 ± 9 nM for glutamate and 8 ± 6 nM for GABA (data not shown). These values were not significantly different from the mean baseline levels during infusion with the AT2R antagonist.

In the group receiving 0.05 μg/μl/h C21 with PD123319, baseline concentrations were 113 ± 17 nM for glutamate (**Figure 1A**) ($n = 4$) and 14 ± 1 nM for GABA (**Figure 1B**) ($n = 5$). Neurotransmitter concentrations during co-infusion of C21 + PD123319 were not significantly different from the mean baseline levels. Co- infusion of the AT2R antagonist, PD123319 (0.05 μg/μl/h) with C21 (0.05 μg/μl/h) thus abolished the C21-evoked increase in GABA concentrations (**Figure 1B**).

Figure 2 shows the AUC values of glutamate and GABA dialysate levels under C21 infusion compared to vehicle infusion. AUC of glutamate levels (**Figure 2A**) ($n = 4$) did not significantly change under C21 (0.05 μg/μl/h) infusion or under C21 + PD123319 (0.05 μg/μl/h) infusion (**Figure 2C**) ($n = 4$). However, GABA levels (**Figure 2B**) ($n = 6$) significantly ($p < 0.05$) increased under C21 (0.05 μg/μl/h) infusion compared to baseline values. This increase in GABA levels mediated by C21 infusion was abolished by co-infusion with PD123319 (**Figure 2D**) ($n = 5$).

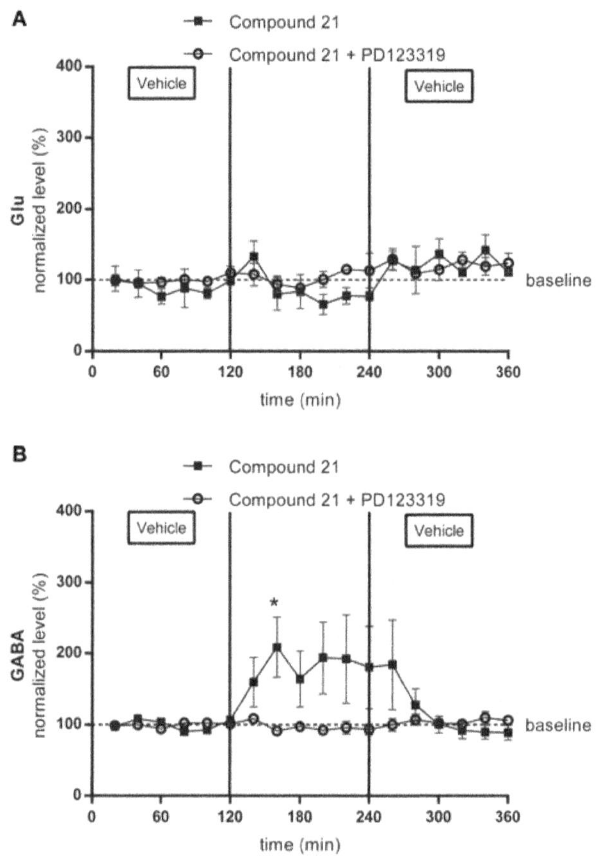

FIGURE 1 | Microdialysis experiment: effect of AT2R stimulation and infusion of the AT2R agonist C21 alone (0.05 μg/μl/h) on the extracellular glutamate (Glu) **(A)** ($n = 4$) and GABA **(B)** ($n = 6$) concentrations and of co-infusion of C21 with the AT2R antagonist PD123319 (0.05 μg/μl/h) on the extracellular glutamate (Glu) **(A)** ($n = 4$) and GABA **(B)** ($n = 5$) concentrations in the RVLM in normotensive freely moving Wistar rats. Dialysates were collected every 20 min. C21 and C21 + PD123319 were dissolved in modified Ringer's solution and administered through the dialysis probe from time 120 to 240 min. Data are presented as the mean percentage of the baseline values (vehicle) ± SEM. Statistical analysis for intragroup differences of the treatment is performed using one-way ANOVA for repeated measures and the Dunnett's multiple comparison test; significant data compared to basal levels are indicated by asterisks (*$p < 0.05$).

Lack of AT2R-Mediated Changes on Neurotransmitter Concentrations in the PVN

Average baseline extracellular concentrations in the microdialysis samples of the PVN were 198 ± 107 nM for glutamate (**Figure 3A**) ($n = 4$) and 5 ± 4 nM for GABA (**Figure 3B**) ($n = 4$). Glutamate and GABA levels were not significantly altered by local infusion of C21 (0.05 μg/μl/h) (**Figures 3A,B**).

AT2R-Mediated MAP Response to C21 Infusion into the RVLM

Baseline MAP in Wistar rats were 96 ± 10 mmHg for the group receiving 0.01 μg/μl/h C21 (data not shown), and 103 ± 8 mmHg for the group receiving 0.05 μg/μl/h C21 (**Figure 4A**) ($n = 6$). Infusion of low dose C21 (0.01 μg/μl/h) within the RVLM did not change MAP (data not shown). Infusion of C21 into the RVLM for 120 min at a dose of 0.05 μg/μl/h significantly lowered MAP (-7 mmHg compared to baseline after 20 min of C21 infusion, $p < 0.01$; −6 mmHg after 40 min, $p < 0.05$) (**Figure 4A**).

Local infusion of PD123319 alone (0.05 μg/μl/h) did not modify the baseline MAP (94 ± 15 mmHg; **Figure 4A**) ($n = 9$).

Baseline MAP in the group of rats receiving co-infusion of C21 with PD123319 were 107 ± 7 mmHg (**Figure 4A**) ($n = 4$). Co-infusion of the AT2R antagonist PD123319 with C21 (0.05 μg/μl/h) abolished the C21 evoked decrease in MAP (**Figure 4A**).

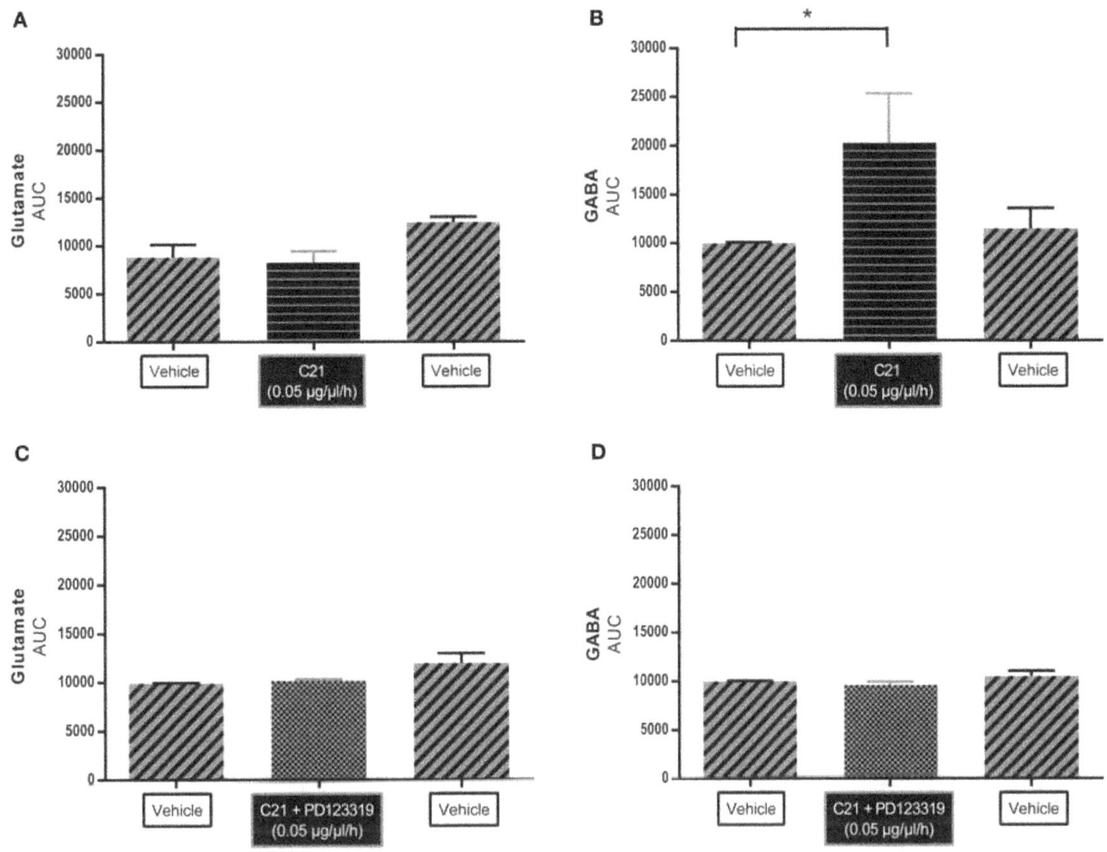

FIGURE 2 | Microdialysis experiment: area under the curve (AUC) values of C21 alone **(A)** ($n = 4$) and **(B)** ($n = 6$) and in co-infusion with PD123319 **(C)** ($n = 4$) and **(D)** ($n = 5$) applied by microdialysis into the RVLM in normotensive freely moving Wistar rats on extracellular levels of glutamate **(A,C)** and GABA **(B,D)**. Data are represented as the mean AUC ± SEM. Statistical analysis for overall differences in neurotransmitter (glutamate and GABA) concentrations between different compounds is performed using Kruskal Wallis test with Dunn's multiple comparison test; significant data are indicated by asterisks (*$p < 0.05$).

Baseline MAP in the group of rats receiving co-infusion of C21 (0.05 μg/μl/h) with bicuculline were 89 ± 9 mmHg (**Figure 4B**) ($n = 7$). Co-infusion of the GABA-A antagonist bicuculline with C21 (0.05 μg/μl/h) abolished the C21 evoked decrease in MAP (**Figure 4B**).

Lack of Blood Pressure Response to C21 Infusion into the PVN

Local infusion of C21 (0.05 μg/μl/h) into the PVN did not change baseline MAP (96 ± 8 mmHg; **Figure 5**; $n = 5$).

DISCUSSION

Although there is increasing evidence for a neuro- and cardioprotective role of the AT2R, several studies have indicated that stimulation of peripheral AT2R does not result in consistent blood pressure lowering effects (Yang et al., 2011; Steckelings et al., 2012; Brouwers et al., 2013; Matavelli and Siragy, 2015; Sumners et al., 2015). However, we recently demonstrated that icv infusion of the selective AT2R agonist C21 evoked a sustained hypotensive response in both normotensive and hypertensive rats, and that this central AT2R mediated hypotensive response is associated with sympatho-inhibition and increased baroreflex sensitivity (Brouwers et al., 2015), confirming and extending earlier results with icv administration of C21 in conscious normotensive Sprague-Dawley rats (Gao et al., 2011). Similar infusions in rats with heart failure also suppress sympathetic outflow by improving baroreflex sensitivity (Gao et al., 2014).

The major novel finding of the present study in male normotensive rats is that the hypotensive response to central administration of the selective non-peptide AT2R agonist C21 appears to be mediated at least in part by stimulation of AT2R located in the RVLM, whereas putative AT2R stimulation in the PVN does not seem to be involved. Indeed, local administration of C21 via microdialysis into the PVN did not alter local extracellular fluid neurotransmitter concentrations and did not reduce blood pressure. However, microdialysis administration of C21 into the RVLM resulted in a consistent blood pressure lowering effect and a significant increase in local GABA concentrations, and tended to decrease local glutamate concentrations. Moreover, these responses to local administration of C21 into the RVLM were abolished by local co-infusion with the selective AT2R antagonist PD123319

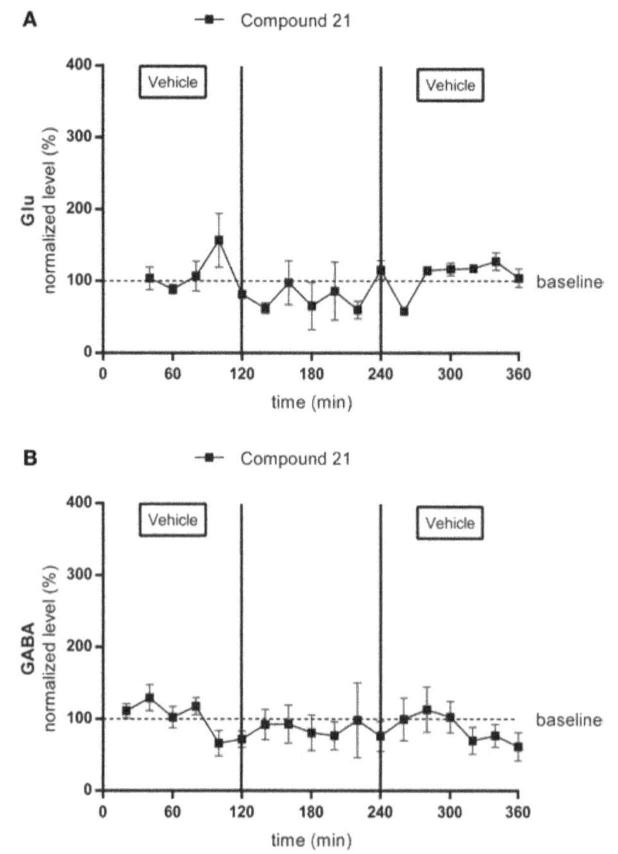

FIGURE 3 | Microdialysis experiment: effect of infusion with the AT2R agonist C21 (0.05 μg/μl/h) on the extracellular glutamate (Glu) **(A)** ($n = 4$) and GABA **(B)** ($n = 4$) concentrations in the PVN in normotensive freely moving Wistar rats. Dialysates were collected every 20 min. C21 was dissolved in modified Ringer's solution and administered through the dialysis probe from time 120 to 240 min. Data are presented as the mean percentage of the baseline values (vehicle) ± SEM. Statistical analysis for intragroup differences of the treatment is performed using one-way ANOVA for repeated measures and the Dunnett's multiple comparison test.

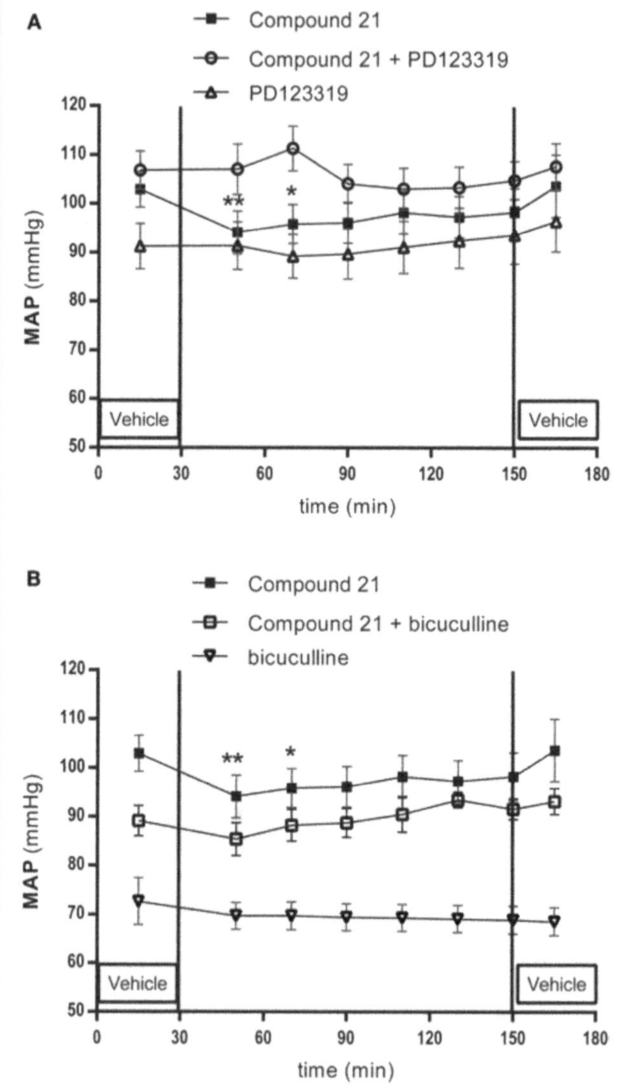

FIGURE 4 | Mean arterial pressure (MAP) measurement experiment: effect of infusion in the RVLM with the AT2R agonist C21 (0.05 μg/μl/h) ($n = 6$), co-infusion of C21 with the AT2R antagonist PD123319 (0.05 μg/μl/h) ($n = 4$) and infusion of PD123319 (0.05 μg/μl/h) alone ($n = 9$) **(A)**; C21 (0.05 μg/μl/h) infusion alone, co-infusion of C21 (0.05 μg/μl/h) with the GABA-A R antagonist bicuculline (100μM) ($n = 7$), or infusion of bicuculline alone ($n = 4$) **(B)** on MAP in normotensive anesthetized Wistar rats. MAP was recorded every 2 s. C21, PD123319 and bicuculline were dissolved in modified Ringer's solution and administered through the dialysis probe from time 30 to 150 min. Data are shown as mean ± SEM. Statistical analysis for intragroup differences of the treatment is performed using one-way ANOVA for repeated measures and the Dunnett's multiple comparison test; significant data compared to the mean of baseline values are indicated by asterisks (*$p < 0.05$; **$p < 0.01$).

confirming that these responses are AT2R-mediated. There was some variation in baseline mean blood pressure between different groups of rats, which is not unusual in anesthetized rats from different batches. However, the reduction in mean blood pressure was very consistent and occurred in all animals at the same moment after starting the infusion of C21, with a return to baseline blood pressure levels after stopping the infusion. The absence of this effect of C21 in animals co-infused with either PD123319 or bicuculline was also consistent in all animals.

It is of interest to note that, whereas the effects of local administration of C21 were abolished by PD123319, indicating that exogenous stimulation of AT2R in the RVLM in normotensive rats results in a hypotensive response, local administration of PD123319 alone had no effect on blood pressure nor on neurotransmitter levels, suggesting that endogenous activation of AT2R in the RVLM is not involved in the regulation of blood pressure under basal conditions. This in line with our previously reported observations after icv infusion of C21 (Brouwers et al., 2015), and with those of Dai et al. (2015, 2016) who also reported that icv infusion of the AT2R antagonist had no effect on basal blood pressure. These authors further suggested that endogenous AT2R activation in the brain protects against the development of DOCA/salt induced hypertension in female, but not in male rats (Dai et al., 2015, 2016).

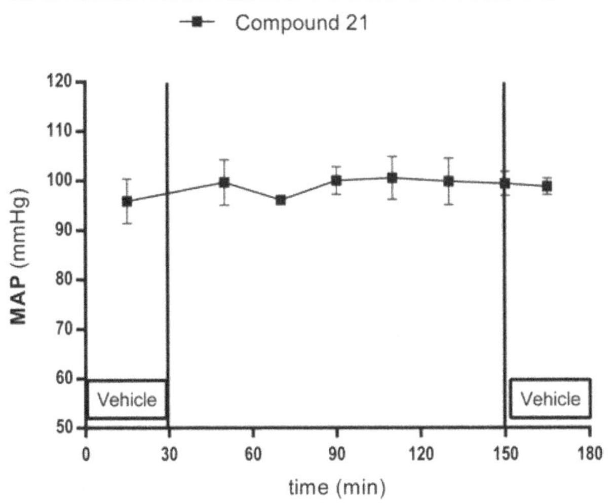

FIGURE 5 | Mean arterial pressure (MAP) measurement experiment: lack of effect of AT2R stimulation and infusion with the AT2R agonist C21(0.05 μg/μl/h) in the PVN on MAP in normotensive anesthetized Wistar rats ($n = 5$). MAP was recorded every 2 s. C21 was dissolved in modified Ringer's solution and administered through the dialysis probe from time 30 to 150 min. Data are shown as mean ± SEM. Statistical analysis for intragroup differences of the treatment is performed using one-way ANOVA for repeated measures and the Dunnett's multiple comparison test.

Most studies on central regulation of blood pressure target the RVLM, the PVN of the hypothalamus and the nucleus tractus solitarii (NTS) (Dampney et al., 2003; Guyenet, 2006; Dupont and Brouwers, 2010). The RVLM receives mainly tonic excitatory signal projections from neurons in the PVN. The RVLM presympathetic neurons, the major source of sympatho-excitatory outflow from the brain, project to sympathetic preganglionic neurons in the spinal cord (Sun et al., 1988; Pan, 2004; Kantzides and Badoer, 2005; Dupont and Brouwers, 2010). The excitatory drive from the RVLM originates from glutamatergic neurons (Ross et al., 1984; Guyenet et al., 2004; Dupont and Brouwers, 2010), which are tonically active under resting conditions but can be modulated by both excitatory and inhibitory synaptic inputs (Dampney et al., 2003). The neuronal activity of the RVLM region is modulated indirectly by input from the NTS, where baroreceptor afferents terminate, by the PVN, and by the caudal ventrolateral medulla (CVLM), which has an inhibitory influence on RVLM neurons (Schreihofer and Guyenet, 2002; Dupont and Brouwers, 2010). Therefore, the RVLM region is considered the most important site in the central regulation of sympathetic tone and blood pressure (Pointer, 2005; Guyenet, 2006; Dupont and Brouwers, 2010).

Several studies have indicated that the hypertensive response and the increased sympathetic tone evoked by central Ang II administration involves the activation of AT1R on spinally projecting glutamatergic vasomotor neurons located in the RVLM, which then further directly or indirectly elevate the sympathetic outflow (Hu et al., 1985; Dupont and Brouwers, 2010).

Although initial studies using receptor binding techniques and autoradiography studies suggested that central nervous system (CNS) cardiovascular control areas in the brainstem such as the RVLM are devoid of or only express low levels of AT2R (Millan et al., 1991; Lenkei et al., 1997; Hu et al., 1985), observations made in earlier functional studies did support a role for AT2R within the RVLM. Gao et al suggested that AT2R in the RVLM exhibit an inhibitory effect on sympathetic outflow and suggested down-regulation of AT2R in the RVLM as a contributory factor in the sympatho-excitation in congestive heart failure (Gao et al., 2008b). The same group further reported that overexpression of AT2R within the RVLM in normotensive rats reduced blood pressure, probably by sympatho-inhibition (Gao et al., 2008a). Further, Tedesco and Ally reported that the pressor and tachycardic responses to static muscle contraction were enhanced by selective blockade of AT2R in the RVLM in anaesthetized rats (Tedesco and Ally, 2009). In addition, electrophysiological studies in AT1Ra knockout mice suggest that AT2R play an antagonistic role against AT1R mediated actions of Ang II through AT2R mediated hyperpolarization and decrease in firing rate in bulbospinal RVLM neurons (Matsuura et al., 2005). The results of the present study in male normotensive rats validate and extend the results of these earlier studies and support the hypothesis that functional AT2R are present within the RVLM of normotensive rats and that their selective stimulation mediates a blood pressure lowering response probably mediated by sympatho-inhibition.

The results are also in line with those of a recent study that used a reporter mouse strain to provide an in-depth analysis of cellular and regional localization of AT2R in the mouse brain (de Kloet et al., 2016b). These investigations showed that AT2R are present in or near different brain sites involved in blood pressure regulation. These authors did not observe AT2R positive neurons within the PVN, which is in line with our observation that local administration of C21 within the PVN had no effect on blood pressure and neurotransmitter levels, confirming the absence of functional AT2R within the PVN. However, they found indications that AT2R are localized on efferents terminating in the PVN and within GABAergic neurons surrounding this nucleus (de Kloet et al., 2016b). They further reported that patch-clamp electrophysiological experiments revealed that selective activation of AT2R not within the PVN but in the peri-PVN area using C21 facilitates inhibitory (i.e., GABAergic) neurotransmission and leads to reduced activity of arginine vasopressin neurons within the PVN (de Kloet et al., 2016a,b).

Although not many AT2R were observed on neuronal cell bodies within the RVLM, de Kloet et al reported that the RVLM (and also the CLVM) are densely populated with AT2R positive nerve terminals/fibers (de Kloet et al., 2016b). It is therefore possible that presynaptic AT2R are expressed on nerve terminals within the RVLM and that their activation may influence neurotransmitter release from these terminals.

Of particular interest is also the observation by de Kloet et al. that AT2R containing neurons in the hindbrain are primarily GABAergic (de Kloet et al., 2016b). This may be important as GABA is known to have potent inhibitory actions within the RVLM (Menezes and Fontes, 2007). Projections of inhibitory GABAergic neurons to the RVLM region decrease its output to the sympathetic preganglionic regions. The CVLM which receives input from the NTS that is stimulated following blood pressure elevation, is one of the important sources of GABA (Blessing and Li, 1989; Dampney et al., 2003; Dupont and Brouwers, 2010). It was previously shown that the tonic excitatory AT1R mediated effect of Ang II on RVLM sympatho-excitatory neurons in normotensive animals is unmasked when tonic inhibitory GABAergic output is blocked (Tagawa et al., 2000). These and other observations suggest that the overall AT1R mediated effect on sympathetic tone of brain Ang II may depend on a balance between the activation of excitatory glutamatergic neurons and the inhibitory GABAergic neurons, which are both known to express AT1R (Dupont and Brouwers, 2010). Pharmacological blockade of GABA-A receptors in the sympathoexcitatory region of the RVLM has previously been shown to almost entirely eliminate the action of caudal inhibitory vasomotor neurons resulting in increased sympathetic tone and blood pressure (Blessing and Li, 1989; Tagawa et al., 2000), whereas GABA-A receptor stimulation in the RVLM lowered blood pressure (Menezes and Fontes, 2007) indicating a functional sympatho-inhibitory role for GABA-A receptors within the RVLM, in contrast to GABA-B receptors, the stimulation of which does not reduce blood pressure (Menezes and Fontes, 2007).

It is therefore tempting to speculate that the hypotensive response to local administration of C21 within the RVLM observed in the present study might be mediated by stimulation of presynaptic AT2R located on inhibitory GABAergic nerve terminals resulting in increased GABA release and subsequent GABA-A receptor-mediated reduction in sympathetic tone. Our observations of a significant increase in local GABA concentration after C21 administration, which was also abolished by co-infusion of the AT2R antagonist, and that the hypotensive response was equally abolished by local administration of the GABA-A receptor antagonist bicuculline, are in line with this hypothesis.

In addition, nitric oxide may also be involved in the observed increase in GABA within the RVLM. Nitric oxide is indeed also an important mediator within the RVLM acting on presynaptic terminals to increase GABA release (Kishi et al., 2001; Shinohara et al., 2012) and impacts on central AT2R mediated modulation of baroreflex regulation (Abdulla and Johns, 2014). This is also in line with our previous observation that the hypotensive and sympatho-inhibitory response to chronic selective stimulation of central AT2R through chronic icv infusion of C21, required a functioning central nitric-oxide pathway (Brouwers et al., 2015).

As mentioned above, we and others found no evidence that endogenous activation of AT2R in the RVLM contributes significantly to the control of blood pressure under basal conditions. This could be due to the dominant Ang II dependent AT1R mediated balance between glutamatergic and GABAergic activity, and may be different in pathologic conditions associated with sympatho-excitation.

Nevertheless, if confirmed by further studies, the presence of AT2R on GABAergic sympatho-inhibitory nerve terminals within the RVLM could open the possibility to develop selective AT2R agonists as a possible new therapy for conditions characterized by increased sympathetic activity. C21 barely crosses the blood-brain-barrier (Shraim et al., 2011), therefore the development of more lipophilic AT2R agonists would be needed to target AT2R within the RVLM as a possible new antihypertensive strategy.

The present study has some limitations. The study was done in normotensive male rats only and some studies have indicated that the role of AT2R in regulating blood pressure may be sex specific (Hilliard et al., 2012; Dai et al., 2015, 2016). Moreover, different or more pronounced responses may be observed in future similar studies in rat models of hypertension.

We observed differences in baseline glutamate and GABA levels between different groups of rats. Such variations in baseline neurotransmitter values, are not unusual and also not a problem, taken into account that the conclusions we drew from our experiments are based on relative changes in transmitter levels in response to the interventions. Our group as well as others previously reported substantial intrastrain differences in for example hippocampal extracellular levels of noradrenalin, dopamine, serotonin, glutamate and GABA (Miller et al., 1968; Portelli et al., 2009). Therefore, we believe that observing intrastrain differences between different batches, even coming from the same vendor, in basal glutamate and GABA levels within the PVN and the RVLM is not unexpected. In addition all rats were outbred, and as described by Yilmazer-Hanke (2008), outbred strains are genetically heterogeneous populations with a high intrastrain variation. Another important factor that needs to be taken into account related to observed variations in our baseline measurements is the yield of a microdialysis probe. Microdialysis does not reflect the absolute values present in the extracellular environment. Indeed, due to the kinetic process of dialysis the yield is not 100%, which is not unusual. However, microdialysis is an excellent tool to measure relative changes in concentrations in function of time after an intervention. There may be variation in probe yields between different experiments, but for each animal the effect (relative increase in GABA) occurred always at the same time (shortly after the start of the C21 administration), and the levels returned again to baseline after withdrawal of the C21 infusion. This relative change from baseline in GABA levels in response to C21 was consistently observed during the same time period in each rat. Moreover, in each rat, GABA levels remained stable when co-infusion with the AT2R antagonist. Further, the results were confirmed when expressed as AUC of GABA values before-during- and after C21 infusion (**Figure 2**).

The fact that we did not observe an increase in blood pressure after bicuculline alone does not exclude a tonic inhibitory GABA output as previously suggested by Smith and Barron (1990). These authors reported an increase in blood pressure after bilateral microinjections of bicuculline. In the present study, we administered bicuculline unilaterally into the left-sided RVLM only, hence leaving the GABA receptors in the RVLM at the other side unaffected. We assume that a blood pressure increase resulting from interruption of a putative tonic inhibitory GABAergic tone can only be detected after bilateral GABA receptor blockade within the RVLM.

It would also be of interest to further explore the effect of local administration of C21 into the NTS which is also known to contain AT2R (de Kloet et al., 2016b).

In conclusion, the results of the present study provide evidence that acute stimulation of AT2R within the RVLM by the non-peptide AT2R agonist C21 lowers blood pressure and increases local GABA release in normotensive rats, and that this hypotensive response requires functional GABA-A receptors.

AUTHOR CONTRIBUTIONS

LL, First author, performed the research and wrote the research paper; SB, Co-promoter and supervisor of practical work and design of the reseach study; IJS, Co-promotor and design of the research study and critical insights in the research paper (Head of Center for Neurosciences, VUB); AD, Promotor Design of the research study and critical insights in the research paper (Head of the department of Clinical Pharmacology and Clinical Pharmacy, UZ Brussel).

FUNDING

This study was supported by Research Council of the Vrije Universiteit Brussel and the department of Pharmaceutical Chemistry, Drug Analysis and Drug Information and the department of Clinical Pharmacology and Clinical Pharmacy, respectively provided to Prof. Dr. Apr. I. J. Smolders and Prof. Dr. A. G. Dupont.

ACKNOWLEDGMENTS

The authors acknowledge the excellent technical assistance of Mrs. R. Berckmans and Mr. G. De Smet.

REFERENCES

Abdulla, M. H., and Johns, E. J. (2014). Nitric oxide impacts on angiotensin AT2 receptor modulation of high-pressure baroreflex control of renal sympathetic nerve activity in anaesthetized rats. *Acta Physiol.* 210, 832–844. doi: 10.1111/apha.12207

Blessing, W. W., and Li, Y. W. (1989). Inhibitory vasomotor neurons in the caudal ventrolateral region of the medulla oblongata. *Prog. Brain Res.* 81, 83–97. doi: 10.1016/S0079-6123(08)62000-2

Brouwers, S., Smolders, I., Massie, A., and Dupont, A. G. (2013). Angiotensin II type 2 receptor-mediated and nitric oxide-dependent renal vasodilator response to compound 21 unmasked by angiotensin-converting enzyme inhibition in spontaneously hypertensive rats *in vivo*. *Hypertension* 62, 920–926. doi: 10.1161/HYPERTENSIONAHA.112.00762

Brouwers, S., Smolders, I., Wainford, R. D., and Dupont, A. G. (2015). Hypotensive and sympathoinhibitory responses to selective central AT2 receptor stimulation in spontaneously hypertensive rats. *Clin. Sci.* 129, 81–92. doi: 10.1042/CS20140776

Butcher, K. S., and Cechetto, D. F. (1998). Receptors in lateral hypothalamic area involved in insular cortex sympathetic responses. *Am. J. Physiol.* 275(2 Pt 2), H689–H696.

Dai, S. Y., Peng, W., Zhang, Y. P., Li, J. D., Shen, Y., and Sun, X. F. (2015). Brain endogenous angiotensin II receptor type 2 (AT2-R) protects against DOCA/salt-induced hypertension in female rats. *J. Neuroinflammation* 12:47. doi: 10.1186/s12974-015-0261-47

Dai, S. Y., Zhang, Y. P., Peng, W., Shen, Y., and He, J. J. (2016). Central infusion of Angiotensin II Type 2 receptor agonist compound 21 attenuates DOCA/NaCl-induced hypertension in female rats. *Oxid. Med. Cell. Longev.* 2016:3981790. doi: 10.1155/2016/3981790

Dampney, R. A., Horiuchi, J., Tagawa, T., Fontes, M. A., Potts, P. D., and Polson, J. W. (2003). Medullary and supramedullary mechanisms regulating sympathetic vasomotor tone. *Acta Physiol. Scand.* 177, 209–218. doi: 10.1046/j.1365-201X.2003.01070.x

de Gasparo, M., Catt, K. J., Inagami, T., Wright, J. W., and Unger, T. (2000). International union of pharmacology. XXIII. The angiotensin II receptors. *Pharmacol. Rev.* 52, 415–472.

de Kloet, A. D., Pitra, S., Wang, L., Hiller, H., Pioquinto, D. J., Smith, J. A., et al. (2016a). Angiotensin Type-2 receptors influence the activity of vasopressin neurons in the paraventricular nucleus of the hypothalamus in male mice. *Endocrinology* 157, 3167–3180. doi: 10.1210/en.2016-1131

de Kloet, A. D., Wang, L., Ludin, J. A., Smith, J. A., Pioquinto, D. J., Hiller, H., et al. (2016b). Reporter mouse strain provides a novel look at angiotensin type-2 receptor distribution in the central nervous system. *Brain Struct. Funct.* 221, 891–912. doi: 10.1007/s00429-014-0943-1

Dupont, A. G., and Brouwers, S. (2010). Brain angiotensin peptides regulate sympathetic tone and blood pressure. *J. Hypertens.* 28, 1599–1610. doi: 10.1097/HJH.0b013e32833af3b2

Gao, J., Zhang, H., Le, K. D., Chao, J., and Gao, L. (2011). Activation of central angiotensin type 2 receptors suppresses norepinephrine excretion and blood pressure in conscious rats. *Am. J. Hypertens.* 24, 724–730. doi: 10.1038/ajh.2011.33

Gao, J., Zucker, I. H., and Gao, L. (2014). Activation of central angiotensin type 2 receptors by compound 21 improves arterial baroreflex sensitivity in rats with heart failure. *Am. J. Hypertens.* 27, 1248–1256. doi: 10.1093/ajh/hpu044

Gao, L., Wang, W., Li, H., Sumners, C., and Zucker, I. H. (2008a). Effects of angiotensin type 2 receptor overexpression in the rostral ventrolateral medulla on blood pressure and urine excretion in normal rats. *Hypertension* 51, 521–527. doi: 10.1161/HYPERTENSIONAHA.107.101717

Gao, L., Wang, W. Z., Wang, W., and Zucker, I. H. (2008b). Imbalance of angiotensin type 1 receptor and angiotensin II type 2 receptor in the rostral ventrolateral medulla: potential mechanism for sympathetic overactivity in heart failure. *Hypertension* 52, 708–714. doi: 10.1161/HYPERTENSIONAHA.108.116228

Gao, L., and Zucker, I. H. (2011). AT2 receptor signaling and sympathetic regulation. *Curr. Opin. Pharmacol.* 11, 124–130. doi: 10.1016/j.coph.2010.11.004

Guyenet, P. G. (2006). The sympathetic control of blood pressure. *Nat. Rev. Neurosci.* 7, 335–346. doi: 10.1038/nrn1902

Guyenet, P. G., Stornetta, R. L., Weston, M. C., McQuiston, T., and Simmons, J. R. (2004). Detection of amino acid and peptide transmitters in physiologically identified brainstem cardiorespiratory neurons. *Auton. Neurosci.* 114, 1–10. doi: 10.1016/j.autneu.2004.06.003

Hatam, M., and Ganjkhani, M. (2012). Effect of GABA(A) receptors in the rostral ventrolateral medulla on cardiovascular response to the activation of the bed nucleus of the stria terminalis in female ovariectomized rats. *Iran J. Med. Sci.* 37, 242–252.

Hilliard, L. M., Jones, E. S., Steckelings, U. M., Unger, T., Widdop, R. E., and Denton, K. M. (2012). Sex-specific influence of angiotensin type 2 receptor stimulation on renal function: a novel therapeutic target for hypertension. *Hypertension* 59, 409–414. doi: 10.1161/HYPERTENSIONAHA.111.184986

Hu, L., Zhu, D. N., Yu, Z., Wang, J. Q., Sun, Z. J., and Yao, T. (1985). Expression of angiotensin II type 1 (AT(1)) receptor in the rostral ventrolateral medulla in rats. *J. Appl. Physiol.* 92, 2153–2161.

Kantzides, A., and Badoer, E. (2005). nNOS-containing neurons in the hypothalamus and medulla project to the RVLM. *Brain Res.* 1037, 25–34. doi: 10.1016/j.brainres.2004.11.032

Kishi, T., Hirooka, Y., Sakai, K., Shigematsu, H., Shimokawa, H., and Takeshita, A. (2001). Overexpression of eNOS in the RVLM causes hypotension and bradycardia via GABA release. *Hypertension* 38, 896–901.

Lenkei, Z., Palkovits, M., Corvol, P., and Llorens-Cortès, C. (1997). Expression of angiotensin type-1 (AT1) and type-2 (AT2) receptor mRNAs in the adult rat brain: a functional neuroanatomical review. *Front. Neuroendocrinol.* 18, 383–439. doi: 10.1006/frne.1997.0155

Li, Y. F., Jackson, K. L., Stern, J. E., Rabeler, B., and Patel, K. P. (2006). Interaction between glutamate and GABA systems in the integration of sympathetic outflow by the paraventricular nucleus of the hypothalamus. *Am. J. Physiol. Heart Circ Physiol.* 291, H2847–H2856. doi: 10.1152/ajpheart.00625.2005

Li, Y., Li, X. H., and Yuan, H. (2012). Angiotensin II type-2 receptor-specific effects on the cardiovascular system. *Cardiovasc. Diagn. Ther.* 2, 56–62. doi: 10.3978/j.issn.2223-3652.2012.02.02

Li, Z., Iwai, M., Wu, L., Shiuchi, T., Jinno, T., Cui, T. X., et al. (2003). Role of AT2 receptor in the brain in regulation of blood pressure and water intake. *Am. J. Physiol. Heart Circ. Physiol.* 284, H116–H121. doi: 10.1152/ajpheart.00515.2002

Matavelli, L. C., and Siragy, H. M. (2015). AT2 receptor activities and pathophysiological implications. *J. Cardiovasc. Pharmacol.* 65, 226–232. doi: 10.1097/FJC.0000000000000208

Matsuura, T., Kumagai, H., Onimaru, H., Kawai, A., Iigaya, K., Onami, T., et al. (2005). Electrophysiological properties of rostral ventrolateral medulla neurons in angiotensin II 1a receptor knockout mice. *Hypertension* 46, 349–354. doi: 10.1161/01.HYP.0000173421.97463.ac

Menezes, R. C., and Fontes, M. A. (2007). Cardiovascular effects produced by activation of GABA receptors in the rostral ventrolateral medulla of conscious rats. *Neuroscience* 144, 336–343. doi: 10.1016/j.neuroscience.2006.08.062

Millan, M. A., Jacobowitz, D. M., Aguilera, G., and Catt, K. J. (1991). Differential distribution of AT1 and AT2 angiotensin II receptor subtypes in the rat brain during development. *Proc. Natl. Acad. Sci. U.S.A.* 88, 11440–11444. doi: 10.1073/pnas.88.24.11440

Miller, F. P., Cox, R. H., and Maickel, R. P. (1968). Intrastrain difference in serotonin and norepinephrine in discrete areas of rat brain. *Science* 162, 463–464. doi: 10.1126/science.162.3852.463

Miyawaki, T., Minson, J., Arnolda, L., Chalmers, J., Llewellyn-Smith, I., and Pilowsky, P. (1996). Role of excitatory amino acid receptors in cardiorespiratory coupling in ventrolateral medulla. *Am. J. Physiol.* 271(5 Pt 2), R1221–R1230.

Namsolleck, P., Recarti, C., Foulquier, S., Steckelings, U. M., and Unger, T. (2014). AT(2) receptor and tissue injury: therapeutic implications. *Curr. Hypertens. Rep.* 16:416. doi: 10.1007/s11906-013-0416-6

Padia, S. H., and Carey, R. M. (2013). AT2 receptors: beneficial counter-regulatory role in cardiovascular and renal function. *Pflugers Arch.* 465, 99–110. doi: 10.1007/s00424-012-1146-3

Pan, H. L. (2004). Brain angiotensin II and synaptic transmission. *Neuroscientist* 10, 422–431. doi: 10.1177/1073858404264678

Paxinos, G., and Watson, S. (1998). *The Rat Brain in Stereotaxic Coordinates, 2nd Edn.* San Diego, CA: Academic Press.

Pointer, M. A. (2005). Is central nitric oxide essential in hypertension? *J. Hypertens.* 23, 1637–1638. doi: 10.1097/01.hjh.0000180352.99042.f3

Portelli, J., Aourz, N., De Bundel, D., Meurs, A., Smolders, I., Michotte, Y., et al. (2009). Intrastrain differences in seizure susceptibility, pharmacological response and basal neurochemistry of Wistar rats. *Epilepsy Res.* 87, 234–246. doi: 10.1016/j.eplepsyres.2009.09.009

Ross, C. A., Ruggiero, D. A., Park, D. H., Joh, T. H., Sved, A. F., Fernandez-Pardal, J., et al. (1984). Tonic vasomotor control by the rostral ventrolateral medulla: effect of electrical or chemical stimulation of the area containing C1 adrenaline neurons on arterial pressure, heart rate, and plasma catecholamines and vasopressin. *J. Neurosci.* 4, 474–494.

Schreihofer, A. M., and Guyenet, P. G. (2002). The baroreflex and beyond: control of sympathetic vasomotor tone by GABAergic neurons in the ventrolateral medulla. *Clin. Exp. Pharmacol. Physiol.* 29, 514–521. doi: 10.1046/j.1440-1681.2002.03665.x

Shinohara, K., Hirooka, Y., Kishi, T., and Sunagawa, K. (2012). Reduction of nitric oxide-mediated gamma-amino butyric acid release in rostral ventrolateral medulla is involved in superoxide-induced sympathoexcitation of hypertensive rats. *Circ. J.* 76, 2814–2821. doi: 10.1253/circj.CJ-12-0399

Shraim, N., Mertens, B., Clinckers, R., Sarre, S., Michotte, Y., and Van Eeckhaut, A. (2011). Microbore liquid chromatography with UV detection to study the *in vivo* passage of compound 21, a non-peptidergic AT_2, receptor agonist, to the striatum in rats. *J. Neurosci. Methods* 202, 137–142. doi: 10.1016/j.jneumeth.2011.06.009

Siragy, H. M., Inagami, T., Ichiki, T., and Carey, R. M. (1999). Sustained hypersensitivity to angiotensin II and its mechanism in mice lacking the subtype-2 (AT2) angiotensin receptor. *Proc. Natl. Acad. Sci. U.S.A.* 96, 6506–6510. doi: 10.1073/pnas.96.11.6506

Smith, J. K., and Barron, K. W. (1990). GABAergic responses in ventrolateral medulla in spontaneously hypertensive rats. *Am. J. Physiol.* 258(2 Pt 2), R450–R456.

Smolders, I., De Klippel, N., Sarre, S., Ebinger, G., and Michotte, Y. (1995a). Tonic GABA-ergic modulation of striatal dopamine release studied by *in vivo* microdialysis in the freely moving rat. *Eur. J. Pharmacol.* 284, 83–91. doi: 10.1016/0014-2999(95)00369-V

Smolders, I., Sarre, S., Michotte, Y., and Ebinger, G. (1995b). The analysis of excitatory, inhibitory and other amino acids in rat brain microdialysates using microbore liquid chromatography. *J. Neurosci. Methods* 57, 47–53. doi: 10.1016/0165-0270(94)00124-Y

Steckelings, U. M., Larhed, M., Hallberg, A., Widdop, R. E., Jones, E. S., Wallinder, C., et al. (2011). Non-peptide AT2-receptor agonists. *Curr. Opin. Pharmacol.* 11, 187–192. doi: 10.1016/j.coph.2010.11.002

Steckelings, U. M., Paulis, L., Namsolleck, P., and Unger, T. (2012). AT2 receptor agonists: hypertension and beyond. *Curr. Opin. Nephrol. Hypertens.* 21, 142–146. doi: 10.1097/MNH.0b013e328350261b

Sumners, C., de Kloet, A. D., Krause, E. G., Unger, T., and Steckelings, U. M. (2015). Angiotensin type 2 receptors: blood pressure regulation and end organ damage. *Curr. Opin. Pharmacol.* 21, 115–121. doi: 10.1016/j.coph.2015.01.004

Sun, M. K., Hackett, J. T., and Guyenet, P. G. (1988). Sympathoexcitatory neurons of rostral ventrolateral medulla exhibit pacemaker properties in the presence of a glutamate-receptor antagonist. *Brain Res.* 438, 23–40. doi: 10.1016/0006-8993(88)91320-0

Tagawa, T., Fontes, M. A., Potts, P. D., Allen, A. M., and Dampney, R. A. (2000). The physiological role of AT1 receptors in the ventrolateral medulla. *Braz. J. Med. Biol. Res.* 33, 643–652. doi: 10.1590/S0100-879X2000000600005

Tasker, J. G., Boudaba, C., and Schrader, L. A. (1998). Local glutamatergic and GABAergic synaptic circuits and metabotropic glutamate receptors in the hypothalamic paraventricular and supraoptic nuclei. *Adv. Exp. Med. Biol.* 449, 117–121. doi: 10.1007/978-1-4615-4871-3_11

Tedesco, A., and Ally, A. (2009). Angiotensin II type-2 (AT2) receptor antagonism alters cardiovascular responses to static exercise and simultaneously changes glutamate/GABA levels within the ventrolateral medulla. *Neurosci. Res.* 64, 372–379. doi: 10.1016/j.neures.2009.04.008

Van Hemelrijck, A., Sarre, S., Smolders, I., and Michotte, Y. (2005). Determination of amino acids associated with cerebral ischaemia in rat brain microdialysates using narrowbore liquid chromatography and fluorescence detection. *J. Neurosci. Methods* 144, 63–71. doi: 10.1016/j.jneumeth.2004.10.013

Wan, Y., Wallinder, C., Plouffe, B., Beaudry, H., Mahalingam, A. K., Wu, X., et al. (2004). Design, synthesis, and biological evaluation of the first selective nonpeptide AT2 receptor agonist. *J. Med. Chem.* 47, 5995–6008. doi: 10.1021/jm049715t

Yang, R., Smolders, I., Vanderheyden, P., Demaegdt, H., Van Eeckhaut, A., Vauquelin, G., et al. (2011). Pressor and renal hemodynamic effects of the novel angiotensin A peptide are angiotensin II type 1A receptor dependent. *Hypertension* 57, 956–964. doi: 10.1161/HYPERTENSIONAHA.110.161836

Yilmazer-Hanke, D. M. (2008). Morphological correlates of emotional and cognitive behaviour: insights from studies on inbred and outbred rodent strains and their crosses. *Behav. Pharmacol.* 19, 403–434. doi: 10.1097/FBP.0b013e32830dc0de

3

Dopamine and the Brainstem Locomotor Networks: From Lamprey to Human

Dimitri Ryczko[1†] and Réjean Dubuc[1,2]*

[1] *Groupe de Recherche sur le Système Nerveux Central, Département de Neurosciences, Université de Montréal, Montréal, QC, Canada,* [2] *Groupe de Recherche en Activité Physique Adaptée, Département des Sciences de l'Activité Physique, Université du Québec à Montréal, Montréal, QC, Canada*

Correspondence:
Réjean Dubuc
rejean.dubuc@gmail.com

†Present Address:
Dimitri Ryczko, Département de Pharmacologie-Physiologie, Université de Sherbrooke, Sherbrooke, QC, Canada

In vertebrates, dopamine neurons are classically known to modulate locomotion via their ascending projections to the basal ganglia that project to brainstem locomotor networks. An increased dopaminergic tone is associated with increase in locomotor activity. In pathological conditions where dopamine cells are lost, such as in Parkinson's disease, locomotor deficits are traditionally associated with the reduced ascending dopaminergic input to the basal ganglia. However, a descending dopaminergic pathway originating from the *substantia nigra pars compacta* was recently discovered. It innervates the mesencephalic locomotor region (MLR) from basal vertebrates to mammals. This pathway was shown to increase locomotor output in lampreys, and could very well play an important role in mammals. Here, we provide a detailed account on the newly found dopaminergic pathway in lamprey, salamander, rat, monkey, and human. In lampreys and salamanders, dopamine release in the MLR is associated with the activation of reticulospinal neurons that carry the locomotor command to the spinal cord. Dopamine release in the MLR potentiates locomotor movements through a D1-receptor mechanism in lampreys. In rats, stimulation of the *substantia nigra pars compacta* elicited dopamine release in the pedunculopontine nucleus, a known part of the MLR. In a monkey model of Parkinson's disease, a reduced dopaminergic innervation of the brainstem locomotor networks was reported. Dopaminergic fibers are also present in human pedunculopontine nucleus. We discuss the conserved locomotor role of this pathway from lamprey to mammals, and the hypothesis that this pathway could play a role in the locomotor deficits reported in Parkinson's disease.

Keywords: locomotion, brainstem, dopamine, mesencephalic locomotor region, *substantia nigra pars compacta*, pedunculopontine nucleus, conservation, Parkinson's disease

ASCENDING DOPAMINERGIC PATHWAY AND LOCOMOTION

Dopaminergic neurons degenerate in patients with Parkinson's disease (PD), resulting in serious motor dysfunctions including locomotor deficits (falls, gait freezing, dysfunctional turning), which constitute major problems in advanced forms of the disease (Stack and Ashburn, 2008, for review see Bloem et al., 2004). These locomotor deficits are traditionally associated with a loss of the ascending dopaminergic projections from the *substantia nigra pars compacta* (SNc) to the basal ganglia (Carlsson et al., 1958; Carlsson, 1959; Sano et al., 1959; Poirier and Sourkes, 1965; Sourkes and Poirier, 1965; Albin et al., 1989; Ehringer and Hornykiewicz, 1998; Kravitz et al., 2010; Roseberry et al., 2016, for review see Fahn, 2015). In turn, the basal ganglia project down to the Mesencephalic Locomotor Region (MLR), a brainstem region that controls locomotion in vertebrates (Shik et al., 1966; for review see Ryczko and Dubuc, 2013, **Figure 1**). The MLR was initially found in cats to initiate locomotion and control its frequency and intensity (Shik et al., 1966). It was later identified in lamprey (Sirota et al., 2000), salamander (Cabelguen et al., 2003), stingray (Bernau et al., 1991), bird (Sholomenko et al., 1991), rat (Garcia-Rill et al., 1987), mouse (Lee et al., 2014; Roseberry et al., 2016), rabbit (Musienko et al., 2008), guinea-pig (Marlinsky and Voitenko, 1991), and monkey (Eidelberg et al., 1981; Karachi et al., 2010; Goetz et al., 2016a). In basal vertebrates, the MLR comprises the laterodorsal tegmental nucleus and the pedunculopontine nucleus (PPN). In mammals, it comprises the PPN, but also the cuneiform nucleus (CnF). In humans, damage to the MLR is associated with locomotor deficits (Masdeu et al., 1994; Kuo et al., 2008; Demain et al., 2014). The MLR is explored as a target for deep brain stimulation to improve locomotor function in Parkinsonian patients (Plaha and Gill, 2005; for review see Hamani et al., 2016a,b).

The ascending dopaminergic projections mostly target the striatum, a major entry of the basal ganglia. These projections favor locomotion initiation by increasing the excitability of D_1-expressing striatal neurons of the direct pathway, and this reduces the tonic inhibition sent by the output stations of the basal ganglia to the MLR. In parallel, dopamine decreases the excitability of D_2-expressing striatal neurons of the indirect pathway. This also contributes to disinhibit the MLR, and initiate movement (Albin

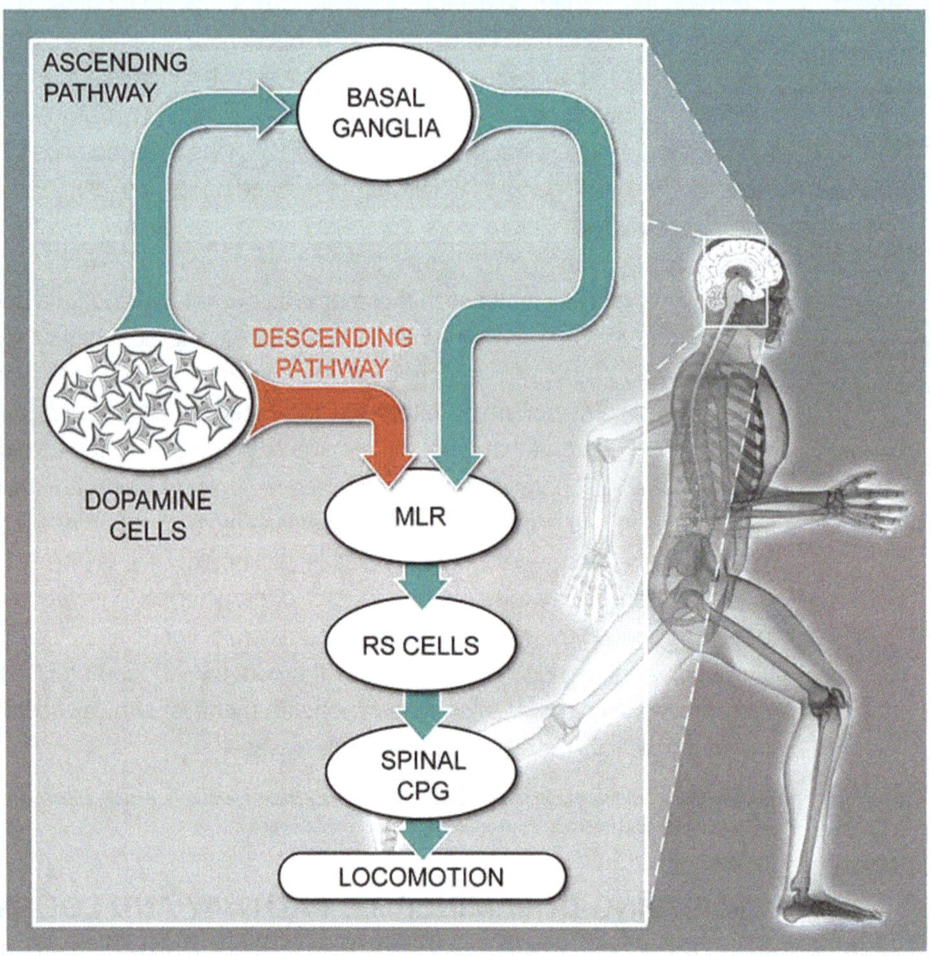

FIGURE 1 | The descending dopaminergic pathway recently uncovered in vertebrates. Schematic representation of the connectivity between the meso-diencephalic dopamine cells, the basal ganglia, the Mesencephalic Locomotor Region (MLR), the reticulospinal cells (RS), and the Central Pattern Generator (CPG) for locomotion. The meso-diencephalic dopamine cells refer to the posterior tuberculum in basal vertebrates and to the *substantia nigra pars compacta* in mammals. For convenience, the well-established direct and indirect pathways within the basal ganglia are not illustrated. (Adapted from (Le Ray et al., 2011). No permission is required for this reproduction).

et al., 1989; Kravitz et al., 2010; Freeze et al., 2013; Roseberry et al., 2016). Such organization is conserved within the basal ganglia from lamprey to mammals (see Grillner and Robertson, 2016). Once disinhibited, the MLR initiates locomotion by sending descending excitatory inputs to reticulospinal neurons, which activate the central pattern generator for locomotion (**Figure 1**, cat: Orlovskii, 1970; Steeves and Jordan, 1980; Garcia-Rill and Skinner, 1987a,b; Noga et al., 1988, 1991; rat: Bachmann et al., 2013; bird: Sholomenko et al., 1991; lamprey: Buchanan and Grillner, 1987; Brodin et al., 1988; Ohta and Grillner, 1989; Brocard and Dubuc, 2003; Le Ray et al., 2003; mouse: Bretzner and Brownstone, 2013; salamander: Ryczko et al., 2016b). MLR glutamatergic neurons are of primary importance to activate reticulospinal neurons and elicit locomotion (lamprey: Brocard and Dubuc, 2003, salamander: Ryczko et al., 2016b, mouse: Lee et al., 2014; Roseberry et al., 2016). MLR cholinergic neurons provide additional excitation to reticulospinal cells (lamprey: Le Ray et al., 2003; Smetana et al., 2010; mouse: Roseberry et al., 2016). The functional significance of this circuitry was elegantly summed in a mouse study, in which it was shown that ascending dopaminergic pathways to the basal ganglia indirectly control MLR glutamatergic cells and locomotion (Roseberry et al., 2016). The loss of the ascending dopaminergic pathway is thus considered the main cause of locomotor deficits in PD.

A NEW DESCENDING DOPAMINERGIC PATHWAY HAS BEEN UNRAVELED

There was some indication in the literature that in addition to their ascending projections, dopaminergic cells also sent direct descending projections to brainstem locomotor networks. In rat, dopamine was detected using radiometric assays or microdialysis in the CnF (Versteeg et al., 1976; Saavedra et al., 1979) and PPN (Steiniger and Kretschmer, 2003) that are both part of the MLR in mammals (see Ryczko and Dubuc, 2013). Moreover, dopaminergic fibers were detected in rat brainstem using immunohistochemistry (Kitahama et al., 2000). In monkey, dopaminergic terminals were found in proximity with cholinergic cells of the PPN and CnF (Rolland et al., 2009). The origin of this dopaminergic projection remained unknown, but tracing studies mentioned a descending projection from the SNc to the PPN in rat (Beckstead et al., 1979; Semba and Fibiger, 1992; Steininger et al., 1992; Ichinohe et al., 2000) and in cat (Edley and Graybiel, 1983). The presence of such descending input was also supported by recordings of short latency antidromic activation of SNc neurons following PPN stimulation in rat (Scarnati et al., 1984, 1987).

We investigated the origin of the dopaminergic innervation of the MLR in vertebrates. In lamprey (Ryczko et al., 2013) and salamander (Ryczko et al., 2016a), dopaminergic fibers were found around MLR cholinergic cells, a conserved landmark of the MLR (see Ryczko and Dubuc, 2013). We identified the origin of this dopaminergic innervation in lamprey (**Figure 2G**, Ryczko et al., 2013; see also Perez-Fernandez et al., 2014) and in salamander (**Figure 2H**, Ryczko et al., 2016a) as a diencephalic dopaminergic region called the posterior tuberculum. This region sends ascending projection to the striatum, and is considered homologous to the mammalian SNc and/or ventral tegmental area (Marin et al., 1997; Pombal et al., 1997; Puelles and Verney, 1998; Smeets et al., 2000; Rink and Wullimann, 2001; Blin et al., 2008; for review see Yamamoto and Vernier, 2011; Wullimann, 2014). We then found that such "new pathway" (**Figure 1**) is conserved in higher vertebrates. In rat, PPN cholinergic cells were innervated by dopaminergic fibers (Ryczko et al., 2016a). Using virogenetic tracing, we found that the dopaminergic innervation of the rat MLR originates from the SNc and to a lesser extent the retrorubral field (**Figure 2I**, Ryczko et al., 2016a). This was confirmed using conventional tracers coupled with immunofluorescence experiments (Ryczko et al., 2016a). While only a few dopamine neurons sent both an ascending projection to the striatum and a descending one to the MLR in lampreys and salamanders, numerous SNc dopamine neurons sent both ascending and descending projections in rats. The proportion of the ascending dopaminergic projection may have increased during evolution due to the expansion of the basal ganglia (see Grillner and Robertson, 2016). We then found in the human brain that PPN cholinergic cells are surrounded by dopaminergic fibers (**Figures 2J–L**, Ryczko et al., 2016a), indicating that the innervation of the MLR is conserved in vertebrates.

The descending dopaminergic pathway was shown to release dopamine in the MLR with fast-scan voltammetry (Ryczko et al., 2016a). Stimulation of the dopaminergic region evoked dopamine release in the MLR *in vitro* in lamprey (**Figures 2A,D**, Ryczko et al., 2013) and in salamander (**Figures 2B,E**, Ryczko et al., 2016a). In rat, SNc stimulation evoked dopamine release in the PPN *in vivo* (**Figures 2C,F**) that was potentiated by intraperitoneal amphetamine injection (Ryczko et al., 2016a). Altogether, these results established that the descending dopaminergic pathway is conserved and functional from basal vertebrates (lampreys, salamanders) to mammals (rats).

The role of the descending dopaminergic pathway in modulating locomotor activity was examined in two basal vertebrates. In lampreys and salamanders, stimulation of the dopamine region evoked dopamine release in the MLR, associated with activation of reticulospinal cells, which carry the locomotor command to the spinal cord (Ryczko et al., 2013, 2016a). There was a precise correlation in time linking MLR dopamine release and the activation of reticulospinal cells. The behavioral role of dopamine release in the MLR was examined in a lamprey semi-intact preparation (Ryczko et al., 2013), where the brain is exposed while the body swims as reported in many studies from our group (Sirota et al., 2000; Viana Di Prisco et al., 2000; Le Ray et al., 2003; Brocard et al., 2005, 2010; Gravel et al., 2007; Menard et al., 2007; Derjean et al., 2010; Smetana et al., 2010; Gariepy et al., 2012; Juvin et al., 2016). Stimulation of the dopaminergic region elicited reticulospinal activity together with locomotion, and microinjections of a D_1 antagonist in the MLR decreased the number of locomotor cycles, the frequency of locomotor movements, and the duration of the locomotor bout (Ryczko et al., 2013). Conversely, microinjection of dopamine in the MLR had an opposite effect (Ryczko et al., 2013). In mammals, whether MLR dopamine release is associated with

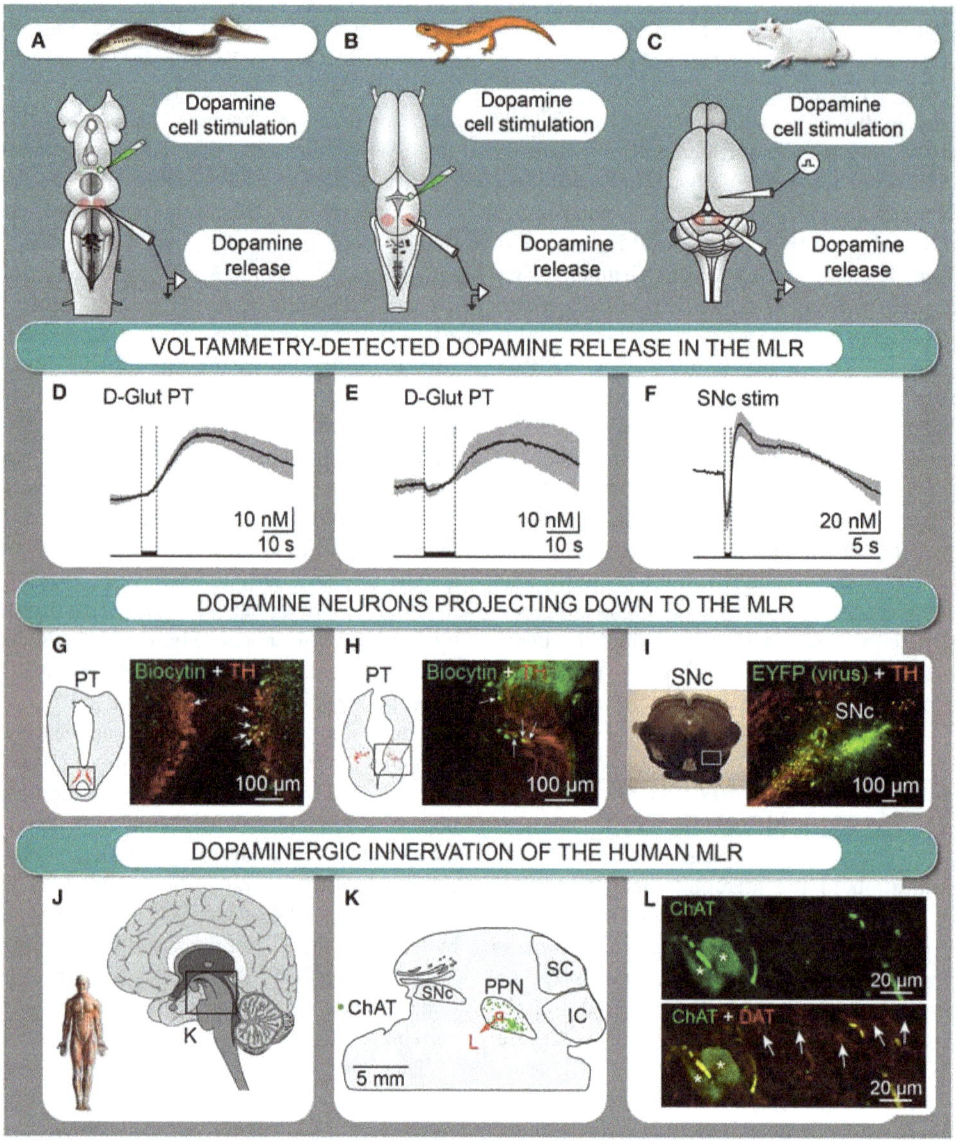

FIGURE 2 | The descending dopaminergic (DA) pathway is conserved from basal vertebrates to mammals. (A–F) Dopamine is released in the MLR after chemical stimulation of DA cells in the posterior tuberculum (PT) of lampreys **(A,D)** or salamanders (*in vitro* isolated brain) **(B,E)**, or after electrical stimulation of the *substantia nigra pars compacta* (SNc) in rats (anesthetized) **(C,F)**. **(D–F)** mean ± sem is illustrated. **(G)** Lamprey tyrosine hydroxylase (TH)-containing cells (red) in the PT and cells projecting to the MLR (green) with arrows indicating double labeled cells. **(H)** Salamander TH-containing cells (red) in the PT and cells projecting to the MLR (green) with arrows indicating double labeled cells. **(I)** DA cells in the SNc retrogradely labeled by an injection of a Cre-dependent adeno-associated virus encoding for the enhanced yellow fluorescent protein (EYFP, green) in the MLR of transgenic rats expressing the Cre-recombinase in TH neurons as shown by immunostaining against TH (red). **(J–L)** DA innervation of the human MLR. **(J–L)** The location of cholinergic cells (choline acetyltransferase-positive, ChAT) of the pedunculopontine nucleus (PPN), part of the MLR, is indicated. **(L)** Fibers containing the dopamine active transporter (DAT, red, highlighted by arrows) in proximity with cholinergic cells (ChAT, green) in the PPN. IC, inferior colliculus; SC, superior colliculus. (Panels **A,D,G** adapted from D. Ryczko, S. Gratsch, F. Auclair, C. Dube, S. Bergeron, M.H. Alpert, J.J. Cone, M.F. Roitman, S. Alford, and R. Dubuc, Forebrain dopamine neurons project down to a brainstem region controlling locomotion. Proceedings of the National Academy of Sciences of the United States of America 110 (2013) E3235–E3242. No permission is required for this reproduction; panels **B,C,E,F,H,I,J–L** adapted from D. Ryczko, J.J. Cone, M.H. Alpert, L. Goetz, F. Auclair, C. Dube, M. Parent, M.F. Roitman, S. Alford, and R. Dubuc, A descending dopamine pathway conserved from basal vertebrates to mammals. Proceedings of the National Academy of Sciences of the United States of America 113 (2016) E2440–E2449. No permission is required for this reproduction).

activation of the locomotor system remains to be addressed. The observation that amphetamine increases dopamine release in the rat MLR (Ryczko et al., 2016a) suggests an involvement of the descending dopaminergic pathway in the well-characterized increase in locomotor activity elicited by dopaminergic drugs (e.g., psychostimulants, L-DOPA).

The mechanisms through which dopamine potentiates MLR cell activity remain to be determined. It is possible that

MLR dopamine enhances locomotor output by potentiating glutamatergic inputs to the MLR. In support of this, stimulation of the dopaminergic region evokes fast excitatory synaptic inputs in MLR cells in lampreys (Gariepy et al., 2012; Ryczko et al., 2013). This fast input could be glutamatergic and monosynaptic according to anatomical and electrophysiological data (Derjean et al., 2010). Future research should determine whether the two transmitters cooperate pre- and/or post-synaptically, and establish the role of dopaminergic inputs on intrinsic properties of MLR cells.

POSSIBLE ROLE OF THE DESCENDING DOPAMINERGIC PATHWAY IN PD

There is accumulating evidence indicating that the MLR plays a similar role in humans as described in animal models. Moreover, it appears that some of the locomotor deficits observed in PD can be attributed to changes in the brainstem locomotor circuitry including the MLR. The PPN and CnF, both parts of the MLR, are activated in healthy individuals when they are asked to imagine that they are walking (Jahn et al., 2008; Snijders et al., 2011; Karachi et al., 2012; Peterson et al., 2014; Tattersall et al., 2014). In Parkinsonian subjects, similar observations were reported (Piallat et al., 2009; Lau et al., 2015; for review see Bohnen and Jahn, 2013). PPN activity increases during walking, and is modulated by L-DOPA with increase in alpha band (5–12 Hz) and decrease in beta (13–35) and gamma (65–90 Hz) bands (Fraix et al., 2013). Gait freezing is associated with a decreased alpha band activity in the PPN (Thevathasan et al., 2012). Motor arrests are associated with decreased blood oxygen levels in the MLR (Shine et al., 2013). Neuronal losses were reported in the PPN of patients with PD or progressive supranuclear palsy (Hirsch et al., 1987; Zweig et al., 1987, 1989; Jellinger, 1988). In PD this includes degeneration of cholinergic (Rinne et al., 2008; Karachi et al., 2010; Pienaar et al., 2013), GABAergic and glycinergic cells (Pienaar et al., 2013). Neuroimaging indicates that locomotor deficits in PD patients are associated with additional MLR abnormalities (notably in the PPN), including altered connectivity between the MLR, thalamus, and motor cortical regions (Fling et al., 2013, 2014), abnormal microstructure (Vercruysse et al., 2015; Youn et al., 2015; Wang et al., 2016), atrophy of the MLR gray matter (Snijders et al., 2011; Fioravanti et al., 2015) and abnormal metabolic activity following a walking task (Tard et al., 2015). Additionally, anatomopathological studies revealed the presence in the MLR of alpha-synuclein immuno-reactive Lewy Bodies (e.g., Seidel et al., 2015), and mitochondrial abnormalities (Pienaar et al., 2013) in PD. The severity of the locomotor deficits increases with the amplitude of PPN damage as captured by neuroimaging (Canu et al., 2015). These data are consistent with those showing that non-Parkinsonian individuals with MLR lesion display locomotor deficits (Masdeu et al., 1994; Kuo et al., 2008; Yeo et al., 2012), and that elderly with high level gait and balance disorders display midbrain gray matter atrophy including in the MLR (Demain et al., 2014). Finally, more and more studies point to the involvement of the PPN in the locomotor improvements related to deep brain stimulation of the subthalamic nucleus (human: Holiga et al., 2015; Knight et al., 2015; Weiss et al., 2015), which sends excitatory glutamatergic input to the PPN (e.g., Breit et al., 2001; Neagu et al., 2013; see Ryczko and Dubuc, 2013).

The benefits of MLR deep brain stimulation on locomotor function in PD (Plaha and Gill, 2005) are variable, from promising to modest (for recent studies, see Schrader et al., 2013; Mazzone et al., 2014; Holiga et al., 2015; Liu et al., 2015; Nosko et al., 2015; Welter et al., 2015) or unsustained benefits over the years (Mestre et al., 2016). This variability could be attributed to degeneration of MLR cells and to the variability of the brainstem anatomy from patient to patient (Mazzone et al., 2013). Reviewing the fast-growing body of literature on this neurosurgical approach is beyond the scope of the present review (for recent reviews, see Collomb-Clerc and Welter, 2015; DeLong and Wichmann, 2015; Fasano et al., 2015; Golestanirad et al., 2016; Rowe et al., 2016; Snijders et al., 2016). Several authors pointed out that adequate control trials and more standardization are needed before concluding on the efficacy of MLR deep brain stimulation (Windels et al., 2015; for review, see Hamani et al., 2016a,b).

The dopaminergic innervation of the PPN and CnF dramatically degenerates in a monkey model of PD (Rolland et al., 2009). The degeneration elicited by MPTP was even more marked in aged monkeys, maybe underlining the increasing fragility of this innervation over lifetime. The loss of dopaminergic innervation in the MLR could contribute to the pathophysiology of PD in several ways. If the role of the descending dopaminergic pathway to the MLR is conserved in higher vertebrates, locomotor deficits in PD may result, at least in part, from the loss of excitatory dopaminergic inputs to the MLR. This would lead to a reduced amplification of descending locomotor commands. Conversely, the descending dopaminergic pathway may improve locomotor function evoked by L-DOPA in people with PD (e.g., Moore et al., 2008; Chastan et al., 2009; Bryant et al., 2011a,b) by increasing the excitability of MLR cells. Importantly, locomotor deficits that are unresponsive to L-DOPA are associated with MLR degeneration (Chastan et al., 2009; Karachi et al., 2010; Snijders et al., 2011). It is thus possible that the beneficial effects of increasing dopamine release in the MLR with L-DOPA, or of stimulating MLR cells with dopaminergic agonists could improve locomotor function before MLR cells are lost in large number.

It is also possible that the loss of dopaminergic inputs to the MLR may disrupt the excitability of MLR cells, causing them to eventually degenerate. Such *transneuronal degeneration* can occur anterogradely or retrogradely and is characterized by a "structural deterioration of areas remote from the initial insult" (Fornito et al., 2015). This phenomenon was shown in the visual (e.g., Hubel and Wiesel, 1970; Herbin et al., 1999) and olfactory systems (e.g., Pinching and Powell, 1971). Transneuronal degeneration was also shown to damage dopaminergic neurons following striatal lesion (Macaya et al., 1994; Marti et al., 1997; El-Khodor and Burke, 2002; Canudas et al., 2005) and was proposed to contribute to PD (Pedersen and Schmidt, 2000). It was also proposed to occur in other neurodegenerative diseases including Alzheimer's disease and amyotrophic lateral sclerosis (see Fornito et al., 2015). The multiple alterations in the MLR in PD are compatible with such phenomenon (see Fornito et al., 2015). The reciprocal projections between the SNc and the PPN (McGeer and McGeer, 1984; Lavoie and Parent, 1994; Ryczko et al., 2013, 2016a; Perez-Fernandez et al., 2014) could also contribute to potentiate the transneuronal degeneration process. Nigral dopamine cell degeneration would cause a loss of the dopaminergic input to the MLR, causing MLR cells to degenerate. In turn, degeneration of PPN cholinergic and glutamatergic cells projecting to the nigral dopamine neurons would contribute to nigral dopamine cell loss. Studies in rat and monkey indicate that destruction of dopamine cells causes degeneration of MLR cholinergic cells (Pienaar et al., 2015b; Bensaid et al., 2016). Conversely, lesion of PPN cholinergic neurons induces a loss of dopaminergic nigral neurons (Bensaid et al., 2016). Finally, lesion of nigral dopaminergic neurons followed by lesion of PPN cholinergic cells induces a more dramatic degeneration of PPN cholinergic cells (Bensaid et al., 2016), suggesting that the two lesions interact to create a transneuronal degeneration loop. Stabilization of the reciprocal interactions between dopamine and cholinergic neurons could be a promising avenue to alleviate degeneration of the two systems. Interestingly, activation of PPN cholinergic cells with designer receptors exclusively activated by designer drugs (DREADDs) improves locomotor function in a rat model of PD (Pienaar et al., 2015a). It would be interesting to determine whether this approach would decrease degeneration of cholinergic and dopaminergic cells.

The descending dopaminergic projections to the PPN could also regulate other important functions such as cognition, sleep (Stefani et al., 2013; Karachi and Francois, 2017), modulation of visual inputs during locomotion (Lee et al., 2014), arousal state (Garcia-Rill et al., 2015a,b; Goetz et al., 2016b), motivation, and reward (Xiao et al., 2016; Yoo et al., 2017). How the descending dopaminergic input to the PPN influences these functions should be the subject of future research. Interestingly, the multifunctional aspects of the MLR, well established in lampreys (i.e., regulation of locomotion, respiration, control of sensory inputs, see Ryczko and Dubuc, 2013), are mirrored by the multifunctionality of the PPN in mammals.

In conclusion, studies carried out in two basal vertebrates (lampreys and salamanders) allowed us to discover a direct dopaminergic projection from the SNc down to the MLR. Several lines of evidence indicate that this new dopaminergic pathway is functional in rats, and could also be present in humans. Future research should address whether the descending dopaminergic pathway potentiates locomotion in mammals as in basal vertebrates, whether it contributes to other PPN functions, and whether this dopaminergic innervation degenerates in PD patients.

AUTHOR CONTRIBUTORS

DR and RD wrote the article.

FUNDING

This work was supported by the Canadian Institutes of Health Research Grant 15129 (to RD); the Natural Sciences and Engineering Research Council of Canada Grant 217435 (to RD); the Great Lakes Fishery Commission Grants 54011, 54021 and 54035 (to RD); the Parkinson Society Canada Grant 2011-11 (to RD); the Fonds de Recherche du Québec—Santé (FRQS: Groupe de Recherche sur le Système Nerveux Central, GRSNC, 5249). DR received fellowships from FRQS and the GRSNC Jasper fellowship.

ACKNOWLEDGMENTS

We thank Danielle Veilleux for her technical assistance and Frédéric Bernard for his help with the graphics.

REFERENCES

Albin, R. L., Young, A. B., and Penney, J. B. (1989). The functional anatomy of basal ganglia disorders. *Trends Neurosci.* 12, 366–375. doi: 10.1016/0166-2236(89)90074-X

Bachmann, L. C., Matis, A., Lindau, N. T., Felder, P., Gullo, M., and Schwab, M. E. (2013). Deep brain stimulation of the midbrain locomotor region improves paretic hindlimb function after spinal cord injury in rats. *Sci. Transl. Med.* 5:208ra146. doi: 10.1126/scitranslmed.3005972

Beckstead, R. M., Domesick, V. B., and Nauta, W. J. (1979). Efferent connections of the substantia nigra and ventral tegmental area in the rat. *Brain Res.* 175, 191–217. doi: 10.1016/0006-8993(79)91001-1

Bensaid, M., Michel, P. P., Clark, S. D., Hirsch, E. C., and Francois, C. (2016). Role of pedunculopontine cholinergic neurons in the vulnerability of nigral dopaminergic neurons in Parkinson's disease. *Exp. Neurol.* 275(Pt 1), 209–219. doi: 10.1016/j.expneurol.2015.11.004

Bernau, N. A., Puzdrowski, R. L., and Leonard, R. B. (1991). Identification of the midbrain locomotor region and its relation to descending locomotor pathways in the Atlantic stingray, Dasyatis sabina. *Brain Res.* 557, 83–94. doi: 10.1016/0006-8993(91)90119-G

Blin, M., Norton, W., Bally-Cuif, L., and Vernier, P. (2008). NR4A2 controls the differentiation of selective dopaminergic nuclei in the zebrafish brain. *Mol. Cell. Neurosci.* 39, 592–604. doi: 10.1016/j.mcn.2008.08.006

Bloem, B. R., Hausdorff, J. M., Visser, J. E., and Giladi, N. (2004). Falls and freezing of gait in Parkinson's disease: a review of two interconnected, episodic phenomena. *Mov. Disord.* 19, 871–884. doi: 10.1002/mds.20115

Bohnen, N. I., and Jahn, K. (2013). Imaging: what can it tell us about parkinsonian gait? *Mov. Disord.* 28, 1492–1500. doi: 10.1002/mds.25534

Breit, S., Bouali-Benazzouz, R., Benabid, A. L., and Benazzouz, A. (2001). Unilateral lesion of the nigrostriatal pathway induces an increase of neuronal activity of the pedunculopontine nucleus, which is reversed by the lesion of the subthalamic nucleus in the rat. *Eur. J. Neurosci.* 14, 1833–1842. doi: 10.1046/j.0953-816x.2001.01800.x

Bretzner, F., and Brownstone, R. M. (2013). Lhx3-Chx10 reticulospinal neurons in locomotor circuits. *J. Neurosci.* 33, 14681–14692. doi: 10.1523/JNEUROSCI.5231-12.2013

Brocard, F., Bardy, C., and Dubuc, R. (2005). Modulatory effect of substance P to the brain stem locomotor command in lampreys. *J. Neurophysiol.* 93, 2127–2141. doi: 10.1152/jn.00401.2004

Brocard, F., and Dubuc, R. (2003). Differential contribution of reticulospinal cells to the control of locomotion induced by the mesencephalic locomotor region. *J. Neurophysiol.* 90, 1714–1727. doi: 10.1152/jn.00202.2003

Brocard, F., Ryczko, D., Fenelon, K., Hatem, R., Gonzales, D., Auclair, F., et al. (2010). The transformation of a unilateral locomotor command into a symmetrical bilateral activation in the brainstem. *J. Neurosci.* 30, 523–533. doi: 10.1523/JNEUROSCI.3433-09.2010

Brodin, L., Tossman, U., Ohta, Y., Ungerstedt, U., and Grillner, S. (1988). The effect of an uptake inhibitor (dihydrokainate) on endogenous excitatory amino acids in the lamprey spinal cord as revealed by microdialysis. *Brain Res.* 458, 166–169. doi: 10.1016/0006-8993(88)90511-2

Bryant, M. S., Rintala, D. H., Hou, J. G., Charness, A. L., Fernandez, A. L., Collins, R. L., et al. (2011a). Gait variability in Parkinson's disease: influence of walking speed and dopaminergic treatment. *Neurol. Res.* 33, 959–964. doi: 10.1179/1743132811Y.0000000044

Bryant, M. S., Rintala, D. H., Hou, J. G., Lai, E. C., and Protas, E. J. (2011b). Effects of levodopa on forward and backward gait patterns in persons with Parkinson's disease. *NeuroRehabilitation* 29, 247–252. doi: 10.3233/NRE-2011-0700

Buchanan, J. T., and Grillner, S. (1987). Newly identified "glutamate interneurons" and their role in locomotion in the lamprey spinal cord. *Science* 236, 312–314. doi: 10.1126/science.3563512

Cabelguen, J. M., Bourcier-Lucas, C., and Dubuc, R. (2003). Bimodal locomotion elicited by electrical stimulation of the midbrain in the salamander *Notophthalmus viridescens. J. Neurosci.* 23, 2434–2439.

Canu, E., Agosta, F., Sarasso, E., Volonte, M. A., Basaia, S., Stojkovic, T., et al. (2015). Brain structural and functional connectivity in Parkinson's disease with freezing of gait. *Hum. Brain Mapp.* 36, 5064–5078. doi: 10.1002/hbm.22994

Canudas, A. M., Pezzi, S., Canals, J. M., Pallas, M., and Alberch, J. (2005). Endogenous brain-derived neurotrophic factor protects dopaminergic nigral neurons against transneuronal degeneration induced by striatal excitotoxic injury. *Brain Res. Mol. Brain Res.* 134, 147–154. doi: 10.1016/j.molbrainres.2004.11.012

Carlsson, A. (1959). The occurrence, distribution and physiological role of catecholamines in the nervous system. *Pharmacol. Rev.* 11, 490–493.

Carlsson, A., Lindqvist, M., Magnusson, T., and Waldeck, B. (1958). On the presence of 3-hydroxytyramine in brain. *Science* 127:471. doi: 10.1126/science.127.3296.471

Chastan, N., Do, M. C., Bonneville, F., Torny, F., Bloch, F., Westby, G. W., et al. (2009). Gait and balance disorders in Parkinson's disease: impaired active braking of the fall of centre of gravity. *Mov. Disord.* 24, 188–195. doi: 10.1002/mds.22269

Collomb-Clerc, A., and Welter, M. L. (2015). Effects of deep brain stimulation on balance and gait in patients with Parkinson's disease: a systematic neurophysiological review. *Neurophysiol. Clin.* 45, 371–388. doi: 10.1016/j.neucli.2015.07.001

DeLong, M. R., and Wichmann, T. (2015). Basal ganglia circuits as targets for neuromodulation in Parkinson disease. *JAMA Neurol.* 72, 1354–1360. doi: 10.1001/jamaneurol.2015.2397

Demain, A., Westby, G. W., Fernandez-Vidal, S., Karachi, C., Bonneville, F., Do, M. C., et al. (2014). High-level gait and balance disorders in the elderly: a midbrain disease? *J. Neurol.* 261, 196–206. doi: 10.1007/s00415-013-7174-x

Derjean, D., Moussaddy, A., Atallah, E., St-Pierre, M., Auclair, F., Chang, S., et al. (2010). A novel neural substrate for the transformation of olfactory inputs into motor output. *PLoS Biol.* 8:e1000567. doi: 10.1371/journal.pbio.1000567

Di Prisco, G. V., Pearlstein, E., Le Ray, D., Robitaille, R., and Dubuc, R. (2000). A cellular mechanism for the transformation of a sensory input into a motor command. *J. Neurosci.* 20, 8169–8176.

Edley, S. M., and Graybiel, A. M. (1983). The afferent and efferent connections of the feline nucleus tegmenti pedunculopontinus, pars compacta. *J. Comp. Neurol.* 217, 187–215. doi: 10.1002/cne.902170207

Ehringer, H., and Hornykiewicz, O. (1998). Distribution of noradrenaline and dopamine (3-hydroxytyramine) in the human brain and their behavior in diseases of the extrapyramidal system. *Parkinsonism Relat. Disord.* 4, 53–57. doi: 10.1016/S1353-8020(98)00012-1

Eidelberg, E., Walden, J. G., and Nguyen, L. H. (1981). Locomotor control in macaque monkeys. *Brain* 104, 647–663. doi: 10.1093/brain/104.4.647-a

El-Khodor, B. F., and Burke, R. E. (2002). Medial forebrain bundle axotomy during development induces apoptosis in dopamine neurons of the substantia nigra and activation of caspases in their degenerating axons. *J. Comp. Neurol.* 452, 65–79. doi: 10.1002/cne.10367

Fahn, S. (2015). The medical treatment of Parkinson disease from James Parkinson to George Cotzias. *Mov. Disord.* 30, 4–18. doi: 10.1002/mds.26102

Fasano, A., Aquino, C. C., Krauss, J. K., Honey, C. R., and Bloem, B. R. (2015). Axial disability and deep brain stimulation in patients with Parkinson disease. *Nat. Rev. Neurol.* 11, 98–110. doi: 10.1038/nrneurol.2014.252

Fioravanti, V., Benuzzi, F., Codeluppi, L., Contardi, S., Cavallieri, F., Nichelli, P., et al. (2015). MRI correlates of Parkinson's disease progression: a voxel based morphometry study. *Parkinson's Dis.* 2015:378032. doi: 10.1155/2015/378032

Fling, B. W., Cohen, R. G., Mancini, M., Carpenter, S. D., Fair, D. A., Nutt, J. G., et al. (2014). Functional reorganization of the locomotor network in Parkinson patients with freezing of gait. *PLoS ONE* 9:e100291. doi: 10.1371/journal.pone.0100291

Fling, B. W., Cohen, R. G., Mancini, M., Nutt, J. G., Fair, D. A., and Horak, F. B. (2013). Asymmetric pedunculopontine network connectivity in parkinsonian patients with freezing of gait. *Brain* 136, 2405–2418. doi: 10.1093/brain/awt172

Fornito, A., Zalesky, A., and Breakspear, M. (2015). The connectomics of brain disorders. *Nat. Rev. Neurosci.* 16, 159–172. doi: 10.1038/nrn3901

Fraix, V., Bastin, J., David, O., Goetz, L., Ferraye, M., Benabid, A. L., et al. (2013). Pedunculopontine nucleus area oscillations during stance, stepping and freezing in Parkinson's disease. *PLoS ONE* 8:e83919. doi: 10.1371/journal.pone.0083919

Freeze, B. S., Kravitz, A. V., Hammack, N., Berke, J. D., and Kreitzer, A. C. (2013). Control of basal ganglia output by direct and indirect pathway projection neurons. *J. Neurosci.* 33, 18531–18539. doi: 10.1523/JNEUROSCI.1278-13.2013

Garcia-Rill, E., Houser, C. R., Skinner, R. D., Smith, W., and Woodward, D. J. (1987). Locomotion-inducing sites in the vicinity of the pedunculopontine nucleus. *Brain Res. Bull.* 18, 731–738. doi: 10.1016/0361-9230(87)90208-5

Garcia-Rill, E., Luster, B., D'Onofrio, S., and Mahaffey, S. (2015a). Arousal, motor control, and parkinson's disease. *Transl. Neurosci.* 6, 198–207. doi: 10.1515/tnsci-2015-0021

Garcia-Rill, E., Luster, B., D'Onofrio, S., Mahaffey, S., Bisagno, V., and Urbano, F. J. (2015b). Pedunculopontine arousal system physiology - Deep brain stimulation (DBS). *Sleep Sci.* 8, 153–161. doi: 10.1016/j.slsci.2015.09.001

Garcia-Rill, E., and Skinner, R. D. (1987a). The mesencephalic locomotor region. I. Activation of a medullary projection site. *Brain Res.* 411, 1–12. doi: 10.1016/0006-8993(87)90675-5

Garcia-Rill, E., and Skinner, R. D. (1987b). The mesencephalic locomotor region. II. Projections to reticulospinal neurons. *Brain Res.* 411, 13–20. doi: 10.1016/0006-8993(87)90676-7

Gariepy, J. F., Missaghi, K., Chevallier, S., Chartre, S., Robert, M., Auclair, F., et al. (2012). Specific neural substrate linking respiration to locomotion. *Proc. Natl. Acad. Sci. U.S.A.* 109, E84–E92. doi: 10.1073/pnas.1113002109

Goetz, L., Piallat, B., Bhattacharjee, M., Mathieu, H., David, O., and Chabardes, S. (2016a). On the role of the pedunculopontine nucleus and mesencephalic reticular formation in locomotion in nonhuman primates. *J. Neurosci.* 36, 4917–4929. doi: 10.1523/JNEUROSCI.2514-15.2016

Goetz, L., Piallat, B., Bhattacharjee, M., Mathieu, H., David, O., and Chabardes, S. (2016b). The primate pedunculopontine nucleus region: towards a dual role in locomotion and waking state. *J. Neural Transm.* 123, 667–678. doi: 10.1007/s00702-016-1577-7

Golestanirad, L., Elahi, B., Graham, S. J., Das, S., and Wald, L. L. (2016). Efficacy and safety of pedunculopontine nuclei (PPN) deep brain stimulation in the treatment of gait disorders: a meta-analysis of clinical studies. *Can. J. Neurol. Sci.* 43, 120–126. doi: 10.1017/cjn.2015.318

Gravel, J., Brocard, F., Gariepy, J. F., Lund, J. P., and Dubuc, R. (2007). Modulation of respiratory activity by locomotion in lampreys. *Neuroscience* 144, 1120–1132. doi: 10.1016/j.neuroscience.2006.10.019

Grillner, S., and Robertson, B. (2016). The basal ganglia over 500 million years. *Curr. Biol.* 26, R1088–R1100. doi: 10.1016/j.cub.2016.06.041

Hamani, C., Aziz, T., Bloem, B. R., Brown, P., Chabardes, S., Coyne, T., et al. (2016a). Pedunculopontine nucleus region deep brain stimulation in Parkinson disease: surgical anatomy and terminology. *Stereotact. Funct. Neurosurg.* 94, 298–306. doi: 10.1159/000449010

Hamani, C., Lozano, A. M., Mazzone, P. A., Moro, E., Hutchison, W., Silburn, P. A., et al. (2016b). Pedunculopontine nucleus region deep brain stimulation in

Parkinson disease: surgical techniques, side effects, and postoperative imaging. *Stereotact. Funct. Neurosurg.* 94, 307–319. doi: 10.1159/000449011

Herbin, M., Boire, D., Theoret, H., and Ptito, M. (1999). Transneuronal degeneration of retinal ganglion cells in early hemispherectomized monkeys. *Neuroreport* 10, 1447–1452. doi: 10.1097/00001756-199905140-00011

Hirsch, E. C., Graybiel, A. M., Duyckaerts, C., and Javoy-Agid, F. (1987). Neuronal loss in the pedunculopontine tegmental nucleus in Parkinson disease and in progressive supranuclear palsy. *Proc. Natl. Acad. Sci. U.S.A.* 84, 5976–5980. doi: 10.1073/pnas.84.16.5976

Holiga, S., Mueller, K., Moller, H. E., Urgosik, D., Ruzicka, E., Schroeter, M. L., et al. (2015). Resting-state functional magnetic resonance imaging of the subthalamic microlesion and stimulation effects in Parkinson's disease: indications of a principal role of the brainstem. *NeuroImage Clin.* 9, 264–274. doi: 10.1016/j.nicl.2015.08.008

Hubel, D. H., and Wiesel, T. N. (1970). The period of susceptibility to the physiological effects of unilateral eye closure in kittens. *J. Physiol.* 206, 419–436. doi: 10.1113/jphysiol.1970.sp009022

Ichinohe, N., Teng, B., and Kitai, S. T. (2000). Morphological study of the tegmental pedunculopontine nucleus, substantia nigra and subthalamic nucleus, and their interconnections in rat organotypic culture. *Anat. Embryol.* 201, 435–453. doi: 10.1007/s004290050331

Jahn, K., Deutschlander, A., Stephan, T., Kalla, R., Wiesmann, M., Strupp, M., et al. (2008). Imaging human supraspinal locomotor centers in brainstem and cerebellum. *Neuroimage* 39, 786–792. doi: 10.1016/j.neuroimage.2007.09.047

Jellinger, K. (1988). The pedunculopontine nucleus in Parkinson's disease, progressive supranuclear palsy and Alzheimer's disease. *J. Neurol. Neurosurg. Psychiatry* 51, 540–543. doi: 10.1136/jnnp.51.4.540

Juvin, L., Gratsch, S., Trillaud-Doppia, E., Gariepy, J. F., Buschges, A., and Dubuc, R. (2016). A specific population of reticulospinal neurons controls the termination of locomotion. *Cell Rep.* 15, 2377–2386. doi: 10.1016/j.celrep.2016.05.029

Karachi, C., Andre, A., Bertasi, E., Bardinet, E., Lehericy, S., and Bernard, F. A. (2012). Functional parcellation of the lateral mesencephalus. *J. Neurosci.* 32, 9396–9401. doi: 10.1523/JNEUROSCI.0509-12.2012

Karachi, C., and Francois, C. (2017). Role of the pedunculopontine nucleus in controlling gait and sleep in normal and parkinsonian monkeys. *J. Neural Transm.* doi: 10.1007/s00702-017-1678-y. [Epub ahead of print].

Karachi, C., Grabli, D., Bernard, F. A., Tande, D., Wattiez, N., Belaid, H., et al. (2010). Cholinergic mesencephalic neurons are involved in gait and postural disorders in Parkinson disease. *J. Clin. Invest.* 120, 2745–2754. doi: 10.1172/JCI42642

Kitahama, K., Nagatsu, I., Geffard, M., and Maeda, T. (2000). Distribution of dopamine-immunoreactive fibers in the rat brainstem. *J. Chem. Neuroanat.* 18, 1–9. doi: 10.1016/S0891-0618(99)00047-2

Knight, E. J., Testini, P., Min, H. K., Gibson, W. S., Gorny, K. R., Favazza, C. P., et al. (2015). Motor and nonmotor circuitry activation induced by subthalamic nucleus deep brain stimulation in patients with parkinson disease: intraoperative functional magnetic resonance imaging for deep brain stimulation. *Mayo Clin. Proc.* 90, 773–785. doi: 10.1016/j.mayocp.2015.03.022

Kravitz, A. V., Freeze, B. S., Parker, P. R., Kay, K., Thwin, M. T., Deisseroth, K., et al. (2010). Regulation of parkinsonian motor behaviours by optogenetic control of basal ganglia circuitry. *Nature* 466, 622–626. doi: 10.1038/nature09159

Kuo, S. H., Kenney, C., and Jankovic, J. (2008). Bilateral pedunculopontine nuclei strokes presenting as freezing of gait. *Mov. Disord.* 23, 616–619. doi: 10.1002/mds.21917

Lau, B., Welter, M. L., Belaid, H., Fernandez Vidal, S., Bardinet, E., Grabli, D., et al. (2015). The integrative role of the pedunculopontine nucleus in human gait. *Brain* 138, 1284–1296. doi: 10.1093/brain/awv047

Lavoie, B., and Parent, A. (1994). Pedunculopontine nucleus in the squirrel monkey: cholinergic and glutamatergic projections to the substantia nigra. *J. Comp. Neurol.* 344, 232–241. doi: 10.1002/cne.903440205

Lee, A. M., Hoy, J. L., Bonci, A., Wilbrecht, L., Stryker, M. P., and Niell, C. M. (2014). Identification of a brainstem circuit regulating visual cortical state in parallel with locomotion. *Neuron* 83, 455–466. doi: 10.1016/j.neuron.2014.06.031

Le Ray, D., Brocard, F., Bourcier-Lucas, C., Auclair, F., Lafaille, P., and Dubuc, R. (2003). Nicotinic activation of reticulospinal cells involved in the control of swimming in lampreys. *Eur. J. Neurosci.* 17, 137–148. doi: 10.1046/j.1460-9568.2003.02417.x

Le Ray, D., Juvin, L., Ryczko, D., and Dubuc, R. (2011). Chapter 4–supraspinal control of locomotion: the mesencephalic locomotor region. *Prog. Brain Res.* 188, 51–70. doi: 10.1016/B978-0-444-53825-3.00009-7

Liu, H. G., Zhang, K., Yang, A. C., and Zhang, J. G. (2015). Deep brain stimulation of the subthalamic and pedunculopontine nucleus in a patient with Parkinson's disease. *J. Korean Neurosurg. Soc.* 57, 303–306. doi: 10.3340/jkns.2015.57.4.303

Macaya, A., Munell, F., Gubits, R. M., and Burke, R. E. (1994). Apoptosis in substantia nigra following developmental striatal excitotoxic injury. *Proc. Natl. Acad. Sci. U.S.A.* 91, 8117–8121. doi: 10.1073/pnas.91.17.8117

Marin, O., Smeets, W. J., and Gonzalez, A. (1997). Basal ganglia organization in amphibians: catecholaminergic innervation of the striatum and the nucleus accumbens. *J. Comp. Neurol.* 378, 50–69.

Marlinsky, V. V., and Voitenko, L. P. (1991). The effect of procaine injection into the medullary reticular formation on forelimb muscle activity evoked by mesencephalic locomotor region and vestibular stimulation in the decerebrated guinea-pig. *Neuroscience* 45, 753–759. doi: 10.1016/0306-4522(91)90287-X

Marti, M. J., James, C. J., Oo, T. F., Kelly, W. J., and Burke, R. E. (1997). Early developmental destruction of terminals in the striatal target induces apoptosis in dopamine neurons of the substantia nigra. *J. Neurosci.* 17, 2030–2039.

Masdeu, J. C., Alampur, U., Cavaliere, R., and Tavoulareas, G. (1994). Astasia and gait failure with damage of the pontomesencephalic locomotor region. *Ann. Neurol.* 35, 619–621. doi: 10.1002/ana.410350517

Mazzone, P., Paoloni, M., Mangone, M., Santilli, V., Insola, A., Fini, M., et al. (2014). Unilateral deep brain stimulation of the pedunculopontine tegmental nucleus in idiopathic Parkinson's disease: effects on gait initiation and performance. *Gait Posture* 40, 357–362. doi: 10.1016/j.gaitpost.2014.05.002

Mazzone, P., Sposato, S., Insola, A., and Scarnati, E. (2013). The clinical effects of deep brain stimulation of the pedunculopontine tegmental nucleus in movement disorders may not be related to the anatomical target, leads location, and setup of electrical stimulation. *Neurosurgery* 73, 894–906; discussion 905–906. doi: 10.1227/neu.0000000000000108

McGeer, E. G., and McGeer, P. L. (1984). Substantia nigra cell death from kainic acid or folic acid injections into the pontine tegmentum. *Brain Res.* 298, 339–342. doi: 10.1016/0006-8993(84)91433-1

Menard, A., Auclair, F., Bourcier-Lucas, C., Grillner, S., and Dubuc, R. (2007). Descending GABAergic projections to the mesencephalic locomotor region in the lamprey Petromyzon marinus. *J. Comp. Neurol.* 501, 260–273. doi: 10.1002/cne.21258

Mestre, T. A., Sidiropoulos, C., Hamani, C., Poon, Y. Y., Lozano, A. M., Lang, A. E., et al. (2016). Long-term double-blinded unilateral pedunculopontine area stimulation in Parkinson's disease. *Mov. Disord.* 31, 1570–1574. doi: 10.1002/mds.26710

Moore, S. T., MacDougall, H. G., Gracies, J. M., and Ondo, W. G. (2008). Locomotor response to levodopa in fluctuating Parkinson's disease. *Exp. Brain Res.* 184, 469–478. doi: 10.1007/s00221-007-1113-y

Musienko, P. E., Zelenin, P. V., Lyalka, V. F., Orlovsky, G. N., and Deliagina, T. G. (2008). Postural performance in decerebrated rabbit. *Behav. Brain Res.* 190, 124–134. doi: 10.1016/j.bbr.2008.02.011

Neagu, B., Tsang, E., Mazzella, F., Hamani, C., Moro, E., Hodaie, M., et al. (2013). Pedunculopontine nucleus evoked potentials from subthalamic nucleus stimulation in Parkinson's disease. *Exp. Neurol.* 250, 221–227. doi: 10.1016/j.expneurol.2013.09.018

Noga, B. R., Kettler, J., and Jordan, L. M. (1988). Locomotion produced in mesencephalic cats by injections of putative transmitter substances and antagonists into the medial reticular formation and the pontomedullary locomotor strip. *J. Neurosci.* 8, 2074–2086.

Noga, B. R., Kriellaars, D. J., and Jordan, L. M. (1991). The effect of selective brainstem or spinal cord lesions on treadmill locomotion evoked by stimulation of the mesencephalic or pontomedullary locomotor regions. *J. Neurosci.* 11, 1691–1700.

Nosko, D., Ferraye, M. U., Fraix, V., Goetz, L., Chabardes, S., Pollak, P., et al. (2015). Low-frequency versus high-frequency stimulation of the pedunculopontine nucleus area in Parkinson's disease: a randomised controlled trial. *J. Neurol. Neurosurg. Psychiatry* 86, 674–679. doi: 10.1136/jnnp-2013-307511

Ohta, Y., and Grillner, S. (1989). Monosynaptic excitatory amino acid transmission from the posterior rhombencephalic reticular nucleus to spinal neurons involved in the control of locomotion in lamprey. *J. Neurophysiol.* 62, 1079–1089.

Orlovskii, G. N. (1970). [Work of reticulo-spinal neurons during locomotion]. *Biofizika* 15, 728–737.

Pedersen, V., and Schmidt, W. J. (2000). The neuroprotectant properties of glutamate antagonists and antiglutamatergic drugs. *Neurotox. Res.* 2, 179–204. doi: 10.1007/BF03033793

Perez-Fernandez, J., Stephenson-Jones, M., Suryanarayana, S. M., Robertson, B., and Grillner, S. (2014). Evolutionarily conserved organization of the dopaminergic system in lamprey: SNc/VTA afferent and efferent connectivity and D2 receptor expression. *J. Comp. Neurol.* 522, 3775–3794. doi: 10.1002/cne.23639

Peterson, D. S., Pickett, K. A., Duncan, R., Perlmutter, J., and Earhart, G. M. (2014). Gait-related brain activity in people with Parkinson disease with freezing of gait. *PLoS ONE* 9:e90634. doi: 10.1371/journal.pone.0090634

Piallat, B., Chabardes, S., Torres, N., Fraix, V., Goetz, L., Seigneuret, E., et al. (2009). Gait is associated with an increase in tonic firing of the sub-cuneiform nucleus neurons. *Neuroscience* 158, 1201–1205. doi: 10.1016/j.neuroscience.2008.10.046

Pienaar, I. S., Elson, J. L., Racca, C., Nelson, G., Turnbull, D. M., and Morris, C. M. (2013). Mitochondrial abnormality associates with type-specific neuronal loss and cell morphology changes in the pedunculopontine nucleus in Parkinson disease. *Am. J. Pathol.* 183, 1826–1840. doi: 10.1016/j.ajpath.2013.09.002

Pienaar, I. S., Gartside, S. E., Sharma, P., De Paola, V., Gretenkord, S., Withers, D., et al. (2015a). Pharmacogenetic stimulation of cholinergic pedunculopontine neurons reverses motor deficits in a rat model of Parkinson's disease. *Mol. Neurodegener.* 10:47. doi: 10.1186/s13024-015-0044-5

Pienaar, I. S., Harrison, I. F., Elson, J. L., Bury, A., Woll, P., Simon, A. K., et al. (2015b). An animal model mimicking pedunculopontine nucleus cholinergic degeneration in Parkinson's disease. *Brain Struct. Funct.* 220, 479–500. doi: 10.1007/s00429-013-0669-5

Pinching, A. J., and Powell, T. P. (1971). Ultrastructural features of transneuronal cell degeneration in the olfactory system. *J. Cell Sci.* 8, 253–287.

Plaha, P., and Gill, S. S. (2005). Bilateral deep brain stimulation of the pedunculopontine nucleus for Parkinson's disease. *Neuroreport* 16, 1883–1887. doi: 10.1097/01.wnr.0000187637.20771.a0

Poirier, L., and Sourkes, T. L. (1965). Influence of the substantia nigra on the catecholamine content of the striatum. *Brain* 88, 181–192. doi: 10.1093/brain/88.1.181

Pombal, M. A., El Manira, A., and Grillner, S. (1997). Afferents of the lamprey striatum with special reference to the dopaminergic system: a combined tracing and immunohistochemical study. *J. Comp. Neurol.* 386, 71–91.

Puelles, L., and Verney, C. (1998). Early neuromeric distribution of tyrosine-hydroxylase-immunoreactive neurons in human embryos. *J. Comp. Neurol.* 394, 283–308.

Rink, E., and Wullimann, M. F. (2001). The teleostean (zebrafish) dopaminergic system ascending to the subpallium (striatum) is located in the basal diencephalon (posterior tuberculum). *Brain Res.* 889, 316–330. doi: 10.1016/S0006-8993(00)03174-7

Rinne, J. O., Ma, S. Y., Lee, M. S., Collan, Y., and Roytta, M. (2008). Loss of cholinergic neurons in the pedunculopontine nucleus in Parkinson's disease is related to disability of the patients. *Parkinsonism Relat. Disord.* 14, 553–557. doi: 10.1016/j.parkreldis.2008.01.006

Rolland, A. S., Tande, D., Herrero, M. T., Luquin, M. R., Vazquez-Claverie, M., Karachi, C., et al. (2009). Evidence for a dopaminergic innervation of the pedunculopontine nucleus in monkeys, and its drastic reduction after MPTP intoxication. *J. Neurochem.* 110, 1321–1329. doi: 10.1111/j.1471-4159.2009.06220.x

Roseberry, T. K., Lee, A. M., Lalive, A. L., Wilbrecht, L., Bonci, A., and Kreitzer, A. C. (2016). Cell-type-specific control of brainstem locomotor circuits by basal ganglia. *Cell* 164, 526–537. doi: 10.1016/j.cell.2015.12.037

Rowe, J., Khan, A., Romanowski, C., Isaac, C., Khan, S., Mair, R., et al. (2016). Clinical experience with pedunculopontine nucleus stimulation in conditions with nigrostriatal disconnection. *World Neurosurg.* 89, 9–18. doi: 10.1016/j.wneu.2015.11.054

Ryczko, D., Auclair, F., Cabelguen, J. M., and Dubuc, R. (2016b). The mesencephalic locomotor region sends a bilateral glutamatergic drive to hindbrain reticulospinal neurons in a tetrapod. *J. Comp. Neurol.* 524, 1361–1383. doi: 10.1002/cne.23911

Ryczko, D., Cone, J. J., Alpert, M. H., Goetz, L., Auclair, F., Dube, C., et al. (2016a). A descending dopamine pathway conserved from basal vertebrates to mammals. *Proc. Natl. Acad. Sci. U.S.A.* 113, E2440–E2449. doi: 10.1073/pnas.1600684113

Ryczko, D., and Dubuc, R. (2013). The multifunctional mesencephalic locomotor region. *Curr. Pharm. Des.* 19, 4448–4470. doi: 10.2174/1381612811319240011

Ryczko, D., Gratsch, S., Auclair, F., Dube, C., Bergeron, S., Alpert, M. H., et al. (2013). Forebrain dopamine neurons project down to a brainstem region controlling locomotion. *Proc. Natl. Acad. Sci. U.S.A.* 110, E3235–E3242. doi: 10.1073/pnas.1301125110

Saavedra, J. M., Kvetnansky, R., and Kopin, I. J. (1979). Adrenaline, noradrenaline and dopamine levels in specific brain stem areas of acutely immobilized rats. *Brain Res.* 160, 271–280. doi: 10.1016/0006-8993(79)90424-4

Sano, I., Gamo, T., Kakimoto, Y., Taniguchi, K., Takesada, M., and Nishinuma, K. (1959). Distribution of catechol compounds in human brain. *Biochim. Biophys. Acta* 32, 586–587. doi: 10.1016/0006-3002(59)90652-3

Scarnati, E., Campana, E., and Pacitti, C. (1984). Pedunculopontine-evoked excitation of substantia nigra neurons in the rat. *Brain Res.* 304, 351–361. doi: 10.1016/0006-8993(84)90339-1

Scarnati, E., Proia, A., Di Loreto, S., and Pacitti, C. (1987). The reciprocal electrophysiological influence between the nucleus tegmenti pedunculopontinus and the substantia nigra in normal and decorticated rats. *Brain Res.* 423, 116–124. doi: 10.1016/0006-8993(87)90831-6

Schrader, C., Seehaus, F., Capelle, H. H., Windhagen, A., Windhagen, H., and Krauss, J. K. (2013). Effects of pedunculopontine area and pallidal DBS on gait ignition in Parkinson's disease. *Brain Stimul.* 6, 856–859. doi: 10.1016/j.brs.2013.05.005

Seidel, K., Mahlke, J., Siswanto, S., Kruger, R., Heinsen, H., Auburger, G., et al. (2015). The brainstem pathologies of Parkinson's disease and dementia with Lewy bodies. *Brain Pathol.* 25, 121–135. doi: 10.1111/bpa.12168

Semba, K., and Fibiger, H. C. (1992). Afferent connections of the laterodorsal and the pedunculopontine tegmental nuclei in the rat: a retro- and antero-grade transport and immunohistochemical study. *J. Comp. Neurol.* 323, 387–410. doi: 10.1002/cne.903230307

Shik, M. L., Severin, F. V., and Orlovskii, G. N. (1966). [Control of walking and running by means of electric stimulation of the midbrain]. *Biofizika* 11, 659–666.

Shine, J. M., Matar, E., Ward, P. B., Bolitho, S. J., Gilat, M., Pearson, M., et al. (2013). Exploring the cortical and subcortical functional magnetic resonance imaging changes associated with freezing in Parkinson's disease. *Brain* 136, 1204–1215. doi: 10.1093/brain/awt049

Sholomenko, G. N., Funk, G. D., and Steeves, J. D. (1991). Avian locomotion activated by brainstem infusion of neurotransmitter agonists and antagonists. II. gamma-Aminobutyric acid. *Exp. Brain Res.* 85, 674–681. doi: 10.1007/BF00231753

Sirota, M. G., Di Prisco, G. V., and Dubuc, R. (2000). Stimulation of the mesencephalic locomotor region elicits controlled swimming in semi-intact lampreys. *Eur. J. Neurosci.* 12, 4081–4092. doi: 10.1046/j.1460-9568.2000.00301.x

Smeets, W. J., Marin, O., and Gonzalez, A. (2000). Evolution of the basal ganglia: new perspectives through a comparative approach. *J. Anat.* 196(Pt 4), 501–517. doi: 10.1046/j.1469-7580.2000.19640501.x

Smetana, R., Juvin, L., Dubuc, R., and Alford, S. (2010). A parallel cholinergic brainstem pathway for enhancing locomotor drive. *Nat. Neurosci.* 13, 731–738. doi: 10.1038/nn.2548

Snijders, A. H., Leunissen, I., Bakker, M., Overeem, S., Helmich, R. C., Bloem, B. R., et al. (2011). Gait-related cerebral alterations in patients with Parkinson's disease with freezing of gait. *Brain* 134, 59–72. doi: 10.1093/brain/awq324

Snijders, A. H., Takakusaki, K., Debu, B., Lozano, A. M., Krishna, V., Fasano, A., et al. (2016). Physiology of freezing of gait. *Ann. Neurol.* 80, 644–659. doi: 10.1002/ana.24778

Sourkes, T. L., and Poirier, L. (1965). Influence of the substantia nigra on the concentration of 5-hydroxytryptamine and dopamine of the striatum. *Nature* 207, 202–203. doi: 10.1038/207202a0

Stack, E., and Ashburn, A. (2008). Dysfunctional turning in Parkinson's disease. *Disabil. Rehabil.* 30, 1222–1229. doi: 10.1080/09638280701829938

Steeves, J. D., and Jordan, L. M. (1980). Localization of a descending pathway in the spinal cord which is necessary for controlled treadmill locomotion. *Neurosci. Lett.* 20, 283–288. doi: 10.1016/0304-3940(80)90161-5

Stefani, A., Peppe, A., Galati, S., Bassi, M. S., D'Angelo, V., and Pierantozzi, M. (2013). The serendipity case of the pedunculopontine nucleus low-frequency brain stimulation: chasing a gait response, finding sleep, and cognition improvement. *Front. Neurol.* 4:68. doi: 10.3389/fneur.2013.00068

Steiniger, B., and Kretschmer, B. D. (2003). Glutamate and GABA modulate dopamine in the pedunculopontine tegmental nucleus. *Exp. Brain Res.* 149, 422–430. doi: 10.1007/s00221-003-1382-z

Steininger, T. L., Rye, D. B., and Wainer, B. H. (1992). Afferent projections to the cholinergic pedunculopontine tegmental nucleus and adjacent midbrain extrapyramidal area in the albino rat. I. Retrograde tracing studies. *J. Comp. Neurol.* 321, 515–543. doi: 10.1002/cne.903210403

Tard, C., Delval, A., Devos, D., Lopes, R., Lenfant, P., Dujardin, K., et al. (2015). Brain metabolic abnormalities during gait with freezing in Parkinson's disease. *Neuroscience* 307, 281–301. doi: 10.1016/j.neuroscience.2015.08.063

Tattersall, T. L., Stratton, P. G., Coyne, T. J., Cook, R., Silberstein, P., Silburn, P. A., et al. (2014). Imagined gait modulates neuronal network dynamics in the human pedunculopontine nucleus. *Nat. Neurosci.* 17, 449–454. doi: 10.1038/nn.3642

Thevathasan, W., Pogosyan, A., Hyam, J. A., Jenkinson, N., Foltynie, T., Limousin, P., et al. (2012). Alpha oscillations in the pedunculopontine nucleus correlate with gait performance in parkinsonism. *Brain* 135, 148–160. doi: 10.1093/brain/awr315

Vercruysse, S., Leunissen, I., Vervoort, G., Vandenberghe, W., Swinnen, S., and Nieuwboer, A. (2015). Microstructural changes in white matter associated with freezing of gait in Parkinson's disease. *Mov. Disord.* 30, 567–576. doi: 10.1002/mds.26130

Versteeg, D. H., Van Der Gugten, J., De Jong, W., and Palkovits, M. (1976). Regional concentrations of noradrenaline and dopamine in rat brain. *Brain Res.* 113, 563–574. doi: 10.1016/0006-8993(76)90057-3

Wang, M., Jiang, S., Yuan, Y., Zhang, L., Ding, J., Wang, J., et al. (2016). Alterations of functional and structural connectivity of freezing of gait in Parkinson's disease. *J. Neurol.* 263, 1583–1592. doi: 10.1007/s00415-016-8174-4

Weiss, P. H., Herzog, J., Potter-Nerger, M., Falk, D., Herzog, H., Deuschl, G., et al. (2015). Subthalamic nucleus stimulation improves Parkinsonian gait via brainstem locomotor centers. *Mov. Disord.* 30, 1121–1125. doi: 10.1002/mds.26229

Welter, M. L., Demain, A., Ewenczyk, C., Czernecki, V., Lau, B., El Helou, A., et al. (2015). PPNa-DBS for gait and balance disorders in Parkinson's disease: a double-blind, randomised study. *J. Neurol.* 262, 1515–1525. doi: 10.1007/s00415-015-7744-1

Windels, F., Thevathasan, W., Silburn, P., and Sah, P. (2015). Where and what is the PPN and what is its role in locomotion? *Brain* 138, 1133–1134. doi: 10.1093/brain/awv059

Wullimann, M. F. (2014). Ancestry of basal ganglia circuits: new evidence in teleosts. *J. Comp. Neurol.* 522, 2013–2018. doi: 10.1002/cne.23525

Xiao, C., Cho, J. R., Zhou, C., Treweek, J. B., Chan, K., McKinney, S. L., et al. (2016). Cholinergic mesopontine signals govern locomotion and reward through dissociable midbrain pathways. *Neuron* 90, 333–347. doi: 10.1016/j.neuron.2016.03.028

Yamamoto, K., and Vernier, P. (2011). The evolution of dopamine systems in chordates. *Front. Neuroanat.* 5:21. doi: 10.3389/fnana.2011.00021

Yeo, S. S., Lee, D. G., Choi, B. Y., Chang, C. H., Jung, Y. J., Kim, S. H., et al. (2012). Neural connectivity of the pedunculopontine nucleus in relation to walking ability in chronic patients with intracerebral hemorrhage. *Eur. Neurol.* 67, 226–231. doi: 10.1159/000335248

Yoo, J. H., Zell, V., Wu, J., Punta, C., Ramajayam, N., Shen, X., et al. (2017). Activation of pedunculopontine glutamate neurons is reinforcing. *J. Neurosci.* 37, 38–46. doi: 10.1523/JNEUROSCI.3082-16.2017

Youn, J., Lee, J. M., Kwon, H., Kim, J. S., Son, T. O., and Cho, J. W. (2015). Alterations of mean diffusivity of pedunculopontine nucleus pathway in Parkinson's disease patients with freezing of gait. *Parkinsonism Relat. Disord.* 21, 12–17. doi: 10.1016/j.parkreldis.2014.10.003

Zweig, R. M., Jankel, W. R., Hedreen, J. C., Mayeux, R., and Price, D. L. (1989). The pedunculopontine nucleus in Parkinson's disease. *Ann. Neurol.* 26, 41–46. doi: 10.1002/ana.410260106

Zweig, R. M., Whitehouse, P. J., Casanova, M. F., Walker, L. C., Jankel, W. R., and Price, D. L. (1987). Loss of pedunculopontine neurons in progressive supranuclear palsy. *Ann. Neurol.* 22, 18–25. doi: 10.1002/ana.410220107

4

A Meta-Analysis of Adenosine A2A Receptor Antagonists on Levodopa-Induced Dyskinesia *In Vivo*

Wen-Wen Wang[1†], Man-Man Zhang[2†], Xing-Ru Zhang[2], Zeng-Rui Zhang[2], Jie Chen[2], Liang Feng[2] and Cheng-Long Xie[2*]*

[1] The Center of Traditional Chinese Medicine, The Second Affiliated Hospital, Yuying Children's Hospital of Wenzhou Medical University, Wenzhou, China, [2] Department of Neurology, The First Affiliated Hospital of Wenzhou Medical University, Wenzhou, China

***Correspondence:**
Liang Feng
fengliangyw@126.com;
Cheng-Long Xie
cl_xie1987@sohu.com

[†]These authors have contributed equally to this work.

Background: Long-term use of levodopa (L-dopa) is inevitably complicated with highly disabling fluctuations and drug-induced dyskinesias, which pose major challenges to the existing drug therapy of Parkinson's disease.

Methods: In this study, we conducted a systematic review and meta-analysis to assess the efficacy of A2A receptor antagonists on reducing L-dopa-induced dyskinesias (LID).

Results: Nine studies with a total of 152 animals were included in this meta-analysis. Total abnormal involuntary movements (AIM) score, locomotor activity, and motor disability were reported as outcome measures in 5, 5, and 3 studies, respectively. Combined standardized mean difference (SMD) estimates were calculated using a random-effects model. We pooled the whole data and found that, when compared to L-dopa alone, A2A receptor antagonists plus L-dopa treatment showed no effect on locomotor activity (SMD −0.00, 95% confidence interval (CI): −2.52 to 2.52, $p = 1.0$), superiority in improvement of motor disability (SMD −5.06, 95% CI: −9.25 to −0.87, $p = 0.02$) and more effective in control of AIM (SMD −1.82, 95% CI: −3.38 to −0.25, $p = 0.02$).

Conclusion: To sum up, these results demonstrated that A2A receptor antagonists appear to have efficacy in animal models of LID. However, large randomized clinical trials testing the effects of A2A receptor antagonists in LID patients are always warranted.

Keywords: adenosine, A2A receptor antagonists, levodopa-induced dyskinesia, Parkinson's disease, meta-analysis

INTRODUCTION

Parkinson's disease (PD) is defined by a set of motor signs and symptoms that are caused by selective degeneration of the dopamine (DA) neurons, which originate in the substantia nigra pars compacta and project into the striatum (1). The most efficacious treatment for PD is the DA precursor levodopa (L-dopa), which not only improves all typical parkinsonian motor symptoms but also increases patients' life expectancy (2). However, the long-term use of L-dopa produces motor complications which include highly disabling fluctuations and L-dopa-induced dyskinesias (LID), representing the major challenges to the existing drug therapy of PD (3, 4). The management of LID includes switching to a controlled-release L-dopa or adding a COMT inhibitor/monoamineoxidase B inhibitor/a longer acting DA agonist (5). However, once LID is established, the increase in dopaminergic load resulted from these strategies can only lead to an aggravation of the condition, not only in the severity but also the duration (6). Moreover, recent researches have revealed that a wide series of non-dopaminergic neurotransmitter systems (glutamatergic, serotoninergic, adrenergic, and cholinergic, etc.) are involved in pre- and postsynaptic changes and thereby contributing to the pathophysiology of LID (5). Based on such therapies, many drugs are available in the market to treat disabling LID, but potential side effects have limited their clinical use (7).

The general pathophysiological interpretation and various hypotheses have been discussed for the genesis and development of LID. However, the exact mechanisms and the molecular targets are still poorly understood (8). Adenosine is believed to play a neuroprotective role in central neurodegenerative disorders and its actions are mediated by different receptors such as A1, A2A, A2B, and A3 (9). It has been suggested that A2A receptors are highly localized to the basal ganglia nuclei of the indirect output pathway, where they are co-localized with DA D2 receptors, and may be capable of influencing motor activity by acting at different levels (10). It is hypothesized that the effects of adenosine A2A receptor antagonists on motor function is attributed to their inhibitory function on neurons of the indirect pathway that expressing both A2A and D2 receptors (10). Moreover, inactivation A2A receptors on striatopallidal neurons of the indirect pathway can produce a parallel behavioral activation by means of mimicking the motor stimulant actions of co-localized D2 receptors on these neurons (11). Preclinical behavioral investigations reported that pharmacological antagonism or genetic knockdown of A2A receptors may be of interest to the management of LID (12). Furthermore, results from clinical studies had also shown that A2A receptor antagonists' significantly reduced off-time as an adjunctive therapy to L-dopa in advanced PD patients with motor fluctuations, also suggesting a possible reduced risk of L-dopa-induced motor complications (13). However, to date, few clinical trials have tested the benefits of A2A antagonists in LID patients. Limited clinical data demonstrate the possibility that in PD patients with established dyskinesia, we might be able to maintain the anti-parkinsonian response and reduce dyskinesia by adding an A2A antagonist and lowering the L-dopa dose, though this remains to be proven (14).

Systematic reviews and meta-analyses of preclinical animal data could facilitate the planning of further investigations and improve the likelihood of success of future clinical trials, also identify where there is a need for further experiment research, preclude unnecessary study replication, and contribute to both reduction and refinement in animal experimentation (15). Therefore, we report a systematic review and meta-analysis of adenosine A2A receptor antagonists in experimental models of PD with LID.

MATERIALS AND METHODS

The whole process and methods of this meta-analysis were performed according to our previous published paper (16) and based on the modified Preferred Reporting Items for Systematic Reviews and Meta-Analyses (PRISMA) Statement.

Search Strategy

We electronically searched three databases (PubMed, Google scholar, and EMBASE database) up to January 2016 for all publications written in English. All searches were limited to studies on animals. Reference lists from the included literature were scrutinized to identify further relevant publications. The search strategy as follows:

1. adenosine
2. adenocard
3. adenoscan
4. or/1–3
5. dyskinesia
6. abnormal
7. involuntary movements
8. hemiballismus
9. or/5–8
10. 4 and 9

Inclusion and Exclusion Criteria

Inclusion criteria:

(1) Test the effects of adenosine A2A receptor antagonists on LID in animal models of PD. Adenosine A2A receptor antagonists are defined as a drug with reported agonism on at least one class of A2A receptor irrespective of actions at other receptor classes.
(2) Use abnormal involuntary movements (AIM) or neurobehavioral score as the outcome measure comparing LID animals receiving combined treatment (both adenosine A2A receptor antagonists and L-dopa) and L-dopa/benserazide or L-dopa/carbidopa alone. AIM ratings were performed as we previously described (17). Briefly, 0 = absent, 1 = present less than 50% of the observation period, 2 = present more than 50% of the observation time, 3 = present all the times but suppressible by external stimuli, and 4 = present all the times and not interfering by external stimuli.
(3) Original data being independent of other studies.

Pre-specified exclusion criteria were: (1) case reports, abstracts, comments, reviews, editorials, and clinical trials; (2) dyskinesia was not developed by long-term L-dopa; (3) not testing the efficacy of adenosine receptor antagonists on LID; and (4) AIM or neurobehavioral score was not the outcome measure.

Data Extraction

From included studies, data listed out as follows were extracted using a comprehensive approach: (1) the first author's name and publication year, experimental models [1-methyl-4-phenyl-1,2,3,6-tetrahydropyridine (MPTP) models or 6-Hydroxydopamine (6-OHDA) models, etc.]; (2) individual data for each animal including number, species, sex, weight, and anesthetic used; (3) information on treatment including route of administration and dosage; and (4) outcome measures and time of assessment of outcomes. If outcomes were presented at different time points, we extracted data from the last one reported. If the data for meta-analysis were missing or only expressed graphically, we tried to contact the authors for further information, or calculate by ourselves using digital ruler software, or excluded the study which we could not get enough information. For each comparison, we extracted data of mean value and standard deviation from treatment and control group, respectively, of each study.

Quality Assessment

Study quality was evaluated based on a six-item modified scale (18): peer-reviewed publication, random allocation to groups, blinded assessment of outcome, sample size calculation, compliance with animal welfare regulations, and a statement of a potential conflict of interest. For the calculation of an aggregate quality score, each item of the six-item modified scale was attributed one point. Two authors (Cheng-Long Xie and Jie Chen) independently extracted data and assessed study quality. Disagreements were solved after discussion on the details of the studies.

Statistical Analysis

We utilized a random-effects model because it took into account the fact that the true treatment effects had likely varied among the included trials. We conceived the main outcome measures as continuous data, and were given an estimate of the combined overall effect sizes using standardized mean difference (SMD) and its standard error, with 95% confidence interval (CI). To pool different scales, we used the SMD as the summary statistic in our meta-analysis as it reveals the effect size of the treatment relative to the variability observed in the same study (19). For the assessment of heterogeneity, the I^2 statistic was used. To assess the stability of the results, a sensitivity analysis was performed by removing each individual study in turn from the total and reanalyzing the remainder. Meanwhile, we performed a stratified meta-analysis with experiments grouped according to different kinds of adenosine A2A receptor antagonists. All the analyses were done with Revman software 5.0. Probability value $p < 0.05$ was considered significant.

RESULTS

Results of the Search

From the electronic search, 621 publications were initially identified, from which we excluded 456 due to repetition. After screening the titles and abstracts, 108 were further excluded because they failed to meet the inclusion criteria. By reading the full text of the remaining 57 articles, 40 studies were excluded as a result of not testing the efficacy of adenosine A2A receptor antagonists on LID ($n = 21$), inappropriate outcome indicators ($n = 14$), and the problem of duplicate data ($n = 7$). Another eight studies were excluded as the dyskinesia presented was not developed by long-term L-dopa. Ultimately, nine eligible studies were identified (12, 20–27) (**Figure 1**).

Study Characteristics

These studies involved 152 animals (A2A receptor antagonists 83, control 69) from three species: Mice ($n = 53$), Sprague-Dawley rats ($n = 67$), and Marmosets ($n = 32$), respectively. The studies varied in size, ranging from 8 to 36 animals. Three out of nine (3/9, 33.3%) studies were MPTP models, while the remaining utilized the 6-OHDA models (6/9, 66.7%). The studies were published between 2000 and 2014. These studies included animals of both sexes ($n = 4$), [22,23,24,25] male only ($n = 3$), [18,19,23] female only ($n = 1$), [21] and gender not reported ($n = 1$) (12). To induce LID in PD model, animals were treated, once parkinsonism was stable, with twice-daily administration of L-dopa (2–25 mg/kg, i.p.) plus benserazide/carbidopa (2.5–15 mg/kg, i.p.) for several weeks, ranging from 16 days to 8 weeks. KW-6002 as the A2A receptor antagonist was reported in four studies (12, 20, 21, 27), ST1535 (22, 23) in two, Caffeine (24, 25) in two, and SCH 412348 (26) in one study. Meanwhile, total AIM score, locomotor activity, and motor disability were reported as a outcome measure in 5, 5, and 3 studies, respectively. The basic characteristics of the nine selected studies are summarized in **Table 1**.

Risk of Bias

Of whom, one study got 6 points (1/9, 11.1%), four studies got 5 (4/9, 44.4%), three studies got 4 (3/9, 33.3%), and one study got 3 (1/9, 11.1%). Only one study described a sample size calculation. Random allocation to a treatment group and blinded assessment of outcome were described in seven studies. Eight studies mentioned the statement of potential conflict of interests. All studies reported compliance with animal welfare regulations (**Table 2**). Generally, all of the included studies were deemed to have a low risk of bias.

Meta-Analyses

All the data for meta-analysis were expressed graphically. We used digital ruler software to calculate the mean and standard error. In the present paper, five studies reported the locomotor activity as the outcome measure with 67 animals were included in the final meta-analyses. We pooled the whole data and found no significant difference between A2A receptor antagonists plus L-dopa treatment and L-dopa alone (SMD −0.00, 95% CI: −2.52 to 2.52, $p = 1.0$, **Figure 2A**). Meanwhile, there was obvious heterogeneity for the analysis of locomotor activity between studies ($Tau^2 = 7.16$, $Chi^2 = 42.62$, $p < 0.00001$, $I^2 = 87\%$, **Figure 2A**). After sequentially excluding each study, the results of heterogeneity and locomotor activity were consistent (I^2 range from 80 to 92%; $p = 0.56$ to $1.53 > 0.05$, respectively). Consequently, we should interpret the pool result prudently.

Three studies reported mild significant effects of A2A receptor antagonists plus L-dopa treatment for improving motor disability compared with L-dopa alone (SMD −5.06, 95% CI: −9.25 to −0.87, $p = 0.02$, **Figure 2B**). Nevertheless, there was severe heterogeneity for the analysis of motor disability between studies ($Tau^2 = 10.90$, $Chi^2 = 10.90$, $p = 0.004$, $I^2 = 82\%$, **Figure 2B**). Removal of the outlier studies (22) led to more homogeneous results ($Tau^2 = 0.00$, $Chi^2 = 0.19$, $p = 0.66$, $I^2 = 0\%$), as well as increased the effect size by −2.18, yielding a still significant pooled SMD of −7.24.

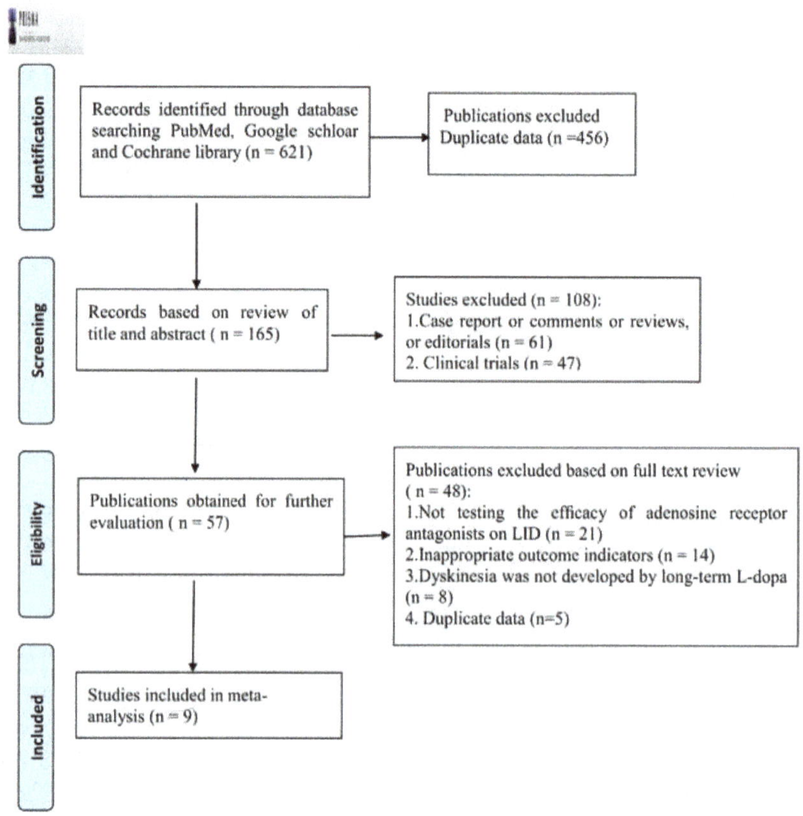

FIGURE 1 | PRISMA 2009 Flow Diagram of trial identification, inclusion, and exclusion. LID, levodopa-induced dyskinesia.

Total AIM was reported by five trials, the result showed a significant difference in the reduction of the score between the A2A receptor antagonists plus L-dopa treatment and L-dopa alone (SMD −1.82, 95% CI: −3.38 to −0.25, $p = 0.02$, **Figure 2C**). Nevertheless, inspection of the data showed that the heterogeneity for the analysis of total AIM between studies was high ($Tau^2 = 2.74$, $Chi^2 = 37.38$, $p < 0.00001$, $I^2 = 89\%$). After sequentially excluding each study, the results of heterogeneity were consistent with the previous result. The remaining four studies (20, 22, 23, 27) failed to enter the pool analysis due to the lack of a Total AIM, one using limb and axial AIM to reflect LID, two using locomotor activity as the outcome measures, and the last one not reporting the criteria to assess the dyskinesia. Funnel plots were not applied to test the publication bias in this paper as the numbers of included studies were small.

Subgroup Analysis

In the subgroup analysis focusing on locomotors activity, the efficacy of KW-6002 was similar with ST1535 (SMD −0.58, 95% CI: −4.85 to 3.69, $p = 0.79$; SMD 0.88, 95% CI: −4.08 to 5.85, $p = 0.73$, respectively, **Figure 3**). Moreover, in terms of total AIM score, efficacy was observed to be higher with the administration of Caffeine than KW-6002 or SCH 412348 (SMD −2.14, 95% CI: −3.86 to −0.41, $p = 0.02 < 0.05$; SMD −2.57, 95% CI: −8.37 to 3.24, $p = 0.39$; SMD −0.55, 95% CI: −1.71 to 0.61, $p = 0.93$, respectively, **Figure 4**).

DISCUSSION

Summary of Main Results

This meta-analysis demonstrated that A2A receptor antagonists substantially reduced total AIM in animal models of LID. Meanwhile, we found A2A receptor antagonists plus L-dopa has similar anti-parkinsonism effects on the locomotors activity and motor disability scores when compared with L-dopa alone. Based on the subgroup analysis, the results showed that effect size of KW-6002 on the locomotors activity in animals was similar with ST1535. Moreover, we found that animals who received Caffeine showed remarkable improvement on the total AIM score compared with KW-6002 or SCH 412348. The improvement in LID behavior without an impact of motor function is highly significant as it differentiates A2A receptor antagonists from the known effects of dopaminergic therapies.

We conducted a preclinical animal meta-analysis for a better understanding and also to facilitate the conversion of experimental evidence to future clinical trials. With such aim, 6-OHDA and MPTP models were chosen as the pathophysiological model as they were closer to human LID. The analysis of A2A receptor

TABLE 1 | Basic characteristics of the included studies.

Reference	Species, weight, anesthetic	Model (Parkinson's disease/L-dopa-induced dyskinesias)	Intervention	Outcome index	*p*-Value
6-0HDA models					
Lundblad et al. (21)	SD rats (female, 9/10), 225 g, NR	Unilateral 6-OHDA (8 μg/3 μl) lesioned; L-dopa (4 mg/kg)/carbidopa (12 mg/kg) for 16 days	KW-6002 (3 and 10 ml/kg, p.o.) for 16 days	1. Rotarod performance 2. Total AIM	1. $p > 0.05$ 2. $p < 0.05$
Danqing (12)	Mice (NR,10/7), NR, avertin	Unilateral 6-OHDA (8 μg/4 μl) lesioned; L-DOPA (2 mg/kg)/benserazide (2 mg/kg) for 21 days	KW-6002 (0.03 mg/kg and 0.3 mg/kg, i.p.) for 21 days	1. Locomotor Activity 2. Total AIM	1. $p > 0.05$ 2. $p < 0.05$
Elisabetta (23)	SD rats (male, 8/8), 275–300 g, chloral hydrate	Unilateral 6-OHDA (8 μg/4 μl) lesioned; L-DOPA (3 mg/kg)/benserazide (6 mg/kg) for 18 days	ST1535 (20 mg/kg, p.o.) for 18 days	1. Locomotor Activity 2. limb and axial AIM	1. $p > 0.05$ 2. $p < 0.05$
Yi-xian (24)	SD rats (male, 10/10), 180–220 g, chloral hydrate	Unilateral 6-OHDA (8 μg/4 μl) lesioned; L-dopa (25 mg/kg)/benserazide (6.25 mg/kg) for 21 days	Caffeine (2.5 mg/kg, i.p.) for 21 days	1. Rotational response 2. Total AIM, limb AIM 3. Orolingual AIM	1. $p > 0.05$ 2. $p < 0.05$ 3. $p < 0.05$
Danqing (25)	Mice (both sex, 24/12), NR, avertin	Unilateral 6-OHDA (10 μg/4 μl) lesioned; L-dopa (2 mg/kg)/benserazide (2 mg/kg) for 21 days	Caffeine (3 and 15 mg/kg, i.p.) for 21 days	1. Total AIM	1. $p < 0.05$
Jones et al. (26)	SD rats (male, 6/6), 350–400 g, NR	Unilateral 6-OHDA (8 μg/4 μl) lesioned; L-dopa (6 mg/kg)/benserazide (15 mg/kg) for 22 days	SCH 412348 (3 mg/kg, i.p.) for 22 days	1. Catalepsy 2. Total AIM	1. $p > 0.05$ 2. $p > 0.05$
MPTP models					
Tomoyuki (20)	Marmosets (both sex, 4/4), 285–420 g, NR	MPTP 2.0 mg/kg sc for 5 days; L-dopa (12.5 mg/kg)/carbidopa (12.5 mg/kg) for 21 days	KW-6002 (10 ml/kg, p.o.) for 21 days	1. Locomotor Activity 2. Motor disability	1. $p > 0.05$ 2. $p < 0.05$
Sarah (22)	Marmosets (both sex, 4/4), 265–437 g, NR	MPTP 2.0 mg/kg sc for 5 days; L-dopa (2.5 mg/kg)/carbidopa (12.5 mg/kg) for 8 weeks	ST1535 (20 mg/kg, p.o.) for 8 weeks	1. Locomotor Activity 2. Motor disability	1. $p > 0.05$ 2. $p < 0.05$
Shin-ichi (27)	Marmosets (both sex, 8/8), 285–420 g, NR	MPTP 2.0 mg/kg sc for 5 days; L-dopa (10 mg/kg)/carbidopa (2.5 mg/kg) for 28 days	KW-6002 (10 mg/kg, p.o.) for 28 days	1. Locomotor Activity 2. Motor disability	1. $p > 0.05$ 2. $p < 0.05$

AIM, abnormal involuntary movements; SD rats, Sprague-Dawley rats; 6-OHDA, 6-hydroxydopamine; NR, no report; MPTP, 1-methyl-4-phenyl-1, 2, 3, 6-tetrahydropyridine; MFB, medial forebrain bundle; L-dopa, levodopa.

TABLE 2 | Risk of bias of included studies.

Reference	Tomoyuki (20)	Lundblad (21)	Danqing (12)	Sarah (22)	Elisabetta (23)	Yi-xian (24)	Danqing (25)	Jones et al. (26)	Shin-ichi (27)
A	Y	Y	Y	Y	Y	Y	Y	Y	Y
B	Y	Y	Y	N	Y	Y	N	Y	Y
C	N	Y	Y	Y	Y	N	Y	Y	Y
D	N	N	Y	N	N	N	N	N	N
E	Y	Y	Y	Y	Y	Y	Y	Y	Y
F	Y	Y	Y	N	Y	Y	Y	Y	Y
Total	4	5	6	3	5	4	4	5	5

Studies fulfilling the criteria of: A: peer-reviewed publication; B: random allocation to group; C: blinded assessment of outcome; D: a sample size calculation; E: compliance with animal welfare regulations; and F: a statement of a potential conflict of interest. Y, yes; N, no.

antagonists in LID could be of great interest for future studies. However, these findings have to be interpreted with caution, because only a few different A2A receptor antagonists' studies were tested in this paper. Nevertheless, the present results reinforced the neuroprotective role of A2A receptor antagonists in experimental LID models, but we did not sure whether it reliably informed human studies. Undoubtedly, further evidence was required to confirm this efficacy in human.

To date, alternative to modification of L-dopa therapy to avoid LID may resort to non-dopaminergic strategies of the indirect pathway of the basal ganglia. One possible strategy is to inactivate the A2A receptors (28). It has been displayed that the expression of adenosine A2A receptors was increased following L-dopa treatment and the appearance of AIM or LID as shown by biochemical, post-mortem, and imaging investigations, suggesting that inhibitation of A2A receptors is helpful for LID. Moreover, numerous preclinical studies have reported that A2A receptor antagonists might hinder the development of LID, which are consistent with this review (29). Moreover, clinical trials have showed that oral administration A2A antagonists increase functional on-time duration in PD patients suffering from wearing-off phenomenon (less effective than DBS or L-dopa continuous infusion), although they may increase dyskinesia in patients with advanced PD (14). Thus, critical aspects of the potential function of A2A antagonists on LID patients are yet to be evaluated.

Interpretation of the Results

The interaction between adenosine A2A and D2 DA receptors has recently attracted much attention as a possible therapeutic target in LID (30). In addition, an increase in adenosine A2A receptor was observed in the striatum of dyskinetic primate's models (31). A2A receptors were reported to adjust the activity of the indirect

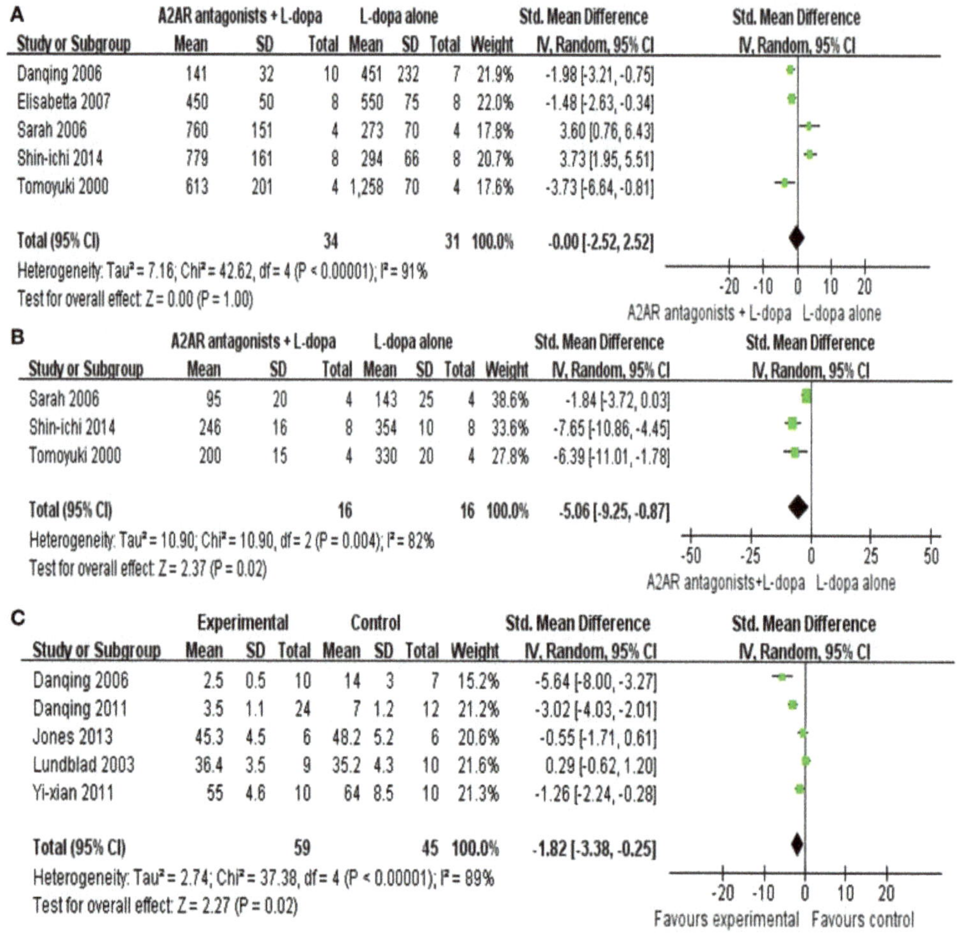

FIGURE 2 | Total effect size of A2A receptor antagonists on locomotor activity score **(A)** reduction including 65 animals in five comparisons, motor disability score outcome **(B)** improvement (32 animals in three comparisons) and total abnormal involuntary movements (AIM) score **(C)** comprising 104 animals in five comparisons.

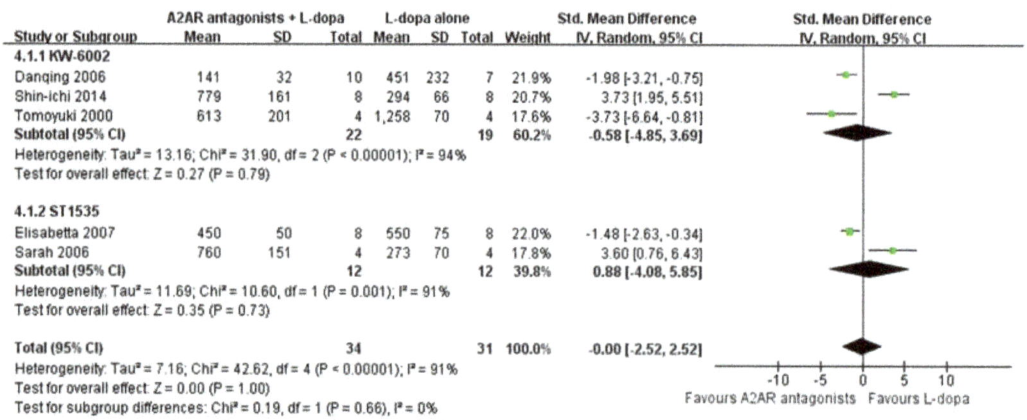

FIGURE 3 | Subgroup analysis: the impact of different classes of A2A receptor antagonists (KW-6002 and ST1535) on the estimate of improvement in locomotor activity score outcome.

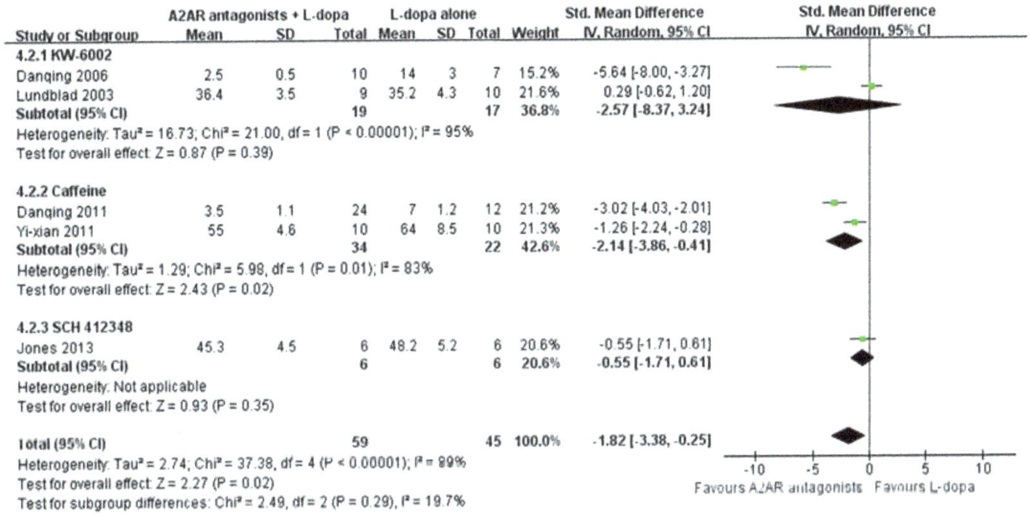

FIGURE 4 | Subgroup analysis: the impact of different classes of A2A receptor antagonists (KW-6002, caffeine and SCH 412348) on the estimate of decrement in total abnormal involuntary movements (AIM) score outcome.

pathway and modulate acetylcholine and glutamate release in the striatum, where they form functional heteromeric complexes with D2 receptors (10). Namely, agonists of A2A receptors inhibit the binding of DA to D2 receptors and have been shown to inhibit D2-mediated neurotransmitter release. On the other hand, evidence shows that A2A receptors antagonists mimic the effects of D2 agonists (29). Interestingly, recent evidence demonstrates that A2A receptors co-localize postsynaptically not only with D2 receptors, but also with the cholinergic interneurons, the cannabinoid receptor and the glutamate receptor, suggesting the existence of important multifunctional interactions between A2A and these receptors (32). In summary, these data strongly indicate that A2A receptors can target a couple of cellular mechanisms involved in the underlying neurodegenerative process, and likely to play a functional role in the modulation of motor behavior in LID.

In our study, caffeine showed more remarkable improvement on the total AIM score when compared with other A2A antagonists. The underlying mechanism by which caffeine attenuates LID remains largely unclear. One previous study reported that chronic administration of L-dopa increased the striatal A2A expression significantly. Nevertheless, co-administration of L-dopa with caffeine not only attenuated the AIM induced by L-dopa, but also lower the level of striatal A2A expression (24). Moreover, Xiao et al. suggested that blocking both A1 and A2A receptors simultaneously, as occurred with caffeine use, might also confer a disease-modifying benefit of reduced risk of disabling LID, suggesting A1 may also play a pivotal role in the function of caffeine (25). On the other hand, SCH 412348 was given concurrently with L-dopa over the course of 19 days of treatment. This treatment paradigm did not reduce the severity of AIM score compared with treatment with L-dopa alone ($p = 0.35$). With regard to KW-6002, our data showed that KW-6002 could not prevent the development of AIM score even when the combined treatment is administered *de novo* ($p = 0.39$).

Limitations

Several limitations of this meta-analysis should be considered. First, there is a chance of overestimation of the efficacy because our paper can only include available data which have been published in some forms, and hence negative studies that are less likely to be published will be missed. Therefore, the inclusion of unpublished studies and the use of trial registries become reasonable means to avoid publication bias (33). Second, a notable feature of the present review is the marked heterogeneity between studies due to the variation in study quality and experimental designs, implying that the overall estimate of efficacy should be interpreted with some caution. Meanwhile, this meta-analysis included a limited number of small studies ($n = 9$) and type-II errors due to chance cannot be entirely excluded as an alternative explanation for our main finding (34), making these findings less robust. Although there is no fixed minimum number of studies required for a meta-analysis, too small a number could lead to an unstable effect size. Therefore, further studies, particularly those of large sample, were warranted to support the drugs' superiority to placebo. Third, our meta-analysis is based on observational research rather than experimental, and thus we are only able to obtain associations rather than causation. Moreover, no study in this meta-analysis using animals with co-morbidities, which is the typical situation in human PD and LID. Finally, as the studies only involved a few classes of A2A receptor antagonists, the majority being KW-6002 ($n = 4$), the results cannot be extrapolated to other A2A receptor antagonist's classes.

Implications for Further Studies

When included in systematic reviews, high-quality studies with lower variance will show larger effects, and improvement in the quality of reporting studies will also help to reduce bias. Therefore, well-designed and high-quality studies would be required to test the efficacy of A2A receptor antagonists on

LID. In the present study, no studies investigated A2A receptor antagonists in LID models with concomitant conditions, such as hypertension, diabetes, dyslipidemia, or aged animals. This lack of information should certainly be addressed in future studies. Our meta-analysis suggested that the efficacy was maximal when Caffeine ($n = 2$, $p = 0.02$) was administered but not KW-6002 ($n = 2$, $p = 0.39$) or SCH 412348 ($n = 1$, $p = 0.35$) in terms of reduced the AIM score. However, the results generated from this subgroup analysis should be interpreted with caution due to the limited studies. We have no sufficient evidence to suggest initiating clinical trials based on these data. Consequently, further studies would be demanded to determine which kinds of A2A receptor antagonists were more effective than others. Moreover, there is currently little accordance on which neurobehavioral tests in rats would offer measures that are predictive of a benefit in clinical patients. In terms of PD, after a few years of L-dopa therapy, most patients will be accompanied with AIM (including movements with dystonic, choreiform, ballistic, or stereotypic features) that appear when plasma and brain levels of L-dopa are high, mimicking the peak-dose variant of human LID (35). It was long assumed that the responsiveness to L-dopa merely could be measured with contralateral rotation test but LID movements was unable to be assessed at all, until Cenci and collaborators first introduced the concept of AIM in 1998 (36). Although contralateral rotations have been used as a measure of LID, it has become increasingly recognized that this neurobehavioral not always correlates with the development of LID (37). Therefore, further studies should use AIM score as an indicator to reflect LID behavior.

CONCLUSION

In summary, we have shown that adenosine A2A receptor antagonists are effective in the management of LID in animal models. Although some factors, such as study quality and total sample sizes, may undermine the validity of the positive findings, A2A receptor antagonists still probably have a potential neuroprotective role in LID models. The systematic review and meta-analysis here provides a framework for an evidence-based approach to the development of new treatments for LID and for the design of future preclinical and clinical studies.

AUTHOR CONTRIBUTIONS

M-MZ and LF conceived and participated in its design, searched databases, extracted and assessed studies, and helped to draft the manuscript. X-RZ, JC, and Z-RZ carried out the statistical analysis and interpretation of data. W-WW and C-LX participated in the conceptualization and design of the review, performed the selection of studies, data extraction and analysis, and drafted the review. All authors read and approved the final manuscript.

FUNDING

The study was supported by the Projects of National Science Foundation of China (No. 81600977), National Key Technology Research and Development Program of the Ministry of Science and Technology of China (grant number: 2015BAI13B01), and Wenzhou Municipal Sci-Tech Bureau Program (Y20160002).

REFERENCES

1. Sharma S, Singh S, Sharma V, Singh VP, Deshmukh R. Neurobiology of l-dopa induced dyskinesia and the novel therapeutic strategies. *Biomed Pharmacother* (2015) 70:283–93. doi:10.1016/j.biopha.2015.01.029
2. Francardo V, Cenci MA. Investigating the molecular mechanisms of L-dopa-induced dyskinesia in the mouse. *Parkinsonism Relat Disord* (2014) 20(Suppl 1): S20–2. doi:10.1016/S1353-8020(13)70008-7
3. Obeso JA, Merello M, Rodriguez-Oroz MC, Marin C, Guridi J, Alvarez L. Levodopa-induced dyskinesias in Parkinson's disease. *Handb Clin Neurol* (2007) 84:185–218. doi:10.1016/S0072-9752(07)84040-1
4. Xie CL, Wang WW, Zhang SF, Gan J, Liu ZG. Continuous dopaminergic stimulation (CDS)-based treatment in Parkinson's disease patients with motor complications: a systematic review and meta-analysis. *Sci Rep* (2014) 4:6027. doi:10.1038/srep06027
5. Schaeffer E, Pilotto A, Berg D. Pharmacological strategies for the management of levodopa-induced dyskinesia in patients with Parkinson's disease. *CNS Drugs* (2014) 28:1155–84. doi:10.1007/s40263-014-0205-z
6. Tokunaga N, Choudhury ME, Nishikawa N, Nagai M, Tujii T, Iwaki H, et al. Pramipexole upregulates dopamine receptor D2 and D3 expression in rat striatum. *J Pharmacol Sci* (2012) 120:133–7. doi:10.1254/jphs.12096SC
7. Bezard E, Brotchie JM, Gross CE. Pathophysiology of levodopa-induced dyskinesia: potential for new therapies. *Nat Rev Neurosci* (2001) 2:577–88. doi:10.1038/35086062
8. Calabresi P, Di Filippo M, Ghiglieri V, Tambasco N, Picconi B. Levodopa-induced dyskinesias in patients with Parkinson's disease: filling the bench-to-bedside gap. *Lancet Neurol* (2010) 9:1106–17. doi:10.1016/S1474-4422(10)70218-0
9. Rivera-Oliver M, Diaz-Rios M. Using caffeine and other adenosine receptor antagonists and agonists as therapeutic tools against neurodegenerative diseases: a review. *Life Sci* (2014) 101:1–9. doi:10.1016/j.lfs.2014.01.083
10. Morelli M, Di Paolo T, Wardas J, Calon F, Xiao D, Schwarzschild MA. Role of adenosine A2A receptors in parkinsonian motor impairment and l-dopa-induced motor complications. *Prog Neurobiol* (2007) 83:293–309. doi:10.1016/j.pneurobio.2007.07.001
11. Kulisevsky J, Poyurovsky M. Adenosine A2A-receptor antagonism and pathophysiology of Parkinson's disease and drug-induced movement disorders. *Eur Neurol* (2012) 67:4–11. doi:10.1159/000331768
12. Xiao D, Bastia E, Xu YH, Benn CL, Cha JH, Peterson TS, et al. Forebrain adenosine A2A receptors contribute to L-3,4-dihydroxyphenylalanine-induced dyskinesia in hemiparkinsonian mice. *J Neurosci* (2006) 26:13548–55. doi:10.1523/JNEUROSCI.3554-06.2006
13. Hauser RA, Shulman LM, Trugman JM, Roberts JW, Mori A, Ballerini R, et al. Study of istradefylline in patients with Parkinson's disease on levodopa with motor fluctuations. *Mov Disord* (2008) 23:2177–85. doi:10.1002/mds.22095
14. Kanda T, Uchida S. Clinical/pharmacological aspect of adenosine A2A receptor antagonist for dyskinesia. *Int Rev Neurobiol* (2014) 119:127–50. doi:10.1016/B978-0-12-801022-8.00006-4
15. Wang WW, Xie CL, Lu L, Zheng GQ. A systematic review and meta-analysis of Baihui (GV20)-based scalp acupuncture in experimental ischemic stroke. *Sci Rep* (2014) 4:3981. doi:10.1038/srep03981
16. Xie CL, Pan JL, Zhang SF, Gan J, Liu ZG. Effect of nicotine on L-dopa-induced dyskinesia in animal models of Parkinson's disease: a systematic review and meta-analysis. *Neurol Sci* (2014) 35:653–62. doi:10.1007/s10072-014-1652-5
17. Xie CL, Wang WW, Zhang SF, Yuan ML, Che JY, Gan J, et al. Levodopa/benserazide microsphere (LBM) prevents L-dopa induced dyskinesia by inactivation of the DR1/PKA/P-tau pathway in 6-OHDA-lesioned Parkinson's rats. *Sci Rep* (2014) 4:7506. doi:10.1038/srep07506
18. Macleod MR, O'Collins T, Howells DW, Donnan GA. Pooling of animal experimental data reveals influence of study design and publication bias. *Stroke* (2004) 35:1203–8. doi:10.1161/01.STR.0000125719.25853.20

19. Vesterinen HM, Sena ES, Egan KJ, Hirst TC, Churolov L, Currie GL, et al. Meta-analysis of data from animal studies: a practical guide. *J Neurosci Methods* (2014) 221:92–102. doi:10.1016/j.jneumeth.2013.09.010
20. Kanda T, Jackson MJ, Smith LA, Pearce RK, Nakamura J, Kase H, et al. Combined use of the adenosine A(2A) antagonist KW-6002 with L-dopa or with selective D1 or D2 dopamine agonists increases antiparkinsonian activity but not dyskinesia in MPTP-treated monkeys. *Exp Neurol* (2000) 162:321–7. doi:10.1006/exnr.2000.7350
21. Lundblad M, Vaudano E, Cenci MA. Cellular and behavioural effects of the adenosine A2a receptor antagonist KW-6002 in a rat model of l-dopa-induced dyskinesia. *J Neurochem* (2003) 84:1398–410. doi:10.1046/j.1471-4159.2003.01632.x
22. Rose S, Jackson MJ, Smith LA, Stockwell K, Johnson L, Carminati P, et al. The novel adenosine A2a receptor antagonist ST1535 potentiates the effects of a threshold dose of L-dopa in MPTP treated common marmosets. *Eur J Pharmacol* (2006) 546:82–7. doi:10.1016/j.ejphar.2006.07.017
23. Tronci E, Simola N, Borsini F, Schintu N, Frau L, Carminati P, et al. Characterization of the antiparkinsonian effects of the new adenosine A2A receptor antagonist ST1535: acute and subchronic studies in rats. *Eur J Pharmacol* (2007) 566:94–102. doi:10.1016/j.ejphar.2007.03.021
24. Huang YX, Luo WF, Li D, Hu WD, Liu CF. CSC counteracts l-dopa-induced overactivity of the corticostriatal synaptic ultrastructure and function in 6-OHDA-lesioned rats. *Brain Res* (2011) 1376:113–21. doi:10.1016/j.brainres.2010.12.070
25. Xiao D, Cassin JJ, Healy B, Burdett TC, Chen JF, Fredholm BB, et al. Deletion of adenosine A(1) or A((2)A) receptors reduces L-3,4-dihydroxyphenylalanine-induced dyskinesia in a model of Parkinson's disease. *Brain Res* (2011) 1367:310–8. doi:10.1016/j.brainres.2010.08.099
26. Jones N, Bleickardt C, Mullins D, Parker E, Hodgson R. A2A receptor antagonists do not induce dyskinesias in drug-naive or L-dopa sensitized rats. *Brain Res Bull* (2013) 98:163–9. doi:10.1016/j.brainresbull.2013.07.001
27. Uchida S, Soshiroda K, Okita E, Kawai-Uchida M, Mori A, Jenner P, et al. The adenosine A2A receptor antagonist, istradefylline enhances anti-parkinsonian activity induced by combined treatment with low doses of L-dopa and dopamine agonists in MPTP-treated common marmosets. *Eur J Pharmacol* (2015) 766:25–30. doi:10.1016/j.ejphar.2015.09.028
28. Pinna A, Pontis S, Borsini F, Morelli M. Adenosine A2A receptor antagonists improve deficits in initiation of movement and sensory motor integration in the unilateral 6-hydroxydopamine rat model of Parkinson's disease. *Synapse* (2007) 61:606–14. doi:10.1002/syn.20410
29. Tomiyama M. Adenosine receptors and dyskinesia in pathophysiology. *Int Rev Neurobiol* (2014) 119:117–26. doi:10.1016/B978-0-12-801022-8.00005-2
30. Chen JF, Moratalla R, Impagnatiello F, Grandy DK, Cuellar B, Rubinstein M, et al. The role of the D(2) dopamine receptor (D(2)R) in A(2A) adenosine receptor (A(2A)R)-mediated behavioral and cellular responses as revealed by A(2A) and D(2) receptor knockout mice. *Proc Natl Acad Sci U S A* (2001) 98:1970–5. doi:10.1073/pnas.98.4.1970
31. Calon F, Dridi M, Hornykiewicz O, Bedard PJ, Rajput AH, Di Paolo T. Increased adenosine A2A receptors in the brain of Parkinson's disease patients with dyskinesias. *Brain* (2004) 127:1075–84. doi:10.1093/brain/awh128
32. Blandini F, Armentero MT. New pharmacological avenues for the treatment of L-dopa-induced dyskinesias in Parkinson's disease: targeting glutamate and adenosine receptors. *Expert Opin Investig Drugs* (2012) 21:153–68. doi:10.1517/13543784.2012.651457
33. Furlan AD, Pennick V, Bombardier C, van Tulder M. 2009 updated method guidelines for systematic reviews in the Cochrane back review group. *Spine* (2009) 34:1929–41. doi:10.1097/BRS.0b013e3181b1c99f
34. Skapinakis P, Bakola E, Salanti G, Lewis G, Kyritsis AP, Mavreas V. Efficacy and acceptability of selective serotonin reuptake inhibitors for the treatment of depression in Parkinson's disease: a systematic review and meta-analysis of randomized controlled trials. *BMC Neurol* (2010) 10:49. doi:10.1186/1471-2377-10-49
35. Iderberg H, Francardo V, Pioli EY. Animal models of L-dopa-induced dyskinesia: an update on the current options. *Neuroscience* (2012) 211:13–27. doi:10.1016/j.neuroscience.2012.03.023
36. Cenci MA, Lee CS, Björklund A. L-dopa-induced dyskinesia in the rat is associated with striatal overexpression of prodynorphin- and glutamic acid decarboxylase mRNA. *Eur J Neurosci* (1998) 10:2694–706. doi:10.1046/j.1460-9568.1998.00285.x
37. Henry B, Crossman AR, Brotchie JM. Characterization of enhanced behavioral responses to L-dopa following repeated administration in the 6-hydroxydopamine-lesioned rat model of Parkinson's disease. *Exp Neurol* (1998) 151:334–42. doi:10.1006/exnr.1998.6819

5

Inspiratory-Activated Airway Vagal Preganglionic Neurones Excited by Thyrotropin-Releasing Hormone via Multiple Mechanisms in Neonatal Rats

Lili Hou[1,2,3], Min Zhang[1], Xingyi Zhang[1], Zhenwei Liu[1], Pengyu Zhang[1], Dongying Qiu[2,4,5], Lei Zhu[3] and Xin Zhou[1]**

[1] Department of Respiratory and Critical Care Medicine, Shanghai General Hospital, Shanghai Jiao Tong University, Shanghai, China, [2] Department of Neurobiology, School of Basic Medical Sciences, Fudan University, Shanghai, China, [3] Department of Respiratory Medicine, Zhongshan Hospital, Fudan University, Shanghai, China, [4] Department of Physiology and Pathophysiology, School of Basic Medical Sciences, Fudan University, Shanghai, China, [5] Department of Gerontology, Zhongshan Hospital, Fudan University, Shanghai, China

***Correspondence:**
Lei Zhu
tfzhu@126.com
Xin Zhou
zhouxin_rm@163.com

The airway vagal preganglionic neurons (AVPNs) providing projections to intrinsic tracheobronchial ganglia are considered to be crucial to modulation of airway resistance in physiological and pathological states. AVPNs classified into inspiratory-activated AVPNs (IA-AVPNs) and inspiratory-inhibited AVPNs (II-AVPNs) are regulated by thyrotropin-releasing hormone (TRH)-containing terminals. TRH causes a direct excitatory current and attenuates the phasic inspiratory glycinergic inputs in II-AVPNs, however, whether and how TRH influences IA-AVPNs remains unknown. In current study, TRH regulation of IA-AVPNs and its mechanisms involved were investigated. Using retrogradely fluorescent labeling method and electrophysiology techniques to identify IA-AVPNs in brainstem slices with rhythmic inspiratory hypoglossal bursts recorded by a suction electrode, the modulation of TRH was observed with patch-clamp technique. The findings demonstrate that under voltage clamp configuration, TRH (100 nM) caused a slow excitatory inward current, augmented the excitatory synaptic inputs, progressively suppressed the inhibitory synaptic inputs and elicited a distinctive electrical oscillatory pattern (OP). Such a current and an OP was independent of presynaptic inputs. Carbenoxolone (100 μM), a widely used gap junction inhibitor, fully suppressed the OP with persistence of TRH-induced excitatory slow inward current and augment of the excitatory synaptic inputs. Both tetrodotoxin (1 μM) and riluzole (20 μM) functioned to block the majority of the slow excitatory inward current and prevent the OP, respectively. Under current clamp recording, TRH caused a slowly developing depolarization and continuously progressive oscillatory firing pattern sensitive to TTX. TRH increased the firing frequency in response to injection of a square-wave current. The results suggest that TRH excited IA-AVPNs via the following multiple mechanisms: (1) TRH enhances the excitatory and depresses the inhibitory inputs; (2) TRH induces an excitatory postsynaptic slow inward current; (3) TRH evokes a distinctive OP mediated by gap junction.

Keywords: thyrotropin-releasing hormone, airway vagal preganglionic neuron, gap junction, oscillation, patch clamp, asthma

INTRODUCTION

Bronchial asthma, a type of common chronic airway disease worldwide, has prominent features of airway hyper-responsiveness, inflammation and excessive activation of cholinergic fibers to the trachea and bronchioles. The mechanisms of neural reflex pathways involved are regarded as very primary points in the process of this disease. In reflex pathways the AVPNs located in medulla oblongata conveying signals from brain to the intrinsic tracheobronchial ganglia are considered to be very crucial for regulating airway function either in diseased conditions or normal states (Haxhiu et al., 2005; McGovern and Mazzone, 2010).

Airway vagal preganglionic neurons have been mainly found in the external compact of nucleus ambiguus (eNA) via application of fluorescent tracer to the extrathoracic tracheal wall (Haselton et al., 1992; Haxhiu and Loewy, 1996; Kc et al., 2004; Chen Y. et al., 2007; Qiu et al., 2011; Chen et al., 2012a,b; Hou et al., 2012, 2015; Zhou et al., 2013; Ge et al., 2015; Guo et al., 2017; Yan et al., 2017). AVPNs in the eNA function as the main neurons which modulate cholinergic tone of airway smooth muscles as well as control the intrapulmonary airway resistance and tracheobronchial caliber (Haselton et al., 1992; Canning and Fischer, 2001; Yan et al., 2017). As shown in previous studies *in vivo* and *in vitro*, postganglionic neurons in intrinsic tracheobronchial ganglia have been identified as "phasic" neurons and "tonic" ones, the former firing in phase with inspiration and primarily projecting to tracheobronchial smooth muscles, and the latter firing tonically during expiration and primarily projecting to the intercartilaginous spaces (Baker, 1986; Mitchell et al., 1987; Myers et al., 1990; Myers, 1998). AVPNs in the eNA also exhibit different rhythmic changes of synaptic inputs in parallel with central inspiratory activities (Chen Y. et al., 2007; Qiu et al., 2011; Chen et al., 2012a,b; Hou et al., 2012, 2015; Zhou et al., 2013; Ge et al., 2015; Guo et al., 2017; Yan et al., 2017). Thus, two types of AVPNs are identified according to their different synaptic control during inspiratory phase: some neurons activated by phasic excitatory inputs are identified as IA-AVPNs, and others inhibited by phasic inhibitory inputs are separated as inspiratory-inhibited airway vagal preganglionic neurons (II-AVPNs) (Chen Y. et al., 2007; Qiu et al., 2011; Chen et al., 2012a,b; Hou et al., 2012; Zhou et al., 2013; Ge et al., 2015; Guo et al., 2017; Yan et al., 2017). Morphological and electrical studies have shown that excitatory and inhibitory synaptic inputs from various brain regions determine the excitability of AVPNs (Haxhiu et al., 1993, 2002, 2003, 2005, 2008; Kc et al., 2006; Wilson et al., 2007; Chen et al., 2012b; Hou et al., 2012; Zhou et al., 2013; Ge et al., 2015; Guo et al., 2017; Yan et al., 2017), although AVPNs are capable of generating synchronous electrical oscillatory pattern (OP), revealed by "activation of NMDA receptors" or "blockade of $GABA_A$ receptors" (Haxhiu et al., 1987, 2005; Moore et al., 2004).

Nerves containing TRH innervate the airway vagal motor neurons in the cNA (Iwase et al., 1992; Sun et al., 1995). Microinjection of TRH, a neuropeptide well-known to excite the respiratory neurons in the PBC, into the NA induces first decrease and then increase of the tracheal pressure (Iwase et al., 1992). TRH affects neurons in the NA of adult guinea pigs by three different ways: depolarization, causing membrane potential oscillations and enhancement of postinhibitory rebound (Johnson and Getting, 1992), indicating that TRH could mediate complex alternations of membrane characteristics in neurons of NA. As demonstrated by the previous study in our laboratory, II-AVPNs were excited by TRH via both postsynaptic and presynaptic mechanisms (Hou et al., 2012). It has been reported that IA-AVPNs differ from II-AVPNs in anatomical location and intrinsic properties (Chen Y. et al., 2007; Chen et al., 2012a). Thus TRH modulation of IA-AVPNs is perhaps distinct from that of II-AVPNs, so how TRH regulates IA-AVPNs still remains elusive. In the current study, IA-AVPNs in the eNA were retrogradely labeled using fluorescent dye and identified in rhythmically active brainstem slices. The influences of TRH on whole-cell current and membrane potential of IA-AVPNs were examined using patch clamp. The current experiment is performed to test the following hypothesis that TRH affects IA-AVPNs via multiple mechanisms in neonatal rats: (1) TRH enhances the excitatory and inhibits the inhibitory synaptic inputs; (2) TRH induces a direct postsynaptic slow inward current; (3) TRH evokes a distinctive OP mediated by gap junction.

Abbreviations: 4V, 4th ventricle; ACSF, artificial cerebral spinal fluid; AMPA, 2-amino-3-(5-methyl-3-oxo-1,2-oxazol-4-yl)propanoic acid; AP_5, D-2-amino-5-phosphonovalerate; CBX, carbenoxolone; AVPNs, airway vagal preganglionic neurons; cNA, the compact formation of the nucleus ambiguous; CNQX, 6-cyano-7-nitroquinoxaline-2,3-dione; DHPG, (RS)-3,5-dihydroxyphenylglycine; DMSO, dimethyl sulfoxide; DMV, dorsal motor nucleus of vagus; eNA, the external formation of the nucleus ambiguous; EPSCs, excitatory postsynaptic currents; EPSPs, excitatory postsynaptic potentials; GABA, γ-aminobutyric acid; IA-AVPNs, inspiratory-activated airway vagal preganglionic neurons; ICSs, inward current spikelets; IO, inferior olive; INaP, persistent sodium currents; K_{ATP}, ATP-sensitive potassium channels; NA, nucleus ambiguous; NMDA, *N*-methyl-D-aspartate; PBC, pre-Bötzinger complex; PY, pyramidal tract; QX314, lidocaine *N*-ethyl bromide; ROb, raphe obscurus nucleus; NTS, nucleus tractus solitarius; sp5, spinal trigeminal tract; Sp5I, spinal trigeminal nucleus, interpolar part; TBOA, DL-threo-β-benzyloxyaspartate; TRH, thyrotropin-releasing hormone; TTX, tetrodotoxin; XIIN, hypoglossal nucleus

MATERIALS AND METHODS

Ethical Approval

The experiments were performed on 120 newborn rats. The protocol was approved by the Ethical Committee of Shanghai Medical College affiliated to Fudan University (No. 20110307-060) and by the Animal Care Committee of Shanghai General Hospital affiliated to Shanghai Jiao Tong University, the research was carried out in line with the guideline of "Guide for the Care and Use of Laboratory Animals" established by the National Institutes of Health.

Retrograde Fluorescent Labeling of AVPNs and Preparation of Brainstem Slices

The 3- to 4-day-old Sprague-Dawley rats (Shanghai Institute for Family Planning and Shanghai General Hospital) were anesthetized with inhalation of halothane (0.5 ml) and hypothermia, and then the AVPNs were labeled retrogradely by rhodamine which have been described in details in our previous studies (Chen Y. et al., 2007; Chen et al., 2012a; Hou et al., 2012). Briefly, the extra thoracic trachea was exposed via a ventral midline incision in the neck. The fluorescent tracer rhodamine (XRITC, Molecular Probes, 1% solution, 0.5 μl) was injected into the tracheal wall between the fourth and eighth tracheal cartilage using a glass pipette of which the tip diameter was 30 μm with a syringe through polyethylene tubing attached. 48 h later, the animal was recovered. Halothane was used again to anesthetize the animal deeply as described above and then was decapitated. The brainstem was dissected out under a dissection microscope and then was submerged into ice-cold (4°C) ACSF which included (in mM) NaCl 124, KCl 3.0, KH_2PO_4 1.2, $CaCl_2$ 2.4, $MgSO_4$ 1.3, $NaHCO_3$ 26, D-glucose 10. The solution was constantly bubbled with 95% O_2–5% CO_2 to keep a pH of 7.4. The final osmolarity of ACSF was adjusted to 320 mosm/L with sucrose. The brainstem was then fixed with a chuck and submerged with the same ACSF in the slicing chamber. The rostral end of the brainstem was set upward; the dorsal surface was glued to an agar block facing the razor. Transverse brainstem slices of 500–800 μm thickness with two hypoglossal rootlets in each side (Smith et al., 1991) were cut using a vibratome (Leica VT 1000S). The brainstem slice with rhythmic inspiratory bursts (Smith et al., 1991) was transferred into the recording chamber (0.6 ml volume) to be superfused with high potassium (10 mM) ACSF at 23 ± 0.5°C. The rostral cutting plane of the slice was set upward to identify fluorescently labeled neurons and record synaptic activities of IA-AVPNs by patch clamp. The flow rate was maintained at 8–11 ml/min.

Electrophysiological Recording

The AVPNs were first identified by their characteristic distribution in the eNA (Chen Y. et al., 2007; Chen et al., 2012a) and by presence of fluorescence with a 40×-water immersion objective lens. The patch pipettes which was filled with K^+ gluconate-dominated internal solution included (in mM): K^+ gluconate 150, HEPES 10, EGTA 10, $CaCl_2$ 1, and $MgCl_2$ 1; pH 7.3; 320 mosm/L. The holding voltage was normally set as −80 mV. In these recording conditions, only excitatory glutamatergic synaptic events were detectable, and the inhibitory synaptic currents mediated by chloride ion were minimized. When the IA-AVPN was clamped at −50 mV, both excitatory synaptic events manifesting inward currents and inhibitory synaptic events showing outward currents were detected. In some experiments, QX314 (lidocaine *N*-ethyl bromide, 2.0 mM) was put into the pipette solution to prevent activation of voltage-dependent sodium currents and slow inward rectifier (I_h) (Marchetti et al., 2003; Sharifullina et al., 2005) of the patched neuron. IA-AVPNs were defined as those that were inspiratorily activated, as manifested by the rhythmic inspiratory discharges under cell-attached configuration (holding voltage 0 mV), by the rhythmic inspiratory bursts of the EPSCs under voltage clamp, or by the rhythmic inspiratory depolarizing EPSPs with superimposed trains of action potentials under current clamp (Chen Y. et al., 2007; Chen et al., 2012a). In each slice experiment was performed only on one IA-AVPN.

To get better recording of spontaneous inhibitory postsynaptic currents (sIPSCs) in some experiments, KCl-dominated internal solution was put into the patch pipette (in mM: KCL, 150; HEPES, 10; EGTA, 2; ATP-Mg, 2; pH 7.3; 320 mosm/L). The patched AVPNs were all clamped at −80 mV. Under this holding potential, both glutamatergic excitatory synaptic currents and sIPSCs in IA-AVPNs as well as sIPSCs in II-AVPNs were recorded as inward currents. In order to separate IA-AVPNs from II-AVPNs, the antagonists of glutamate receptors (CNQX and AP5) were topically applied to the patched neurons with the PV830 Pneumatic Picopump pressure delivery system (World Precision Instruments, Sarasota, FL, United States). IA-AVPNs were identified as those whose inspiratory inward currents could be abolished reversibly by CNQX and AP5.

The patch-clamp signal was amplified with an Axopatch 700B amplifier (10 kHz sampling frequency; 3 kHz filter frequency), digitized with 1322A digidata, and collected with Clampex 9.2 software (Axon Instruments, United States). The inspiratory hypoglossal bursts were recorded from hypoglossal rootlets using a suction electrode, amplified with a BMA-931 bioamplifier (5 kHz sampling frequency; 10–1,000 HZ band pass; 20,000 times), and electronically integrated (τ = 200 ms) with an MA-1000 Moving Averager (CWE Inc., Ardmore, PA, United States) before recording in the computer.

Drug Application

Carbenoxolone and glibenclamide were dissolved in DMSO to make fresh stock solution of 100 mM and diluted to 100 μM in the bath to block gap junctions and inhibit ATP-sensitive potassium channels (K_{ATP}), respectively. TRH affects the neural activity of inspiratory neurons and increases the discharging frequency of hypoglossal nerves in newborn mouse brainstem slices at the concentration of 1–5 μM (Rekling et al., 1996). In nucleus ambiguus neurons, 100 nM TRH induced membrane potential oscillations (Johnson and Getting, 1992). Thus two concentrations of TRH (1 μM and 100 nM) were used in this study at first. Because there were no significant differences between the effects of TRH on IA-AVPNs at these two concentrations, 100 nM was then used in this study. TRH was applied normally in the bath at 100 nM for 3–5 min. Strychnine (1 μM) and picrotoxin (40 μM) were used to block glycine receptors and $GABA_A$ (γ-aminobutyric acid) receptors, respectively. CNQX (50 μM) and D-2-amino-5-phosphonovalerate (AP_5; 50 μM) were used to block non-NMDA and NMDA-type glutamate receptors, respectively. When KCL-dominated internal solution was used to record synaptic currents, CNQX and AP5 were first topically applied to distinguish IA-AVPNs from II-AVPNs, and then were added into the perfusate to block EPSCs. In some experiments, TTX (1 μM) was included in the bath to prevent action potential generation and polysynaptic effects; riluzole (20 μM), to block persistent sodium currents (INaP). ACSF flowing into the chamber was all fresh and was not recycled. The drugs were purchased from Sigma-Aldrich (St. Louis, MO, United States).

Data Analysis

The hypoglossal bursts and the TRH-evoked fast oscillatory currents (FOCs) in IA-AVPNs were analyzed with Clampfit 9.2 (Axon Instrument, United States). Spontaneous or miniature synaptic currents, as well as the ICSs phase-locked to the rapid inward phase of FOCs, were analyzed with MiniAnalysis (version 4.3.1, Synaptosoft), with a minimally acceptable amplitude at 10 pA. Regression analysis was performed with Origin 8.0 (OriginLab Corporation, Northampton, MA, United States). The results were presented as means ± SEM, and statistically compared with paired or independent Student's *t*-test when appropriate. The significant difference was set at $P < 0.05$.

RESULTS

Identification of Inspiratory-Activated Airway Vagal Preganglionic Neurons (IA-AVPNs)

Inspiratory-activated airway vagal preganglionic neurons were first identified by the presence of fluorescence and by their characteristic distribution in the eNA, which is in the close ventral, ventrolateral and ventromedial vicinity of the cNA (Chen Y. et al., 2007; Chen et al., 2012a) (**Figures 1A,B**).

Inspiratory-activated airway vagal preganglionic neurons were defined as those that were activated during inspiratory phase and were manifested by the rhythmic inspiratory-related discharges under cell-attached configuration (**Figure 1C**), by the rhythmic bursts of EPSCs during inspiratory phase under voltage clamp recording (**Figures 2A,D**) or by the rhythmic inspiratory-related depolarizing EPSPs superimposed by trains of action potentials under current clamp recording data not shown. Inspiratory inhibited AVPNs (II-AVPNs) were further defined as those that were inspiratorily inhibited and were manifested by the rhythmic bursts of the inhibitory (outward) postsynaptic currents (IPSCs) during inspiratory phase at holding voltages more positive than −50 mV or by the rhythmic hyperpolarizing inhibitory postsynaptic potentials (IPSPs) during inspiratory phase under current clamp recording (Chen Y. et al., 2007; Chen et al., 2012a). IA-AVPNs were mostly found in the close ventrolateral vicinity and II-AVPNs were mostly found in the near ventral or ventral medial vicinity of the cNA. From 120 slices, a total of 136 AVPNs were identified and tested, of which 120 were IA-AVPNs (88.2%) and 16 were II-AVPNs (11.8%).

TRH Caused an Excitatory Slow Inward Current and Fast Oscillatory Currents (FOCs) in IA-AVPNs

Under voltage clamp, TRH (100 nM) increased baseline current noise and caused a slowly developing excitatory inward current (**Figure 2A**), which peaked within 3 min, with an average amplitude of 55.3 ± 19.7 pA (from 12 neurones). As the excitatory slow inward current developed, the baseline current generated a fast oscillatory change with respect to a steady level reached by TRH. This change was readily recognizable during the inspiratory intervals in all the 12 IA-AVPNs examined from 12 slices (**Figures 2B,C**), with an average cycle length of 201.2 + 18.5 ms. In some (eight of twelve) IA-AVPNs, the change was also identifiable during the inspiratory phase (**Figures 2D,E**), with a significantly shorter cycle length of 90.1 ± 6.2 ms ($P < 0.05$ compared with the value during inter-inspiratory intervals; $n = 8$). The amplitude of this FOCs was relatively consistent in individual neurones, with an average of 38.3 ± 4.1 pA ($n = 12$). Each oscillatory cycle was composed of a rapid inward phase and a slower outward phase (**Figure 2C**). The rapid inward phase of each oscillatory cycle was superimposed by a bursting of EPSCs (**Figure 2C**), and the slower outward phase was superimposed by sporadically occurring EPSCs that were either relatively more frequent (**Figure 2C**) or very scarce (data not shown) in individual neurons. During TRH application the tonic EPSCs increased in the frequency (4.7 ± 0.9 HZ vs. 18.9 ± 2.6 HZ, $P < 0.05$, $n = 12$, Student's paired *t*-test, **Figures 2C,F**) and showed a rhythmic-like change synchronized with FOCs (**Figure 2C**). TRH increased the frequency of the inspiratory inward currents from 3.9 ± 0.6 to 7.6 ± 0.9 bursts/min ($P < 0.05$, $n = 12$, Student's paired *t*-test, **Figures 2A,G**) but bell-shaped inspiratory inward currents became very irregular due to TRH-induced FOCs, which made the amplitude and area incomparable with that in the absence of TRH (**Figure 2H**). Additionally, TRH significantly increased the frequency, peak amplitude and area of the hypoglossal inspiratory bursts (Rekling et al., 1996; Hou et al., 2012). The effects of TRH usually disappeared in about 5 min upon wash, and a second application of TRH at 10–20 min interval caused comparable responses.

Tetrodotoxin (TTX) Inhibited the TRH-Induced Excitatory Slow Inward Current and Prevented the Oscillatory Pattern

In five of the twelve IA-AVPNs examined above, TRH was also applied in the presence of TTX (1 μM) (**Figure 3A**). TTX abolished hypoglossal respiratory bursts and the phasic EPSCs during inspiratory bursts in IA-AVPNs, and significantly inhibited tonic EPSCs in both the frequency

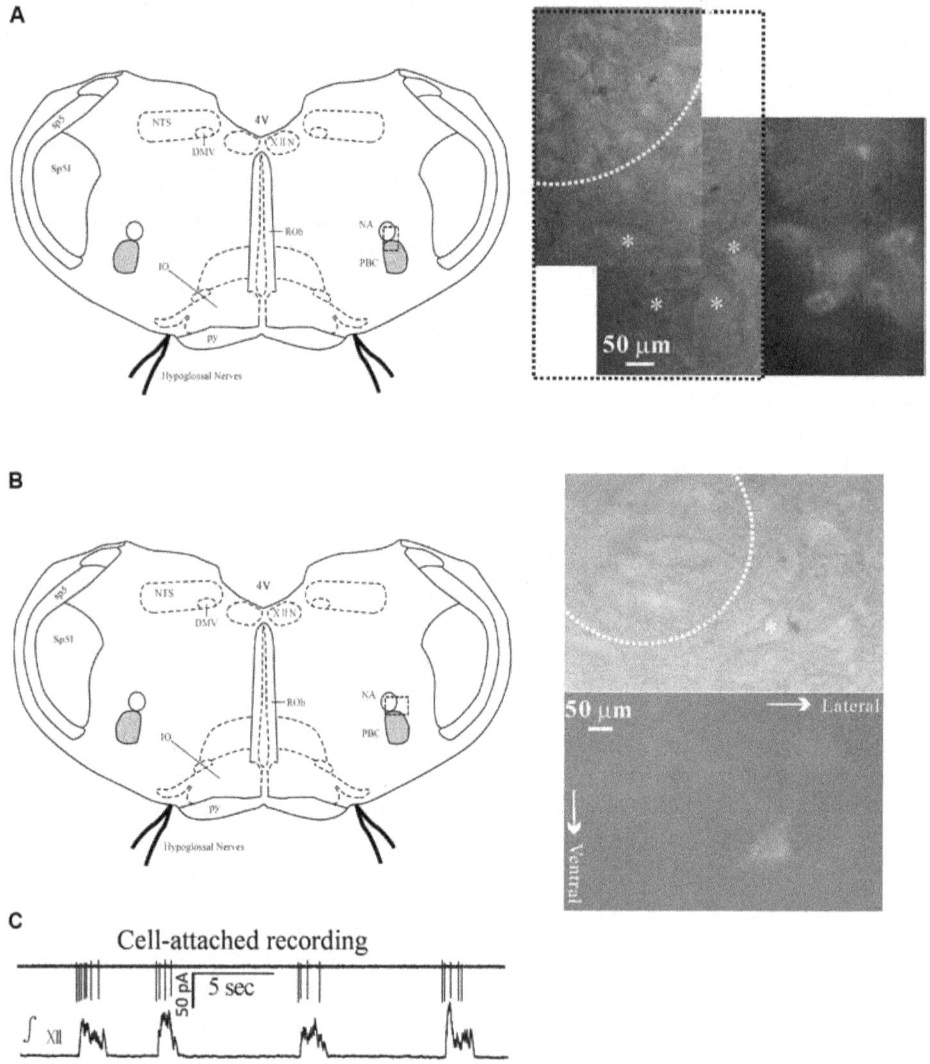

FIGURE 1 | Identification of inspiratory-activated airway vagal preganglionic neurons (IA-AVPNs) in the external formation of NA. **(A,B)** After application of rhodamine into extra-thoracic tracheal wall fluorescently labeled IA-AVPNs (marked by *) in the ventrolateral medulla were mostly in the ventrolateral, and occasionally in the ventral or ventromedial vicinity (not shown) of the compact portion (dashed circle) of the nucleus ambiguus (NA). Note these cells were larger in size compared with those within the compact portion of the NA, and were typically multipolar or spindle-like. The dashed frames in the schematic figures of the medullary slices indicate the areas from which photos were taken under infrared or fluorescent illumination. **(C)** IA-AVPNs in the ventrolateral vicinity of the NA mostly exhibited trains of inspiratory-related discharges under cell-attached configuration and were identified as inspiratory IA-AVPNs. ∫ XII, integrated hypoglossal activity; XIIN, hypoglossal nucleus; NTS, nucleus tractus solitarius; DMV, dorsal motor nucleus of vagus; sp5, spinal trigeminal tract; Sp5I, spinal trigeminal nucleus, interpolar part; PBC, pre-Bötzinger complex; ROb, raphe obscurus nucleus; py, pyramidal tract; 4V, 4th ventricle.

(from 6.9 ± 2.2 to 0.7 ± 0.03 Hz; $P < 0.05$, $n = 5$; pared Student's t-test) and the amplitude (from 61.1 ± 7.3 to 43.7 ± 1.5 pA; $P < 0.05$, $n = 5$; pared Student's t-test). Under this condition TRH did not cause any change of miniature EPSCs (mEPSCs), neither in the frequency nor in the amplitude (**Figures 3B–F**), and did not cause FOCs in any of these five IA-AVPNs (**Figure 3B**). The TRH-induced excitatory slow inward current was significantly inhibited (**Figure 3B**), from a control of 61.9 ± 16.2 pA to 19.0 ± 7.2 pA in the presence of TTX ($P < 0.05$; $n = 5$). All the mEPSCs were abolished by CNQX (50 μM) at the end of the experiments.

The TRH-Induced Excitatory Slow Inward Current and the Oscillatory Pattern (OP) in the IA-AVPNs Were Largely Independent of Their Inputs From Chemical Synapses

Tetrodotoxin blocked the TRH-induced enhancement of tonic EPSCs, significantly reduced the amplitude of the excitatory slow inward current and prevented the FOCs. These results raised such possibilities as in the absence of TTX TRH-induced enhancement of EPSCs might be critical in the generation of FOCs and might also contribute to the significantly larger

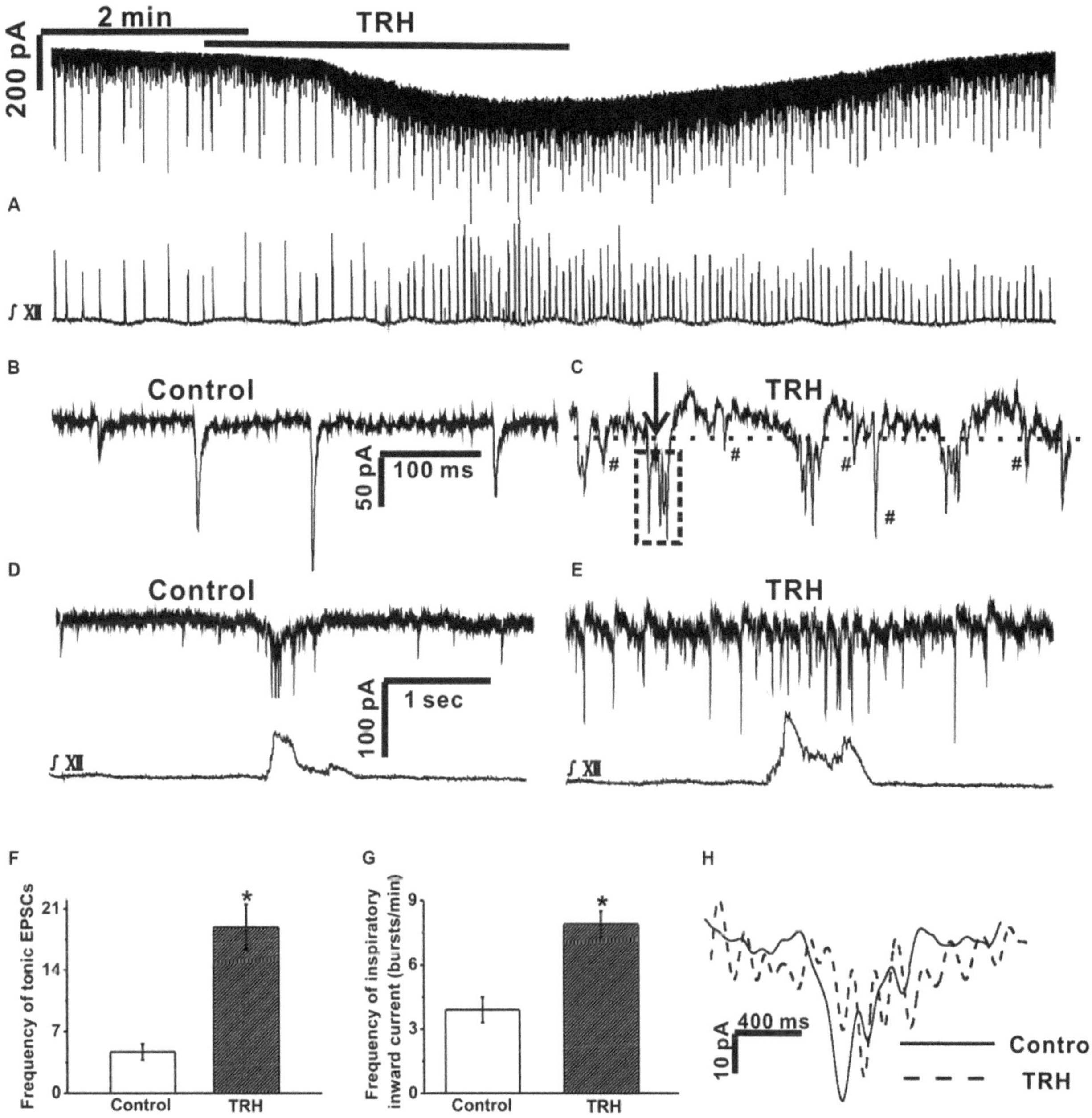

FIGURE 2 | TRH caused an excitatory slow inward current and fast oscillatory currents in the inspiratory-activated airway vagal preganglionic neurons (IA-AVPNs). **(A)** Simultaneous recording of an IA-AVPN under voltage clamp (upper panel) and the hypoglossal respiratory bursts (lower panel), showing that TRH application caused a slow excitatory inward current in this IA-AVPN and increased the frequency and the intensity of the hypoglossal respiratory bursts. **(B,C)** Selected traces of the tonic EPSCs captured from **(A)** during control **(B)** and during TRH application **(C)** are shown in an enlarged scale. The dashed horizontal line in **(C)** indicates the range of the slower outward phase and the arrow shows a typical rapid inward phase of FOCs. The tonic EPSCs show a rhythmic-like change (the box in dashed line) synchronous with the FOCs during TRH application **(C)**. EPSCs (marked by #) occurred during the slower outward phase. The scale bars in **(B)** also applies to **(C)**. **(D,E)** The phasic EPSCs during control **(D)** and TRH-induced FOCs in a different IA-AVPN were also identifiable during inspiratory phase **(E)** with a shorter cycle length. The scale bars in **(D)** also applies to **(E)**. **(F)** Summarized data for the frequency of tonic EPSCs in average ($n = 12$). **(G)** Summarized data for the frequency of phasic inspiratory inward currents in average ($n = 12$). **(H)** Comparison of bell-shaped inspiratory inward currents in **(D)** (during control) and in **(E)** (during application of TRH). $^*P < 0.05$, Student's paired t-test.

excitatory slow inward current via summation. To test these possibilities, TRH was applied to IA-AVPNs pre-exposed to CNQX (50 μM) and AP_5 (50 μM) (**Figure 4A**). CNQX and AP5 blocked all the EPSCs and abolished hypoglossal respiratory bursts (**Figures 4B,C**). Under this condition TRH (100 nM) caused an excitatory slow inward current of 54.4 ± 11.9 pA ($n = 36$), which was not significantly different from that obtained in the twelve IA-AVPNs unexposed to CNQX and

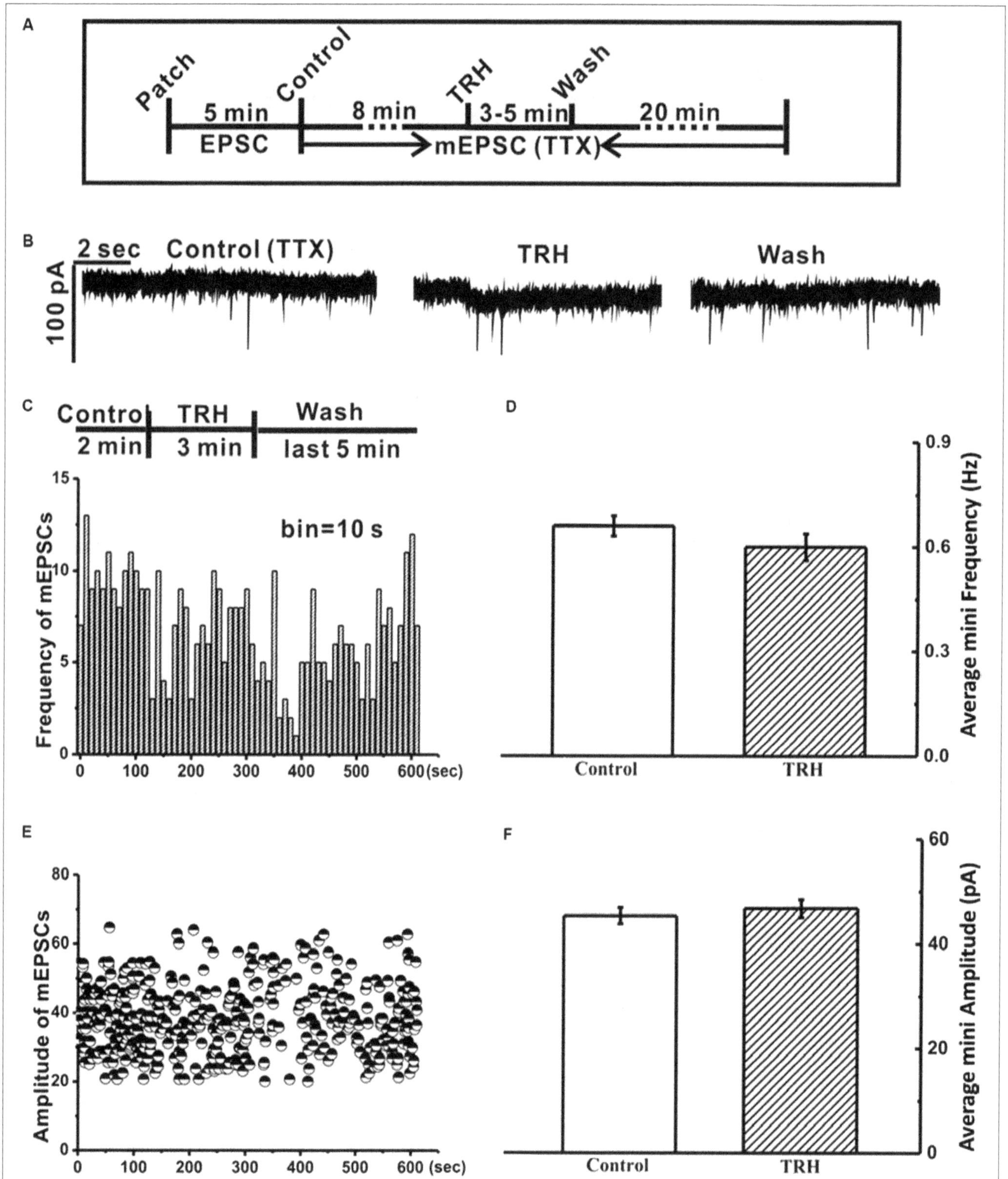

FIGURE 3 | Tetrodotoxin (TTX) inhibited the TRH-induced excitatory slow inward current and prevented generation of FOCs in IA-AVPNs. **(A)** A time axis in this experimental protocol. After TTX was applied for 8 min, TRH was globally applied into the bath for 3–5 min, followed by a 20 min wash with ACSF including TTX. **(B)** Representative mEPSCs recorded under control (left panel), during application of TRH (middle panel), and after 20 min wash (right panel) from an IA-AVPN. **(C,E)** Frequency histogram **(C)** and running amplitude of mEPSCs **(E)** in a representative IA-AVPN, showing TRH caused little alteration in both frequency and amplitude of mEPSCs. **(D,F)** Summarized data of the frequency **(D)** and amplitude **(F)** of mEPSCs in average in IA-AVPNs (n = 5).

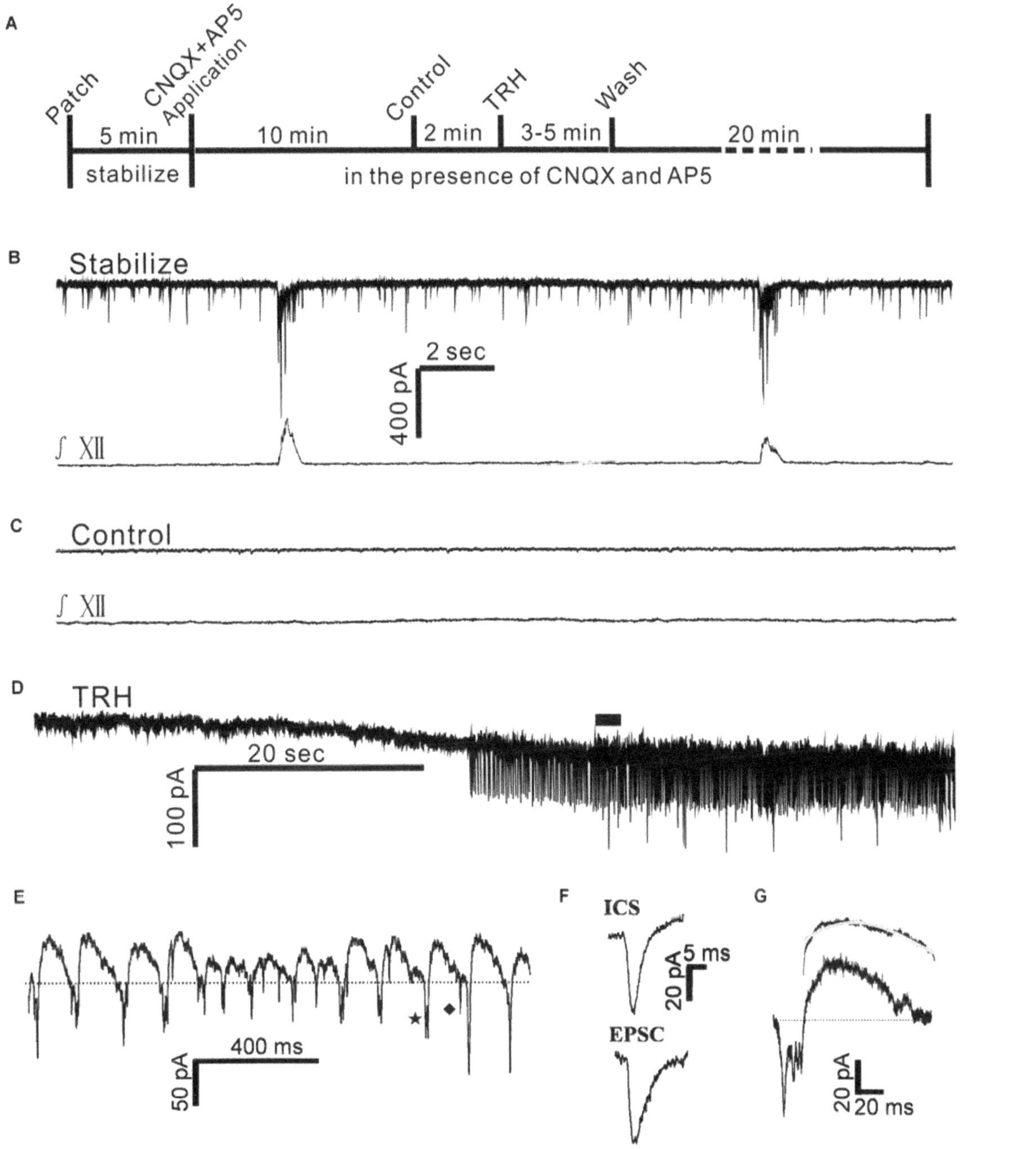

FIGURE 4 | TRH induced an excitatory slow inward current and oscillatory pattern (OP) in IA-AVPNs in the pre-incubation of CNQX and AP5. **(A)** A time axis in this experimental protocol. TRH was globally applied to the patched neuron for 3–5 min after control recording in the presence of CNQX and AP5, followed by a 20 min wash with ACSF including CNQX and AP5. **(B,C)** A representative stabilized recording trace of IA-AVPNs before **(B)** and during bath application of CNQX and AP5 **(C)**. **(D)** TRH induced the excitatory slow inward current and OPs in the presence of CNQX and AP5. **(E)** OPs indicated in **(D)** by the filled bar. Dashed line shows the slower outward phase superimposed by inward current spikelets (ICSs, a typical one indicated by ♦) and the rapid inward phase of FOCs coincident with single or multiple phase-locked ICSs (a typical one indicated by ★). **(F)** Comparison of the kinetics of the ICSs with the EPSCs, showing that the EPSCs had a longer decay time. **(G)** The time course of an oscillatory cycle, showing a rapid inward phase coincident with multiple ICSs and a slower outward phase. The bi-exponential outward phase averaged from 120 oscillatory cycles and the fitted curve (gray) is shown on the top.

AP5 ($P > 0.05$; independent Student's t-test). Interestingly, in all these 36 IA-AVPNs pre-incubation of CNQX and AP5, TRH still exclusively triggered the FOCs (**Figures 4D,E**). Moreover, the rapid inward phase of each oscillatory cycle was still accompanied by single or multiple phase-locked ICSs, and the slower outward phase was also superimposed by sporadically occurring ICSs (**Figure 4E**). FOCs and ICSs formed the OP. Noteworthily, our finding showed that TRH caused an initial increase (three neurons, as is exemplified in **Figure 5B**) or no changes (one neuron, data not shown) in the frequency and/or amplitude of sIPSCs (**Figure 5A**). However, TRH caused progressive declination of sIPSCs in the frequency and amplitude with its prolonged application, which was accompanied by the occurrence of OPs in all the examined neurons (**Figures 5B–F**). TRH caused no changes in the frequency and amplitude of mIPSCs (data not shown). In order to investigate the effect of IPSCs in the generation of OP, in 13 of these 36 IA-AVPNs, picrotoxin (40 μM) and strychnine (1 μM) were also added into the bath to block sIPSCs before TRH application. Importantly, neither the cycle length nor the amplitude of the TRH-evoked oscillatory currents in these 13 neurones was significantly different from those obtained in IA-AVPNs untreated with

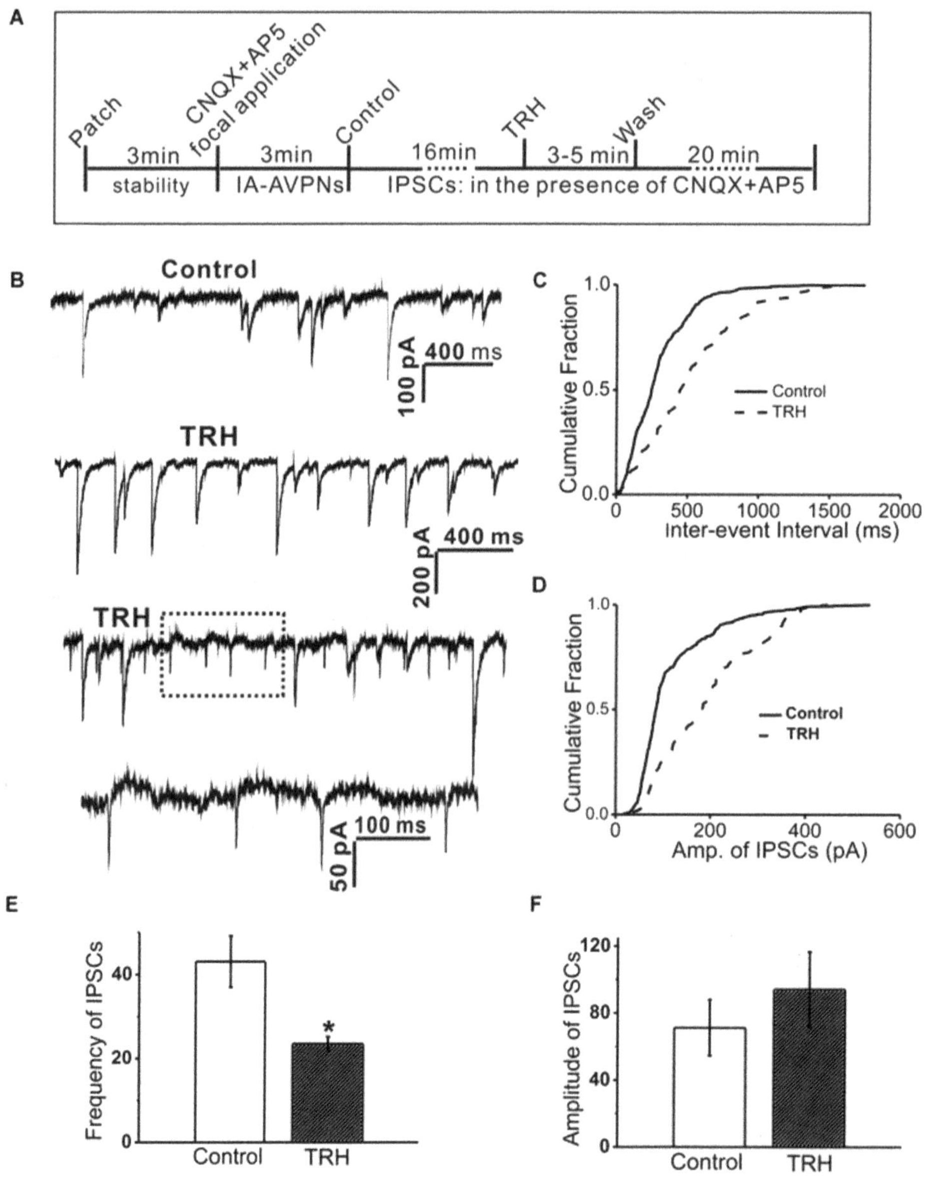

FIGURE 5 | TRH inhibited the frequency and amplitude of spontaneous inhibitory postsynaptic currents (sIPSCs) in IA-AVPNs and simultaneously induced OPs. **(A)** A time axis in this experimental protocol. After IA-AVPN was identified by focal application of CNQX and AP5, the baseline control was recorded in the bath application of CNQX and AP5. TRH was then globally applied to the patched neuron for 3–5 min, followed by a 20 min wash with ACSF including CNQX and AP5. **(B)** A representative recording of control (the first trace) and during application of TRH (the second and third trace), showing that TRH caused an initial increase in the frequency and amplitude (the second trace), and then decreased the frequency and amplitude accompanied by the occurrence of OPs (the third trace). The dashed box in the third trace is shown in an enlarged time scale (the fourth trace). The scale bars in the first trace also applicable to the third trace. **(C,D)** Cumulative plots of IPSCs intervals **(C)** and amplitude **(D)** of IPSCs during control (solid line) and the period of TRH-induced OPs (dashed line; plotted from the same IA-AVPN in **B**). Note that TRH induced a rightward shift in both the inter-event interval and the amplitude distribution curve, indicating decreases in the frequency and increases in the amplitude, respectively. **(E,F)** Summarized data for the frequency **(E)** and amplitude **(F)** of IPSCs in average (n = 4). *P < 0.05, Student's paired t-test.

picrotoxin and strychnine (n = 23). The data were thus pooled together when analyzed. These results demonstrated that the inputs from the chemical synapses were less likely to be involved in the generation of TRH-induced OP and suggest that the summation of the TRH-enhanced tonic EPSCs might contribute little, if any, to the TRH-induced excitatory slow inward current.

In the presence of CNQX and AP_5 both the cycle length and the amplitude of the TRH-evoked FOCs were quite consistent in the individual neurones. Among different neurones, the frequency ranged from 3.8 to 9.5 Hz (6.4 ± 0.2 Hz; n = 36), and the amplitude ran from 20 to 50 pA (meanly 40.4 ± 2.7 pA; n = 36). The average amplitude of the TRH-induced FOCs in the IA-AVPNs pre-exposed to CNQX and AP_5 (n = 36) was not significantly different from that in those unexposed to CNQX and AP_5 (n = 12; P > 0.05). Furthermore, the rapid inward phase of the FOCs was usually accompanied by one to four ICSs, of which the amplitude was relatively consistent in individual neurons but ranged from 20 to 120 pA (46.5 ± 2.3 pA; n = 36) among different neurones. Compared with the tonic EPSCs during control recording, ICSs had a comparable rise time (1.3 ± 0.1 ms for ICSs, n = 12; 1.4 ± 0.2 ms for EPSCs, n = 6; P > 0.05, independent Student's t-test), and a significantly shorter decay time (2.4 ± 0.1 ms for ICSs, n = 12; 4.9 ± 0.4 ms for EPSCs, n = 6; P < 0.05, independent Student's t-test). A comparison was made by average of the difference in the kinetics of ICSs and tonic EPSCs (**Figure 4F**). The outward phase of the FOCs presented a bi-exponential time course, as indicated in the inset to the top of **Figure 4G**, in which a comparison was made of the average (n = 120) and the bi-exponentially fitted outward currents (gray). Properties of EPSCs in the absence of TRH during the inspiratory intervals and the inward phase of FOCs as well as ICSs induced by TRH in the presence of CNQX and AP5 were compared in **Table 1**.

In the majority (21 out of 36) of IA-AVPNs to which TRH was applied in the pre-incubation of CNQX and AP5, QX-314 (2 mM) was included in the pipette solution to block activation of voltage-dependent sodium currents and I_h. The cycle length and amplitude of the TRH-evoked FOCs, as well as the amplitude of the TRH-induced excitatory slow inward current in these neurones, was not significantly different from those obtained IA-AVPNs without intracellular QX-314 (values not shown). These data were thus pooled together when analyzed. The results suggested that the blockade of the voltage-dependent sodium channels from the inside of individual neurones under recording cannot prevent the occurrence of the FOCs as well as the concurrent ICSs, and has little effect on the excitatory slow inward current. Thus, it is likely that TRH-induced OP in IA-AVPNs are synchronized group activity, other than the activity of those under recording.

TRH-Induced OPs Were Insensitive to Membrane Potential

To test if TRH-induced FOCs as well as the coincident ICSs in IA-AVPNs were network-based activities, holding potential was changed under voltage-clamp recording. In the four IA-AVPNs examined from four slices, once the slow inward current evoked by TRH was in a steady level, the membrane potential was shifted from −100 mV to +30 mV. The cycle length of FOCs and the amplitude of ICSs were both unaltered at four different levels of membrane potentials (n = 4, **Figure 6**). Moreover, OPs couldn't be reversed by the very positive commanded potential of +30 mV in the presence of CNQX, AP5, picrotoxin and strychnine. In this experiment, the pipette solution contained QX-314. Similar voltage shifts didn't induce OPs in the absence of TRH (data not shown, n = 8).

The TRH-Induced OP Were Prevented by Gap Junction Blocker Carbenoxolone (CBX)

Since inspiratory motor neurones in the NA have been reported to be gap junction coupled (Rekling and Feldman, 1997), TRH-induced FOCs as well as the coincident ICSs in IA-AVPNs might be related to gap junction. To test this possibility CBX (100 μM) was added in the bath after the first TRH application, both in the normally perfused IA-AVPNs (n = 5) and in those pre-exposed to CNQX and AP_5 (n = 7). Under both circumstances, 30 min presence of CBX prevented completely the occurrence of the OPs during a subsequent TRH application. However, CBX did not significantly alter the amplitude of the TRH-induced excitatory slow inward current, neither in the normally perfused IA-AVPNs (63.6 ± 17.9 before vs. 56.8 ± 19.3 pA after CBX; P > 0.05; n = 5) nor in the IA-AVPNs pre-exposed to CNQX and AP_5 (55.8 ± 20.9 before vs. 56.6 ± 26.1 pA after CBX; P > 0.05; n = 7). A comparison was made of the TRH-induced excitatory slow inward current in a representative IA-AVPN in the absence and in the presence of CBX (**Figures 7A,B**)

In the normally perfused IA-AVPNs, CBX application inhibited gradually, and abolished finally the hypoglossal inspiratory bursts in a 3–60 min period, and also eventually abolished the bursting EPSCs. TRH was usually applied within the initial 10 min after the disappearance of the bursting EPSCs, under which TRH increased the frequency of the tonic EPSCs from 1.2 ± 0.3 to 5.6 ± 1.4 Hz (P < 0.05; n = 5), and also increased the amplitude from 32.2 ± 2.4 to 56.1 ± 4.4 pA (P < 0.05; n = 5). In three of these five IA-AVPNs, TRH caused rhythmic bursting of EPSCs (**Figures 7C–E**), which were coincident with the temporarily restored hypoglossal inspiratory bursts (not shown). At the end of the experiment, EPSCs induced by TRH in the presence of CBX were abolished by CNQX and AP5. These results indicated that TRH is capable of enhancing the EPSCs in IA-AVPNs, and that in the TRH-application experiments performed in the normally perfused IA-AVPNs without CBX, TRH-enhanced EPSCs include both those caused by enhanced glutamate release and those of ICSs coincident with the FOCs.

Additionally, the tonic EPSCs were slowly decreased in frequency and amplitude during CBX application. Since CBX was applied before the second application of TRH at varied time lengths, the CBX-induced gradual changes of tonic EPSCs were not statistically compared.

TABLE 1 | Comparision of properties of FOCs, ICSs and glutamatergic EPSCs in IA-AVPNs in the presence of CNQX, AP5, strychnine and picrotoxin.

	Amplitude (pA)	Rise time (ms)	Decay time (ms)	Frequency (Hz)	*n*
EPSCs	39.5 ± 1.3	1.4 ± 0.2	4.9 ± 0.4	6.2 ± 1.2 Hz	6
ICSs	41.5 ± 4.3	1.3 ± 0.1	2.4 ± 0.1*	6.9 ± 3.2 Hz	12
FOCs	41.9 ± 3.7	2.07 ± 0.3$	3.22 ± 0.4☆	4.7 ± 0.3 Hz$	12

**P* < 0.05 from EPSCs, $*P* < 0.05 from EPSCs or ICSs, ☆*P* < 0.05 from ICSs.*

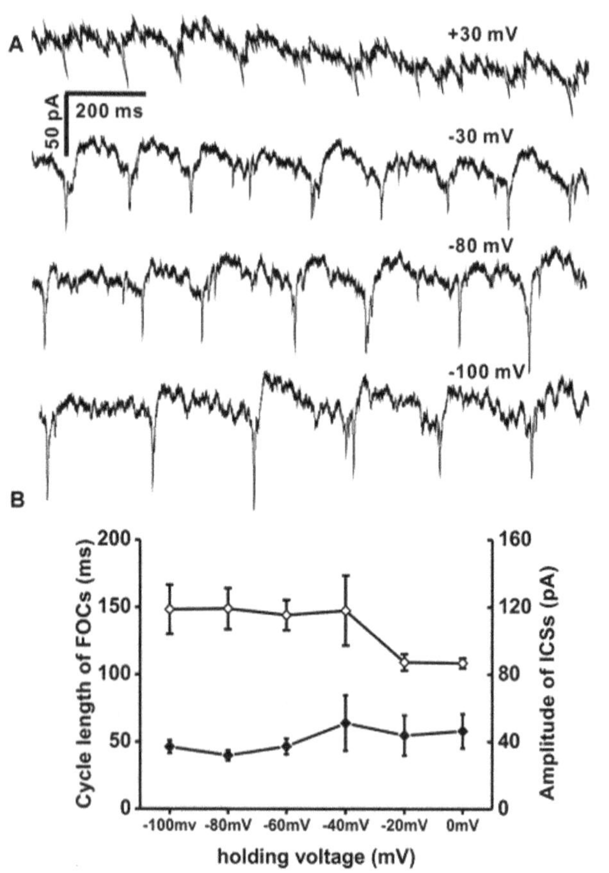

FIGURE 6 | OPs induced by TRH were insensitive to membrane potential. **(A)** A representative recording of OPs recorded at four different levels of holding voltage (values showed above each recording trace) of the same IA-AVPN in the presence of CNQX, AP5, strychnine and picrotoxion, showing that insensitivity of OP cycle length as well as amplitude in ICSs to membrane potential. Pipette solution included QX314 (2 mM). **(B)** Average plots of cycle length of FOCs (◊; left vertical scale; *n* = 4) and amplitude of ICSs (♦; right vertical scale, *n* = 4). QX314 was put into the electrodes in the process of recording.

Riluzole Decreased the Amplitude of TRH-Induced Excitatory Slow Inward Current and Prevented OPs

Since the summation of TRH-enhanced EPSCs contributed little to the TRH-induced excitatory slow inward current, its inhibition by TTX might be mediated by a direct postsynaptic mechanism, possibly via blockade of the persistent sodium current (INaP), because the blockade of voltage-gated sodium transient with intracellular QX-314 exerted little effect on this current. To test the mechanism, riluzole (20 μM) was added in the bath after the first TRH application to the IA-AVPNs pre-exposed to CNQX and AP$_5$; consequently, riluzole alone caused no change of the baseline current in IA-AVPNs. However, 10 min presence of riluzole inhibited significantly the TRH-induced excitatory slow inward current from 51.1 ± 24.3 pA of control to 19.3 ± 10.6 pA (P < 0.05; n = 7). In four of seven IA-AVPNs, the excitatory slow inward current was actually abolished by riluzole (**Figures 7F,G**). Interestingly, riluzole also completely prevented the occurrence of OPs in these seven IA-AVPNs (**Figure 7G**). These results suggested that activation of INaP might be involved in the generation of both the excitatory slow inward current and the OPs during TRH application.

Importantly, K_{ATP} inhibitor glybenclamide was reported to block the oscillatory currents triggered by the activation of metabotrophic glutamate receptors in hypoglossal motor neurones (Sharifullina et al., 2005). In the current study, therefore, the effect of glybenclamide (100 μM) was tested on the TRH-induced changes in the IA-AVPNs pre-exposed to CNQX and AP$_5$; consequently, glybenclamide had no effect neither on the TRH-evoked OPs nor on the excitatory slow inward current (n = 3; data not shown).

TRH Depolarized IA-AVPNs, Causing Continuous or Synchronized Firing Under Current Clamp, Both in the Absence and in the Pre-incubation of CNQX and AP$_5$

To test how TRH affects the firing behavior of IA-AVPNs, TRH was also applied under current clamp, both in normally perfused IA-AVPNs and in those pre-exposed to CNQX and AP5. Under current clamp configuration, the IA-AVPNs showed rhythmic depolarization and action potential firing during inspiratory phase under normal perfusion. Application of 100 nM TRH induced a slowly developing depolarization of 5–25 mV (14.2 ± 3.1 mV; n = 5), and the discharge of the IA-AVPNs became continuous, with significantly decreased action potential amplitude (from 70.4 ± 3 mV to 53.1 ± 5 mV; P < 0.05, n = 5) and significantly increased action potential duration (from 4.7 ± 0.1 to 6.2 ± 0.2 ms; P < 0.05, n = 5). A typical experiment is exhibited in **Figures 8A–D**. In the pre-incubation of CNQX and AP5, which silenced all the IA-AVPNs (**Figure 9A**), TRH application (100 nM) caused a similar slowly developing depolarization, and exclusively caused continuous discharge (n = 5). A typical experiment is exhibited in **Figure 8F**.

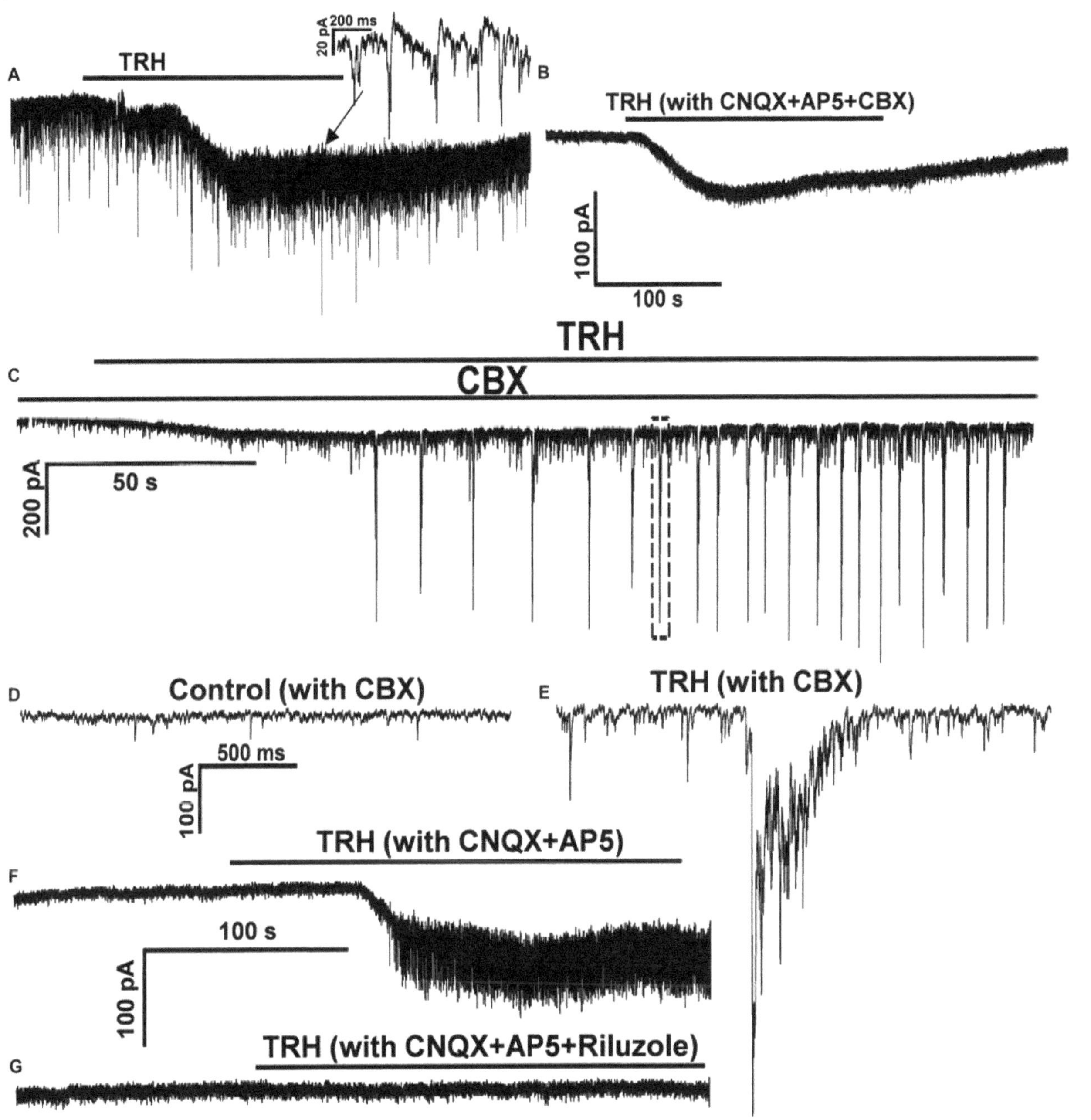

FIGURE 7 | CBX prevented the TRH-evoked oscillatory pattern, and TRH enhanced the EPSCs in the presence of CBX. **(A)** In a representative IA-AVPNs under normal perfusion TRH caused an excitatory slow inward current and evoked OPs. OPs was also evoked in this neurone in the pre-incubation of CNQX and AP5 (not shown). **(B)** In the same neurone in **(A)** CBX prevented OPs without altering the excitatory slow inward current. **(C)** In the presence of CBX, TRH increased the frequency and the amplitude of the tonic EPSCs, and evoked rhythmic bursts of the EPSCs that were coincident with the restored hypoglossal bursts (not shown). **(D,E)** The EPSCs captured from **(C)** before **(D)** and during (**E**: from the dashed box in **C**) TRH application are shown in an enlarged scale. **(F,G)** In a representative IA-AVPNs the TRH-induced OPs and the excitatory slow inward current **(F)** were completely blocked by pre-incubation of 20 μM riluzole **(G)**.

In two IA-AVPNs when the membrane potential was depolarized to a level more positive than −30 mV, the discharge ceased both under normally perfused condition and in the pre-incubation of CNQX and AP_5. The cessation of discharge was obviously because of the inactivation of the voltage-gated sodium channels by over depolarization. When the membrane potential was manually repolarised to a level equal or more negative to the level before TRH application, via injection of a hyperpolarizing current of 10–50 pA, the shape of the action potentials became relatively normal. Under the manually re-polarized condition, moreover, the IA-AVPNs showed fast oscillatory depolarizing potentials, and sporadic action potentials was loaded on the

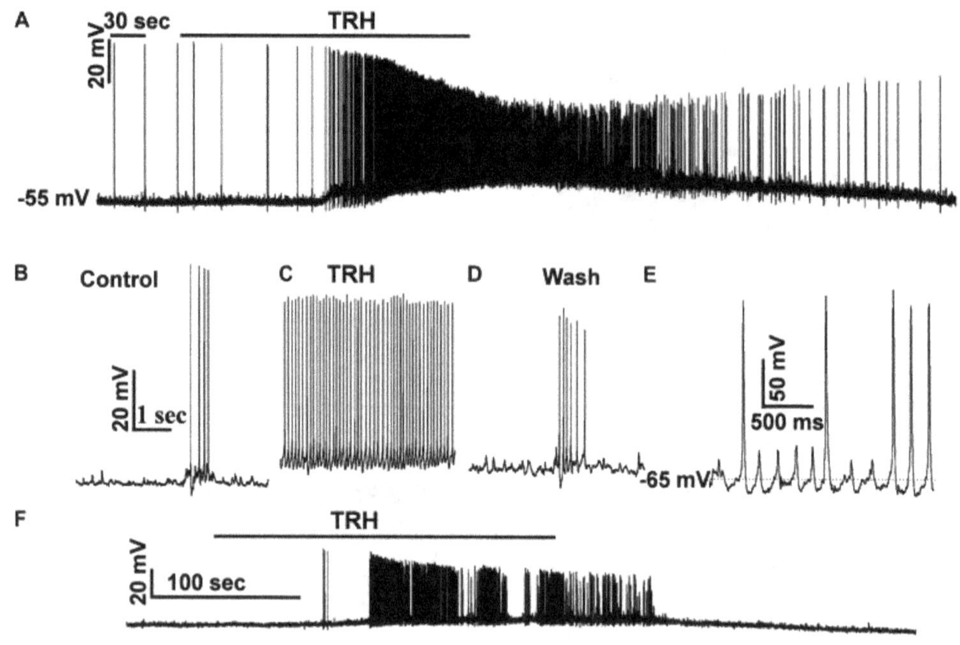

FIGURE 8 | TRH caused continuous firing of the IA-AVPNs and induced increases in firing frequency under current clamp. **(A)** TRH caused depolarization and continuous firing in a representative IA-AVPN. Note the amplitude decrease of action potentials. **(B–D)** Recording of the same IA-AVPN as in **(A)** in an enlarged scale, showing the rhythmic inspiratory depolarization and the superimposed trains of action potentials during control **(B)**, the continuous firing during TRH application **(C)**, and recovery **(D)**. **(E)** The rhythmic oscillatory potentials and the superimposed action potentials when the IA-AVPNs were manually re-polarized during TRH application. **(F)** TRH caused depolarization and continuous firing in a representative IA-AVPN pre-exposed to CNQX and AP_5.

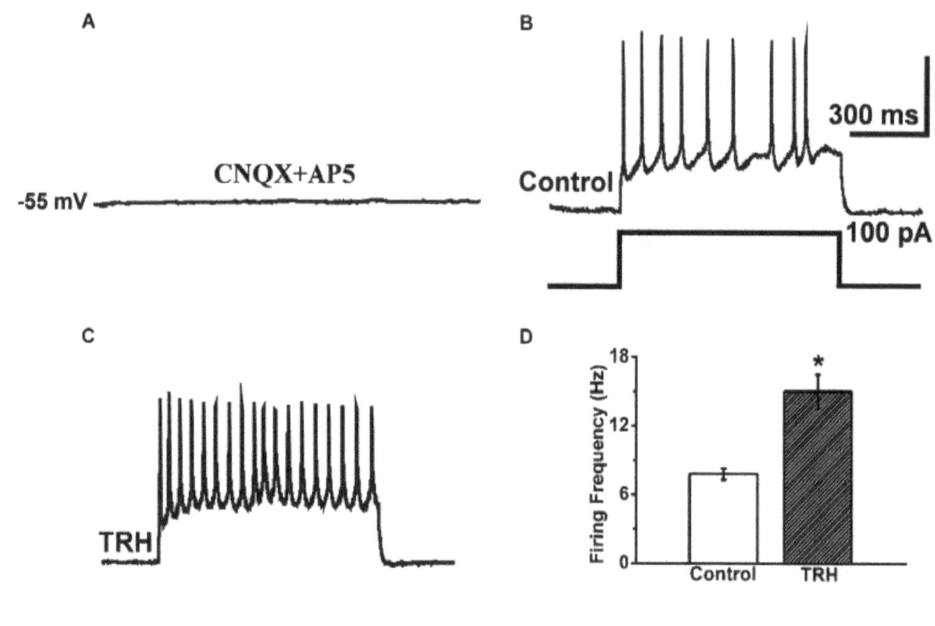

FIGURE 9 | TRH induced increases in instantaneous firing frequency responses to 100 pA depolarizing current. **(A)** In the pre-exposed to CNQX and AP5, an IA-AVPN was silent. **(B)** Injection of 100 pA current induced repetitive instantaneous firing. **(C)** Application of TRH increased the firing frequency in the same neuron in **(B)**. **(D)** Summarized data for the frequency of firing frequency (n = 4). *$P < 0.05$, Student's paired t-test.

peak of some of these fast oscillatory depolarizing potentials (**Figure 8E**), of which the cycle length was identical to that of FOCs under voltage clamp.

In the pre-incubation of CNQX and AP5, the IA-AVPN was silent (**Figure 9A**), and injection of a square-wave current (100 pA) induced repetitive firing (**Figure 9B**). Under this condition, TRH significantly increased firing frequency from 7.75 ± 0.48 Hz to 15 ± 1.47 Hz (n = 4) (**Figures 9C,D**). In the pre-incubation of TTX, TRH didn't cause any significant depolarization and failed to elicit firing behavior of IA-AVPNs. Under such circumstances, injection of a depolarizing current didn't trigger oscillatory depolarizing potentials (n = 3, data not shown).

DISCUSSION

The current study exhibits seven main findings:, (1) TRH caused an excitatory slow inward current and the OPs in IA-AVPNs, which were largely independent of their presynaptic inputs; (2) gap junction blocker CBX prevented the TRH-evoked OPs, but had little impact on the excitatory slow inward current; (3) in the presence of CBX, which blocked the hypoglossal respiratory rhythm and inspiratory bursting EPSCs, TRH enhanced the tonic EPSCs and restored the hypoglossal respiratory bursts in some slices; (4) TRH progressively decreased the frequency of the tonic sIPSCs coincident with the occurrence of OPs and had no influence on mIPSCs; (5) TRH-induced OPs were insensitive to membrane potential; (6) TTX and riluzole completely prevented the TRH-evoked OPs in IA-AVPNs, each of them also inhibiting a large proportion of the excitatory slow inward current; and (7) TRH depolarized IA-AVPNs, causing continuous or synchronized discharge under current clamp, both with and without perfusion of CNQX and AP_5; TRH increased firing frequency responses to input wave-forms.

In general, alterations of a baseline current in the pre-incubation of TTX reveal a postsynaptic mechanism. In IA-AVPNs, an excitatory slow inward current that was inhibited but not completely prevented by TTX during perfusion of TRH, suggesting that TRH had a postsynaptic effect. These results demonstrate that IA-AVPNs have TRH receptors, supporting the previous findings that TRH-containing terminals projected to respiratory motor neurons in NA (Iwase et al., 1992; Sun et al., 1995). In IA-AVPNs, TRH triggered a CBX-sensitive OPs, which was consistent with a previous report that inspiratory motor neurons in NA were coupled by gap junctions (Rekling et al., 2000). The finding also suggests that the generation of the TRH-evoked OPs in IA-AVPNs is a network-based, other than a single-neuron-based, behavior. TRH increased the frequency and the amplitude of the tonic EPSCs in IA-AVPNs in the presence of CBX, and in some slices restored the hypoglossal respiratory bursts and bursting EPSCs that had been abolished by CBX. These results suggest that TRH can have an excitatory stimulation on the glutamatergic inputs of IA-AVPNs, possibly via actions on the pre-terminal sites of the precedent glutamatergic neurons; and that TRH might also be of crucial importance in the respiratory rhythmogenesis via actions on glutamatergic rhythmogenesis neurons.

Thyrotropin-releasing hormone decreased the frequency of sIPSCs accompanied by the occurrence of OPs but didn't affect mIPSCs, indicating that presynaptic release of inhibitory transmitters was inhibited, in which perhaps two mechanisms involved. One possibility is that the propagation of action potential in the inhibitory neurons preceding the IA-AVPNs determines the presynaptic release of inhibitory transmitters. Once TTX eliminated action potentials mentioned above, TRH had no impact on the release of inhibitory transmitters by just targeting at the terminals of these inhibitory neurons. The other possibility is that OPs induced by TRH affect presynaptic release of inhibitory transmitters. Combined with enhancement of excitatory synaptic inputs induced by TRH, the possible significance of these findings lie in unveiling not only the imbalance of excitatory and inhibitory activities (Moore et al., 2004; Haxhiu et al., 2005) but also the generation of OPs contributes to abnormal activation of IA-AVPNs.

Blockade of chemical synaptic inputs of the IA-AVPNs could not prevent the TRH-evoked OPs. Nicotine and arginine vasopressin applied to the normally perfused IA-AVPNs enhanced the tonic EPSCs and the inspiratory bursting EPSCs, but did not evoke the OPs (Zhou et al., 2013; Yan et al., 2017). These findings suggest that presynaptic inputs are not the underlying cause for the TRH-evoked OP. However, in the normally perfused IA-AVPNs the TRH-evoked OPs had a significantly shorter cycle length during the inspiratory phase compared with that during inspiratory intervals. This finding suggests that the inspiratory-enhanced glutamate release, although cannot trigger the OP alone during inspiratory intervals, might have a promoting effect on this pattern during the inspiratory phase.

Oscillatory currents have been reported to be evoked in the hypoglossal motoneurons by NMDA, nicotine, TBOA (a selective blocker of glutamate transporter), or DHPG (an agonist of group I metabotropic glutamate receptors) (Sharifullina et al., 2008; Cifra et al., 2009). In the current study, TRH-evoked OPs shared some similar properties with the oscillatory currents evoked in the hypoglossal motoneurons, such as blockade by CBX or riluzole, and they also showed some quite different properties, as indicated by the evidence that TRH-evoked OP was independent of the inputs from chemical synapses, sensitive to TTX and resistant to glybenclamide. Whereas the oscillatory currents in the hypoglossal motoneurons evoked by nicotine, DHPG, or TBOA were enhanced by AMPA and blocked by CNQX and K_{ATP} inhibitors (Sharifullina et al., 2005; Cifra et al., 2009). Additionally, both the hypoglossal motoneurons and respiratory rhythmogenesis neurons have been reported to be linked by gap junctions (Rekling and Feldman, 1997; Rekling et al., 2000; Sharifullina et al., 2005). In the current study, TRH caused continuous discharge in IA-AVPNs, while the rhythm of the hypoglossal bursts was maintained. These results suggest that neither in the respiratory rhythmogenesis neurons nor in the hypoglossal motoneurons TRH caused persisted or oscillatory-like excitation, and OPs in IA-AVPNs is a rather specific response of these neurons to TRH. Gap junction couplings existed in the IA-AVPNs are of critical importance in the generation of OPs. This was supported by previous studies that gap junctions were identified between AVPNs in the rostral nucleus ambiguous (Rekling and Feldman, 1997) and were recorded in single IA-AVPNs located in eNA (Chen Y.H. et al., 2007). In the propagation of oscillatory currents, gap junction coupling involves a few HMs (Mazza et al., 1992; Sharifullina et al., 2005).

Perhaps gap junctions in IA-AVPNs also involve several neurons in the propagation of TRH-induced OPs. As a limitation, the current study doesn't use the method of paired patch clamp recording of two IA-AVPNs to clarify it, although CBX inhibits OPs on all the examined single-recorded neurons.

Thyrotropin-releasing hormone increased the bell-shaped inspiratory inward currents in the frequency and induced OPs during inspiratory bursts. In view of the rhythmic activation of inspiratory EPSCs, obviously IA-AVPNs receive synaptic inputs from neuronal network of inspiratory rhythmic generation, e.g., pre-BötC (PBC), or the synaptic inputs mentioned above happen to be the rhythm-generated origin. These are consistent with previous studies that TRH activated respiratory neurons in PBC (Rekling et al., 1996; Ruangkittisakul et al., 2006). In our recent study, gap junction couplings could also be activated by central inspiratory activity during inspiratory phase (Hou et al., unpublished paper). The location of the IA-AVPNs in this study are eNA region, within which the PBC neurons locate. Thus, it makes sense to postulate that gap junctions between IA-AVPNs and PBC neurons might contribute to the generation of OPs during inspiratory phase. Future studies are required to address the question as to whether IA-AVPNs are coupled via gap junctions with PBC neurons. Although we couldn't provide precise morphological locus of gap junctions at present, it seems that gap junctions here don't locate at axo-axonal coupling (Schmitz et al., 2001; Sharifullina et al., 2005). This view is supported by the current finding that the cycle length of FOCs is insensitive to membrane potential in a single recorded IA-AVPN in this study. The spikelets induced in hippocampal slice neurons originating from axo-axonal electrical coupling would be inhibited by hyperpolarizing the soma (Schmitz et al., 2001), which was inconsistent with the present findings. Therefore, it is reasonable to infer gap junctions here might locate on somatic-dendritic couplings. Additionally, although we can't completely rule out the probability that the generation of OPs originates from currents of nearby unclamped neurons, the resistance of input resistance to depolarization or hyper-polarization (from -100 mV to $+30$ mV) makes it impossible.

Both excitatory slow inward current and OPs induced by TRH were depressed by riluzole (20 μM). This finding indicates that persistent sodium current might play a crucial role in the generation of OPs due to its high sensitivity to riluzole (<10 μM) (Bellingham, 2011). However, riluzole was reported to have a wide-ranging neural effects (Bellingham, 2011), including inhibition of voltage-gated Ca^{2+} current (Bellingham, 2013) and augment of Ca^{2+}-dependent potassium current (Beltran-Parrazal and Charles, 2003), etc. It is unlikely that riluzole in this study suppresses presynaptic glutamate release (He et al., 2002; Pace et al., 2007; Rammes et al., 2008; Bellingham, 2013) or blocks ionotropic glutamate receptor postsynaptically (Bellingham, 2013) as OPs evoked by TRH is independent of chemical synapses, although other non-specific effects couldn't be excluded at present.

It is noted that AVPNs involved in the modulation of lower airway caliber experience developmental changes (Kohn et al., 2009). Especially, as a very crucial factor in the generation of TRH-induced OPs, gap junctions exist not only in inspiratory motoneurons of newborn mouse (Rekling and Feldman, 1997) and neonatal rats (Chen Y.H. et al., 2007), but also in vagal motoneurons in the nucleus ambiguus of adult animals (Lewis, 1994). To our knowledge, gap junction is made up of connexins (Cx). Cx 26 and Cx32, two important components of Cx, were expressed in PBC neurons, and both of them exhibit developmental variations (Solomon et al., 2001). Unfortunately, there is very little information on the expression and developmental changes of gap junctions in IA-AVPNs in the previous literatures. Therefore, it is not known whether OPs in this study could be induced by TRH in adult rats. This issue needs further investigations.

The inspiratory oscillations have been proved in previous studies to play significant roles in facilitating neural output at respiratory motor neurons levels (Huang et al., 1996; Funk and Parkis, 2002; Parkis et al., 2003). In this study, current clamp experiments showed that the IA-AVPNs were overall excited by TRH. Obviously, OPs contributed to increasing firing frequency of IA-AVPNs via the rapid inward phase of FOCs and multiple ICSs. ICSs in this study are likely to be caused by gap-junction communication among neighboring neurons due to their properties and sensitivity to CBX. Increase of such gap-junction communication involve in the synchronization of motor neurons (Kepler et al., 1990; Haxhiu et al., 2005; Sharifullina et al., 2005), although electrical coupling is also demonstrated to reduce motor-neural synchrony in the previous study (Bou-Flores and Berger, 2001). Thus ICSs are likely to play vital roles in the synchronization of IA-AVPNs. Funk et al. documented that the oscillations, especially high frequency oscillations of motor neurons, have high correlations with that of their respective nerves (Funk and Parkis, 2002). Accordingly, it makes reasonable to infer that OPs of IA-AVPNs are possibly synchronized with the oscillations of vagus nerves or airway smooth muscles they innervate. Therefore, OPs of IA-AVPNs might form functional basis for synchronous activation of airway smooth muscles. In addition, because the cycle length of FOCs was insensitive to membrane potentials, the neuronal output was likely to be constrained to the cycle length. Consequently, the emergence of this kind of fast oscillatory depolarizing potentials under current clamp might prevent excessive excitation of IA-AVPNs.

It is not exactly known how TRH induced the excitatory inward current and triggered FOCs in the IA-AVPNs. Based on the current findings, it is likely that TRH first activated of INaP and then opened gap junctions in IA-AVPNs. It seems that INaP contribute to the excitatory slow inward current. The slow outward phase of FOCs might due to the activation of some potassium channels, although TRH could inhibit acid-sensitive TASK channels in locus coeruleus noradrenergic neurons (Ishibashi et al., 2009). Once IA-AVPNs were depolarized to the threshold they fired action potentials, which were then synchronized by opened gap junctions and were detected as OPs in individual IA-AVPNs. The ion channel mechanisms of mediating the rapid inward phase and slow outward phase merit further investigations.

The physiological or pathological significance of the TRH-induced OPs in IA-AVPNs remains unknown. It has been demonstrated that activation of AVPNs by antidiuretic hormone might participate in psychological stress-induced asthma exacerbations in our previous study (Hou et al., 2017). In the previous animal experiment, the central release of TRH after cold stress was seven folds of the control level (Fiedler et al., 2006). Since cold stress is a well-recognized factor in inducing or accelerating asthma, it is likely that the TRH-induced OPs in IA-AVPNs contributes to the genesis or exacerbation of asthma. Network-based OPs mediated by gap junction in this study might be very crucial in the synchronization of IA-AVPNs. Changes in central mechanisms affecting such synchronization might lead to bronchoconstrictive asynchrony. For example, the imbalance of such synchronization might result in a fact that some bronchial branches nearly totally closed but others stay normal when asthma attacks. Alleviation of airway inflammation and airway hyperactivity by inhaled CBX had also been reported (Ram et al., 2009). Thus, ion channel blockers that can inhibit the TRH-induced the slow excitatory currents and block the triggering of the OP might function as promising candidates to prevent and treat asthma.

CONCLUSION

In current study, TRH enhances the excitatory inputs, decreases the inhibitory inputs, induces a slow postsynaptic excitatory inward current and triggers an OP mediated by gap junction, all of which contribute to the excitation of IA-AVPNs.

AUTHOR CONTRIBUTIONS

LH, LZ, and XZo designed the research. LH, MZ, XZa, ZL, PZ, and DQ performed the research. LH, MZ, XZa, LZ, and XZo analyzed the data. LH wrote the paper. LH, LZ, and XZo revised the paper.

FUNDING

This study was supported by the NSFC grant (81300020) to LH, the Young Physician Assistant Training Program of Shanghai and the Excellent Young Physician Assistant Training Program of Shanghai General Hospital affiliated to Shanghai Jiao Tong University to LH.

REFERENCES

Baker, D. G. (1986). Parasympathetic motor pathways to the trachea: recent morphologic and electrophysiologic studies. *Clin. Chest Med.* 7, 223–229.

Bellingham, M. C. (2011). A review of the neural mechanisms of action and clinical efficiency of riluzole in treating amyotrophic lateral sclerosis: what have we learned in the last decade? *CNS Neurosci. Ther.* 17, 4–31. doi: 10.1111/j.1755-5949.2009.00116.x

Bellingham, M. C. (2013). Pre- and postsynaptic mechanisms underlying inhibition of hypoglossal motor neuron excitability by riluzole. *J. Neurophysiol.* 110, 1047–1061. doi: 10.1152/jn.00587.2012

Beltran-Parrazal, L., and Charles, A. (2003). Riluzole inhibits spontaneous Ca2 + signaling in neuroendocrine cells by activation of K + channels and inhibition of Na + channels. *Br. J. Pharmacol.* 140, 881–888. doi: 10.1038/sj.bjp.0705491

Bou-Flores, C., and Berger, A. J. (2001). Gap junctions and inhibitory synapses modulate inspiratory motoneuron synchronization. *J. Neurophysiol.* 85, 1543–1551. doi: 10.1152/jn.2001.85.4.1543

Canning, B. J., and Fischer, A. (2001). Neural regulation of airway smooth muscle tone. *Respir. Physiol.* 125, 113–127. doi: 10.1016/S0034-5687(00)00208-5

Chen, Y., Hou, L., Zhou, X., Qiu, D., Yuan, W., Zhu, L., et al. (2012a). Inspiratory-activated and inspiratory-inhibited airway vagal preganglionic neurons in the ventrolateral medulla of neonatal rat are different in intrinsic electrophysiological properties. *Respir. Physiol. Neurobiol.* 180, 323–330. doi: 10.1016/j.resp.2011.12.014

Chen, Y., Li, M., Liu, H., and Wang, J. (2007). The airway-related parasympathetic motoneurones in the ventrolateral medulla of newborn rats were dissociated anatomically and in functional control. *Exp. Physiol.* 92, 99–108. doi: 10.1113/expphysiol.2006.036079

Chen, Y., Wang, L., Zhou, X., Ge, D., Yuan, W., and Wang, J. (2012b). Agonist of 5-HT1A/7 receptors but not that of 5-HT2 receptors disinhibits tracheobronchial-projecting airway vagal preganglionic neurons of rats. *Neuroscience* 207, 78–87. doi: 10.1016/j.neuroscience.2012.01.047

Chen, Y. H., Hou, L. L., and Wang, J. J. (2007). Selective revealing of gap junction currents in single inspiratory tracheal motor neurons. *Sheng Li Xue Bao* 59, 770–776.

Cifra, A., Nani, F., Sharifullina, E., and Nistri, A. (2009). A repertoire of rhythmic bursting produced by hypoglossal motoneurons in physiological and pathological conditions. *Philos. Trans. R. Soc. Lond. B. Biol. Sci.* 364, 2493–2500. doi: 10.1098/rstb.2009.0071

Fiedler, J., Jara, P., Luza, S., Dorfman, M., Grouselle, D., Rage, F., et al. (2006). Cold stress induces metabolic activation of thyrotrophin-releasing hormone-synthesising neurones in the magnocellular division of the hypothalamic paraventricular nucleus and concomitantly changes ovarian sympathetic activity parameters. *J. Neuroendocrinol.* 18, 367–376. doi: 10.1111/j.1365-2826.2006.01427.x

Funk, G. D., and Parkis, M. A. (2002). High frequency oscillations in respiratory networks: functionally significant or phenomenological? *Respir. Physiol. Neurobiol.* 131, 101–120. doi: 10.1016/S1569-9048(02)00041-1

Ge, D., Yan, X., Guo, Y., Chen, X., Guan, R., Chen, Y., et al. (2015). Activation of alpha1-adrenoceptors facilitates excitatory inputs to medullary airway vagal preganglionic neurons. *J. Appl. Physiol.* 119, 686–695. doi: 10.1152/japplphysiol.00045.2015

Guo, Y., Yan, X., Chen, X., He, D., Zeng, M., Chen, Y., et al. (2017). Corticotropin-releasing hormone modulates airway vagal preganglionic neurons of Sprague-Dawley rats at multiple synaptic sites via activation of its type 1 receptors: implications for stress-associated airway vagal excitation. *Neuroscience* 355, 101–112. doi: 10.1016/j.neuroscience.2017.04.049

Haselton, J. R., Solomon, I. C., Motekaitis, A. M., and Kaufman, M. P. (1992). Bronchomotor vagal preganglionic cell bodies in the dog: an anatomic and functional study. *J. Appl. Physiol.* 73, 1122–1129. doi: 10.1152/jappl.1992.73.3.1122

Haxhiu, M. A., Deal, E. C. Jr., Norcia, M. P., van Lunteren, E., and Cherniack, N. S. (1987). Effect of N-methyl-D-aspartate applied to the ventral surface of the medulla on the trachea. *J. Appl. Physiol.* 63, 1268–1274. doi: 10.1152/jappl.1987.63.3.1268

Haxhiu, M. A., Jansen, A. S., Cherniack, N. S., and Loewy, A. D. (1993). CNS innervation of airway-related parasympathetic preganglionic neurons: a transneuronal labeling study using pseudorabies virus. *Brain Res.* 618, 115–134. doi: 10.1016/0006-8993(93)90435-p

Haxhiu, M. A., and Loewy, A. D. (1996). Central connections of the motor and sensory vagal systems innervating the trachea. *J. Auton. Nerv. Syst.* 57, 49–56. doi: 10.1016/0165-1838(95)00092-5

Haxhiu, M. A., Kc, P., Balan, K. V., Wilson, C. G., and Martin, R. J. (2008). Modeling of sleep-induced changes in airway function: implication for nocturnal worsening of bronchial asthma. *Adv. Exp. Med. Biol.* 605, 469–474. doi: 10.1007/978-0-387-73693-8_82

Haxhiu, M. A., Kc, P., Moore, C. T., Acquah, S. S., Wilson, C. G., Zaidi, S. I., et al. (2005). Brain stem excitatory and inhibitory signaling pathways regulating bronchoconstrictive responses. *J. Appl. Physiol.* 98, 1961–1982. doi: 10.1152/japplphysiol.01340.2004

Haxhiu, M. A., Kc, P., Neziri, B., Yamamoto, B. K., Ferguson, D. G., and Massari, V. J. (2003). Catecholaminergic microcircuitry controlling the output of airway-related vagal preganglionic neurons. *J. Appl. Physiol.* 94, 1999–2009. doi: 10.1152/japplphysiol.01066.2002

Haxhiu, M. A., Yamamoto, B. K., Dreshaj, I. A., and Ferguson, D. G. (2002). Activation of the midbrain periaqueductal gray induces airway smooth muscle relaxation. *J. Appl. Physiol.* 93, 440–449. doi: 10.1152/japplphysiol.00752.2001

He, Y., Zorumski, C. F., and Mennerick, S. (2002). Contribution of presynaptic Na(+) channel inactivation to paired-pulse synaptic depression in cultured hippocampal neurons. *J. Neurophysiol.* 87, 925–936. doi: 10.1152/jn.00225.2001

Hou, L., Zhou, X., Chen, Y., Qiu, D., Zhu, L., and Wang, J. (2012). Thyrotropin-releasing hormone causes a tonic excitatory postsynaptic current and inhibits the phasic inspiratory inhibitory inputs in inspiratory-inhibited airway vagal preganglionic neurons. *Neuroscience* 202, 184–191. doi: 10.1016/j.neuroscience.2011.12.003

Hou, L., Zhou, X., Zhang, M., Liu, Z., and Zhang, G. (2015). Effects of Methyleugenol on central respiratory drive to inspiratory-activated airway vagal preganglionic neurons. *Zhonghua Yi Xue Za Zhi* 95, 933–937. doi: 10.3760/cma.j.issn.0376-2491.2015.12.014

Hou, L., Zhu, L., Zhang, M., Zhang, X., Zhang, G., Liu, Z., et al. (2017). Participation of antidiuretic hormone (adh) in asthma exacerbations induced by psychological stress via pka/pkc signal pathway in airway-related vagal preganglionic neurons (AVPNs). *Cell. Physiol. Biochem.* 41, 2230–2241. doi: 10.1159/000475638

Huang, W. X., Cohen, M. I., Yu, Q., See, W. R., and He, Q. (1996). High-frequency oscillations in membrane potentials of medullary inspiratory and expiratory neurons (including laryngeal motoneurons). *J. Neurophysiol.* 76, 1405–1412. doi: 10.1152/jn.1996.76.3.1405

Ishibashi, H., Nakahata, Y., Eto, K., and Nabekura, J. (2009). Excitation of locus coeruleus noradrenergic neurons by thyrotropin-releasing hormone. *J. Physiol.* 587, 5709–5722. doi: 10.1113/jphysiol.2009.181420

Iwase, M., Shioda, S., Nakai, Y., Iwatsuki, K., and Homma, I. (1992). TRH regulation of tracheal tension through vagal preganglionic motoneurons. *Brain Res. Bull.* 29, 821–829. doi: 10.1016/0361-9230(92)90150-V

Johnson, S. M., and Getting, P. A. (1992). Excitatory effects of thyrotropin-releasing hormone on neurons within the nucleus ambiguus of adult guinea pigs. *Brain Res.* 590, 1–5. doi: 10.1016/0006-8993(92)91074-O

Kc, P., Karibi-Ikiriko, A., Rust, C. F., Jayam-Trouth, A., and Haxhiu, M. A. (2006). Phenotypic traits of the hypothalamic PVN cells innervating airway-related vagal preganglionic neurons. *Respir. Physiol. Neurobiol.* 154, 319–330. doi: 10.1016/j.resp.2006.01.006

Kc, P., Mayer, C. A., and Haxhiu, M. A. (2004). Chemical profile of vagal preganglionic motor cells innervating the airways in ferrets: the absence of noncholinergic neurons. *J. Appl. Physiol.* 97, 1508–1517. doi: 10.1152/japplphysiol.00282.2004

Kepler, T. B., Marder, E., and Abbott, L. F. (1990). The effect of electrical coupling on the frequency of model neuronal oscillators. *Science* 248, 83–85. doi: 10.1126/science.2321028

Kohn, A. Z., Hoxha, Z., Balan, K. V., Martin, R. J., Haxhiu, M. A., Wilson, C. G., et al. (2009). Developmental changes in brainstem neurons regulating lower airway caliber. *Pediatr. Res.* 65, 509–513. doi: 10.1203/PDR.0b013e31819da270

Lewis, D. I. (1994). Dye-coupling between vagal motoneurones within the compact region of the adult rat nucleus ambiguus, in-vitro. *J. Auton. Nerv. Syst.* 47, 53–58. doi: 10.1016/0165-1838(94)90065-5

Marchetti, C., Taccola, G., and Nistri, A. (2003). Distinct subtypes of group I metabotropic glutamate receptors on rat spinal neurons mediate complex facilitatory and inhibitory effects. *Eur. J. Neurosci.* 18, 1873–1883. doi: 10.1046/j.1460-9568.2003.02924.x

Mazza, E., Núñez-Abades, P. A., Spielmann, J. M., and Cameron, W. E. (1992). Anatomical and electrotonic coupling in developing genioglossal motoneurons of the rat. *Brain Res.* 598, 127–137. doi: 10.1016/0006-8993(92)90176-A

McGovern, A. E., and Mazzone, S. B. (2010). Characterization of the vagal motor neurons projecting to the Guinea pig airways and esophagus. *Front. Neurol.* 1:153. doi: 10.3389/fneur.2010.00153

Mitchell, R. A., Herbert, D. A., Baker, D. G., and Basbaum, C. B. (1987). In vivo activity of tracheal parasympathetic ganglion cells innervating tracheal smooth muscle. *Brain Res.* 437, 157–160. doi: 10.1016/0006-8993(87)91537-X

Moore, C. T., Wilson, C. G., Mayer, C. A., Acquah, S. S., Massari, V. J., and Haxhiu, M. A. (2004). A GABAergic inhibitory microcircuit controlling cholinergic outflow to the airways. *J. Appl. Physiol.* 96, 260–270. doi: 10.1152/japplphysiol.00523.2003

Myers, A. C. (1998). Ca2+ and K+ currents regulate accommodation and firing frequency in guinea pig bronchial ganglion neurons. *Am. J. Physiol.* 275, L357–364. doi: 10.1152/ajplung.1998.275.2.L357

Myers, A. C., Undem, B. J., and Weinreich, D. (1990). Electrophysiological properties of neurons in guinea pig bronchial parasympathetic ganglia. *Am. J. Physiol.* 259, L403–409. doi: 10.1152/ajplung.1990.259.6.L403

Pace, R. W., Mackay, D. D., Feldman, J. L., and Del Negro, C. A. (2007). Role of persistent sodium current in mouse preBotzinger Complex neurons and respiratory rhythm generation. *J. Physiol.* 580, 485–496. doi: 10.1113/jphysiol.2006.124602

Parkis, M. A., Feldman, J. L., Robinson, D. M., and Funk, G. D. (2003). Oscillations in endogenous inputs to neurons affect excitability and signal processing. *J. Neurosci.* 23, 8152–8158. doi: 10.1523/JNEUROSCI.23-22-08152.2003

Qiu, D., Hou, L., Chen, Y., Zhou, X., Yuan, W., Rong, W., et al. (2011). Beta-asarone inhibits synaptic inputs to airway preganglionic parasympathetic motoneurons. *Respir. Physiol. Neurobiol.* 177, 313–319. doi: 10.1016/j.resp.2011.05.010

Ram, A., Singh, S. K., Singh, V. P., Kumar, S., and Ghosh, B. (2009). Inhaled carbenoxolone prevents allergic airway inflammation and airway hyperreactivity in a mouse model of asthma. *Int. Arch. Allergy Immunol.* 149, 38–46. doi: 10.1159/000176305

Rammes, G., Zieglgansberger, W., and Parsons, C. G. (2008). The fraction of activated N-methyl-D-aspartate receptors during synaptic transmission remains constant in the presence of the glutamate release inhibitor riluzole. *J. Neural Transm.* 115, 1119–1126. doi: 10.1007/s00702-008-0059-y

Rekling, J. C., Champagnat, J., and Denavit-Saubie, M. (1996). Thyrotropin-releasing hormone (TRH) depolarizes a subset of inspiratory neurons in the newborn mouse brain stem in vitro. *J. Neurophysiol.* 75, 811–819. doi: 10.1152/jn.1996.75.2.811

Rekling, J. C., and Feldman, J. L. (1997). Bidirectional electrical coupling between inspiratory motoneurons in the newborn mouse nucleus ambiguus. *J. Neurophysiol.* 78, 3508–3510. doi: 10.1152/jn.1997.78.6.3508

Rekling, J. C., Shao, X. M., and Feldman, J. L. (2000). Electrical coupling and excitatory synaptic transmission between rhythmogenic respiratory neurons in the preBotzinger complex. *J. Neurosci.* 20:RC113. doi: 10.1523/JNEUROSCI.20-23-j0003.2000

Ruangkittisakul, A., Schwarzacher, S. W., Secchia, L., Poon, B. Y., Ma, Y., Funk, G. D., et al. (2006). High sensitivity to neuromodulator-activated signaling pathways at physiological [K+] of confocally imaged respiratory center neurons in on-line-calibrated newborn rat brainstem slices. *J. Neurosci.* 26, 11870–11880. doi: 10.1523/JNEUROSCI.3357-06.2006

Schmitz, D., Schuchmann, S., Fisahn, A., Draguhn, A., Buhl, E. H., Petrasch-Parwez, E., et al. (2001). Axo-axonal coupling: a novel mechanism for ultrafast neuronal communication. *Neuron* 31, 831–840. doi: 10.1016/S0896-6273(01)00410-X

Sharifullina, E., Ostroumov, K., Grandolfo, M., and Nistri, A. (2008). N-methyl-D-aspartate triggers neonatal rat hypoglossal motoneurons in vitro to express rhythmic bursting with unusual Mg2+ sensitivity. *Neuroscience* 154, 804–820. doi: 10.1016/j.neuroscience.2008.03.010

Sharifullina, E., Ostroumov, K., and Nistri, A. (2005). Metabotropic glutamate receptor activity induces a novel oscillatory pattern in neonatal rat hypoglossal motoneurones. *J. Physiol.* 563, 139–159. doi: 10.1113/jphysiol.2004.079509

Smith, J. C., Ellenberger, H. H., Ballanyi, K., Richter, D. W., and Feldman, J. L. (1991). Pre-Botzinger complex: a brainstem region that may generate respiratory rhythm in mammals. *Science* 254, 726–729. doi: 10.1126/science.1683005

Solomon, I. C., Halat, T. J., El-Maghrabi, R., and O'Neal, M. H. III. (2001). Differential expression of connexin26 and connexin32 in the pre-Botzinger complex of neonatal and adult rat. *J. Comp. Neurol.* 440, 12–19. doi: 10.1002/cne.1366

Sun, Q. J., Pilowsky, P., and Llewellyn-Smith, I. J. (1995). Thyrotropin-releasing hormone inputs are preferentially directed towards respiratory motoneurons in rat nucleus ambiguus. *J. Comp. Neurol.* 362, 320–330. doi: 10.1002/cne.903620303

Wilson, C. G., Akhter, S., Mayer, C. A., Kc, P., Balan, K. V., Ernsberger, P., et al. (2007). Allergic lung inflammation affects central noradrenergic control of cholinergic outflow to the airways in ferrets. *J. Appl. Physiol.* 103, 2095–2104. doi: 10.1152/japplphysiol.01182.2006

Yan, X., Chen, X., Guo, Y., He, D., Chen, Y., Xia, C., et al. (2017). Arginine vasopressin alters both spontaneous and phase-locked synaptic inputs to airway vagal preganglionic neuron via activation of v1a receptor: insights into stress-related airway vagal excitation. *Front. Cell. Neurosci.* 11:12. doi: 10.3389/fncel.2017.00012

Zhou, X., Chen, Y., Ge, D., Yuan, W., and Wang, J. (2013). Nicotine enhances both excitatory and inhibitory synaptic inputs to inspiratory-activated airway vagal preganglionic neurons. *Exp. Physiol.* 98, 67–80. doi: 10.1113/expphysiol.2012.066589

6

Neuronal Correlates of Functional Coupling between Reach -and Grasp-Related Components of Muscle Activity

Shashwati Geed[1,2†], Martha L. McCurdy[1] and Peter L. E. van Kan[1]*

[1] *Motor Systems Physiology Laboratory, Department of Kinesiology, University of Wisconsin–Madison, Madison, WI, USA,*
[2] *Department of Rehabilitation Medicine, Georgetown University Medical Center, Washington, DC, USA*

Correspondence:
Shashwati Geed
sg1075@georgetown.edu

Coordinated reach-to-grasp movements require precise spatiotemporal synchrony between proximal forelimb muscles (shoulder, elbow) that transport the hand toward a target during reach, and distal muscles (wrist, digit) that simultaneously preshape and orient the hand for grasp. The precise mechanisms through which the redundant neuromuscular circuitry coordinates reach with grasp, however, remain unclear. Recently, Geed and Van Kan (2016) demonstrated, using exploratory factor analysis (EFA), that limited numbers of global, template-like transport/preshape- and grasp-related muscle components underlie the complexity and variability of intramuscular electromyograms (EMGs) of up to 21 distal and proximal muscles recorded while monkeys performed reach-to-grasp tasks. Importantly, transport/preshape- and grasp-related muscle components showed invariant spatiotemporal coupling, which provides a potential mechanism for coordinating forelimb muscles during reach-to-grasp movements. In the present study, we tested whether ensemble discharges of forelimb neurons in the cerebellar nucleus interpositus (NI) and its target, the magnocellular red nucleus (RNm), a source of rubrospinal fibers, function as neuronal correlates of the transport/preshape- and grasp-related muscle components we identified. EFA applied to single-unit discharges of populations of NI and RNm neurons recorded while the same monkeys that were used previously performed the same reach-to-grasp tasks, revealed neuronal components in the ensemble discharges of both NI and RNm neuronal populations with characteristics broadly similar to muscle components. Subsets of NI and RNm neuronal components were strongly and significantly cross-correlated with subsets of muscle components, suggesting that similar functional units of reach-to-grasp behavior are expressed by NI and RNm neuronal populations and forelimb muscles. Importantly, like transport/preshape- and grasp-related muscle components, their NI and RNm neuronal correlates showed invariant spatiotemporal coupling. Clinical and lesion studies have reported disruption of coupling between reach and grasp following cerebellar damage; the present results expand on those studies by identifying a neuronal mechanism that may underlie cerebellar contributions to spatiotemporal coordination of distal and proximal limb muscles during reaching to grasp. We conclude that finding similar functional units of behavior expressed at multiple levels of information processing along interposito-rubrospinal pathways and forelimb muscles supports the hypothesis that functionally related populations of NI and RNm neurons act synergistically in the control of complex coordinated motor behaviors.

Keywords: reach to grasp, cerebellum, magnocellular red nucleus, coordination, nucleus interpositus

INTRODUCTION

Reach-to-grasp movements require precisely coordinated activation of shoulder, elbow, wrist, and digit muscles such that while shoulder and elbow muscles transport the hand toward a target during reach, wrist and digit muscles preshape and orient the hand for grasp. Psychophysical studies of reach-to-grasp movements have demonstrated functional coupling between reach and grasp such that the wrist follows a largely bell-shaped velocity profile during reach and attains peak velocity at approximately 70% of the transport trajectory (Jeannerod, 1984). Peak wrist velocity during the transport phase coincides in time with attainment of maximal grip aperture (i.e., distance between the thumb and index finger), which characterizes hand opening prior to closing the hand in anticipation of grasp (Jeannerod, 1981, 1984). Furthermore, perturbation of target location, which directly impacts the reach, also influences grasp (Paulignan et al., 1991b; Roy et al., 2006), and perturbation of target size or orientation (Paulignan et al., 1991a, 1997; Roy et al., 2006), which directly impacts grasp, also influences the reach. Recently, Geed and Van Kan (2016) demonstrated, using exploratory factor analysis (EFA), invariant spatiotemporal coupling between transport/preshape- and grasp-related components of forelimb muscle activity in monkeys performing reach-to-grasp tasks, consistent with the observed functional coupling between reach and grasp movements.

Reaching to grasp critically depends on cerebellar function. Cerebellar damage causes a specific breakdown in coupling of reach and grasp movement components (Bastian and Thach, 1995; Bastian et al., 1996, 2000; Mason et al., 1998; Lang and Bastian, 1999; Cooper et al., 2000; Rand et al., 2000; Zackowski et al., 2002). Although cerebellar output targets many, if not all, neural structures involved in movement production, its most direct influences are exerted via the pathway from nucleus interpositus (NI), the sole output of intermediate cerebellum, to the magnocellular red nucleus (RNm). RNm receives its dominant input from NI (Humphrey and Rietz, 1976; Kennedy et al., 1986; Houk et al., 1988), and RNm neurons terminate as rubrospinal fibers on spinal interneurons, or directly on motoneurons that innervate digit muscles (Kuypers et al., 1962; Lawrence and Kuypers, 1968a,b; Kuypers, 1982; McCurdy et al., 1987; Holstege et al., 1988; Ralston et al., 1988; McCurdy et al., 1992). In keeping with influences on distal limb muscles, rubrospinal fibers show promise for prehensile recovery following stroke (Carmel et al., 2013; Takenobu et al., 2014), and following experimental lesions of the pyramidal tract in monkeys (Belhaj-Saif and Cheney, 2000). Therefore, studying the role of interposito-rubrospinal (NI-RNm) circuitry in the control of coordinated reach-to-grasp movements is not only important for understanding cerebellar function in general but is also important for potential neuromodulation and rehabilitation post-stroke, which is in line with recent investigations in other subcortical pathways (Baker, 2011; Bradnam et al., 2013; Cunningham et al., 2015).

Although a mechanistic understanding of how NI-RNm circuits contribute to control of spatiotemporal coordination of reach and grasp movement components has remained elusive, several lines of evidence indicate that NI-RNm circuitry is important to this process. First, forelimb NI and RNm neurons discharge consistently and at high rates when monkeys reach to grasp objects (NI: Gibson et al., 1994; Van Kan et al., 1994; Van Kan and McCurdy, 2001, 2002a,b), RNm: (Gibson et al., 1994; Van Kan et al., 1994; Van Kan and McCurdy, 2001, 2002a,b), and the high discharge rates of NI and RNm neurons are associated with coordinating the hand in the context of whole-limb reaching movements (Miller et al., 1993; Van Kan et al., 1994; Van Kan and McCurdy, 2001). Second, behavioral studies indicate that lesioning or inactivating NI or RNm (NI: Mason et al., 1998; Cooper et al., 2000); RNm: (Sybirska and Gorska, 1980; Gibson et al., 1994) profoundly and specifically affect coordination of reach and grasp movement components. Third, anatomical investigations have demonstrated that NI-RNm circuitry projects (through rubrospinal pathways) to interneuronal and motoneuronal pools that innervate forelimb muscles crucial for coordinated reach-to-grasp movements (Kuypers et al., 1962; Lawrence and Kuypers, 1968a,b; Kuypers, 1982; McCurdy et al., 1987; Holstege et al., 1988; Ralston et al., 1988; McCurdy et al., 1992). The combined results of electrophysiological, behavioral, and anatomic studies support strongly the hypothesis that NI-RNm circuitry serves as a potential neuronal correlate of reaching to grasp.

The primary objective of the current study was to test whether EFA, applied to ensembles of single-unit discharges of populations of NI and RNm neurons recorded while the same monkeys that were used previously (Geed and Van Kan, 2016) performed the same reach-to-grasp tasks, would reveal neuronal components with characteristics broadly similar to the muscle components identified. Our results demonstrate that EFA did indeed reveal 5–7 NI or RNm neuronal components in each monkey, which, while explaining a large proportion of the variance in the ensemble discharges of the NI and RNm neurons recorded, showed significant correlations with the transport/preshape- or grasp-related muscle components identified. Importantly, in both NI and RNm populations, invariant spatiotemporal coupling between transport/preshape-

and grasp-related neuronal components closely resembled the coupling observed between transport/preshape- and grasp-related muscle components. The results of the present study significantly strengthen our hypothesis that the combined output from NI-RNm circuitry reflects a neuronal correlate of the functional coupling between reach and grasp movement components.

MATERIALS AND METHODS

Two rhesus macaques (Macaca mulatta, male, 7–10 kg) were trained to perform reach-to-grasp movements. Animal care and experimental procedures complied with the United States Public Health Service Policy on Humane Care and Use of Laboratory Animals, conformed to the National Institutes of Health, "Guide for the Care and Use of Laboratory Animals," and were approved by the Institutional Animal Care and Use Committee of the University of Wisconsin – Madison. A more detailed description of behavioral paradigms, surgical implantation of EMG electrodes, and data collection procedures has been provided in earlier publications (Van Kan and McCurdy, 2001, 2002a). Brief reports of these results have appeared in abstract form (Geed et al., 2011, 2013).

Experimental Protocol

The two monkeys (*W*, *B*) performed reach-to-grasp tasks with their right forelimb while seated upright in a primate chair with their backs and feet supported. A neck collar and waist plate loosely restrained the animals while seated. The reaching forelimb and head were unrestrained. The animals were trained to reach and grasp a cereal reward (Kellogg's® *Froot Loops*® Cereal, thickness: ~6 mm; diameter: ~19 mm) using either a precision or whole-hand grasp from a target assembly located in the parasagittal plane through the shoulder of the animal's reaching limb, 56° above the horizontal plane through the shoulder. The cereal reward was dispensed in a horizontally oriented narrow slot (height: 6 mm, width: 25 mm, depth: 25 mm), which necessitated apposition of the index finger and thumb in a precision grasp, or a 50-ml glass beaker (clear, diameter: 32 mm, tilted at a 45° angle toward the animal), which required concerted use of all digits in a whole-hand grasp.

A typical reach-to-grasp trial began with the animal holding a handle at the waist for a variable inter-trial interval of 3-5 *s*, which minimized anticipatory muscle activity prior to movement onset. During the inter-trial interval, the animal received water reward for holding the handle steady at the waist. To initiate a reaching movement, a computer-controlled air cylinder dispensed the cereal reward into either the beaker or narrow slot, and a light-emitting diode (LED) next to the receptacle with the cereal reward lit up cueing the animal to initiate its reach-to-grasp movement as well as instructing whether to reach to the beaker (for whole-hand grasp) or slot (for precision grasp). Upon illumination of the LED, the monkey released the handle at the start location, reached toward the target assembly, retrieved the cereal reward from the beaker or slot as instructed, returned its hand to the mouth to eat the cereal reward, and finally, moved its hand back to the starting position to grasp the handle. The next trial was initiated following the variable inter-trial interval. The cereal reward was presented in the narrow slot or beaker in a pseudorandom fashion, controlled by custom software running in LabVIEW (National Instruments, LabVIEW 7.1).

Data Recording and Preprocessing

Behavioral event time data, intramuscular EMGs, and single-unit discharges from RNm and NI neurons were recorded in both monkeys. EMG recording sessions were carried out separately from the single-unit recording sessions although EMGs and neuronal data were recorded from the same two monkeys performing the same reach-to-grasp tasks.

Behavioral Event Markers

Behavioral event times were recorded with contact sensors on the handle at the starting location, on the slot, and on the beaker's rim at the target locations. Reach onset and offset were defined as the times of breaking contact with the handle and making contact with the slot or beaker, respectively. Grasp onset and offset were defined as the times of making and breaking contact with the slot or beaker, respectively. Behavioral event times were used to normalize the durations of transport and grasp intervals over trials and to align trials.

Intramuscular Electromyograms (EMGs)

The complete sets of muscles implanted in both monkeys, as well as the frequency of recording sessions in a given muscle is shown in **Table 1**. We recorded activity from 14 (monkey *W*) and 20 (monkey *B*) forelimb muscles in sets of 9 muscles/recording session on different days in close succession while the monkeys performed precision and whole-hand reach-to-grasp tasks. EMG signals were rectified, integrated (time constant: 10 ms), band-pass filtered (30 Hz – 3 kHz), and digitized at 167 Hz by A/D computer inputs (CED 1401 *plus*, Cambridge Electrical Design). Rectified, integrated, and band-pass filtered EMG signals were low-pass filtered using a fourth-order zero-lag Butterworth filter with a cut-off frequency of 15 Hz.

Neural Recordings

Discharges of forelimb RNm and NI neurons were recorded with epoxylite-coated tungsten microelectrodes (exposed tip of microelectrodes: 15–25 μm) as monkeys performed the precision or whole-hand reach-to-grasp tasks. We recorded from 33 and 34 forelimb RNm neurons in monkey *W* and monkey *B*, respectively; and from 30 and 48 forelimb NI neurons in monkey *W* and monkey *B*, respectively. Microelectrodes were inserted through the dura mater with a microdrive (Narishige MO-97), modified to include a stainless-steel guide tube assembly, which allowed the microelectrode tip to traverse the dura without being damaged. The microdrive was covered by a lightweight cylinder (diameter: 100 mm), which prevented the animal access to the microdrive. Single-unit discharges were monitored visually on an oscilloscope, filtered (half-amplitude band-pass at 100 Hz and 10 kHz ± 3dB), and fed into a window discriminator circuit that produced a standard pulse for each action potential.

TABLE 1 | Forelimb muscles recorded in each monkey.

	Muscle	Abbreviation	Recording frequency	
			Monkey *W*	Monkey *B*
Digits	Extensor digitorum communis	EDC	7/7	3/5
	Extensor digitorum two and three	ED23		3/5
	Extensor digitorum four and five	ED45	2/7*	1/5
	Flexor digitorum superficialis	FDS	6/7	1/5
	Flexor digitorum profundus	FDP	3/7	2/5
	Extensor pollicis longus	EPL		1/5
	Abductor pollicis longus	APL	7/7	2/5
	Palmaris longus	PL	3/7	3/5
Wrist	Extensor carpii radialis	ECR	6/7	3/5
	Extensor carpii ulnaris	ECU		3/5
	Flexor carpii radialis	FCR	6/7	3/5
	Flexor carpii ulnaris	FCU	2/7	4/5
Elbow	Brachioradialis	BR		2/5
	Biceps	BIC	2/7	2/5
	Triceps	TRI	4/7	2/5
Shoulder	Acromion deltoid	AcDLT	5/7	2/5
	Spino deltoid	SpDLT	4/7	2/5
	Cleido deltoid	CIDLT		2/5
	Pectoralis	PEC	4/7	2/5
	Teres major	TM		2/5
	Latissimus dorsii	LAT	2/7	

*EMGs were recorded in 12 sessions (1 session/day) over a 2–3-week period. Seven sessions were conducted in monkey W, 5 in monkey B. In a given session, EMGs of combinations of 9 muscles were recorded simultaneously. Numerical entries indicate recording frequency, i.e., (number of sessions in which EMGs of a given muscle were recorded) / (total number of sessions). *EMGs of ED45 in monkey W were not included in the analyses because of technical difficulties. EMGs, intramuscular electromyograms.*

Discriminated pulses were used as computer clock triggers to collect interspike intervals with 100 μs precision. **Figure 1B** shows representative spike trains recorded from an individual RNm neuron over 12 reach-to-grasp trials of the precision task in monkey *W*.

Data Preprocessing

Each neuron's discharge frequency was computed from the interspike interval record by averaging the neuron's discharge rate over consecutive 6-ms periods taking into account fractional interspike intervals. Task-related modulations in discharge rate during individual trials were quantified by calculating the average discharge rate over a 100-ms window that was moved, 6 ms at a time, between the times of reach onset and grasp offset. This created a record of the neuron's discharge frequency throughout the reach-to-grasp trial. **Figure 1A** shows records of discharge frequency computed from neural spikes recorded from a single RNm neuron recorded over 12 reach-to-grasp trials. Additional time intervals of 500 ms preceding reach onset, and 250 ms following grasp offset were also included to account for neural activity before reach onset and during the early part of the hand's return to the mouth.

Outlier Removal

Trials with outlier durations of the transport or grasp phase were removed using Rosner's Many Outliers Procedure (Rosner, 1983). A trial was removed if the duration of either the transport or grasp phase was determined to be an outlier. Most outlier trials had unusually long durations. The number of reach-to-grasp trials removed from EMGs ranged from 0/40 (0%) to 6/44 (13.6%) in monkey *B*, and from 1/87 (1.1%) to 6/84 (7.1%) in monkey *W*. The number of reach-to-grasp trials removed from RNm data ranged from 8/223 (3.6%) in monkey *B* to 21/187 (11.2%) in monkey *W*. The number of outlier trials removed in NI data ranged from 40/741 (5.4%) in monkey *B* to 21/209 (10%) in monkey *W*.

Trial Alignment

The transport and the grasp phase of each trial was time normalized to the mean duration of transport or grasp phase in a given monkey. Time-normalized trials were aligned on reach onset and averaged across trials. Thus, all precision reach-to-grasp data from different EMG recording sessions were averaged across trials to give a single dataset with time-normalized, trial-averaged values of the activation amplitudes of 14 muscles in monkey *W* (or 20 muscles in monkey *B*). Similarly, there was a single dataset with time-normalized, trial-averaged values of the 33 RNm neurons, and 30 NI neurons in monkey *W* (or 34 RNm neurons, and 48 NI neurons in monkey *B*). Each of the EMG, RNm, and NI datasets were standardized to have zero mean and unit standard deviation as required for subsequent factor analysis. **Figure 1C** shows the time-normalized, trial-averaged, standardized activity of a representative set of RNm neurons.

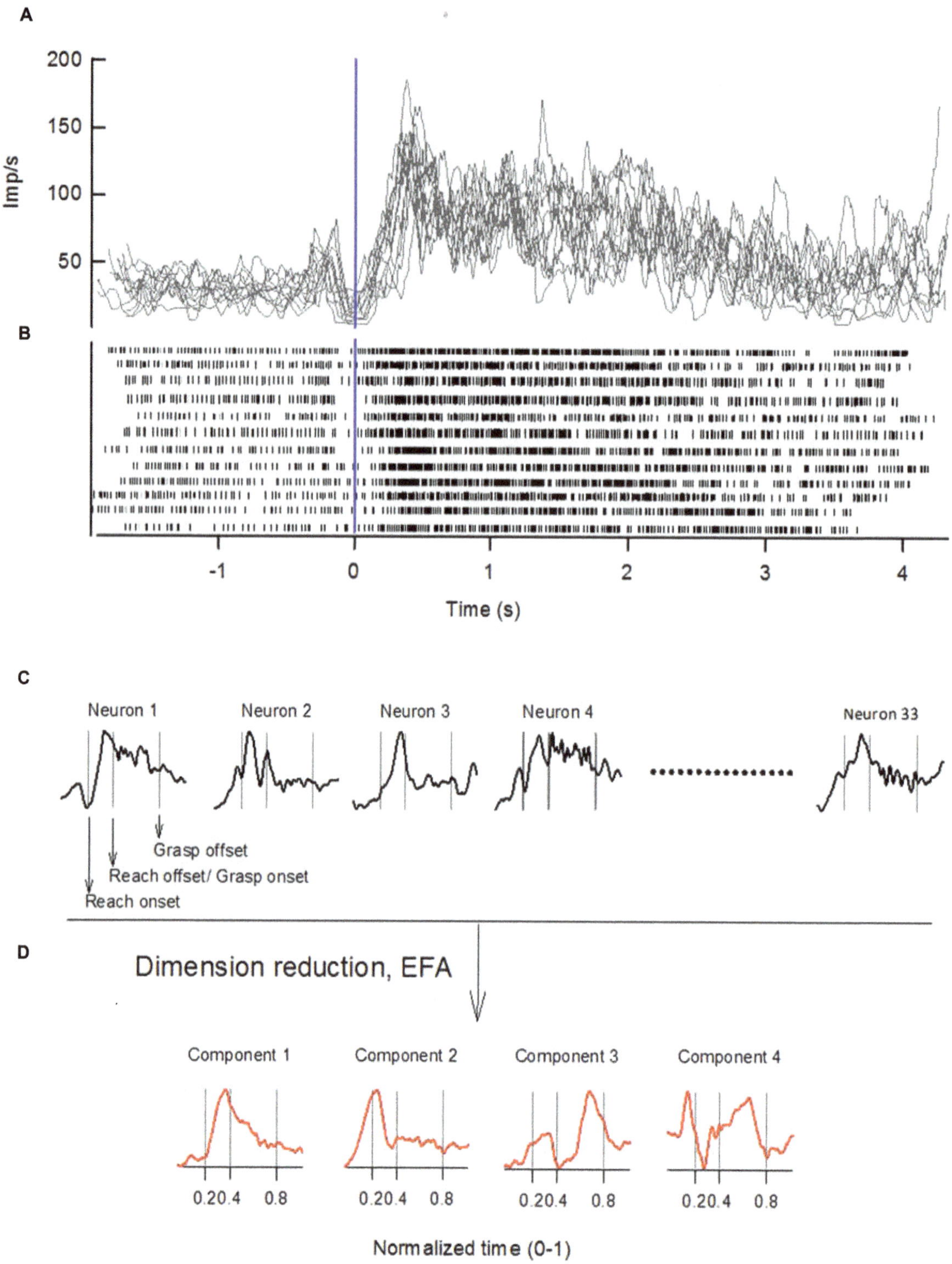

FIGURE 1 | Sequence of steps for extracting neuronal components by applying EFA to ensembles of single-unit discharges of NI and RNm neurons. **(A)** Records of discharge frequency of a single RNm neuron, computed from interspike intervals, are overplotted for 12 representative reach-to-grasp trials of the precision task in monkey *W*. Records are aligned on reach onset (Time 0, vertical line). **(B)** Spike-raster of neural discharge showing the same 12 reach-to-grasp trials as in **(A)**. **(C)** Records of discharge frequency of each neuron were time normalized, standardized, and trial-averaged to yield a dataset of the population of neurons with $n = 1, 2, \ldots$ n (here $n = 33$). EFA with *varimax* factor rotation was applied to the correlation matrix of this neuronal dataset to derive a low-dimensional representation of the data. **(D)** A limited number of neuronal components was retained following EFA. Behavioral event times are indicated by vertical lines in **(C,D)**: reach onset, reach offset/grasp onset, grasp offset respectively.

Data Analysis

Exploratory Factor Analysis on Muscle and Neuronal Data

Exploratory factor analysis with varimax factor rotation was applied to the correlation matrices of time-normalized, trial-averaged, standardized EMGs, RNm, and NI data separately to derive a low-dimensional representation of the data. The low-dimensional representation retained the variance of muscle or neuronal data while allowing for computationally simpler comparisons between groups of 14 or 20 muscles, and the combined output of 33 or 34 RNm neurons, and 30 or 48 NI neurons in monkey W and monkey B, respectively.

The goal of applying EFA is to represent "D" number of muscles (or neurons in case of neuronal components) as a linear combination of N components with N < D such that:

$$m(t) = \sum_{i=1}^{N} c_i(t) w_i$$

Here *m(t)* is a D-dimensional vector that specifies the activation of each muscle (or neuron) at time t. $c_i(t)$, referred to as the component's temporal scaling coefficient is a time-varying scaling coefficient for the *i*-th component. w_i (D × N matrix) represents the weighting coefficients of the i-th component, the relative strength of activation of the muscle (or neuron) in a given component. The weighting coefficients range between +1 and −1, with strong increased activation of a muscle (or neuron) in the component represented by a value close to +1 and strong decreased activation represented by a value close to −1. $c_i(t)$, which is a (N × t) matrix, represents the time-varying temporal scaling coefficient of the i-th component throughout the reach-to-grasp movement. **Figure 1D** shows the temporal scaling coefficients from a representative set of RNm neuronal components.

The number of muscle or neuronal components to retain following EFA was based on *(1)* Kaiser criteria (Kaiser, 1974), and *(2)* Scree plot of the extracted components and amounts of variance explained (Cattell, 1966). The combined criteria ensured that the components retained in the factor analysis contributed to meaningful interpretation of muscle and neuronal activity in the context of reaching to grasp, and captured a sizable amount of variance in the data whereas components that accounted for relatively small contributions to the variance of the collected sample were excluded. EFA was carried out using SPSS version 20 (SPSS IBM, New York).

Characterizing the Functional Contributions of Muscle Components

Detailed criteria for characterizing a muscle component as predominantly transport/preshape- or grasp-related have been described previously (Geed and Van Kan, 2016). Briefly, a muscle component was characterized as either transport/preshape- or grasp-related based on the combination of two criteria: *(1)* combinations of muscles showing weighting coefficient values greater than 0.4 ($w_i > 0.4$), and *(2)* timing of maximal contribution of the temporal scaling coefficient during the reach-to-grasp trial. Cross-referencing the temporal scaling coefficients with weighting coefficients is critical to determine the functional contribution of a given muscle component because the weighting coefficients reflect the relative ratios of activation of a combination of muscles in the component, and the temporal scaling coefficients reflect the activation profile of the combination of muscles in a component over time. Taken together, the weighting and temporal scaling coefficients indicate a component's functional contribution during reach-to-grasp movements. Based on these criteria, cross-referencing showed that muscle components 1 and 2 contributed predominantly during the transport/preshape phase in both monkeys. Muscle components 3 and 4 (4 only in monkey *W*) contributed predominantly during grasp in both monkeys.

Comparison of Neuronal and Muscle Components

The cross-correlation function was used to compare temporal scaling coefficients of muscle components with RNm and NI neuronal components. We hypothesized that if NI and RNm discharges represent neuronal correlates of coordinated reach-to-grasp muscle activity, we would find broad similarities between the temporal scaling coefficients of muscle, RNm, and NI components. Pair-wise cross-correlation magnitudes between each of the muscle-RNm, and muscle-NI component pairs were computed using Matlab® (MathWorks). The highest cross-correlation magnitude within a predefined −50 to +30 normalized time-bin window defined the best-matching muscle-neuronal component pair. The next highest cross-correlation defined the next best-matching muscle-neuronal component pair and so on, until there were no more unpaired components left in either the neuronal or muscle datasets.

Negative cross-correlation lags signify that a neuronal component occurs earlier than the muscle component on the normalized time scale, whereas positive lags signify that a neuronal component lags the muscle component on the normalized time scale. The loss of the absolute durations of individual trials was a drawback of time normalizing each trial for further analysis to compare the forelimb muscle activity and neuronal activities in low-dimensional space; however, we predefined a relative duration of −50 to +30 bins as the relevant time-window for meaningful neuronal-muscle signal interaction. This duration was chosen in accordance with Miller et al. (1993), who have reported that relatively analogous time lag windows (−150 to 200 ms) capture approximately 85% of the significant cross-correlation peaks between activity of single RNm neurons and EMGs recorded during free-form forelimb movements in monkeys. Before time normalization, each bin represented 6-ms worth of EMG or neuronal data, and so our predefined time window of −50 to +30 bins of normalized time captures the majority of the neuronal-muscle interactions of interest. We considered relatively short positive lags as meaningful too because small positive lags may signify parallel descending inputs to muscle components, to which NI-RNm components contribute only partially or at particular times during the entire duration of the reach-to-grasp movement.

Significance tests for cross-correlations are not well defined. Therefore, Monte Carlo simulations were used to determine the probability that the cross-correlation peak at a given time lag would occur by chance. The muscle component signal was randomly shuffled, and cross-correlations were computed between this randomly shuffled muscle component signal and the neuronal component signal. This process was repeated 10,000 times for each muscle-neuronal component pair to generate a distribution of peak cross-correlation values between the 10,000 randomly shuffled muscle components and the neuronal component. The 0.5th and 99.5th percentiles for this distribution served as the upper and lower bounds of significance for the cross-correlation (i.e., $p \leq 0.01$). If peak cross-correlations between muscle and neuronal components occurred due to chance, values would fall between the upper and lower bounds; however, statistically significant cross-correlation values would be outside the confidence interval allowing us to reject the null hypothesis that muscle and neuronal components were uncorrelated. Significance testing of the cross-correlations using Monte Carlo simulations was performed offline using custom programs in MATLAB® (MathWorks).

Temporal Coupling between Transport/Preshape- and Grasp-Related Neuronal Correlates

Transport/preshape- and grasp-related muscle components show invariant spatiotemporal coupling during reach-to-grasp movements irrespective of the type of grasp or the target location in the workspace (Geed and Van Kan, 2016). The time of peak activation of the transport/preshape-related muscle component occurs simultaneously with the time of peak slope of activation of the grasp-related muscle component. In the present study, we tested the hypothesis that NI and RNm components represent the neuronal correlates of the invariant spatiotemporal coupling between transport/preshape- and grasp-related muscle components. Slope (M) of the grasp-related component was computed using the following equation,

$$M = \frac{(y_2 - y_1)}{(x_2 - x_1)}$$

where (x_1, y_1), and (x_2, y_2) are points on the grasp-related component of interest. A paired-samples t-test was used to determine if the NI and RNm neuronal correlates of the transport/preshape- and grasp-related muscle components showed similar functional coupling as reported for muscle components.

RESULTS

Two monkeys performed reach-to-grasp tasks that required either a precision or whole-hand grasp to retrieve cereal reward. This report is based on single-unit discharges of task-related forelimb NI and magnocellular red nucleus (RNm) neurons (NI: $n = 30$ and $n = 48$, RNm: $n = 33$ and $n = 34$, in monkey *W* and monkey *B*, respectively), and intramuscular EMGs of forelimb muscles ($n = 14$ and $n = 20$ in monkey *W* and monkey *B*, respectively, **Table 1**). Data from the RNm neurons have been included in previous reports (Van Kan and McCurdy, 2001, 2002a,b). EMGs included in the present report are a subset of those included in Geed and Van Kan (2016). EMGs were recorded during reach-to-grasp movements to only one target location ("up") of the four locations included in the previous report.

For each task condition, EFA was used to determine whether a limited number of components is able to explain a large amount of variance in the ensemble discharges of the NI and RNm neurons of our sample. Scree plots (**Figure 2**, left ordinates, black) show the progressive decrease in eigenvalues of extracted factors as the number of factors selected increases. The first 7 factors (NI, **Figure 2A**) or 5 factors (RNm, **Figure 2B**) extracted had eigenvalues > 1, which fulfills the Kaiser criteria for retaining factors as components (see Materials and Methods). Plots of percent variance accounted for (% VAF) as a function of the number of factors (**Figure 2**, right ordinates, red) demonstrate that the first 7 components (NI, **Figure 2A**) or 5 components (RNm, **Figure 2B**) accounted for >85% of the variance in the ensemble discharges of NI and RNm neurons for both precision (solid lines) and whole-hand tasks (dotted lines). **Table 2** summarizes % VAF by NI and RNm neuronal components, and muscle components. Percent VAF by muscle components was taken from Geed and Van Kan (2016). Supplementary Table 1 shows cumulative variances accounted for by each of the neuronal and muscle components in the two monkeys during precision and whole-hand tasks. In summary, EFA revealed that 7-5 NI and RNm neuronal components accounted for >85% of the variance in ensemble discharges of the NI and RNm neurons of our sample, and 4–6 muscle components accounted for >85% of the variance in EMGs of the forelimb muscles we sampled.

Neuronal Correlates of Muscle Components

In a recent study, Geed and Van Kan (2016) reported that muscle components extracted using EFA were functionally aligned with transport/preshape- or grasp-related aspects of reach-to-grasp movements. In the following sections, we demonstrate similarities in characteristics of the NI, RNm, and muscle components we identified. Pairwise cross-correlations quantified similarities between temporal scaling coefficients $c_i(t)$ of the best-matching NI and RNm neuronal components and those of their corresponding transport/preshape- or grasp-related muscle components. Of note, each muscle component contributed throughout the reach-to-grasp movement; however, components were characterized as mainly transport/preshape- or grasp-related in order to simplify the expression of muscle activity of up to 21 forelimb muscles, and to evaluate relations between muscle components and neuronal components extracted from ensemble discharges of NI and RNm neurons.

Neuronal Correlates of Transport/Preshape-Related Muscle Components

Figure 3 shows correlations between the best-matching NI and RNm neuronal components and transport/preshape-related muscle component 1. Muscle component 1 increased activity at or prior to reach onset, attained peak amplitude during the transport/preshape phase prior to (**Figure 3B**, monkey *W*) or at the time the hand made contact with the target (**Figure 3F**, monkey *B*), and sharply decreased activity during the latter half of the transport/preshape phase (**Figure 3B**) or early in the grasp

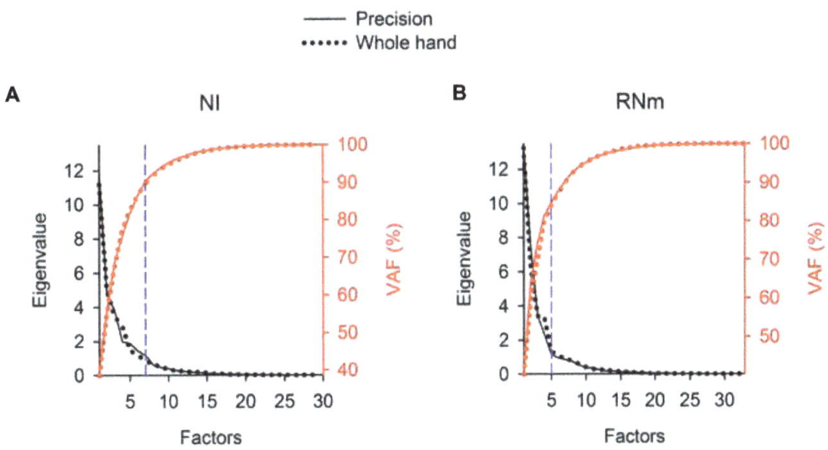

FIGURE 2 | Eigenvalues and percent variance accounted for (%VAF) of NI (A) and RNm (B) neuronal components in Monkey *W*. Scree plots (left ordinates, black) illustrate the progressive decrease in eigenvalues of extracted neuronal components as the number of components selected increases. The first 7 (in NI) or 5 (in RNm) components had eigenvalues > 1, which fulfills the Kaiser criteria for retaining factors as components. The "elbow" in the Scree plots (dashed, vertical blue lines) marks the cut off for retaining the first 7 (NI) or 5 (RNm) factors as neuronal components. Plots of %VAF (right ordinates, red) as a function of the number of factors demonstrate that the first 7 (or 5 in RNm) accounted for >85% of the variance in NI or RNm data. Solid lines show data for the precision task, dotted lines show data for the whole-hand task.

TABLE 2 | Variance accounted for by NI, RNm, and muscle components.

	Monkey *W*		Monkey *B*	
	Whole-hand	**Precision**	**Whole-hand**	**Precision**
NI	89.7 (7)	90.4 (7)	92.9 (6)	93.4 (7)
RNm	87.0 (6)	85.0 (5)	91.9 (6)	89.9 (5)
Muscle	90.1 (4)	86.9 (4)	93.0 (6)	91.8 (5)

Values represent percent variance accounted for (% VAF) by the number of components (n) in parentheses.

phase (**Figure 3F**). Component 1 was characterized by strong contributions from proximal muscles with coactivation of wrist and digit muscles (**Figure 3A**, monkey *W*; **Figure 3E**, monkey *B*).

The best-matching NI components (NI component 1 in monkey *W*; NI component 3 in monkey *B*) were strongly correlated with transport/preshape-related muscle component 1 in both animals (**Figure 3C**, $r = 0.62$, precision task in monkey *W*; **Figure 3G**, $r = 0.78$, whole-hand task in monkey *B*). The best-matching NI components explained 23.2 and 19.9% of the variance in the ensemble discharges of the 30 and 48 forelimb NI neurons in monkey *W* and monkey *B*, respectively. The best matching RNm components (component 2 in monkey *W*, precision task; and component 1 in monkey *B*, whole-hand task) were strongly correlated with transport/preshape-related muscle component 1 (**Figure 3D**, $r = 0.83$, precision task in monkey *W*; **Figure 3H**, $r = 0.83$, whole-hand task in monkey *B*). RNm component 2 explained 24.3% and component 1 explained 26.8% of the variance in the ensemble discharges of the 33 and 34 forelimb RNm neurons in monkey *W* and monkey *B*, respectively.

Figure 4 shows correlations between the best-matching NI and RNm neuronal components and transport/preshape-related muscle component 2. Muscle component 2 (**Figure 4B**, monkey *W*; **Figure 4G**, monkey *B*) attained peak activation amplitude during the transport/preshape phase and sharply decreased activity around grasp onset. A second, relatively smaller peak of activation was attained in the latter third of the grasp phase or early during the return phase when the hand moved back to the mouth to ingest the food reward. Muscle component 2 showed combined activity of shoulder, wrist, and digit muscles (**Figure 4A**, monkey *W*; **Figure 4F**, monkey *B*).

The best matching NI neuronal components (NI component 4 in monkey *W*; NI component 1 in monkey *B*) were strongly correlated with transport/preshape-related muscle component 2 (**Figure 4C**, $r = 0.73$, precision task in monkey *W*; **Figure 4H**, $r = 0.76$, whole-hand task in monkey *B*). The best-matching NI components explained 11.3%, and 29.2% of the variance in the ensemble discharges of the 30 and 48 forelimb NI neurons recorded in monkey *W* and monkey *B*, respectively. The best matching RNm components (RNm components 3 and 4 in monkey *W*; RNm component 5 in monkey *B*) were moderately correlated with transport/preshape-related muscle component 2 (**Figure 4D**, $r = 0.52$; **Figure 4E**, $r = 0.41$). The RNm neuronal components explained 12.4% and 8.7% of the variance in the ensemble discharges of the 33 RNm neurons in monkey *W*. RNm component 5 in monkey *B* was moderately correlated with transport/preshape-related muscle component 2 (**Figure 4I**, $r = 0.51$, whole-hand task) and explained 11.1% of the variance in the ensemble discharges of the 34 RNm neurons in monkey *B*.

In summary, a considerable amount of variance in the ensemble discharges within both the NI and RNm populations was directed toward transport/preshape-related aspects of reach-to-grasp movements in both animals during performance of both tasks. In addition, the transport/preshape-related NI and RNm neuronal components showed strong to moderate correlations with the transport/preshape-related muscle components.

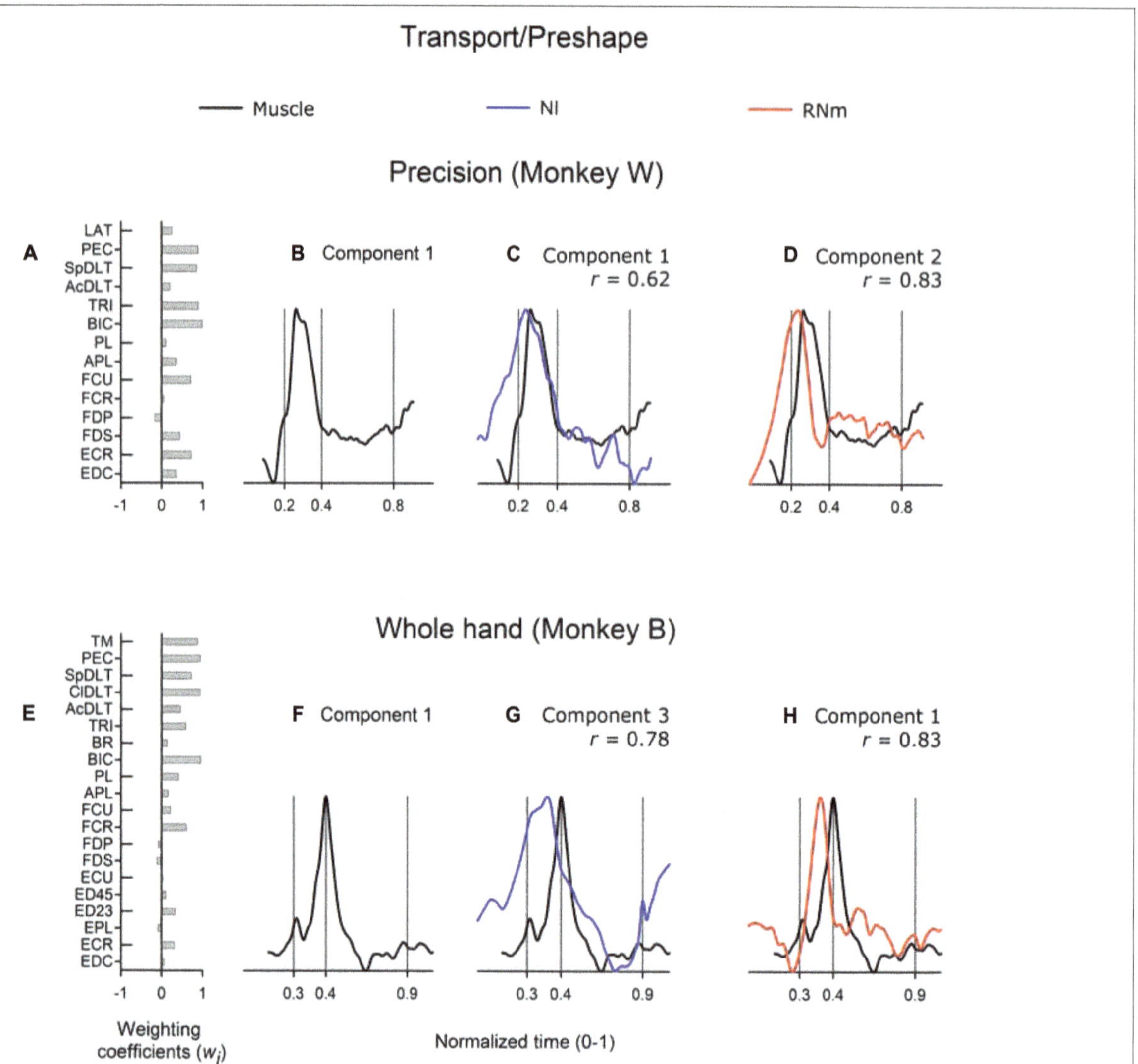

FIGURE 3 | Best-matching NI and RNm neuronal correlates of transport/preshape-related muscle component 1. (A,E) Weighting coefficients of transport/preshape-related muscle component 1 in precision **(A)** and whole-hand **(E)** task in monkey *W* and monkey *B*, respectively. **(B,F)** Temporal scaling coefficients of transport/preshape-related muscle component 1. Temporal scaling coefficients shown in **(B,F)** specify activation of all muscles included in the muscle component according to their corresponding weighting coefficients shown in **(A,E)**, respectively. **(C,G)** Temporal scaling coefficients of the NI components that best matched with transport/preshape-related muscle component 1 shown in **(B,F)**, respectively. **(D,H)** Temporal scaling coefficients of the RNm components that best matched with transport/preshape-related muscle component 1 shown in **(B,F)** respectively. Cross-correlation magnitude between NI or RNm and muscle components is indicated by *r*. Behavioral event times are indicated by vertical lines: reach onset, reach offset/grasp onset, grasp offset respectively. Ordinate scales are arbitrary but uniform throughout. Time scale is normalized (0–1) across neuronal and EMG reach-to-grasp data to allow neuronal-muscle comparisons.

Neuronal Correlates of Grasp-Related Muscle Components

Figure 5 shows correlations between the best-matching RNm and NI neuronal components and grasp-related muscle component 3. Grasp-related muscle component 3 attained peak amplitude early in the grasp phase, near the time the hand contacted the target, and remained active at a relatively high amplitude throughout the first two-thirds (**Figure 5B**, precision task in monkey *W*) or first half (**Figure 5F**, whole-hand task in monkey *B*) of the grasp phase. Grasp-related muscle component 3 included combinations of proximal and distal muscles: EDC, FDP, AcDLT, and SpDLT in monkey *W* (**Figure 5A**, precision task) and various wrist and digit flexor and extensor muscles in combination with BR in monkey *B* (**Figure 5E**, whole-hand task).

The best matching NI neuronal components (NI component 2 in both monkeys) were strongly correlated with grasp-related muscle component 3 in both monkeys (**Figure 5C**, $r = 0.79$, precision task in monkey *W*; **Figure 5G**, $r = 0.76$, whole-hand task in monkey *B*). The best matching NI neuronal components accounted for 19.6 and 20.3% of the variance in the ensemble discharges of the 30 and 48 NI neurons in monkey *W* and monkey *B*, respectively. The best matching RNm neuronal component in monkey *W* (RNm component 1) was strongly correlated with grasp-related muscle component

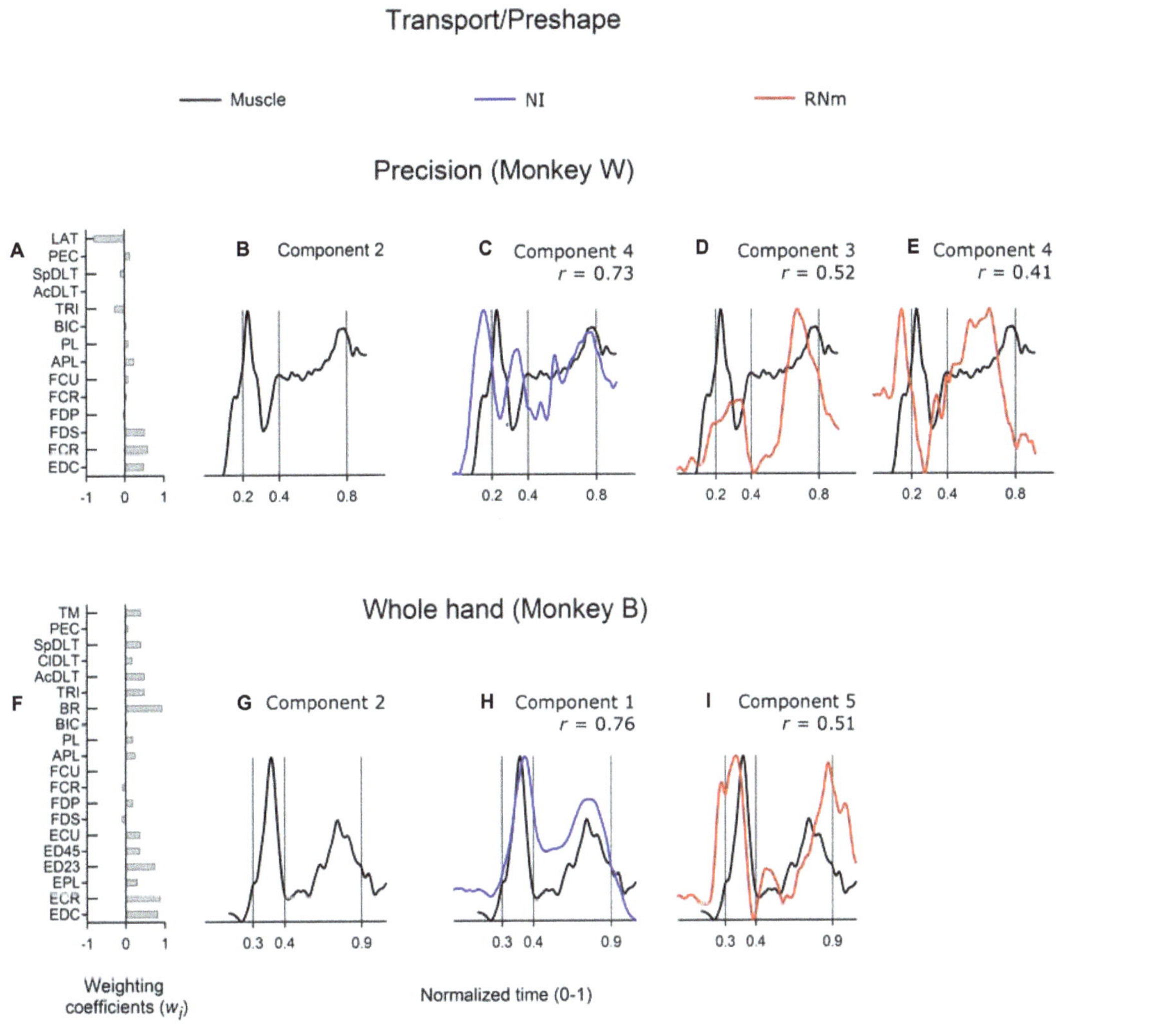

FIGURE 4 | Best-matching NI and RNm neuronal correlates of transport/preshape-related muscle component 2. (A,F) Weighting coefficients of transport/preshape-related muscle component 2 in precision **(A)** and whole-hand **(F)** task in monkey *W* and monkey *B*, respectively. **(B,G)** Temporal scaling coefficients of transport/preshape-related muscle component 2. Temporal scaling coefficients shown in **(B,G)** specify activation of all muscles included in the muscle component according to their corresponding weighting coefficients shown in **(A,F)**, respectively. **(C,H)** Temporal scaling coefficients of the NI components that best matched with transport/preshape-related muscle component 2 shown in **(B,G)**, respectively. **(D,E,I)** Temporal scaling coefficients of the RNm components that best matched with transport/preshape-related muscle component 2 shown in **(B,G)** respectively. Format as in **Figure 3**.

3 (**Figure 5D**, $r = 0.87$), whereas correlations were moderate in monkey *B* (**Figure 5H**, $r = 0.52$). The best matching RNm components accounted for 32.8 and 12.8% of the variance in the ensemble discharges of the 33 and 34 forelimb RNm neurons in monkey *W* and monkey *B*, respectively. Thus, grasp-related components of NI and RNm neuronal populations showed strong to moderate correlations with grasp-related muscle component 3 in both monkeys but explained relatively variable amounts of the variance in the ensemble discharges of RNm versus NI neurons.

Higher-Order Muscle Components

Figure 6 illustrates correlations between best matching neuronal components and higher-order muscle components. Grasp-related muscle component 4 was identified in both precision and whole-hand tasks in monkey W and included wrist and digit flexors (**Figure 6A**). The temporal scaling coefficient (**Figure 6B**) was characterized by a sharp and brief peak in the pre-movement phase when the monkey grasped the device handle prior to reach onset. A second, smaller peak occurred at grasp onset, and a third rapid increase in amplitude occurred during the return phase when the monkey, having grasped the cereal reward, started to move the hand toward the mouth in order to ingest the cereal reward. The best-matching NI component was moderately correlated (**Figure 6C**, $r = 0.46$) and accounted for 2.5% of the variance in ensemble discharges of the 30 forelimb NI neurons in monkey *W*. No best-matching RNm neuronal correlate of grasp-related muscle component 4 was identified.

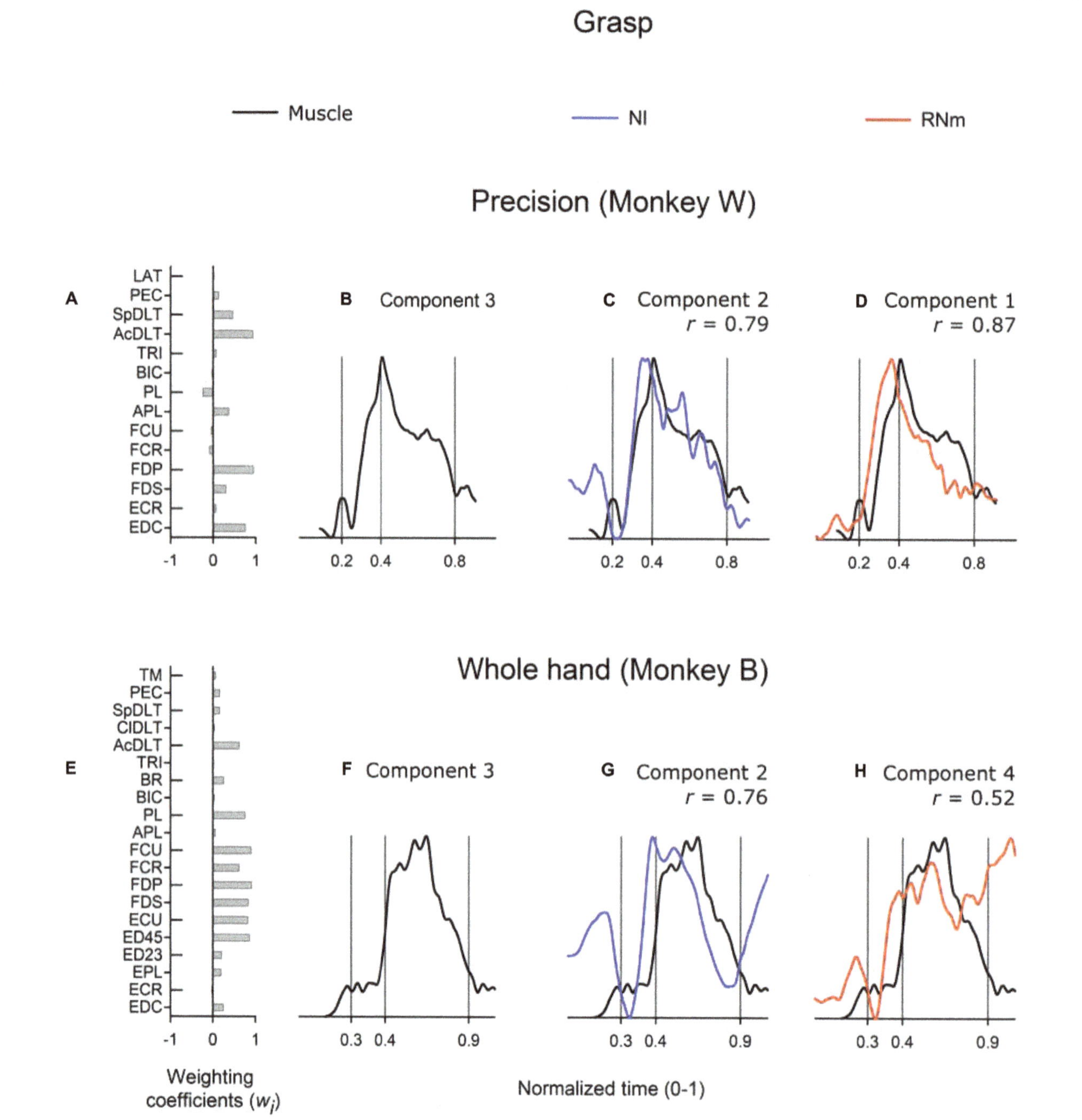

FIGURE 5 | Best-matching NI and RNm neuronal correlates of grasp-related muscle component 3. (A,E) Weighting coefficients of grasp-related muscle component 3 in precision **(A)** and whole-hand **(E)** task in monkey *W* and monkey *B* respectively. **(B,F)** Temporal scaling coefficients of grasp-related muscle component 3. Temporal scaling coefficients shown in **(B,F)** specify activation of all muscles included in the muscle component according to their corresponding weighting coefficients shown in **(A,E)**, respectively. **(C,G)** Temporal scaling coefficient of the NI components that best matched with grasp-related muscle component 3 shown in **(B,F)**, respectively. **(D, H)** Temporal scaling coefficient of the RNm components that best matched with grasp-related muscle component 3 shown in **(B,F)**, respectively. Format as in **Figure 3**.

Muscle components 4 and 5 in monkey *B* were not formally classified as transport/preshape- or grasp-related given our predefined criteria for selection of a factor as a muscle component (eigenvalue > 1, scree-plot criteria; Geed and Van Kan, 2016). Nevertheless, these components were compared with neuronal components extracted from the ensemble discharges of NI or RNm neurons because previous studies have reported that higher-order muscle components carry

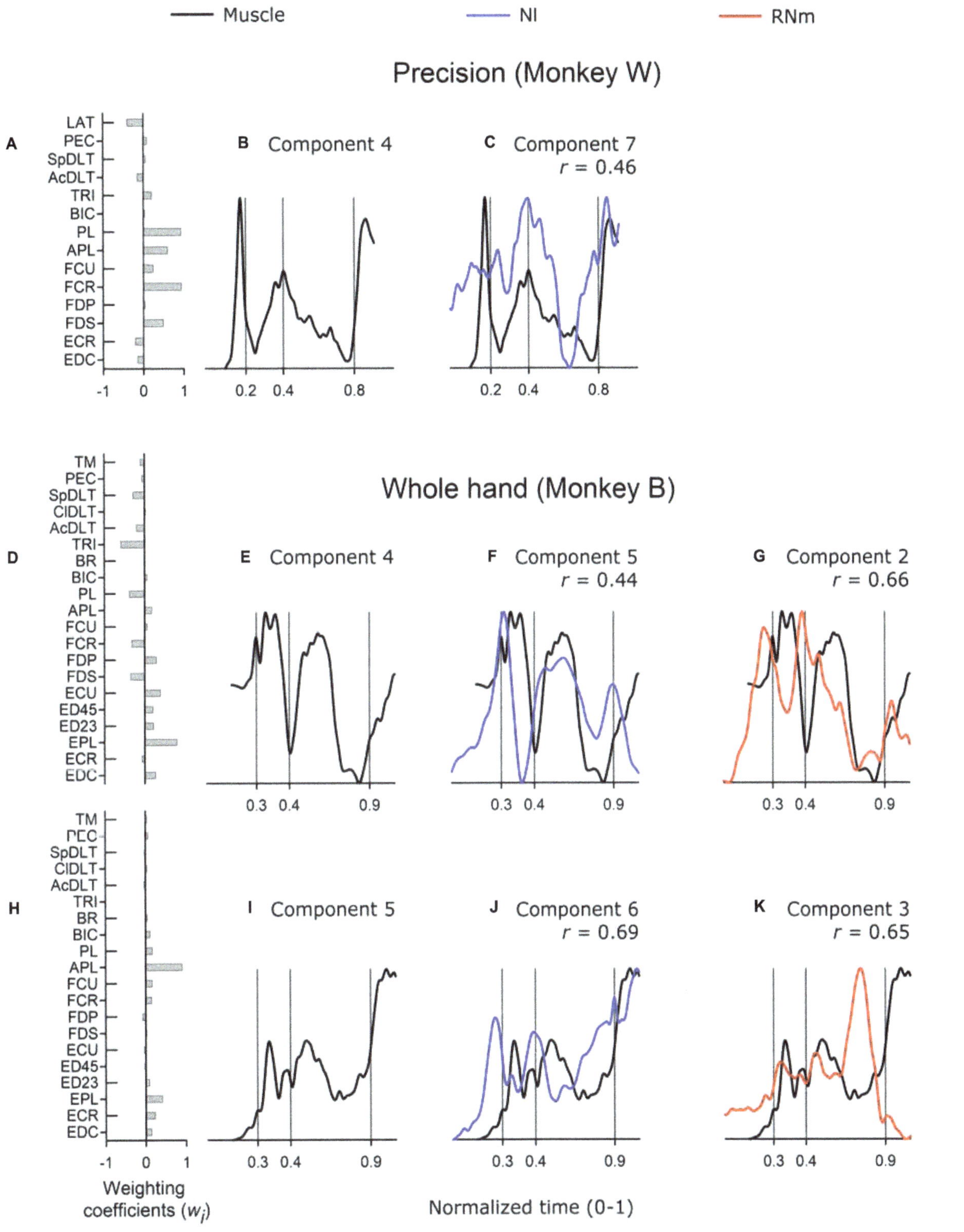

FIGURE 6 | Best-matching NI and RNm neuronal correlates of higher-order muscle components. (A) Weighting coefficients of grasp-related muscle component 4 in precision task in monkey *W*. **(B)** Temporal scaling coefficient of muscle component 4 specifies activation all muscles included in the muscle component according to their corresponding weighting coefficients shown in **(A)**. **(C)** Temporal scaling coefficient of the NI component that best matched with grasp-related muscle component 4 shown in **(A,B)**. **(D,E)** and **(H,I)** Show weighting coefficients and temporal scaling coefficients of muscle components in whole-hand task in monkey *B*. **(F,G)** and **(J,K)** Temporal scaling coefficient of best-matching NI and RNm neuronal components in the whole-hand task in monkey *B*. Format as in **Figure 3**.

meaningful control information (Brochier et al., 2004). Muscle component 4 and 5 were characterized by strong contribution of EPL (**Figure 6D**) or APL (**Figure 6H**) and small contributions from many other forelimb muscles. Muscle components 4 and 5 accounted for relatively small amounts of variance in EMGs (9.6 and 5.8% for components 4 and 5, respectively). The best-matching NI component to muscle component 4 (**Figure 6F**) was moderately correlated ($r = 0.44$) and accounted for 7.8% of the variance in the ensemble discharges of the 48 NI neurons in monkey *B*. The best matching RNm component to muscle component 4 (**Figure 6G**) was strongly correlated ($r = 0.66$) and accounted for 17.4% of the variance in the ensemble discharges of the 34 RNm neurons in monkey *B*. The best matching neuronal correlates to muscle component 5 showed strong correlations (NI, **Figure 6J**, $r = 0.69$; RNm, **Figure 6K**, $r = 0.65$), and accounted for 7.2 and 17.4% of the variance in the ensemble discharges of the 48 NI and 34 RNm neurons in monkey *B*, respectively. Thus, NI and RNm neuronal correlates were identified even for higher-ordered muscle components, which explained relatively small amounts of variance in EMGs.

In summary, a considerable amount of variance in the ensemble discharges within both the NI and RNm populations sampled is directed toward both transport/preshape-related and grasp-related aspects of reach-to-grasp movements in both animals during performance of both tasks. The results of cross-correlating NI and RNm neuronal components and muscle components support the view that the ensemble discharges of populations of NI and RNm neurons are part of the neural substrate underlying coordinated reach-to-grasp behaviors.

Temporal Coupling between Transport/Preshape- and Grasp-Related Neuronal and Muscle Components

Geed and Van Kan (2016) recently demonstrated that transport/preshape- and grasp-related muscle components are spatiotemporally coupled such that peak activation of the transport/preshape-related component is precisely synchronized in time with the peak slope of activation of its corresponding grasp-related component. **Figures 7A,B** (precision task) and **Figures 7G,H** (whole-hand task) illustrate the temporal synchrony between transport/preshape-related muscle component 1 (**Figures 7A,G**, black) and grasp-related muscle component 3 (**Figures 7B,H**) in monkey *B*. Records of the slope of activation amplitudes of grasp-related muscle components as a function of time were calculated (Methods) and are overplotted (**Figures 7A,G**, green) on activation amplitudes of the corresponding transport/preshape-related muscle component (**Figures 7A,G**, black). Analogous to the invariant temporal coupling between transport/preshape- and corresponding grasp-related muscle components, **Figures 7C,D** (precision task) and **Figures 7I,J** (whole-hand task) show similar spatiotemporal coupling between NI neuronal correlates of transport/preshape-related and corresponding grasp-related muscle components. **Figures 7E,F** (precision task) and **Figures 7K,L** (whole-hand task) show similar spatiotemporal coupling between RNm neuronal correlates of transport/preshape-related and corresponding grasp-related muscle components.

Table 3 summarizes the times of peak amplitude of transport/preshape-related components and the times of peak slope of activation of the corresponding grasp-related components in NI, RNm, and muscle domains for precision and whole-hand tasks in both monkeys. Consistent with our hypothesis, the neuronal correlates of transport/preshape- and grasp-related muscle components are temporally coupled such that times of peak activation of transport/preshape-related NI and RNm neuronal correlates are precisely synchronized with times of peak slope of activation of the corresponding grasp-related NI and RNm neural correlates. A paired-samples t-test showed no significant difference [$t(11) = -0.64, p = 0.54$] between the times of peak activation of the transport/preshape-related components and the times of peak slope of activation of the corresponding grasp-related components in NI, RNm, and muscle domains.

In summary, the results presented in this section provide evidence for invariant spatiotemporal coupling between NI and RNm neuronal correlates of transport/preshape- and grasp-related muscle components that is qualitatively and quantitatively similar to the invariant spatiotemporal coupling observed between corresponding muscle components.

DISCUSSION

Our results demonstrate that neuronal components, extracted from the ensemble of single-unit discharges of populations of NI and RNm neurons recorded while monkeys performed reach-to-grasp tasks, are strongly, consistently, and systematically correlated with transport/preshape- and grasp-related muscle components. Importantly, as was found for transport/preshape- and grasp-related muscle components (Geed and Van Kan, 2016), both NI and RNm neuronal correlates show invariant spatiotemporal coupling, suggesting that during reach-to-grasp movements, ensembles of neurons within NI and RNm distribute their variances along the functional dimensions of transport/preshape or grasp such that the timing of activation of transport/preshape is invariantly coupled with the timing of activation of grasp. These results add mechanistic insight to data from clinical and lesion studies that have reported decoupling between reach and grasp following cerebellar lesions. Overall, the results provide strong support for the hypothesis that interposito-rubrospinal (NI-RNm) circuitry underlies spatiotemporal coordination of complex reach-to-grasp behaviors.

Similar Units of Behavior Are Expressed in Neural and Muscle Signals

Our result of finding similar functional units of behavior at three successive levels (NI, RNm, and EMGs) of information

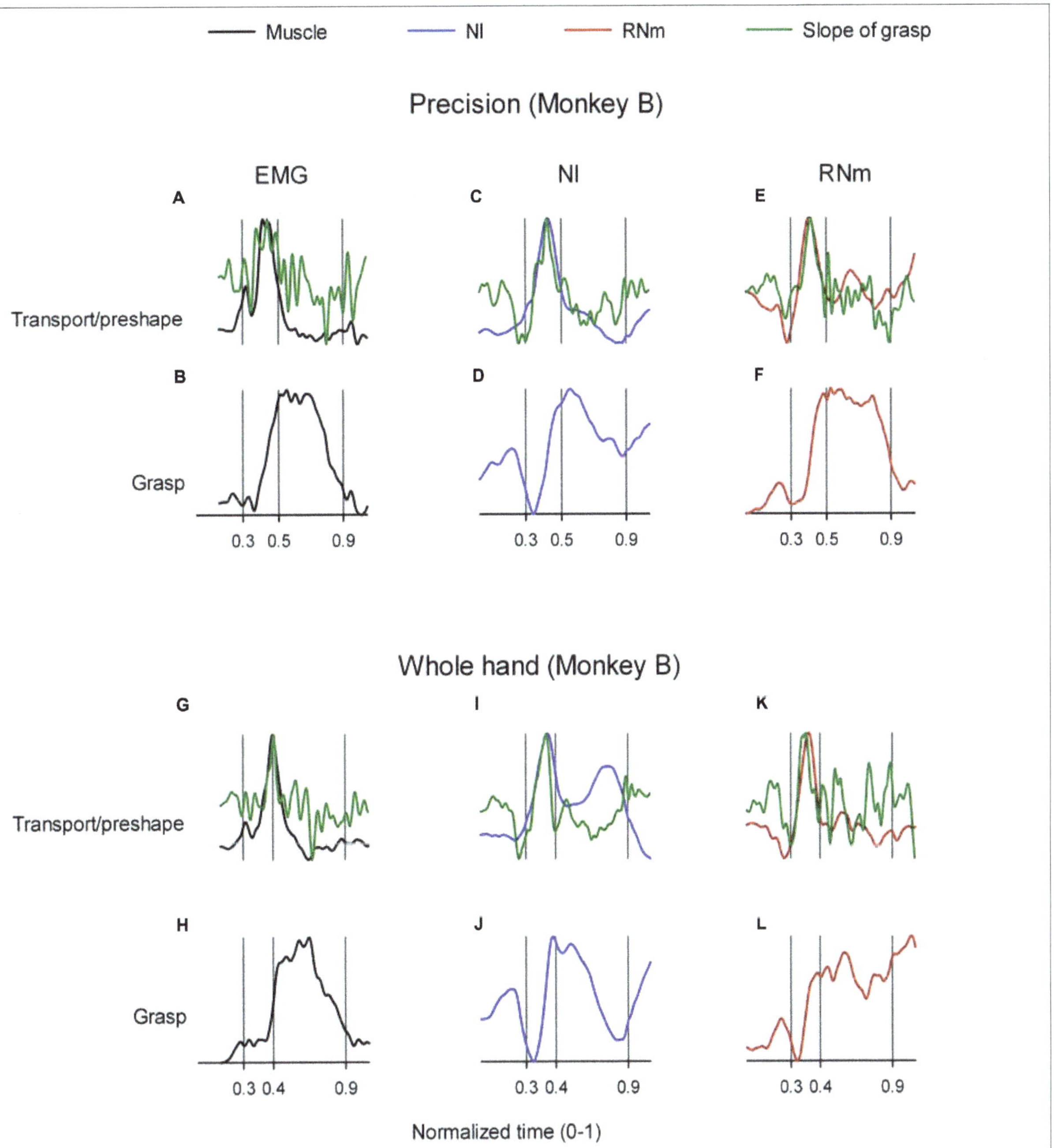

FIGURE 7 | Temporal coupling between transport/preshape- and grasp-related muscle and neuronal components. **(A,C,E)** and **(G,I,K)** show temporal scaling coefficients of transport/preshape-related muscle (black), NI (blue), and RNm (red) components in monkey *B* during precision **(A,C,E)** and whole-hand **(G,I,K)** tasks. **(B,D,F)** and **(H,J,L)** show temporal scaling coefficients of the grasp-related components that correspond to the transport/preshape-related components shown in **(A,C,E)** and **(G,I K)** respectively. Slope of grasp-related components (green) is overplotted on the temporal scaling coefficient of the corresponding transport/preshape-related components to highlight synchronicity between peak activation of transport/preshape-related components and peak slope of corresponding grasp-related components. For example, **(C,D)** illustrate temporal coupling between transport/preshape- and grasp-related NI neuronal components in monkey *B* during performance of the precision task. Temporal scaling coefficients of the transport/preshape- and the corresponding grasp-related component are plotted (blue) in **(C,D)**, respectively. The slope of the grasp-related component was calculated (see Materials and Methods) and is overplotted (green) on the temporal scaling coefficients of the preshape/transport-related component in *C*.

processing in the NI-RNm circuitry supports the view that intermediate cerebellar output engages synergistic groups of neurons and muscles to coordinate reach-to-grasp movements. The neuronal components we identified provide a weighting of each neuron's contribution to the ensemble average based on the neuron's correlation pattern with all other neurons in the dataset. Each neuron contributes portions of its variance to each of the neuronal components in a neuron-specific, weighted fashion,

TABLE 3 | Temporal coupling between transport/preshape- and grasp-related NI, RNm, and muscle components.

	Whole-hand		Precision	
	$T_{transport}$	T_{grasp}	$T_{transport}$	T_{grasp}
Monkey *W*				
NI	0.29	0.28	0.31	0.32
RNm	0.31	0.32	0.25	0.27
Muscle	0.29	0.28	0.28	0.29
Monkey *B*				
NI	0.39	0.39	0.40	0.40
RNm	0.38	0.35	0.38	0.39
Muscle	0.44	0.44	0.39	0.42

Values represent normalized time (0–1). $T_{transport}$, time of peak activation of transport/preshape-related component. T_{grasp}, time of peak slope of activation of corresponding grasp-related component.

and linear combinations of these neural weights, scaled by the neuronal component's temporal scaling coefficients, account for a large proportion of the variance in the ensemble discharges of the neuronal population. Neuronal components thus distill motor control information distributed across a population of neurons into limited numbers of discrete motor command signals.

The EFA-based neuronal components we identified are comparable with previous reports on information processing in M1 and RNm. For instance, Miller et al. (1993) proposed that groups of mutually correlated RNm neurons may contribute control signals in muscle space that are summed in the spinal cord, in line with the neuronal component framework where linear combinations of a few neuronal components may specify the activation parameters of synergistic groups of muscles. M1 and RNm neurons have been shown to process information in muscle-based "functional linkage vectors (FLVs)" (Miller et al., 1993; Holdefer and Miller, 2002). Krouchev and Drew (2013) demonstrated that a limited number of sparse muscle synergies explained substantial proportions of the variance in cat forelimb EMGs, and they proposed, based on their previously recorded data in cat motor cortex during the same behaviors (Drew, 1993; Drew et al., 1996, 2008), that multiple populations of pyramidal tract neurons (PTNs) may be involved in regulating each of the specific sparse muscle synergies.

Neuronal components, FLVs, and sparse synergies share the conceptual premise that populations of neurons contribute to activity of functionally-related muscle groups; however, the different algorithms underlying cluster and factor analyses result in small differences. FLVs involve correlated activity between individual neurons and groups of muscles, which are then clustered to identify the sub-populations of neurons that share relatively similar correlation patterns with groups of muscles. In contrast, EFA-based neuronal components provide a weighting of each neuron's contribution to the population average according to its pattern of correlation with all other neurons in the sample. Our approach of identifying a neural basis of muscle components thus adopts a relatively direct population-based view of interrelationships within the neuronal ensemble in order to identify how groups of neurons may specify activation parameters to control groups of muscles as synergistic units. Further, clustering of FLVs leads to a model in which each neuron contributes exclusively to a given muscle "synergy" because clustering algorithms group variables (neurons) so that the variance within a cluster is minimized while the variance between clusters is maximized. In our EFA-based approach, each neuron contributes portions of its variance toward each of the components in the model in a weighted fashion. The same set of neurons may thus apportion their variances differently across each of the components to give rise to a flexible and diverse range of motor behaviors. This mechanism is consistent with recent findings from ICMS-evoked cortical "synergies" where each unit (neuron) appeared to also encode synergies other than the "most evoked synergy" (Overduin et al., 2014, 2015).

Our finding of limited numbers of neuronal components underlying the ensemble activity of forelimb NI and RNm neurons is significant because it demonstrates for the first time that NI-RNm circuitry may specify motor commands in the same low-dimensional space as found for muscle components underlying naturally-occurring reach-to-grasp behaviors in monkeys. In particular, finding neuronal correlates of higher-order muscle components (shown in **Figure 6**) indicates that similar functional units of reach-to-grasp behaviors are isolated from ensemble discharges of neurons and EMGs even if the muscle components account for relatively small amounts of variance in the EMGs. Thus, higher-order components of reach-to-grasp muscle activity may transmit meaningful information with respect to behavior, which is consistent with the findings of Brochier et al. (2004) that higher-order muscle components were able to discriminate between grasp types in their reach-to-grasp task. Evidence consistent with our findings has also come from transcranial magnetic stimulation (TMS) (Gentner and Classen, 2006) and intracortical microstimulation (ICMS) (Overduin et al., 2012, 2014, 2015) of various motor cortical sites in human and non-human primates, respectively. TMS- or ICMS-evoked digit movements demonstrate similar muscle synergies as identified during naturally-occurring digit movements, such as grasping either imagined (Gentner and Classen, 2006) or differently shaped objects (Overduin et al., 2012). Whereas the TMS- or ICMS-based studies support the hypothesis of building blocks underlying voluntary motor control in the motor cortex, our framework of neuronal components in NI-RNm circuitry supports and expands previous findings by proposing a mechanism and additional substrates by which neuromotor circuitry may organize functional building blocks of behavior.

Cerebello-Rubrospinal Circuitry and Spatiotemporal Coupling of Reach and Grasp

Transport/preshape- and grasp-related muscle components show invariant temporal coupling with each other such that the time at which the temporal scaling coefficient of a given transport/preshape-related muscle component attains peak activity during transport coincides exactly with the time of peak slope of activation of the corresponding grasp-related muscle component (Geed and Van Kan, 2016). This relationship was preserved in monkeys preforming reach-to-grasp movements irrespective of the type of grasp or target location in the workspace, indicating that the temporal coupling may reflect a central mechanism to coordinate transport/preshape-related muscle activity with grasp-related muscle activity. The findings in the present study support and extend this hypothesis. NI and RNm neuronal correlates of transport/preshape- and grasp-related muscle components were temporally coupled such that the times of peak activation of transport/preshape-related neuronal correlates coincided with the times of peak slope of activation of corresponding grasp-related neuronal correlates. The invariant spatiotemporal coupling was not a function of the orthogonal relationship between components as a result of the varimax rotation in our factor analysis algorithm because non-orthogonal rotation of extracted factors (promax rotation) yielded similar temporal scaling coefficients and coupling, suggesting that the spatiotemporal coupling did not depend on specific rotation of extracted factors.

Muscle components reflect synchronous activation of functionally-related groups of muscles as synergistic units. Muscles included in a given component are activated in precise ratios with respect to each other as defined by the component weighting coefficients w_i. The temporal scaling coefficients specify the activation amplitude of a muscle component throughout the movement. Thus, a muscle component gives rise to precise spatiotemporal coupling between muscles included in the component. Temporal coupling between muscle components thus enforces a higher-level of structure on how combinations of muscles included in the respective components are activated. Temporal coupling between activation waveform of transport, and slope of activation waveform of grasp, implies that neuromotor circuitry activates transport/preshape-related muscle components in direct relation to corresponding grasp-related muscle components.

Significantly, strong to moderate correlation between neuronal and muscle components suggests that populations of NI and RNm neurons process information about synergistic groups of forelimb muscles. This view is supported by findings that mossy fiber *inputs* to intermediate cerebellum show high joint specificity (Van Kan et al., 1993a,b) whereas even at the hierarchical level of single NI neurons, which represents the sole *output* of intermediate cerebellum, information processing pertains to combinations of multiple forelimb joints (Van Kan et al., 1993b). The transformation of highly joint-specific cerebellar afferent input through mossy fibers into broad whole-limb based neuromotor information in cerebellar output through NI is consistent with our results that the ensemble output from NI reflects control signals for coordinating groups of transport/preshape- and grasp-related muscles synergistically.

Further, NI projects to two extra-cerebellar targets: indirectly, via ventrolateral (VL) thalamus, to primary motor cortex (Rispal-Padel and Latreille, 1974; Jorntell and Ekerot, 1999) and directly to contralateral RNm neurons (Flumerfelt et al., 1973; Asanuma et al., 1983a,b). RNm neurons give rise to descending projections which, via the rubrospinal tract (Shinoda et al., 1977; Shinoda et al., 1982; Holstege et al., 1988; Shinoda et al., 1988; Pong et al., 2002), target interneurons and motoneurons of forelimb muscles (McCurdy et al., 1987; Holstege et al., 1988; Ralston et al., 1988). Converging evidence from behavioral neurophysiology in NI and RNm (Van Kan et al., 1994; Gibson et al., 1996; Van Kan and McCurdy, 2001, 2002a,b), lesion studies in NI (Mason et al., 1998; Cooper et al., 2000; Martin et al., 2000; Johnson et al., 2001), and clinical data from patients with cerebellar lesions (Bastian and Thach, 1995; Bastian, 1997, 2002; Bastian et al., 2000; Zackowski et al., 2002; Morton and Bastian, 2004, 2007) support the view that NI-RNm circuitry plays an important role in the coordination of proximal and distal forelimb muscles during whole-limb multi-joint movements. Thus, physiologically, NI-RNm circuitry is well placed to specify coordination between synergistic groups of proximal and distal forelimb muscles, consistent with the invariant spatiotemporal coupling identified between the functional domains of transport/preshape and grasp.

CONCLUSION

The results provide evidence for the hypothesis that ensemble discharges of forelimb neurons in NI and RNm function as neuronal correlates of synergistic, functionally-related groups of proximal and distal forelimb muscles in monkeys performing natural reach-to-grasp movements. The NI and RNm neuronal correlates of transport/preshape- and grasp-related muscle components show precise and invariant spatiotemporal coupling, which is essential for coordinated activation of forelimb muscles during reach to-grasp behaviors.

AUTHOR CONTRIBUTIONS

SG, MM, and PvK contributed to design, acquisition, analysis, and interpretation of data for this work. SG wrote the draft for the manuscript and prepared all figures. SG, MM, and PvK revised and edited the manuscript. SG, MM, and PvK approved the final draft of the manuscript, and agree to be accountable for all aspects of the work.

FUNDING

Research reported in this publication was supported by National Institutes of Neurological Disorders and Stroke Grant NS43317 (PI: PvK), by the Graduate School of the University of Wisconsin-Madison (PvK and SG), by National institutes of Neurological Disorders and Stroke Grant 1U10NS086513-01 (NIH StrokeNet awarded to SG; PI: Alexander W. Dromerick, and Amie Hsia, MedStar National Rehabilitation Hospital), by the National Institute on Disability, Independent Living, and Rehabilitation Research (NIDILRR) Advanced Rehabilitation Research Training

(ARRT) Grant H133P100015 (awarded to SG, PI: Barbara S. Bregman, MedStar National Rehabilitation Hospital and Georgetown University), and the National Center For Advancing Translational Sciences of the National Institutes of Health under Award Number TL1TR001431 (NIH-TL1, awarded to SG). The content is solely the responsibility of the authors and does not necessarily represent the official views of the National Institutes of Health.

ACKNOWLEDGMENTS

We thank Robert P. Scobey for design and construction of experimental equipment and Janet L. Ruhland for assistance in data collection. We thank Barbara S. Bregman, Michelle L. Harris-Love, Peter S. Lum, Sahana Kukke, and Susan Ryerson for valuable discussions and feedback on the manuscript. This research was conducted in the Motor Systems Physiology Laboratory at the University of Wisconsin-Madison in partial fulfillment of SG Ph.D. degree.

REFERENCES

Asanuma, C., Thach, W. T., and Jones, E. G. (1983a). Brainstem and spinal projections of the deep cerebellar nuclei in the monkey, with observations on the brainstem projections of the dorsal column nuclei. *Brain Res. Rev.* 5, 299–322. doi: 10.1016/0165-0173(83)90017-6

Asanuma, C., Thach, W. T., and Jones, E. G. (1983b). Distribution of cerebellar terminations and their relation to other afferent terminations in the ventral lateral thalamic region of the monkey. *Brain Res.* 286, 237–265. doi: 10.1016/0165-0173(83)90015-2

Baker, S. N. (2011). The primate reticulospinal tract, hand function and functional recovery. *J. Physiol.* 589, 5603–5612. doi: 10.1113/jphysiol.2011.215160

Bastian, A. J. (1997). Mechanisms of ataxia. *Phys. Ther.* 77, 672–675.

Bastian, A. J. (2002). Cerebellar limb ataxia: abnormal control of self-generated and external forces. *Ann. N. Y. Acad. Sci.* 978, 16–27. doi: 10.1111/j.1749-6632.2002.tb07552.x

Bastian, A. J., Martin, T. A., Keating, J. G., and Thach, W. T. (1996). Cerebellar ataxia: abnormal control of interaction torques across multiple joints. *J. Neurophysiol.* 76, 492–509.

Bastian, A. J., and Thach, W. T. (1995). Cerebellar outflow lesions: a comparison of movement deficits resulting from lesions at the levels of the cerebellum and thalamus. *Ann. Neurol.* 38, 881–892. doi: 10.1002/ana.410380608

Bastian, A. J., Zackowski, K. M., and Thach, W. T. (2000). Cerebellar ataxia: torque deficiency or torque mismatch between joints? *J. Neurophysiol.* 83, 3019–3030.

Belhaj-Saif, A., and Cheney, P. D. (2000). Plasticity in the distribution of the red nucleus output to forearm muscles after unilateral lesions of the pyramidal tract. *J. Neurophysiol.* 83, 3147–3153.

Bradnam, L. V., Stinear, C. M., and Byblow, W. D. (2013). Ipsilateral motor pathways after stroke: implications for non-invasive brain stimulation. *Front. Hum. Neurosci.* 7:184. doi: 10.3389/fnhum.2013.00184

Brochier, T., Spinks, R. L., Umilta, M. A., and Lemon, R. N. (2004). Patterns of muscle activity underlying object-specific grasp by the macaque monkey. *J. Neurophysiol.* 92, 1770–1782. doi: 10.1152/jn.00976.2003

Carmel, J. B., Kimura, H., Berrol, L. J., and Martin, J. H. (2013). Motor cortex electrical stimulation promotes axon outgrowth to brain stem and spinal targets that control the forelimb impaired by unilateral corticospinal injury. *Eur. J. Neurosci.* 37, 1090–1102. doi: 10.1111/ejn.12119

Cattell, R. B. (1966). The scree test for the number of factors. *Multivariate Behav. Res.* 1, 245–276. doi: 10.1207/s15327906mbr0102_10

Cooper, S. E., Martin, J. H., and Ghez, C. (2000). Effects of inactivation of the anterior interpositus nucleus on the kinematic and dynamic control of multijoint movement. *J. Neurophysiol.* 84, 1988–2000.

Cunningham, D. A., Potter-Baker, K. A., Knutson, J. S., Sankarasubramanian, V., Machado, A. G., and Plow, E. B. (2015). Tailoring brain stimulation to the nature of rehabilitative therapies in stroke: a conceptual framework based on their unique mechanisms of recovery. *Phys. Med. Rehabil. Clin. N. Am.* 26, 759–774. doi: 10.1016/j.pmr.2015.07.001

Drew, T. (1993). Motor cortical activity during voluntary gait modifications in the cat. I. Cells related to the forelimbs. *J. Neurophysiol.* 70, 179–199.

Drew, T., Jiang, W., Kably, B., and Lavoie, S. (1996). Role of the motor cortex in the control of visually triggered gait modifications. *Can. J. Physiol. Pharmacol.* 74, 426–442. doi: 10.1139/cjpp-74-4-426

Drew, T., Kalaska, J., and Krouchev, N. (2008). Muscle synergies during locomotion in the cat: a model for motor cortex control. *J. Physiol.* 586, 1239–1245. doi: 10.1113/jphysiol.2007.146605

Flumerfelt, B. A., Otabe, S., and Courville, J. (1973). Distinct projections to the red nucleus from the dentate and interposed nuclei in the monkey. *Brain Res.* 50, 408–414. doi: 10.1016/0006-8993(73)90742-7

Geed, S., Mccurdy, M. L., and Van Kan, P. L. E. (2011). Primate magnocellular red nucleus (RNm) encodes muscle synergies during reaching to grasp. *Soc. Neurosci. Abstr.* 37.

Geed, S., Mccurdy, M. L., and Van Kan, P. L. E. (2013). Contribution of interposito-rubrospinal pathway to muscle synergies underlying reaching to grasp. *Soc. Neurosci. Abstr.* 39.

Geed, S., and Van Kan, P. L. E. (2016). Grasp-Based Functional Coupling Between Reach- and Grasp-Related Components of Forelimb Muscle Activity. *J. Mot. Behav.* 48, 1–17. doi: 10.1080/00222895.2016.1204265

Gentner, R., and Classen, J. (2006). Modular organization of finger movements by the human central nervous system. *Neuron* 52, 731–742. doi: 10.1016/j.neuron.2006.09.038

Gibson, A. R., Horn, K. M., Stein, J. F., and Van Kan, P. L. E. (1996). Activity of interpositus neurons during a visually guided reach. *Can. J. Physiol. Pharmacol.* 74, 499–512. doi: 10.1139/y96-039

Gibson, A. R., Horn, K. M., and Van Kan, P. L. E. (1994). "Chapter 5 Grasping Cerebellar Function," in *Advances in Psychology*, eds M. B. B. Keree and C. Umberto (Cambridge, MA: Academic Press), 85–108.

Holdefer, R. N., and Miller, L. E. (2002). Primary motor cortical neurons encode functional muscle synergies. *Exp. Brain Res.* 146, 233–243. doi: 10.1007/s00221-002-1166-x

Holstege, G., Blok, B. F., and Ralston, D. D. (1988). Anatomical evidence for red nucleus projections to motoneuronal cell groups in the spinal cord of the monkey. *Neurosci. Lett.* 95, 97–101. doi: 10.1016/0304-3940(88)90639-8

Houk, J. C., Gibson, A. R., Harvey, C. F., Kennedy, P. R., and Van Kan, P. L. E. (1988). Activity of primate magnocellular red nucleus related to hand and finger movements. *Behav. Brain Res.* 28, 201–206. doi: 10.1016/0166-4328(88)90097-6

Humphrey, D. R., and Rietz, R. R. (1976). Cells of origin of corticorubral projections from the arm area of primate motor cortex and their synaptic actions in the red nucleus. *Brain Res.* 110, 162–169. doi: 10.1016/0006-8993(76)90217-1

Jeannerod, M. (1981). "Intersegmental coordination during reaching at natural visual objects," in *Attention and Performance IX*, eds J. Long and A. Baddeley (Hillsdale, NJ: Erlbaum), 153–169.

Jeannerod, M. (1984). The timing of natural prehension movements. *J. Mot. Behav.* 16, 235–254. doi: 10.1080/00222895.1984.10735319

Johnson, M. T. V., Mason, C. R., and Ebner, T. J. (2001). Central processes for the multiparametric control of arm movements in primates. *Curr. Opin. Neurobiol.* 11, 684–688. doi: 10.1016/S0959-4388(01)00269-0

Jorntell, H., and Ekerot, C. F. (1999). Topographical organization of projections to cat motor cortex from nucleus interpositus anterior and forelimb skin. *J. Physiol.* 514(Pt 2), 551–566. doi: 10.1111/j.1469-7793.1999.551ae.x

Kaiser, H. (1974). An index of factorial simplicity. *Psychometrika* 39, 31–36. doi: 10.1007/BF02291575

Kennedy, P. R., Gibson, A. R., and Houk, J. C. (1986). Functional and anatomic differentiation between parvicellular and magnocellular regions of red nucleus in the monkey. *Brain Res.* 364, 124–136. doi: 10.1016/0006-8993(86)90993-5

Krouchev, N., and Drew, T. (2013). Motor cortical regulation of sparse synergies provides a framework for the flexible control of precision walking. *Front. Comput. Neurosci.* 7:83. doi: 10.3389/fncom.2013.00083

Kuypers, H. G., Fleming, W. R., and Farinholt, J. W. (1962). Subcorticospinal projections in the rhesus monkey. *J. Comp. Neurol.* 118, 107–137. doi: 10.1002/cne.901180109

Kuypers, H. G. J. M. (1982). "A new look at the organization of the motor system," in *Progress in Brain Research*, eds H. G. J. M. Kuypers and G. F. Martin (Amsterdam: Elsevier), 381–403.

Lang, C. E., and Bastian, A. J. (1999). Cerebellar subjects show impaired adaptation of anticipatory EMG during catching. *J. Neurophysiol.* 82, 2108–2119.

Lawrence, D. G., and Kuypers, H. G. (1968a). The functional organization of the motor system in the monkey. I. The effects of bilateral pyramidal lesions. *Brain* 91, 1–14.

Lawrence, D. G., and Kuypers, H. G. (1968b). The functional organization of the motor system in the monkey. II. The effects of lesions of the descending brain-stem pathways. *Brain* 91, 15–36.

Martin, J. H., Cooper, S. E., Hacking, A., and Ghez, C. (2000). Differential effects of deep cerebellar nuclei inactivation on reaching and adaptive control. *J. Neurophysiol.* 83, 1886–1899.

Mason, C. R., Miller, L. E., Baker, J. F., and Houk, J. C. (1998). Organization of reaching and grasping movements in the primate cerebellar nuclei as revealed by focal muscimol inactivations. *J. Neurophysiol.* 79, 537–554.

McCurdy, M. L., Gibson, A. R., and Houk, J. C. (1992). Spatial overlap of rubrospinal and corticospinal terminals with input to the inferior olive. *Neuroimage* 1, 23–41. doi: 10.1016/1053-8119(92)90005-8

McCurdy, M. L., Hansma, D. I., Houk, J. C., and Gibson, A. R. (1987). Selective projections from the cat red nucleus to digit motor neurons. *J. Comp. Neurol.* 265, 367–379. doi: 10.1002/cne.902650306

Miller, L. E., Van Kan, P. L. E., Sinkjaer, T., Andersen, T., Harris, G. D., and Houk, J. C. (1993). Correlation of primate red nucleus discharge with muscle activity during free-form arm movements. *J. Physiol.* 469, 213–243. doi: 10.1113/jphysiol.1993.sp019812

Morton, S. M., and Bastian, A. J. (2004). Cerebellar control of balance and locomotion. *Neuroscientist* 10, 247–259. doi: 10.1177/1073858404263517

Morton, S. M., and Bastian, A. J. (2007). Mechanisms of cerebellar gait ataxia. *Cerebellum* 6, 79–86. doi: 10.1080/14734220601187741

Overduin, S. A., D'avella, A., Carmena, J. M., and Bizzi, E. (2012). Microstimulation activates a handful of muscle synergies. *Neuron* 76, 1071–1077. doi: 10.1016/j.neuron.2012.10.018

Overduin, S. A., D'avella, A., Carmena, J. M., and Bizzi, E. (2014). Muscle synergies evoked by microstimulation are preferentially encoded during behavior. *Front. Comput. Neurosci.* 8:20. doi: 10.3389/fncom.2014.00020

Overduin, S. A., D'avella, A., Roh, J., Carmena, J. M., and Bizzi, E. (2015). Representation of muscle synergies in the primate brain. *J. Neurosci.* 35, 12615–12624. doi: 10.1523/JNEUROSCI.4302-14.2015

Paulignan, Y., Frak, V. G., Toni, I., and Jeannerod, M. (1997). Influence of object position and size on human prehension movements. *Exp. Brain Res.* 114, 226–234. doi: 10.1007/PL00005631

Paulignan, Y., Jeannerod, M., Mackenzie, C., and Marteniuk, R. (1991a). Selective perturbation of visual input during prehension movements. 2. The effects of changing object size. *Exp. Brain Res.* 87, 407–420.

Paulignan, Y., Mackenzie, C., Marteniuk, R., and Jeannerod, M. (1991b). Selective perturbation of visual input during prehension movements. 1. The effects of changing object position. *Exp. Brain Res.* 83, 502–512.

Pong, M., Horn, K. M., and Gibson, A. R. (2002). Spinal projections of the cat parvicellular red nucleus. *J. Neurophysiol.* 87, 453–468.

Ralston, D. D., Milroy, A. M., and Holstege, G. (1988). Ultrastructural evidence for direct monosynaptic rubrospinal connections to motoneurons in *Macaca mulatta*. *Neurosci. Lett.* 95, 102–106. doi: 10.1016/0304-3940(88)90640-4

Rand, M. K., Shimansky, Y., Stelmach, G. E., Bracha, V., and Bloedel, J. R. (2000). Effects of accuracy constraints on reach-to-grasp movements in cerebellar patients. *Exp. Brain Res.* 135, 179–188. doi: 10.1007/s002210000528

Rispal-Padel, L., and Latreille, J. (1974). The organization of projections from the cerebellar nuclei to the contralateral motor cortex in the cat. *Exp. Brain Res.* 19, 36–60. doi: 10.1007/BF00233394

Rosner, B. (1983). Percentage points for a generalized ESD many-outlier procedure. *Technometrics* 25, 165–172. doi: 10.1080/00401706.1983.10487848

Roy, A. C., Paulignan, Y., Meunier, M., and Boussaoud, D. (2006). Prehension movements in the macaque monkey: effects of perturbation of object size and location. *Exp. Brain Res.* 169, 182–193. doi: 10.1007/s00221-005-0133-8

Shinoda, Y., Futami, T., Mitoma, H., and Yokota, J. (1988). Morphology of single neurones in the cerebello-rubrospinal system. *Behav. Brain Res.* 28, 59–64. doi: 10.1016/0166-4328(88)90076-9

Shinoda, Y., Ghez, C., and Arnold, A. (1977). Spinal branching of rubrospinal axons in the cat. *Exp. Brain Res.* 30, 203–218.

Shinoda, Y., Yokota, J.-I., and Futami, T. (1982). Morphology of physiologically identified rubrospinal axons in the spinal cord of the cat. *Brain Res.* 242, 321–325. doi: 10.1016/0006-8993(82)90316-X

Sybirska, E., and Gorska, T. (1980). Effects of red nucleus lesions on forelimb movements in the cat. *Acta Neurobiol. Exp. (Wars)* 40, 821–841.

Takenobu, Y., Hayashi, T., Moriwaki, H., Nagatsuka, K., Naritomi, H., and Fukuyama, H. (2014). Motor recovery and microstructural change in rubro-spinal tract in subcortical stroke. *Neuroimage* 4, 201–208. doi: 10.1016/j.nicl.2013.12.003

Van Kan, P. L. E., Gibson, A. R., and Houk, J. C. (1993a). Movement-related inputs to intermediate cerebellum of the monkey. *J. Neurophysiol.* 69, 74–94.

Van Kan, P. L. E., Houk, J. C., and Gibson, A. R. (1993b). Output organization of intermediate cerebellum of the monkey. *J. Neurophysiol.* 69, 57–73.

Van Kan, P. L. E., Horn, K. M., and Gibson, A. R. (1994). The importance of hand use to discharge of interpositus neurones of the monkey. *J. Physiol.* 480(Pt 1), 171–190. doi: 10.1113/jphysiol.1994.sp020351

Van Kan, P. L. E., and McCurdy, M. L. (2001). Role of primate magnocellular red nucleus neurons in controlling hand preshaping during reaching to grasp. *J. Neurophysiol.* 85, 1461–1478.

Van Kan, P. L. E., and McCurdy, M. L. (2002a). Contribution of primate magnocellular red nucleus to timing of hand preshaping during reaching to grasp. *J. Neurophysiol.* 87, 1473–1487.

Van Kan, P. L. E., and McCurdy, M. L. (2002b). Discharge of primate magnocellular red nucleus neurons during reaching to grasp in different spatial locations. *Exp. Brain Res.* 142, 151–157. doi: 10.1007/s00221-001-0924-5

Zackowski, K. M., Thach, W. T. Jr., and Bastian, A. J. (2002). Cerebellar subjects show impaired coupling of reach and grasp movements. *Exp. Brain Res.* 146, 511–522. doi: 10.1007/s00221-002-1191-9

7

Parameter Optimization Analysis of Prolonged Analgesia Effect of tDCS on Neuropathic Pain Rats

*Hui-Zhong Wen[1], Shi-Hao Gao[1], Yan-Dong Zhao[1], Wen-Juan He[2], Xue-Long Tian[3] and Huai-Zhen Ruan[1]**

[1]Department of Neurobiology, College of Basic Medical Science, Chongqing Key Laboratory of Neurobiology, Third Military Medical University, Chongqing, China, [2]Department of Pathophysiology and High Altitudepathology, College of High Altitude Military Medicine, Third Military Medical University, Chongqing, China, [3]Bioengineering College, Chongqing University, Chongqing, China

***Correspondence:**
Huai-Zhen Ruan
hzruan163@163.com

Background: Transcranial direct current stimulation (tDCS) is widely used to treat human nerve disorders and neuropathic pain by modulating the excitability of cortex. The effectiveness of tDCS is influenced by its stimulation parameters, but there have been no systematic studies to help guide the selection of different parameters.

Objective: This study aims to assess the effects of tDCS of primary motor cortex (M1) on chronic neuropathic pain in rats and to test for the optimal parameter combinations for analgesia.

Methods: Using the chronic neuropathic pain models of chronic constriction injury (CCI), we measured pain thresholds before and after anodal-tDCS (A-tDCS) using different parameter conditions, including stimulation intensity, stimulation time, intervention time and electrode located (ipsilateral or contralateral M1 of the ligated paw on male/female CCI models).

Results: Following the application of A-tDCS over M1, we observed that the antinociceptive effects were depended on different parameters. First, we found that repetitive A-tDCS had a longer analgesic effect than single stimulus, and both ipsilateral-tDCS (ip-tDCS) and contralateral-tDCS (con-tDCS) produce a long-lasting analgesic effect on neuropathic pain. Second, the antinociceptive effects were intensity-dependent and time-dependent, high intensities worked better than low intensities and long stimulus durations worked better than short stimulus durations. Third, timing of the intervention after injury affected the stimulation outcome, early use of tDCS was an effective method to prevent the development of pain, and more frequent intervention induced more analgesia in CCI rats, finally, similar antinociceptive effects of con- and ip-tDCS were observed in both sexes of CCI rats.

Conclusion: Optimized protocols of tDCS for treating antinociceptive effects were developed. These findings should be taken into consideration when using tDCS to produce analgesic effects in clinical applications.

Keywords: transcranial direct current stimulation, tDCS, chronic constriction injury, neuropathic pain, intervention time, parameter optimization

INTRODUCTION

Chronic neuropathic pain is a common and severely disabling state that typically develops when peripheral nerves are damaged due to surgery, bone compression in cancer, diabetes or infection (Dworkin et al., 2013). Recent studies indicate increased activation of descending modulatory circuits (both descending facilitation and inhibition) in chronic neuropathic pain syndrome, and these circuit changes reflect long-lasting changes in synaptic efficacy (Zhuo, 2008, 2013). An increasing number of investigators hold the view that non-invasive brain stimulation techniques can be used to treat chronic neuropathic pain (O'Connell et al., 2011; Volz et al., 2012). The aim of brain stimulation in managing of pain is to reduce pain symptoms by altering activity in brain areas that are involved in processing painful stimuli (Nguyen et al., 2011; Mylius et al., 2012; Woods et al., 2016).

Repetitive transcranial magnetic stimulation (rTMS) and transcranial direct current stimulation (tDCS) are two typical and common techniques of non-invasive brain stimulation techniques (Woods et al., 2016). Relative to invasive stimulation, non-invasive stimulation requires no surgical procedure and is therefore easier and safer to administer. However, there are several advantages of tDCS over rTMS, such as lower cost, increased portability, and more convincing sham conditions (Zaghi et al., 2009). TDCS is considered as a neuromodulatory intervention for the brain (Nitsche et al., 2008) which modulates the membrane potential dependently by type of electrode's application. Anode-tDCS (A-tDCS) is able to facilitate the depolarization of neurons and increase the cortical excitability. However, cathode-tDCS (C-tDCS) hyperpolarizes the resting membrane potential and reduces the cortical excitability (Nitsche et al., 2008; Mylius et al., 2012). Numerous clinical studies have concluded that A-tDCS is an effective method for pain modulations, which is helpful at reducing both fibromyalgia and spinal cord injury related-pain (Fregni et al., 2006; Roizenblatt et al., 2007; Soler et al., 2010). There are also studies showing effects of A-tDCS in inflammatory and neuropathic pain in animals (Laste et al., 2012; Spezia Adachi et al., 2012; Cioato et al., 2016; Filho et al., 2016).

Sensory-motor cortex has been reported to decrease pain sensation and to increase pain threshold (Xie et al., 2009; Ossipov et al., 2010). As a result, the primary motor cortex (M1) is regarded as the location for stimulation electrode placement in the vast majority of trials in patients (Ferrucci et al., 2015; Woods et al., 2016), but there was little research testing the location of the stimulation electrode in animal research, the stimulation electrodes of those studies were placed on the middle of the scalp of rat rather than on a particular location (Ferrucci et al., 2015; Woods et al., 2016). There are three location modes for electrodes as related to the region of pain: contralateral M1, bilateral M1 and ipsilateral M1 to the injured region. A-tDCS delivered to contralateral M1 and bilateral M1 have been reported to have an antinociceptive effect in a number of patients with chronic pain (Ngernyam, 2014; O'Neill et al., 2015; Woods et al., 2016), whereas few studies of tDCS of ipsilateral M1 have been reported.

Beside the location of the stimulation electrode, physical parameters and practical applications of tDCS are important factors in treating neuropathic pain in animal and clinical experiments (Nitsche et al., 2008; Nitsche and Paulus, 2011; Stagg and Nitsche, 2011). Therefore, tDCS protocols should state current intensity, electrode size, stimulation duration and other parameters to aid in assessing comparability among studies (Nitsche et al., 2008). Originally, tDCS was believed to follow simple rules: the more electric charge flowing through the electrode, the stronger the analgesic effect would be (Nitsche et al., 2008; Nitsche and Paulus, 2011). However, the safety and side effects of tDCS on participants should be precisely calculated, because high current density can cause tissue damage (Nitsche et al., 2008; Liebetanz et al., 2009). Another important parameter of tDCS is the intervention time, which involves the time when stimulation is administered in relation to the course of pain processing and how many times tDCS is delivered. According to previous findings, repetitive stimulation has been proven to enhance efficacy and prolong after-effects of tDCS during specific time intervals (Nitsche et al., 2008). In addition, because the course of neuropathic pain is fairly long and easy to be targeted repeatedly (Dworkin et al., 2013), it will be significant if the patient can be treated when the pain is onset with negligible side effects.

Therefore, a combination of tDCS stimulation parameters including current intensity as well as stimulation time, interval and position need to be studied systematically in clinical and animal experiments. However, due to the limitation of choosing suitable parameters in clinical studies, optimal protocol characteristics have not been explored systematically (Ngernyam, 2014). In this article, we conducted studies to explore the optimal physical parameters and practical applications of A-tDCS in treating chronic neuropathic pain in both male and female rats.

MATERIALS AND METHODS

Experimental Animals

Experiments were carried out on adult Sprague–Dawley rats (8–10 weeks old weighing 220–250 g), which were purchased from the Center of Laboratory Animal, Third Military Medical University, Chongqing, China. The SD rats were housed in plastic cages with soft bedding under controlled temperature settings (24 ± 1°C), humidity (60 ± 5%) and a 12-h light/dark cycle. The study, animal care and handling procedures were in strict accordance with the recommendations of International Association for the Study of Pain's ethical guidelines (Zimmermann, 1983), and the protocol was also approved by the Ethical Committee for Animal Research of Third Military Medical University.

Animal Model of Neuropathic Pain

A typical neuropathic pain model was established through chronic constriction injury (CCI) of the sciatic nerve (Bennett and Xie, 1988).The right sciatic nerve of rats was tied with four 4-0 chromic gut ligatures 1 mm apart under 4% chloral hydrate-anesthesia (10 ml/kg, i.p.). The sutures were not tied so tight that blood flow was affected. The overlying muscle was sutured and the skin wound was sealed with topical antibiotics. Rats with right sciatic nerve exposed without chromic gut ligature served as sham CCI controls.

Transcranial Direct Current Stimulation

We improved the previously implanted electrode protocol by optimizing the internal structural stability and by decreasing the contact impedance of the electrode (Liebetanz et al., 2006; Yu et al., 2015). Three days before CCI or sham CCI surgery, a saline soaked sponge was placed at the end of a plastic tube (inner diameter: 2 mm; length: 1 cm; **Figures 1A,B**). A copper wire was inserted into the sponge and held in place inside the tube with polyacrylate adhesive. Next, the tube was fixed with glass ionomer cement onto the cranium over M1 as a stimulation electrode using a stereotaxic apparatus; ipsilateral tDCS (ip-tDCS) refers to a stimulation electrode being fixed overlying the ipsilateral M1 to the ligated hind paw, and contralateral tDCS (con-tDCS) refers to stimulation electrode fixed overlying the contralateral M1 to the ligated hind paw (**Figure 1A**). A far larger conventional sponge electrode (10 cm^2) was placed on the ventral thorax with a corset and served as a reference electrode (**Figure 1B**).

As described below, constant current was applied via the stimulation electrode as A-tDCS at the schedule times (1st, 7th or 14th days after CCI; **Figure 1C**). For sham tDCS, the stimulation electrode was placed in the same positions as for real stimulation, but stimulation duration of 10 s was used as described above (Yu et al., 2015). Meanwhile, at the beginning and end of tDCS, current was ramped up and down for 10 s to prevent damage to the brain tissues by suddenly changing current (Bindman et al., 1964; Yu et al., 2015). Saline was injected continuously into the sponge through the hole that we left on the top of the tube during the DC stimulation in order to reduce contact impedance when stimulating (Yu et al., 2015). Notably, animals were not anesthetized during tDCS or sham tDCS.

Experimental Protocols

The experiment was composed by seven series (**Figure 1C**, Supplementary Table S1):

- **Series 1**: changes of pain thresholds after CCI. Thirty-three male rats were randomly divided into three groups: control (CT), sham CCI (SC) and CCI. Pain thresholds were tested 1 day before the CCI surgery and at days 1, 3, 7, 10, 14, 21 and 28 after CCI surgery.
- **Series 2**: changes of pain thresholds after single A-tDCS on CCI rats. On day 14 after CCI surgery, contralateral or ipsilateral A-tDCS was delivered in a single session of 20 min with stimulation current intensity of 100/200 μA. Male rats were divided into 12 groups: SC, sham CCI + sham 200 μA ip-tDCS (SCSIT), sham CCI + 200 μA sham con-tDCS (SCSCT), sham CCI + 200 μA ip-tDCS (SCIT), sham CCI + 200 μA con-tDCS (SCCT), CCI, CCI + sham 200 μA ip-tDCS (CSIT), CCI + sham 200 μA con-tDCS (CSCT), CCI + 100 μA ip-tDCS (CIT100), CCI + 200 μA ip-tDCS (CIT200), CCI + 100 μA con-tDCS (CCT100) and CCI + 200 μA con-tDCS (CCT200; n = 11 per group, of which were observed before, and 30 min, 2 h and 24 h after A-tDCS or sham A-tDCS).
- **Series 3**: changes of pain thresholds after processed with repetitive ip-tDCS and con-tDCS on CCI rats. Daily A-tDCS (20 min/200 μA) was applied over five sessions over the contralateral or ipsilateral M1 from the 7th day after CCI. In this series, male rats were divided into four groups: SC, CCI, CIT and CCT.
- **Series 4**: observation of pain thresholds changes after repetitive contralateral A-tDCS with different intensities. Five times daily A-tDCS with different intensities was applied for 20 min on the contralateral M1 from the 7th day after CCI. In this series, male rats were divided into six groups: SC, CCI, CCI + 15 μA con-tDCS (CCT15), CCI + 50 μA con-tDCS (CCT50), CCI + 100 μA con-tDCS (CCT100), and CCI + 200 μA con-tDCS (CCT200).
- **Series 5**: observation of pain thresholds changes after repetitive contralateral A-tDCS with different times. Daily 200 μA A-tDCS was applied on five sessions over the contralateral M1 from the 7th day after CCI. In this series, male rats were divided into six groups: SC, CCI, CCI + 5 min con-tDCS (CCT200-5), CCI + 10 min con-tDCS (CCT200-10), CCI + 20 min con-tDCS (CCT200-20), and CCI + 30 min con-tDCS (CCT200-30).
- **Series 6**: changes in the pain thresholds after A-tDCS on CCI model with different intervention time and sessions. In this series, CCI rats were given with five sessions of repetitive contralateral A-tDCS (20 min/200 μA) on the 1st day (5CCI-1), 7th day (5CCI-7) and 14th day (5CCI-14) after CCI surgery. Other rats were given 10 sessions of repetitive tDCS (20 min/200 μA) starting on the 1st day (10CCT-1) after CCI surgery. Male rats were divided into six groups: SC, CCI, 5CCT-1, 5CCT-7, 5CCT-14, and 10CCT-1.
- **Series 7**: changes in the pain thresholds after repetitive A-tDCS on female rats of the CCI model. Fifty-five female rats were divided into five groups: CT, SC, CCI, CCT and CIT, and daily A-tDCS (20 min/200 μA) was applied on five sessions over the contralateral or ipsilateral M1 from the 7th day after CCI.
- **Series 2–7**: pain thresholds were tested 1 day before CCI surgery and on days 1, 3, 7, 10, 14, 21 and 28 after CCI surgery (n = 11, per group).

Radiant Heat Test

The radiant heat test was carried out to estimate the thermal withdrawal latency (TWL; Hargreaves et al., 1988). After an adaptation period of 30 min, the rats were placed into the test cage with a glass plate under which a light was located; 52 ± 0.2°C radiant heat was applied to the plantar surface of the right hind-paw. The latency period was recorded in response to the thermal hyperalgesia by lifting hind-paw licking, flicking or commences jumping. To avoid tissue injury, the cut-off limit was set at 60 s (Hargreaves et al., 1988). Each hind-paw was measured for three times alternately at a 5 min interval. The mean was recorded as TWL.

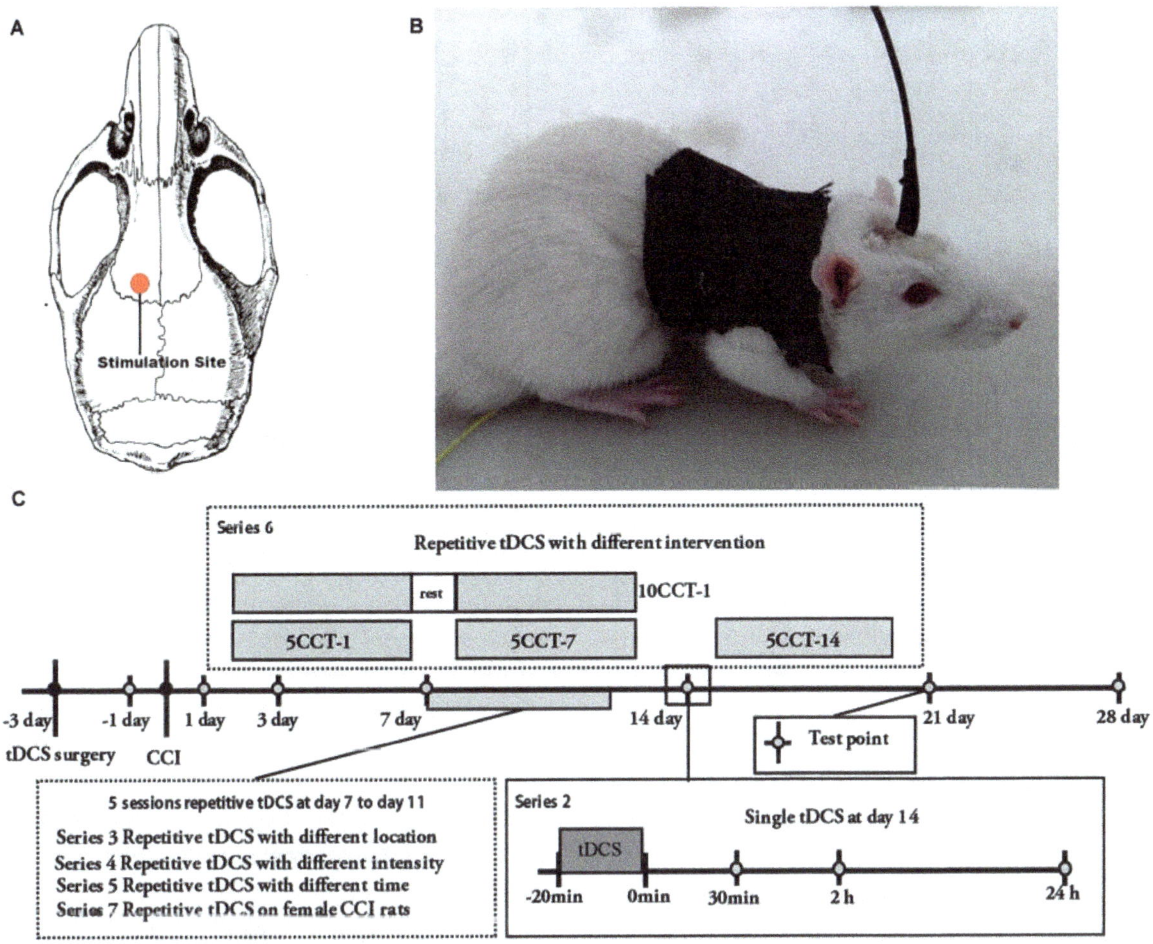

FIGURE 1 | (A) Schematic diagram displaying the location of the stimulation electrode in the rat brain model. **(B)** Electrode configurations in rat. Two electrodes were applied during transcranial direct current stimulation (tDCS). The stimulation electrode was fixed onto the skull and a reference electrode was attached onto the thorax. **(C)** Schematic diagram of the experiment protocol schedule. 5CCT-1/5CCT-7/5CCT-14 means five times daily contralateral-tDCS (con-tDCS) started on day 1, 7, or 14 following chronic constriction injury (CCI), respectively; 10CCT-1 means 10 times con-tDCS at 2 weeks. Test point was the day to test the mechanical allodynia and thermal hyperalgesia on the hind paw of CCI.

Von Frey Filaments Test

The von Frey filaments test using an up-down method was performed to estimate the 50% system mechanical withdrawal threshold (MWT) with bending forces at a range of 0.3–20.3 g von Frey hairs (vFh; Chaplan et al., 1994). Each rat was placed inside a transparent acrylic cage (18 cm × 12 cm × 12 cm) with wire mesh floor with 60 min of acclimatization. The test was initiated with 4.10 g vFh. The filament was applied to the ventral surface of each right hind-paw for 4–6 s, hind paw withdrawal was considered as a positive response. When a positive result was noted, then the filament was decremented by one step size. If a negative result occurs, the filament was increased. The test continues until four measurements have been made after the first change in direction.

Statistical Analysis

Analyses were done with the SPSS software package (version 19). All data are expressed as the mean ± SD. The pain thresholds were evaluated by one way (**Figure 2**) or two-way (except **Figure 2**) repeated measure analysis of variance (ANOVA), when significant differences were observed, a *post hoc* test was made via Tukey's test. In all cases, $p < 0.05$ was considered to be statistically significant.

RESULTS

Changes of Pain Thresholds in CCI Rats

Significant mechanical allodynia and thermal hyperalgesia were elicited in surgical hind paw CCI rats (**Figure 2**). Two-way repeated measures ANOVA showed a significant main effect of group on the MWT (main effect of group $F_{(2,30)} = 663.718$, $p = 0.000$) and TWL ($F_{(2,30)} = 828.857$, $p = 0.000$). The values of MWT and TWL were decreased starting 1 day after CCI surgery, and the most severe stage appeared around day 14 (MWT: 1.03 ± 0.21 g, TWL: 8.61 ± 0.44 s) and then began

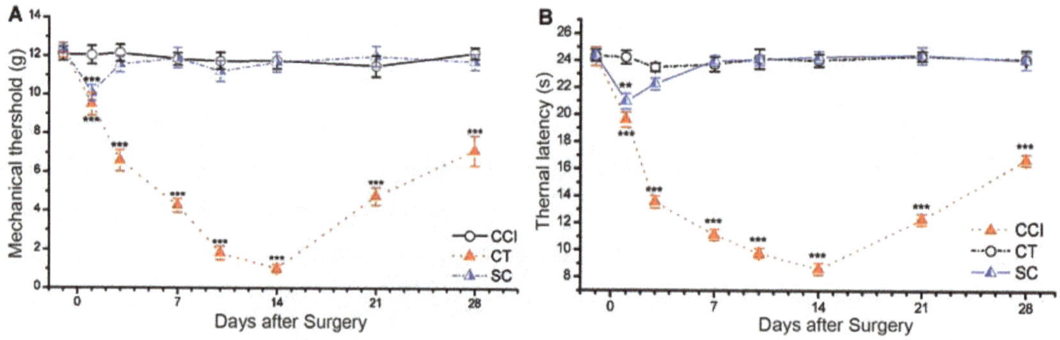

FIGURE 2 | CCI induced significant mechanical allodynia and thermal hyperalgesia in rat. **(A)** Mechanical withdrawal threshold (MWT). **(B)** Thermal withdrawal latency (TWL). Control (CT); sham CCI (SC). All behavior tests were examined 1 day before the CCI surgery and on days 1, 3, 7, 10, 14, 21 and 28 after CCI surgery. Statistical significance was analyzed by two-way analysis of variance (ANOVA) followed by Tukey's *post hoc* test. The data are shown as mean ± SEM; $^{**}p < 0.01$, $^{***}p < 0.001$ vs. CT group.

to recover on the following day (**Figure 2**). This trend was in line with our previous studies (Xiao et al., 2010; Ou et al., 2011; He et al., 2012). There was no significant difference in the thermal latency and mechanical threshold between control and sham CCI groups (p = 0.259 of TWL, p = 0.128 of MWT).

Effects of Single tDCS Treatment Disappeared within 24 h after Stimulation

We chose the 14th day after CCI to test the duration of antinociceptive effects after one time tDCS.

No difference was found in TWL and MWT among SC, SCSIT, SCSCT, SCIT and SCCT groups at all test points (one-way ANOVA, all $p > 0.05$). Sham tDCS (both SCSCT and SCSIT) had no impact on behaviors of Sham CCI rats, and the tDCS (both SCIT and SCCT) also did not have impact on behaviors of sham CCI rats (one-way ANOVA, all $p > 0.05$; **Figure 3**).

Compared with CCI, single con-tDCS (both CCT100 and CCT200) sharply increased TWL and MWT after one session of A-tDCS that ended 30 min before behavioral tests (one-way ANOVA, all p = 0.000). The effects were gradually diminished in the following 2 h (one-way ANOVA, TWL: p = 0.000 for CCT100, p = 0.000 for CCT200; MWT: p = 0.001 for CCT100, p = 0.000 for CCT200 vs. CCI). After 24 h, the antinociceptive effects were almost completely gone and there were no differences compared with the CCI group (one-way ANOVA, all $p > 0.05$). Moreover, we also observed a better recovery of pain in CCT200 than CCT100 (one-way ANOVA, TWL: p = 0.044 for 30 min, p = 0.004 for 2 h, p = 0.490 for 24 h; MWT: p = 0.037 for 30 min, p = 0.009 for 2 h, p = 0.523 for 24 h).

Similarly, single ip-tDCS (CIT100 and CIT200) also showed analgesia effects on CCI rats (one-way ANOVA, 30 min: all p = 0.000 vs. CCI). However, compared to the effects observed with con-tDCS, the antinociceptive effects decreased in the following 2 h (one-way ANOVA, TWL: p = 0.005 for CIT100 and p = 0.000 for CIT200; MWT: p = 0.010 for CIT100 and p = 0.000 for CIT200) and disappeared after 24 h with ip-tDCS (one-way ANOVA, all $p > 0.05$; **Figure 3**). We also observed increased pain recovery in the CIT200 group compared to the CIT100 group (one-way ANOVA, TWL: p = 0.000 for 30 min, p = 0.006 for 2 h, p = 1.000 for 24 h; MWT: p = 0.001 for 30 min, p = 0.028 for 2 h, p = 0.582 for 24 h; **Figure 3**).

However, we did not observed changes in pain thresholds of sham tDCS (both CSIT and CSCT) in CCI rats (one-way ANOVA, all $p > 0.05$; **Figure 3**).

Both ip- and con-Repetitive tDCS Had Long-Term Antinociceptive Effects in CCI Rats

Repetitive A-tDCS had long-term antinociceptive effects, significant increases in TWL and MWT were observed not only during the stimulation process, but also 1 or more weeks following A-tDCS (**Figures 4A,C**). Five sessions of repetitive A-tDCS had similar antinociceptive effects in both CIT and CCT groups; similar effects were observed in surgical hind paw of CCI rats (two-way repeated measures ANOVA: TWL: $F_{(3,40)}$ = 480.888, p = 0.000; MWT: $F_{(3,40)}$ = 150.201, p = 0.000. Tukey's test of groups: all p = 0.000 vs. CCI). Moreover, the values of TWL and MWT in the CCT group were slightly higher than those in the CIT group at every test point, but the differences did not reach statistical significance (Tukey: TWL: p = 0.226, MWT: p = 0.051).

We also normalized the values of TWL and MWT (% of control) and observed the significant analgesia effect during and after tDCS in CIT and CCT groups (**Figures 4B,D**).

Intensity-Dependent Antinociceptive Effects of Repetitive tDCS in CCI Rats

After confirming the location of stimulation electrode in the above studies, we chose different stimulation intensities and simulation times to determine the most effective stimulation current.

Increasing stimulation current intensity resulted in an intensity-dependent increase in TWL of the ipsilateral

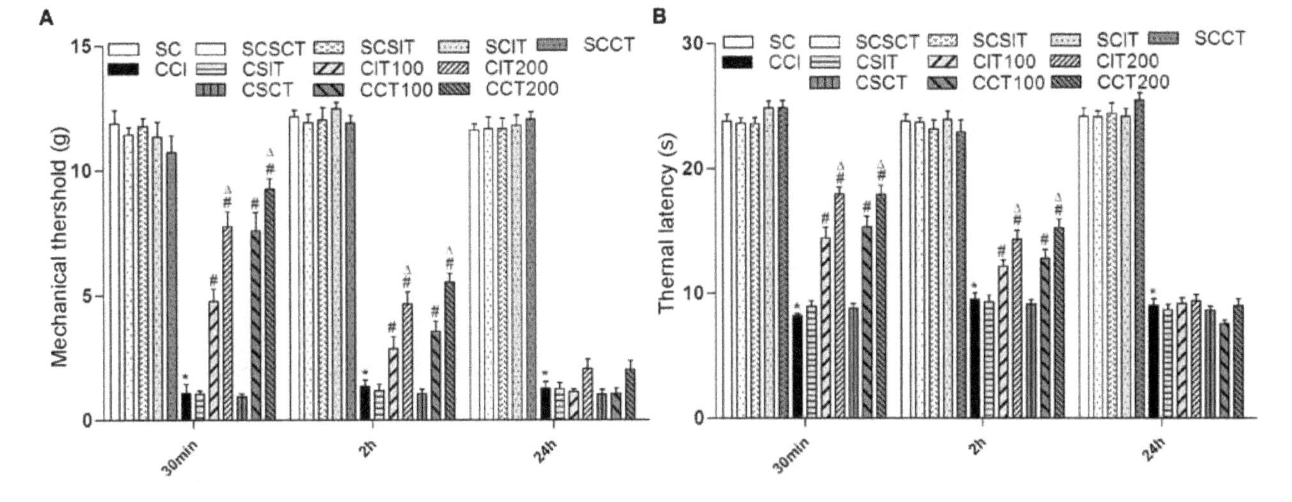

FIGURE 3 | Effects of single tDCS on mechanical allodynia and thermal hyperalgesia. All behavior tests were examined before, and then 30 min, 2 h and 24 h after tDCS. Administration of tDCS started on day 14 after CCI surgery. Experimental groups include, sham CCI (SC); CCI; sham CCI + sham 200 μA ip-tDCS (SCSIT); sham CCI + sham 200 μA con-tDCS (SCSCT), sham CCI + 200 μA ip-tDCS (SCIT); sham CCI + 200 μA con-tDCS (SCCT); CCI + sham 200 μA ip-tDCS (CSIT); CCI + sham 200 μA con-tDCS (CSCT); CCI + 100 μA ip-tDCS (CIT100); CCI + 200 μA ip-tDCS (CIT200); CCI + 100 μA con-tDCS (CCT100); CCI + 200 μA con-tDCS (CCT200). **(A)** MWT. **(B)** TWL. Group analysis was performed by one-way ANOVA followed by Tukey's test. In all three test phases, there were no difference between SC and SCSIT, SCSCT, SCIT, SCCT groups, and there was also no difference between CCI and CSCT, CSIT groups. However, there were significant differences between SC, SCSIT, SCSCT, SCIT, SCCT and CCI groups (all $^{*}p < 0.05$ vs. CCI group). 30 min: the CIT and CCT groups (both 100 μA and 200 μA) differ from the CCI, CSIT and CSCT groups; 2 h: the CIT and CCT groups (both 100 μA and 200 μA) differ from the CCI, CSIT and CSCT groups; 24 h: there is no significant difference from CCI, CSIT, CSST, CIT and CCT groups ($^{\#}p < 0.05$ compared with CCI group, and $^{\Delta}p < 0.05$ compared with CIT100 or CCT100 group).

hind paw after five repetitive A-tDCS (two-way repeated measures ANOVA: TWL: $F_{(5,60)} = 336.733$, $p = 0.000$; MWT: $F_{(5,60)} = 172.656$, $p = 0.000$; **Figure 5**). Compared to the CCI group, the CCT50, CCT100 and CCT200 induced significant increases in TWL and MWT during and after stimulation (Tukey's test of groups: TWL and MWT: all $p = 0.000$), but the CCT15 did not induced analgesia effect (TWL: CCT15 $p = 0.320$; MWT: $p = 0.833$), The analgesic effects were higher in high intensity groups as compared to low intensity groups (Tukey's test of groups: TWL: CCT50 vs. CCT15 $p = 0.009$, CCT100 vs. CCT50 $p = 0.000$, CCT200 vs. CCT100 $p = 0.009$; MWT: CCT50 vs. CCT15 $p = 0.018$, CCT100 vs. CCT50 $p = 0.000$, CCT200 vs. CCT100 $p = 0.589$; **Figure 5**).

Time-Dependent Antinociceptive Effects of Repetitive tDCS in CCI Rats

We observed time-dependent increases in pain thresholds in the ligated hind paw after five daily 200 μA con-tDCS, time points used were 5 min, 10 min, 20 min and 30 min (two-way repeated measures ANOVA: TWL: $F_{(5,60)} = 347.503$, $p = 0.000$; MWT: $F_{(5,60)} = 132.278$, $p = 0.000$; **Figure 6**). The CCT200-5, CCT200-10, CCT200-20 and CCT200-30 groups increased the pain values sharply during the test periods (Tukey's test of groups: TWL and MWT: all $p = 0.000$). We also observed time-dependent increases in pain thresholds (Tukey's test of groups: TWL: CCT200-5 vs. CCT200-10 $p = 0.000$, CCT200-10 vs. CCT200-20 $p = 0.000$, CCT200-20 vs. CCT200-30 $p = 0.681$; MWT: CCT200-5 vs. CCT200-10 $p = 0.000$, CCT200-10 vs. CCT200-20 $p = 0.030$, CCT200-20 vs. CCT200-30 $p = 0.967$).

Proper Intervention Time Enhanced the Long-Term Antinociceptive Effects of Repetitive tDCS in CCI Rats

Intervention time also played a role in the antinociceptive effects following repetitive tDCS, the after-effects were different depending on the time of intervention of tDCS (two-way repeated measures ANOVA: TWL: $F_{(5,60)} = 258.796$, $p = 0.000$; MWT: $F_{(5,60)} = 160.171$, $p = 0.000$; **Figures 7A,C**).

When intervention was performed at 1 day after CCI (5CCT-1), repetitive A-tDCS maintained pain thresholds of the MWT and the TWL in the days following tDCS (Tukey's test of groups: all: $p = 0.000$ vs. CCI). Given tDCS 7 days after CCI (5CCT-7) reversed the development of pain thresholds which gradually approached normal (Tukey's test of groups: all: $p = 0.000$ vs. CCI). Pain thresholds were began to recover 14 days after CCI, and giving A-tDCS at this time point (5CCT-14) greatly reduced the recovery time and increased pain thresholds (Tukey's test of groups: TWL: $p = 0.000$, MWT: $p = 0.639$ vs. CCI). We also observed using twice the number of stimulation sessions (10CCT-1) was helpful in reducing mechanical allodynia and thermal hyperalgesia (Tukey's test of groups: all: $p = 0.000$ vs. CCI). The antinociceptive effects of 10CCT-1 was greater than those observed in the 5CCT-7 group following thermal hyperalgesia (TWL: $p = 0.000$: MWT: $p = 0.379$ vs. 5CCT-7; **Figures 7A,C**). Moreover, we found that inter-quartile range in the 10CCT-1 group was more centralized than that for other groups on 14th day following CCI, which reflected the spread of the threshold data (one-way measures ANOVA: TWL: $F_{(4,50)} = 122.89$, $p = 0.000$; MWT: $F_{(4,50)} = 75.96$, $p = 0.000$; **Figures 7B,D**).

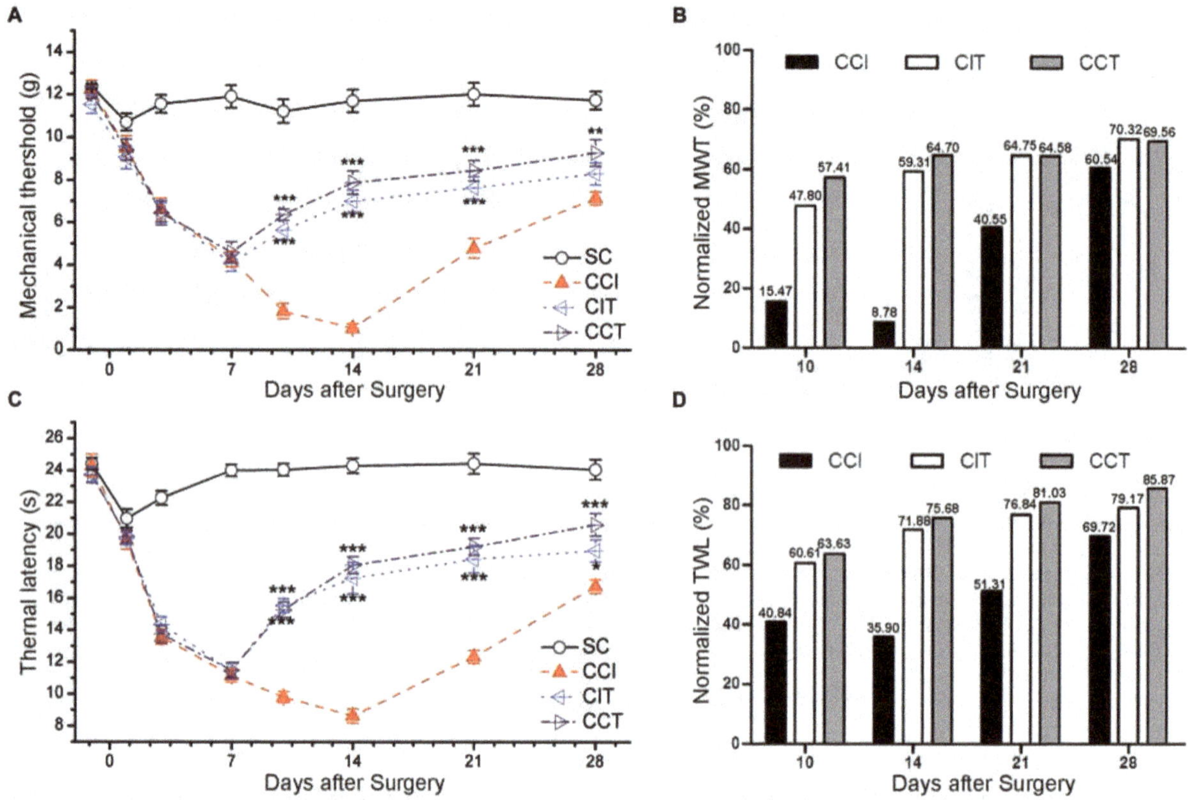

FIGURE 4 | Effects of repetitive tDCS on mechanical allodynia and thermal hyperalgesia with different electrode locations. **(A)** MWT. **(B)** Normalized of MWT. **(C)** TWL. **(D)** Normalized of TWL. Five sessions daily of tDCS (200 μA, 20 min) were administered starting on day 7 after CCI surgery. SC (sham CCI); CCI + ip-tDCS (CIT); CCI + con-tDCS (CCT). CIT and CCT treatments significantly increased the values of TWL and MWT. All behavior tests were tested 1 day before the CCI surgery and on days 1, 3, 7, 10, 14, 21 and 28 after CCI surgery. Statistical significance was analyzed by two-way ANOVA followed by Tukey's *post hoc* test. $^{*}p < 0.05$, $^{**}p < 0.01$, $^{***}p < 0.001$ vs. CCI group.

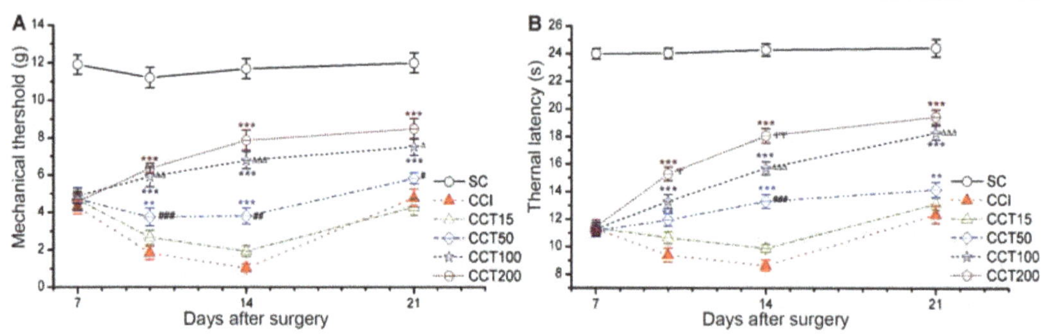

FIGURE 5 | Effects of repetitive tDCS on mechanical allodynia and thermal hyperalgesia with different stimulation intensities. **(A)** MWT. **(B)** TWL. Five sessions daily of con-tDCS (20 min) with different intensity administrations started on day 7 after CCI surgery. Sham CCI (SC); CCI + 15 μA con-tDCS treatment (CCT15); CCI + 50 μA con-tDCS treatmen (CCT50); CCI + 100 μA con-tDCS treatment (CCT100); CCI + 200 μA con-tDCS treatment (CCT200). All behavior tests were examined at days 7, 10, 14, and 21 after CCI surgery. Statistical significance was analyzed by two-way ANOVA followed by Tukey's *post hoc* test. $^{**}p < 0.01$, $^{***}p < 0.001$ vs. CCI group; $^{\#}p < 0.05$, $^{\#\#}p < 0.01$, $^{\#\#\#}p < 0.001$ vs. CCT15 group; $^{\Delta}p < 0.05$, $^{\Delta\Delta}p < 0.01$, $^{\Delta\Delta\Delta}p < 0.001$ vs. CCT50 group; $^{\Psi}p < 0.05$, $^{\Psi\Psi}p < 0.01$ vs. CCT100 group.

Antinociceptive Effects in Female Rats after Repetitive tDCS

A similar pain tend was observed in female rats compared to male rats following CCI, the TWL and MWT were significantly decreased in CCI rats compared to CT rats (Tukey's test of groups: TWL and MWT: all $p = 0.000$; **Figure 8**). Consecutive sessions of tDCS (both CIT and CCT) induced antinociceptive effects which lasted for at least 1 week after stimulation in

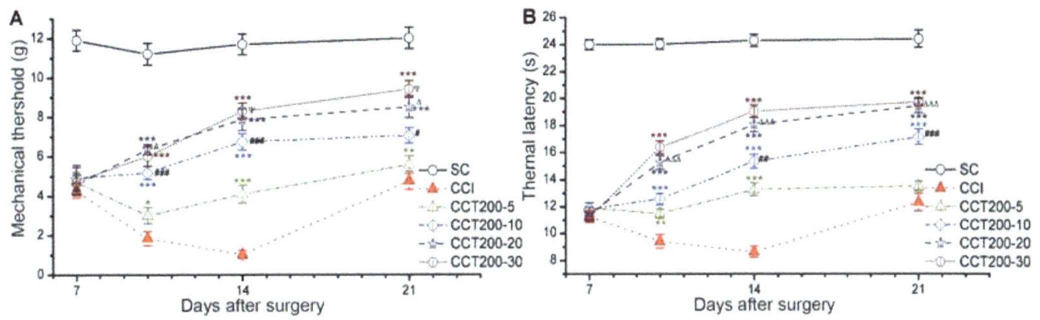

FIGURE 6 | Effects of repetitive tDCS on mechanical allodynia and thermal hyperalgesia with different stimulation times. **(A)** MWT. **(B)** TWL. Five sessions daily of con-tDCS (200 μA) with different time administrations started on day 7 after CCI surgery. Sham CCI (SC); CCI + 5 min con-tDCS treatment (CCT200-5); CCI + 10 min con-tDCS treatment (CCT200-10); CCI + 20 min con-tDCS treatment (CCT200-20); CCI + 30 min con-tDCS treatment (CCT200-30). All behavior tests were examined at days 7, 10, 14 and 21 after CCI surgery. Statistical significance was analyzed by two-way ANOVA followed by Tukey's *post hoc* test. $^{**}p < 0.01$, $^{***}p < 0.001$ vs. CCI group; $^{\#}p < 0.05$, $^{\#\#}p < 0.01$, $^{\#\#\#}p < 0.001$ vs. CCT200-5 group; $^{\Delta}p < 0.05$, $^{\Delta\Delta\Delta}p < 0.001$ vs. CCT200-10 group; $^{\Psi}p < 0.05$ vs. CCT200-20 group.

female CCI rats (two-way repeated measures ANOVA: TWL: $F_{(4,50)} = 248.424$, $p = 0.000$; MWT: $F_{(4,50)} = 136.015$, $p = 0.000$). Compared to the CCI group, A-tDCS significantly increased the pain values to a high level in both CIT group (Tukey's test of groups: TWL and MWT: all $p = 0.000$) and CCT group (Tukey's test of groups: TWL and MWT: all $p = 0.000$). We also observed that the mechanical allodynia and thermal hyperalgesia of the CCT group were mildly increased compared to the CIT group, but the differences did not reach statistical significance (Tukey's test of groups: TWL: $p = 0.074$; MWT: $p = 0.093$; **Figure 8**). We also normalized the values of TWL and MWT (% of control) and observed the significant analgesia effect during and after tDCS (**Figures 8B,D**).

DISCUSSION

Clinical treatment of neuropathic pain is still a major challenge because of its long duration and difficulty in managing (Brunoni et al., 2012). As a non-invasive electrical stimulation treatment, tDCS technology has been used for many years in clinical settings (Gandiga et al., 2006; Brunoni et al., 2012). Radiological and clinical practice have proven that tDCS can play a role in the plasticity of CNS regulation and serve as a treatment for neuronal abnormalities (Borckardt et al., 2012; Brunoni et al., 2012; DosSantos et al., 2014; Woods et al., 2016). However, as systematical basic research is lacking, clinical effects are inconsistent and critical stimulus parameters are uncertain (Lee et al., 2015; Dedoncker et al., 2016). In this article, we choose a rat CCI model as the neuropathic pain model, which is the most common pain model that could finely simulate the clinical chronic neuropathic pain as reported by previous studies (Xiao et al., 2010; Ou et al., 2011; He et al., 2012). The pain threshold of MWT and TWL were evaluated at the different times after CCI.

Previous clinical studies chose the M1 cerebral cortex as the stimulus location because of its roles in the modulation of chronic pain, as it receives pain-related information from the thalamus and the somatosensory cortex (Nguyen et al., 2011; Mylius et al., 2012). Earlier findings indicated that the neural activity of contralateral M1 to an injured paw was increased after CCI (Ooi et al., 2006), and contralateral M1 stimulation has been used as a clinical treatment of chronic pain with the use of transdural motor cortex stimulation (MCS) and rTMS (Lefaucheur, 2006; Fontaine et al., 2009; Young et al., 2014). However, previous work has also reported that M1 stimulation with MCS or rTMS ipsilateral to injury could also significantly suppress pain-related responses in rats and human (Nahmias et al., 2009; Lucas et al., 2011; Viisanen et al., 2012), but there have been no extensive experimental study testing tDCS. In our study, the anode stimulation electrode was mounted contralateral or ipsilateral to the injured paw to measure the antinociceptive effect of tDCS, and our results demonstrated that both locations of A-tDCS led to significant decreases in pain. Our study supplements previous experiments in which the location of the electrode was not taken into consideration (Cioato et al., 2016; Filho et al., 2016). A possible mechanism of these results is supra-spinal antinociceptive activities via multiple parallel pathways (Pertovaara and Wei, 2003). Recent studies had found that M1 stimulation can also active the adjacent regions, including the periaqueductal gray, anterior cingulate cortex and amygdale (Nguyen et al., 2011). Further experiments have shown that rTMS enhances the corticospinal inhibitory system which might in turn mediate M1 stimulation-induced spinal antinociception (Rojas-Piloni et al., 2010; Dall Agnol et al., 2014). The transduction mechanism of antinociception release needs further study in the future.

We observed that the effects of A-tDCS on reducing hyperalgesia and allodynia depended on stimulus intensity and time. Stronger intensities or longer duration correlates with more charged input to the cortex (Nitsche and Paulus, 2011), and a better after-effect on relieving pain (Nitsche et al., 2008). In Series 2, we found the analgesic effect of single tDCS was diminished following 2 h, but repetitive tDCS prolongs the duration of analgesic effect (Series 3). We found that greater charge inputs given 1 week after original stimulation maintained high pain thresholds when

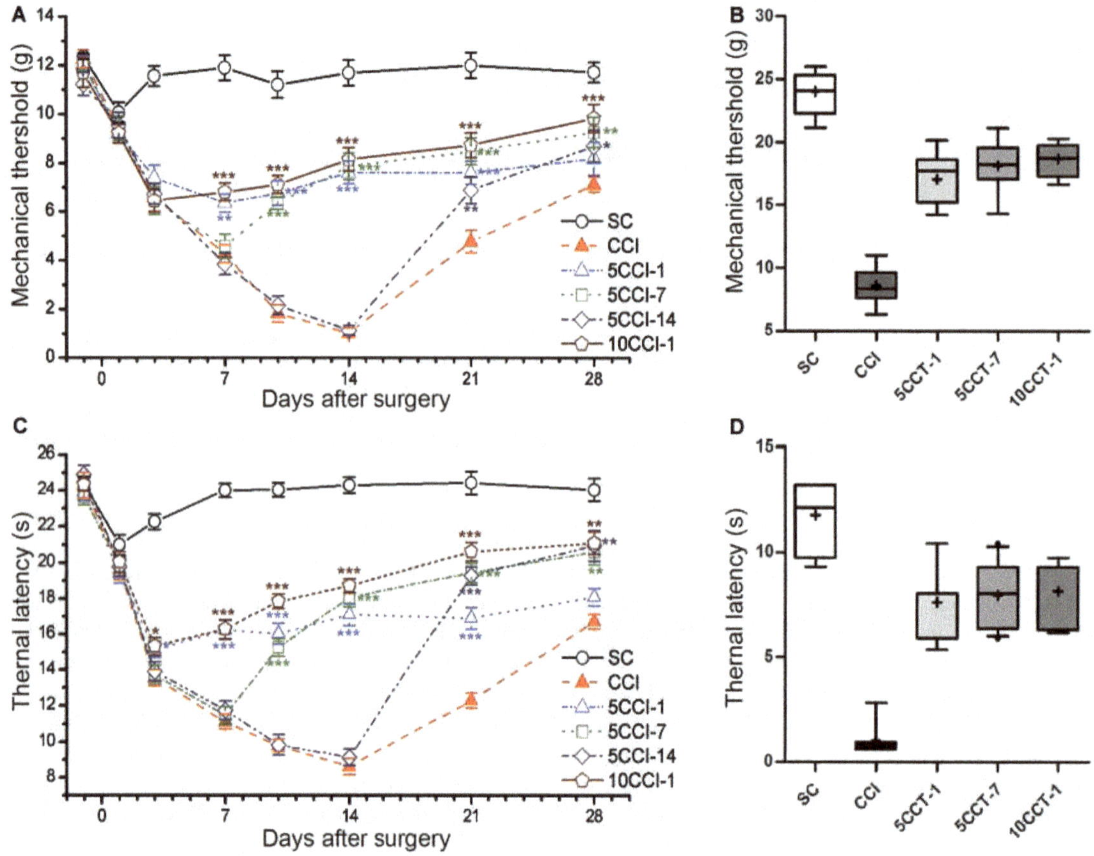

FIGURE 7 | Effects of repetitive tDCS on mechanical allodynia and thermal hyperalgesia with different intervention times. **(A)** MWT. **(B)** Boxplot graph of MWT at day 14 after CCI. **(C)** TWL. **(D)** Boxplot graph of TWL at day 14 after CCI. Five or 10 sessions repetitive tDCS (20 min and 200 μA) with different intervention times were administered started on days 1, 7 and 14 following CCI surgery, respectively. Sham CCI (SC); CCI plus five sessions daily con-tDCS from day 1 after CCI (5CCT-1); CCI plus five sessions daily con-tDCS from day 7 after CCI (5CCT-7); CCI plus five sessions daily con-tDCS from day 14 after CCI (5CCT-14); CCI plus 10 sessions con-tDCS from day 1 after CCI (10CCT-1). All behavior tests were tested 1 day before the CCI surgery and at days 1, 3, 7, 10, 14, 21 and 28 after CCI surgery. Statistical significance was analyzed by two-way ANOVA followed by Tukey's *post hoc* test. $^{*}p < 0.05$, $^{**}p < 0.01$, $^{***}p < 0.001$ vs. CCI group.

re-assessed on days 21 and 28 following CCI. Therefore, to create more effective and long-lasting after-effects, we should increase the stimulation duration and the current intensity. In the last few decades, there has been consensus that increasing stimulation duration prolongs the occurrence and duration of after-effects in humans and animals (Nitsche et al., 2008), which we verified in our study. However, increasing of duration and intensity has limitations. Considering the safety of tDCS, we choose 200 μA as the highest intensity because in our preliminary experiments we observed transient tremors if the intensity was over 220 μA. On the other hand, we found that there were no statistical differences in pain thresholds between CCT200-30 and CCT200-20 groups (**Figure 6**), suggesting that the antinociceptive effects of tDCS may be saturated after 20 min of tDCS at 200 μA. As such, it is necessary to determine the best intervention time if the stimulation intensity and duration cannot be further increased to continue prolonging the after-effects of tDCS.

CCI was first reported by Bennett and Xie (1988) and was regarded as a typical model in neuropathic pain research. The duration of neuropathic pain was divided into two parts (**Figure 2**). Part one was described as the "progression period" and referred to days 1 through 14 following CCI, peaking between days 10 and 14; part two was described as "recovery period" and referred to the period following day 14 in which the sensitivity to pain decreased daily. We chose two time points (1 and 7 days after surgery) in the progression period and one point in the recovery period (14 days after surgery) for delivering tDCS. There were substantial signs of recovery in each treatment group compared to the CCI group: (1) repetitive A-tDCS reversed the decreased thresholds observed in CCI rats at every time point; (2) early intervention prevented the sharp decrease in the pain threshold, but did not restore the threshold to its normal level; (3) as chronic pain worsened, the degree of antinociception following tDCS decreased and the after-effect were not well maintained; (4) antinociceptive effects were present when tDCS was delivered throughout the progressed

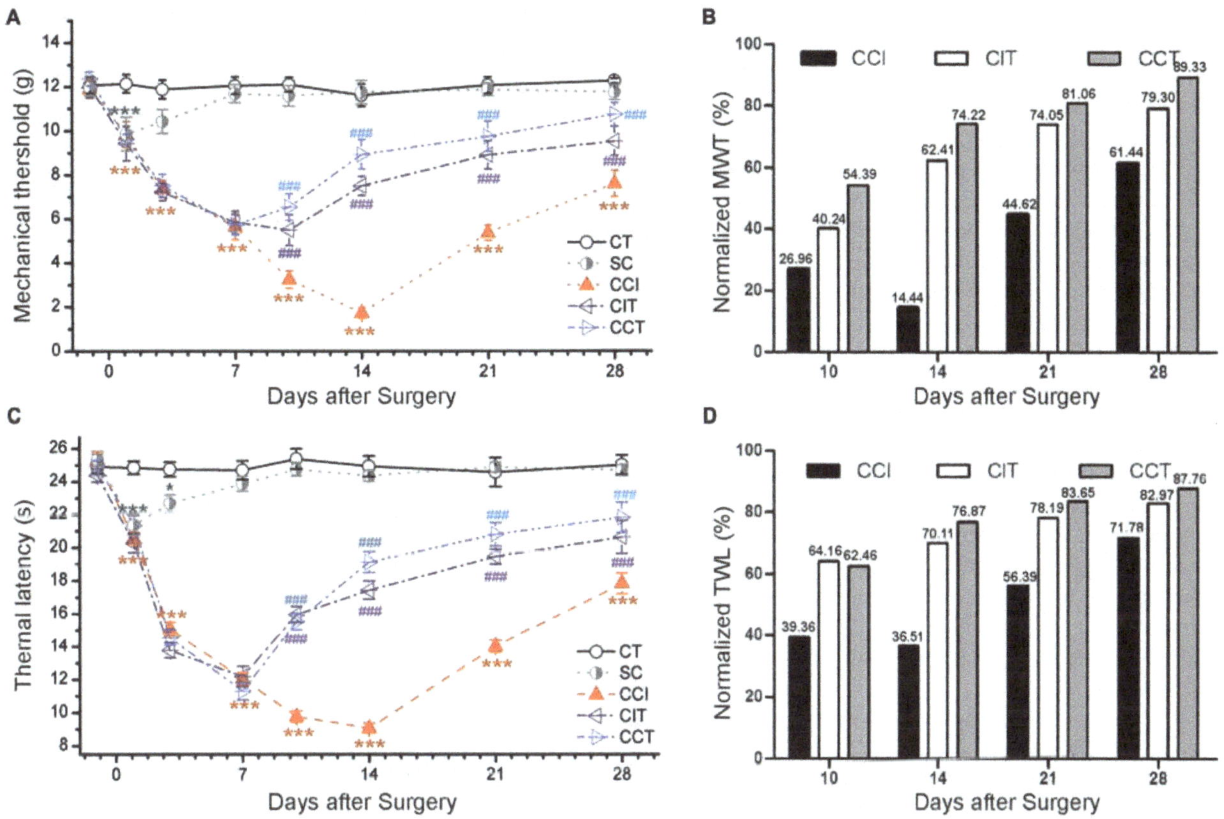

FIGURE 8 | Effects of repetitive tDCS on mechanical allodynia and thermal hyperalgesia with different locations in female rats. **(A)** MWT. **(B)** Normalized of MWT. **(C)** TWL. **(D)** Normalized of TWL. Five sessions daily of tDCS (200 μA, 20 min) were administration started on day 7 following CCI surgery. CT (control); SC (sham CCI); CIT (CCI + ip-tDCS treatment); CCT (CCI + con-tDCS treatment). CIT and CCT treatments significantly increased the values of TWL and MWT. All behavior tests were tested 1 day before the CCI surgery and on days 1, 3, 7, 10, 14, 21 and 28 after CCI surgery. Statistical significance was analyzed by two-way ANOVA followed by Tukey's *post hoc* test. *$p < 0.05$, ***$p < 0.001$ vs. CT group, ###$p < 0.001$ vs. CCI group.

period; and (5) pain thresholds significantly improved when tDCS were given at the beginning of the recovery period (**Figure 7**).

To the best of our knowledge, we are the first to discover that intervention time is another key factor that influences the efficacy of stimulation. With the same intensity and duration, the efficacy of analgesia was prolonged and consolidated by choosing the right time points when stimulation is participated in the pain processing and extending the original session of tDCS.

Clinically, A-tDCS is widely used in chronic pain treatment, an intensity of 2 mA and duration of 20 min with five or seven daily repetitions are usually chosen, parameters that have proven effects (Mori et al., 2010; Ngernyam, 2014). However, other researchers have also been obtained in which A-tDCS was ineffective in the treatment of chronic pain using the same conditions (Ihle et al., 2014; Nardone et al., 2014) The patient described in this study had stable chronic pain for at least 6 months with a high VAS scores before the stimulation, however, intervention time was not considered during therapy. A proper intervention time, the number of session and the length of stimulus duration should be considered and may be dependent on different states and causes of illness (Ihle et al., 2014). Our results suggest that clinicians should consider personalized treatment in patients with chronic neuropathic pain, pay attention to specific stimulus parameters and disease characteristics.

Furthermore, brain lesions were reported when the current density was greater than 142.9 A/m^2 in rat experiments. Our studies used a maximum current density of 63.69 A/m^2 (200 $\mu A/3.14\ mm^2$) which is not associated with any tissue injure after tDCS (Liebetanz et al., 2009).

Futhermore, we examined the effect of tDCS in female rats. Previous work found gender-related differences in utilitarian behavior after tDCS with greater effects in females as compared to males (Chaieb et al., 2008). For CCI rats, the chronic nociceptive processing was similar in both sexes, but male rats responded more quickly than females to a thermal nociceptive stimulus, and the stimulus elicited less robust thermal hyperalgesic symptoms in males than in females (Tall et al., 2001). In our study, we also found hyperalgesia and allodynia in female CCI rats. Both ip- and con-tDCS had the similar antinociceptive effects in female CCI rats. However, the hormonal fluctuate could be interfere in the nociceptive response

(Tall et al., 2001) and the mechanism of gender difference needs further study in the future.

There is increasing evidence that the after-effects of tDCS are not only driven by the regulation of inhibition and excitation, but also by the modification of synapses (Nguyen et al., 2011; Stagg and Nitsche, 2011). Another view is that tDCS does not only elicit that rapid depolarization required to produce action potentials in neurons, but also may produces long-lasting changes in cortical excitability and activity (Mylius et al., 2012). Consistent with this, another key hypothesis holds that chronic pain is likely to employ highly selective synaptic connections and molecular signaling pathways within pain-related cortical areas (Zhuo, 2008, 2013), resulting in cortical plasticity in both the descending and ascending systems. In the rat with peripheral injured, bilateral M1 receives pain-related information from the thalamus and the somatosensory cortex that maps to the injured paw (Xie et al., 2009; Ossipov et al., 2010). Stimulation of M1 might induce plasticity changes and reorganizations in the expression of neurotransmitter receptors (Lefaucheur et al., 2010; Stagg and Nitsche, 2011) which might include tonic activation of NMDA receptors (Pertovaara and Wei, 2003; Nguyen et al., 2011) and an enhanced anti-hypersensitivity effect in dopamine receptors (Viisanen et al., 2012). We observed increased NMDA receptors in bilateral M1 regions in CCI rats after repetitive tDCS (unpublished results). Therefore, the changes in NMDA receptors after tDCS might decrease the function of brain areas related to pain management through long-term potentiation (LTP) synaptic efficacy, thereby inducing cortical reorganization and CNS network processing. These affects are likely to reintroduce an optimal excitation/inhibition balance that allows for optimal homeostatic plasticity (Nitsche and Paulus, 2011; Stagg and Nitsche, 2011; Krause et al., 2013; Ngernyam, 2014).

The present study demonstrates the antinociceptive effect of tDCS in the male and female CCI rats. Both ip-DCS and con-tDCS produce a long-lasting analgesic effect on neuropathic pain, and the optimal stimulation parameters of tDCS are future studied. These dates may be helpful for the clinical applications of tDCS in pain control. More investigations on the synaptic mechanisms of tDCS should be conducted in the future.

AUTHOR CONTRIBUTIONS

H-ZR and H-ZW conceived and designed the study. H-ZW wrote the manuscript. S-HG, Y-DZ and W-JH carried out the animals' experiments. H-ZW and X-LT participated in the treatment of tDCS. H-ZW and S-HG participated in data analyses and arranged the figures. All authors have read and approved the final manuscript.

ACKNOWLEDGMENTS

This work was supported by the National Natural Science Foundation of China (Grant number 31171069, 2011).

REFERENCES

Bennett, G. J., and Xie, Y. K. (1988). A peripheral mononeuropathy in rat that produces disorders of pain sensation like those seen in man. *Pain* 33, 87–107. doi: 10.1016/0304-3959(88)90209-6

Bindman, L. J., Lippold, O. C. J., and Redfearn, J. W. (1964). The action of brief polarizing currents on the cerebral cortex of the rat (1) during current flow and (2) in the production of long-lasting after-effects. *J. Physiol.* 172, 369–382. doi: 10.1113/jphysiol.1964.sp007425

Borckardt, J. J., Bikson, M., Frohman, H., Reeves, S. T., Datta, A., Bansal, V., et al. (2012). A pilot study of the tolerability and effects of high-definition transcranial direct current stimulation (HD-tDCS) on pain perception. *J. Pain* 13, 112–120. doi: 10.1016/j.jpain.2011.07.001

Brunoni, A. R., Nitsche, M. A., Bolognini, N., Bikson, M., Wagner, T., Merabet, L., et al. (2012). Clinical research with transcranial direct current stimulation (tDCS): challenges and future directions. *Brain Stimul.* 5, 175–195. doi: 10.1016/j.brs.2011.03.002

Chaieb, L., Antal, A., and Paulus, W. (2008). Gender-specific modulation of short-term neuroplasticity in the visual cortex induced by transcranial direct current stimulation. *Vis. Neurosci.* 25, 77–81. doi: 10.1017/s0952523808080097

Chaplan, S. R., Bach, F. W., Pogrel, J. W., Chung, J. M., and Yaksh, T. L. (1994). Quantitative assessment of tactile allodynia in the rat paw. *J. Neurosci. Methods* 53, 55–63. doi: 10.1016/0165-0270(94)90144-9

Cioato, S. G., Medeiros, L. F., Marques Filho, P. R., Vercelino, R., de Souza, A., Scarabelot, V. L., et al. (2016). Long-lasting effect of transcranial direct current stimulation in the reversal of hyperalgesia and cytokine alterations induced by the neuropathic pain model. *Brain Stimul.* 9, 209–217. doi: 10.1016/j.brs.2015.12.001

Dall Agnol, L., Medeiros, L. F., Torres, I. L. S., Deitos, A., Brietzke, A., Laste, G., et al. (2014). Repetitive transcranial magnetic stimulation increases the corticospinal inhibition and the brain-derived neurotrophic factor in chronic myofascial pain syndrome: an explanatory double-blinded, randomized, sham-controlled trial. *J. Pain* 15, 845–855. a doi: 10.1016/j.jpain.2014.05.001

Dedoncker, J., Brunoni, A. R., Baeken, C., and Vanderhasselt, M. (2016). A Systematic review and meta-analysis of the effects of transcranial direct current stimulation (tDCS) over the dorsolateral prefrontal cortex in healthy and neuropsychiatric samples: influence of stimulation parameters. *Brain Stimul.* 9, 501–517. doi: 10.1016/j.brs.2016.04.006

DosSantos, M. F., Martikainen, I. K., Nascimento, T. D., Love, T. M., DeBoer, M. D., Schambra, H. M., et al. (2014). Building up analgesia in humans via the endogenous mu-opioid system by combining placebo and active tDCS: a preliminary report. *PLoS One* 9:e102350. doi: 10.1371/journal.pone.0102350

Dworkin, R. H., O'Connor, A. B., Kent, J., Mackey, S. C., Raja, S. N., Stacey, B. R., et al. (2013). Interventional management of neuropathic pain: NeuPSIG recommendations. *Pain* 154, 2249–2261. doi: 10.1016/j.pain.2013.06.004

Ferrucci, R., Cortese, F., and Priori, A. (2015). Cerebellar tDCS: how to do it. *Cerebellum* 14, 27–30. doi: 10.1007/s12311-014-0599-7

Filho, P. R. M., Vercelino, R., Cioato, S. G., Medeiros, L. F., de Oliveira, C., Scarabelot, V. L., et al. (2016). Transcranial direct current stimulation (tDCS) reverts behavioral alterations and brainstem BDNF level increase induced by neuropathic pain model: long-lasting effect. *Prog. Neuropsychopharmacol. Biol. Psychiatry* 64, 44–51. doi: 10.1016/j.pnpbp.2015.06.016

Fontaine, D., Hamani, C., and Lozano, A. (2009). Efficacy and safety of motor cortex stimulation for chronic neuropathic pain: critical review of the literature. *J. Neurosurg.* 110, 251–256. doi: 10.3171/2008.6.17602

Fregni, F., Boggio, P. S., Lima, M. C., Ferreira, M. J. L., Wagner, T., Rigonatti, S. P., et al. (2006). A sham-controlled, phase II trial of transcranial direct current stimulation for the treatment of central pain in traumatic spinal cord injury. *Pain* 122, 197–209. doi: 10.1016/j.pain.2006.02.023

Gandiga, P. C., Hummel, F. C., and Cohen, L. G. (2006). Transcranial DC stimulation (tDCS): a tool for double-blind sham-controlled clinical studies in brain stimulation. *Clin. Neurophysiol.* 117, 845–850. doi: 10.1016/j.clinph.2005.12.003

Hargreaves, K., Dubner, R., Brown, F., Flores, C., and Joris, J. (1988). A new and sensitive method for measuring thermal nociception in cutaneous hyperalgesia. *Pain* 32, 77–88. doi: 10.1016/0304-3959(88)90026-7

He, W., Cui, J., Du, L., Zhao, Y., Burnstock, G., Zhou, H., et al. (2012). Spinal P2X7 receptor mediates microglia activation-induced neuropathic pain in the sciatic nerve injury rat model. *Behav. Brain Res.* 226, 163–170. doi: 10.1016/j.bbr.2011.09.015

Ihle, K., Rodriguez-Raecke, R., Luedtke, K., and May, A. (2014). tDCS modulates cortical nociceptive processing but has little to no impact on pain perception. *Pain* 155, 2080–2087. doi: 10.1016/j.pain.2014.07.018

Krause, B., Márquez-Ruiz, J., and Cohen Kadosh, R. C. (2013). The effect of transcranial direct current stimulation: a role for cortical excitation/inhibition balance? *Front. Hum. Neurosci.* 7:602. doi: 10.3389/fnhum.2013.00602

Laste, G., Caumo, W., Adachi, L. N. S., Rozisky, J. R., de Macedo, I. C., Filho, P. R. M., et al. (2012). After-effects of consecutive sessions of transcranial direct current stimulation (tDCS) in a rat model of chronic inflammation. *Exp. Brain Res.* 221, 75–83. doi: 10.1007/s00221-012-3149-x

Lee, M., Kim, Y. H., Im, C. H., Kim, J. H., Park, C. H., Chang, W. H., et al. (2015). What is the optimal anodal electrode position for inducing corticomotor excitability changes in transcranial direct current stimulation? *Neurosci. Lett.* 584, 347–350. doi: 10.1016/j.neulet.2014.10.052

Lefaucheur, J., Holsheimer, J., Goujon, C., Keravel, Y., and Nguyen, J. (2010). Descending volleys generated by efficacious epidural motor cortex stimulation in patients with chronic neuropathic pain. *Exp. Neurol.* 223, 609–614. doi: 10.1016/j.expneurol.2010.02.008

Lefaucheur, J. P. (2006). The use of repetitive transcranial magnetic stimulation (rTMS) in chronic neuropathic pain. *Neurophysiol. Clin.* 36, 117–124. doi: 10.1016/j.neucli.2006.08.002

Liebetanz, D., Fregni, F., Monte-Silva, K. K., Oliveira, M. B., Amâncio-dos-Santos, A., Nitsche, M. A., et al. (2006). After-effects of transcranial direct current stimulation (tDCS) on cortical spreading depression. *Neurosci. Lett.* 398, 85–90. doi: 10.1016/j.neulet.2005.12.058

Liebetanz, D., Koch, R., Mayenfels, S., König, F., Paulus, W., and Nitsche, M. A. (2009). Safety limits of cathodal transcranial direct current stimulation in rats. *Clin. Neurophysiol.* 120, 1161–1167. doi: 10.1016/j.clinph.2009.01.022

Lucas, J. M., Ji, Y., and Masri, R. (2011). Motor cortex stimulation reduces hyperalgesia in an animal model of central pain. *Pain* 152, 1398–1407. doi: 10.1016/j.pain.2011.02.025

Mori, F., Codecà, C., Kusayanagi, H., Monteleone, F., Buttari, F., Fiore, S., et al. (2010). Effects of anodal transcranial direct current stimulation on chronic neuropathic pain in patients with multiple sclerosis. *J. Pain* 11, 436–442. doi: 10.1016/j.jpain.2009.08.011

Mylius, V., Borckardt, J. J., and Lefaucheur, J. (2012). Noninvasive cortical modulation of experimental pain. *Pain* 153, 1350–1363. doi: 10.1016/j.pain.2012.04.009

Nahmias, F., Debes, C., de Andrade, D. C., Mhalla, A., and Bouhassira, D. (2009). Diffuse analgesic effects of unilateral repetitive transcranial magnetic stimulation (rTMS) in healthy volunteers. *Pain* 147, 224–232. doi: 10.1016/j.pain.2009.09.016

Nardone, R., Höller, Y., Leis, S., Höller, P., Thon, N., Thomschewski, A., et al. (2014). Invasive and non-invasive brain stimulation for treatment of neuropathic pain in patients with spinal cord injury: a review. *J. Spinal Cord Med.* 37, 19–31. doi: 10.1179/2045772313Y.0000000140

Ngernyam, N. (2014). Transcranial direct current stimulation in neuropathic pain. *J. Pain Relief* s3:1. doi: 10.4172/2167-0846.1000s3-001

Nguyen, J. P., Nizard, J., Keravel, Y., and Lefaucheur, J. P. (2011). Invasive brain stimulation for the treatment of neuropathic pain. *Nat. Rev. Neurol.* 7, 699–709. doi: 10.1038/nrneurol.2011.138

Nitsche, M. A., Cohen, L. G., Wassermann, E. M., Priori, A., Lang, N., Antal, A., et al. (2008). Transcranial direct current stimulation: state of the art 2008. *Brain Stimul.* 1, 206–223. doi: 10.1016/j.brs.2008.06.004

Nitsche, M. A., and Paulus, W. (2011). Transcranial direct current stimulation—update 2011. *Restor. Neurol. Neurosci.* 29, 463–492. doi: 10.3233/RNN-2011-0618

O'Connell, N. E., Wand, B. M., Marston, L., Spencer, S., and Desouza, L. H. (2011). Non-invasive brain stimulation techniques for chronic pain. A report of a Cochrane systematic review and meta-analysis. *Eur. J. Phys. Rehabil. Med.* 47, 309–326.

O'Neill, F., Sacco, P., and Nurmikko, T. (2015). Evaluation of a home-based transcranial direct current stimulation (tDCS) treatment device for chronic pain: study protocol for a randomised controlled trial. *Trials* 16:186. doi: 10.1186/s13063-015-0710-5

Ooi, Y., Satomura, Y., Seki, J., Yanagida, T., and Seiyama, A. (2006). Optical coherence tomography reveals *in vivo* cortical plasticity of adult mice in response to peripheral neuropathic pain. *Neurosci. Lett.* 397, 35–39. doi: 10.1016/j.neulet.2005.12.010

Ossipov, M. H., Dussor, G. O., and Porreca, F. (2010). Central modulation of pain. *J. Clin. Invest.* 120, 3779–3787. doi: 10.1172/JCI43766

Ou, S., Zhao, Y., Xiao, Z., Wen, H., Cui, J., and Ruan, H. (2011). Effect of lappaconitine on neuropathic pain mediated by P2X3 receptor in rat dorsal root ganglion. *Neurochem. Int.* 58, 564–573. doi: 10.1016/j.neuint.2011.01.016

Pertovaara, A., and Wei, H. (2003). A dissociative change in the efficacy of supraspinal versus spinal morphine in the neuropathic rat. *Pain* 101, 237–250. doi: 10.1016/s0304-3959(02)00320-2

Roizenblatt, S., Fregni, F., Gimenez, R., Wetzel, T., Rigonatti, S. P., Tufik, S., et al. (2007). Site-specific effects of transcranial direct current stimulation on sleep and pain in fibromyalgia: a randomized, sham-controlled study. *Pain Pract.* 7, 297–306. doi: 10.1111/j.1533-2500.2007.00152.x

Rojas-Piloni, G., Martínez-Lorenzana, G., Condés-Lara, M., and Rodríguez-Jiménez, J. (2010). Direct sensorimotor corticospinal modulation of dorsal horn neuronal C-fiber responses in the rat. *Brain Res.* 1351, 104–114. doi: 10.1016/j.brainres.2010.06.010

Soler, M. D., Kumru, H., Pelayo, R., Vidal, J., Tormos, J. M., Fregni, F., et al. (2010). Effectiveness of transcranial direct current stimulation and visual illusion on neuropathic pain in spinal cord injury. *Brain* 133, 2565–2577. doi: 10.1093/brain/awq184

Spezia Adachi, L. N., Caumo, W., Laste, G., Fernandes Medeiros, L., Ripoll Rozisky, J., de Souza, A., et al. (2012). Reversal of chronic stress-induced pain by transcranial direct current stimulation (tDCS) in an animal model. *Brain Res.* 1489, 17–26. doi: 10.1016/j.brainres.2012.10.009

Stagg, C. J., and Nitsche, M. A. (2011). Physiological basis of transcranial direct current stimulation. *Neuroscientist* 17, 37–53. doi: 10.1177/1073858410386614

Tall, J. M., Stuesse, S. L., Cruce, W. L. R., and Crisp, T. (2001). Gender and the behavioral manifestations of neuropathic pain. *Pharmacol. Biochem. Behav.* 68, 99–104. doi: 10.1016/s0091-3057(00)00461-5

Viisanen, H., Ansah, O. B., and Pertovaara, A. (2012). The role of the dopamine D2 receptor in descending control of pain induced by motor cortex stimulation in the neuropathic rat. *Brain Res. Bull.* 89, 133–143. doi: 10.1016/j.brainresbull.2012.08.002

Volz, M. S., Volz, T. S., Brunoni, A. R., de Oliveira, J. P. V. T., and Fregni, F. (2012). Analgesic effects of noninvasive brain stimulation in rodent animal models: a systematic review of translational findings. *Neuromodulation* 15, 283–295. doi: 10.1111/j.1525-1403.2012.00478.x

Woods, A. J., Antal, A., Bikson, M., Boggio, P. S., Brunoni, A. R., Celnik, P., et al. (2016). A technical guide to tDCS, and related non-invasive brain stimulation tools. *Clin. Neurophysiol.* 127, 1031–1048. doi: 10.1016/j.clinph.2015.11.012

Xiao, Z., Ou, S., He, W., Zhao, Y., Liu, X., and Ruan, H. (2010). Role of midbrain periaqueductal gray P2X3 receptors in electroacupuncture-mediated endogenous pain modulatory systems. *Brain Res.* 1330, 31–44. doi: 10.1016/j.brainres.2010.03.030

Xie, Y.-F., Huo, F.-Q., and Tang, J.-S. (2009). Cerebral cortex modulation of pain. *Acta Pharmacol. Sin.* 30, 31–41. doi: 10.1038/aps.2008.14

Young, N. A., Sharma, M., and Deogaonkar, M. (2014). Transcranial magnetic stimulation for chronic pain. *Neurosurg. Clin. N. Am.* 25, 819–832. doi: 10.1016/j.nec.2014.07.007

Yu, X., Li, Y., Wen, H., Zhang, Y., and Tian, X. (2015). Intensity-dependent effects of repetitive anodal transcranial direct current stimulation on learning and memory in a rat model of Alzheimer's disease. *Neurobiol. Learn. Mem.* 123, 168–178. doi: 10.1016/j.nlm.2015.06.003

Zaghi, S., Heine, N., and Fregni, F. (2009). Brain stimulation for the treatment of pain: a review of costs, clinical effects, and mechanisms of treatment for three different central neuromodulatory approaches. *J. Pain Manag.* 2, 339–352.

Zhuo, M. (2008). Cortical excitation and chronic pain. *Trends Neurosci.* 31, 199–207. doi: 10.1016/j.tins.2008.01.003

Zhuo, M. (2013). Long-term potentiation in the anterior cingulate cortex and chronic pain. *Philos. Trans. R. Soc. Lond. B Biol. Sci.* 369:20130146. doi: 10.1098/rstb.2013.0146

Zimmermann, M. (1983). Ethical guidelines for investigations of experimental pain in conscious animals. *Pain* 16, 109–110. doi: 10.1016/0304-3959(83)90201-4

8

Modulation of Neurogenesis through the Promotion of Energy Production Activity is behind the Antidepressant-Like Effect of Colonial Green Alga, *Botryococcus braunii*

*Kazunori Sasaki[1,2], Mahmoud B. Othman[3], Mikihide Demura[4], Makoto Watanabe[4,5] and Hiroko Isoda[3,5]**

[1] Interdisciplinary Research Center for Catalytic Chemistry, National Institute of Advanced Industrial Science and Technology, Tsukuba, Japan, [2] Faculty of Pure and Applied Sciences, University of Tsukuba, Tsukuba, Japan, [3] Alliance for Research on North Africa, University of Tsukuba, Tsukuba, Japan, [4] Algal Biomass and Energy System R&D Center, University of Tsukuba, Tsukuba, Japan, [5] Faculty of Life and Environmental Sciences, University of Tsukuba, Tsukuba, Japan

***Correspondence:**
Hiroko Isoda
isoda.hiroko.ga@u.tsukuba.ac.jp

Algae have been recognized as important resources providing functional components due to their capacity to exert beneficial effects on health. Therefore, there is increasing interest in investigating the biological activity of algae. In this study, we evaluated the antidepressant-like effect of the administration of 100 mg/kg/day of the ethanol extract of colonial green alga *Botryococcus braunii* (EEB) for 14 consecutive days in the forced swimming test (FST)-Induced depression in imprinting control region (ICR) mice. Imipramine, a commercial antidepressant drug, was used as a positive control. In addition, we investigated the molecular mechanisms underlying the effect of EEB by measuring ATP production and by assessing any change in gene expression at the end of the treatment using real-time polymerase chain reaction (PCR) and microarray assays. We showed that the immobility time in the water-administered control (FST stress) group gradually increased from day 1 to day 14. However, treatment with EEB caused a significant decrease of immobility time in the FST compared with that in the FST stress group. Microarray and real-time PCR results revealed that EEB treatment induced variation in the expression of several genes associated with neurogenesis, energy metabolism, and dopamine synthesis. Interestingly, we revealed that only EEB treatment enhanced the promotion of energy production, while treatment with imipramine was ineffective. Our study provides the first evidence that *B. braunii* enhances energy production, which may contribute to the modulation of neurogenesis and to the enhancement of dopaminergic function, in turn potentially underlying the antistress- and antidepressant-like effects that we observed.

Keywords: microalgae, *Botryococcus braunii*, depression, forced swimming test, dopamine synthesis, energy promotion activity, neurogenesis

INTRODUCTION

Stress is a part of everyday life and particularly prevalent in modern societies. There are various sources of stress in people's lives, and excessive or prolonged exposure to such stress factors has a significant impact on our wellbeing, ultimately leading to emotional and behavioral changes, together with reduced cognitive function and physical illness. Therefore, it is not surprising that stress remains a top health concern, particularly in developed countries. The damaging effect of stress on cells is well-documented; in particular, stress affects neuronal cells and may lead to the induction of neurodegenerative disorders, such as Alzheimer's disease, Parkinson's disease, and major depression. Depression is a psychiatric disorder commonly characterized by a sense of prostration; in its most severe forms, it can be life-threatening. This disorder has a worldwide prevalence of ~17% (Liu et al., 2013). Depression, which is the most common type of affective disorders, is caused by a combination of biological, psychological, social, and other factors. Depressive syndrome is characterized by significant and lasting low mood (Lu et al., 2015). In clinical practice, drug classes used for the treatment of depression include monoamine oxidase inhibitors, selective serotonin noradrenaline reuptake inhibitors (SNRIs), selective serotonin reuptake inhibitors, and tricyclic antidepressants (Bouvier et al., 2003; Fava, 2003; Shen and Liang, 2007). However, these drugs can cause a variety of adverse effects, including nausea, headaches, and nerve pain. Therefore, new and safer antidepressants, which are derived from natural products and lack side effects, need to be developed.

Algae are photosynthetic organisms that mainly inhabit the hydrosphere. They form a large and diverse group within which over 40,000 species have been described so far. However, the total number of algal species is estimated to exceed 10 million, including those that remain undiscovered and undescribed (Norton et al., 1996). Some algae and particularly microalgae have served as important sources of functional materials, such as n-3 polyunsaturated fatty acids (PUFA), vitamins, minerals, polysaccharides, and bioactive compounds (Shahidi and Janak Kamil, 2001). Moreover, microalgae are known to exhibit various biological and physiological activities, including antioxidant, anticoagulant, antiviral, and antitumoral effects (Pangestuti and Kim, 2011). Therefore, we speculated that microalgae have the potential to be a valuable natural resource of novel bioactive compounds and focused on the colonial green alga *Botryococcus braunii* Kützing (Trebouxiophyceae, Chlorophyta), which is found worldwide in freshwater and brackish lakes, reservoirs, and ponds. *B. braunii* produces large amounts of hydrocarbons, which are excreted from cells and accumulate in its colonies. Therefore, it is considered to have great potential as a renewable source of chemical products and is useful for searching for new antidepressant drugs. Moreover, to the best of our knowledge, few reports on studies exploring the physiological effects of *B. braunii* have been published.

The objectives of this study were to evaluate the antidepressant-like effect of ethanol extract of *B. braunii* (EEB), using the forced swimming test (FST) to obtain a rodent model of depression by inducing stress in imprinting control region (ICR) mice, and to understand the molecular mechanism behind the antidepressant-like effect of EEB. We also focused our attention on changes in expression levels for genes associated with neurogenesis, energy promotion activity, and dopamine synthesis. In addition, we analyzed the neuroprotective effect of EEB using rat pheochromocytoma PC12 cells.

MATERIALS AND METHODS

Preparation of Ethanol Extract of *B. braunii* (EEB)

A dried sample of *B. braunii* was provided by ABES, the University of Tsukuba, Japan. The dried sample was extracted using 99.5% ethanol, in the dark, and at room temperature for 2 weeks, with shaking of the mixture occurring at least once a day. At the end of the procedure, the liquid fraction (EEB) was collected, filtered through a 0.22-μm filter (Merck Millipore, Billerica, MA, USA), and used in the *in vitro* assays. For animal dosing in the *in vivo* assay, EEB was concentrated using SpeedVac (Thermo Fisher Scientific, Waltham, MA, USA) and the dried EEB was dissolved in MilliQ water.

Animals

Male ICR mice (Charles River Laboratories Japan Inc., Yokohama, Kanagawa, Japan), 5 weeks old, weighing 35–40 g, were used for *in vivo* experiments. The animals were kept individually in cages and maintained with free access to water and food *ad libitum*, under a 12/12-h light/dark cycle. All of the experiments were carried out between 09:00 and 16:00, and the animals had been acclimatized for 7 days to the laboratory conditions ahead of the experiment. This animal experiment was approved by the Ethics Animal Care and Use Committee of the University of Tsukuba.

Administration of Ethanol Extract of *B. braunii* (EEB) to ICR Mice

After 1 week of acclimatization to the laboratory conditions, mice were assigned to three groups: a control group ($n = 8$), a group administered 20 mg/kg imipramine daily ($n = 8$), and a group administered 100 mg/kg EEB daily ($n = 8$). EEB dissolved in drinking water was administered orally using a tube and a syringe for 14 consecutive days. The control group was administered an equivalent volume of tap water.

Imipramine, an SNRI antidepressant drug that selectively increases dopamine and noradrenaline levels in the synaptic cleft, was used as a positive control. Imipramine was freshly dissolved in distilled water and orally administered to mice at a dose of 20 mg/kg, as reported in our previous study (Ben Othman et al., 2013).

Forced Swimming Test

The FST was conducted as previously described by Ben Othman et al. (2013) To carry out the FST, we used a cylindrical jar (14 cm in diameter × 25 cm in height) filled from the bottom with 19 cm of water at 25 ± 1°C. The FST was performed at 1, 2, 6, 10, and 14 d during the period of the oral administration of EEB. Each mouse was placed gently into the water and allowed to swim freely for 5 min. The mouse was considered immobile when it showed disparity and became motionless in the water. Periods of immobility were defined as when mice only made those movements that were necessary to keep their head above the water. The duration of immobility was recorded and analyzed off-line over the last 4 min of the test.

RNA Isolation from Mouse Brain

Following the last FST at day 14, all mice were sacrificed by dislocation of the cervical spine and their brains were isolated. A small amount (0.1 mg) of cerebral tissue was removed and washed with ice-cold phosphate-buffered solution (PBS). The total RNA was extracted from it using the ISOGEN kit (Nippon Gene Co. Ltd., Toyama, Japan), as we reported previously (Sasaki et al., 2013). Total RNA was quantified and assessed for its quality with the NanoDrop 2000 spectrophotometer (Thermo Scientific, Wilmington, DE, USA).

DNA Microarray Analysis

DNA microarray analysis was conducted on isolated RNA samples from brains treated with EEB. DNA microarray analysis was performed as reported previously (Isoda et al., 2012; Samet et al., 2015). Double-stranded cDNA was synthesized from 100 ng of total RNA with the GeneAtlas 3′ IVT Express Kit (Affymetrix Inc., Santa Clara, CA, USA). Biotin-labeled amplified RNA (aRNA) was synthesized by *in vitro* transcription using the GeneChip 3′ IVT Express Kit (Affymetrix Inc., Santa Clara, CA, USA). A total of 9.4 mg of purified aRNA was fragmented using the GeneAtlas 3′ IVT Express Kit and was hybridized for 16 h at 45°C using GeneChip MG-430 PM microarray (Affymetrix Inc., Santa Clara, CA, USA). The chip was washed and stained in the Gene Atlas Fluidics Station 400 (Affymetrix Inc., Santa Clara, CA, USA) and then the resulting image was scanned using the GeneAtlas Imaging Station (Affymetrix Inc., Santa Clara, CA, USA). Data analysis was performed using the Partek Express software (Partek Inc., St. Louis, MO, USA) provided by Affymetrix as part of their GeneAtlas system. Compared with the control (water-treated group), fold change in expression in the imipramine- or EEB-treated group was calculated and converted to log 2 data.

Taqman Quantitative RT-PCR Analysis of Gene Expression in Mouse Brain

Based on the microarray analysis, reverse transcription reactions were carried out with the SuperScript III Reverse Transcriptase (RT) kit (Invitrogen, Carlsbad, CA, USA). In accordance with the manufacturer's instructions, 1 μg of total RNA and 1 μl of oligo$(dT)_{12-18}$ primers were denatured at 65°C for 5 min and subsequently chilled at 4°C. After the addition of SuperScript III RT (200 U), the reaction mix was incubated at 42°C for 60 min, followed by another 10 min at 70°C. All primer sets and TaqMan probes for experimental genes were from Applied Biosystems (Foster City, CA, USA): mouse tyrosine hydroxylase (TH) (Mm00447557_m1), mouse pyruvate carboxylase (PC) (Mm00500992_m1), mouse brain-derived neurotrophic factor (BDNF) (Mm04230607_s1), and mouse GAPDH (Mm99999915_g1). For the quantification of mRNA, TaqMan Real Time-PCR amplification reactions were carried out using an AB 7500 Fast Real-Time PCR system (Applied Biosystems). Amplifications were performed in a final volume of 20 μl, using 10 μl of TaqMan Universal PCR Master Mix UNG (Applied Biosystems), 1 μl of the corresponding primer/probe mix, and 9 μl of template cDNA (final concentration 100 ng/20 μl). Cycling conditions were as follows: 2 min at 50°C, 10 min at 95°C, and 40 cycles at 95°C for 15 s followed by 60°C for 1 min.

Measurement of Brain ATP Content

ATP levels in the bupropion tissues were measured with firefly bioluminescence using a luminescence luciferase assay kit (TOYO Ink, Tokyo, Japan). A small amount (0.1 mg) of cerebral tissue was homogenized with 10 mL of ice-cold homogenate buffer (0.25 M sucrose, 10 mM HEPES-NaOH, pH 7.4). After centrifugation, the supernatant was collected and 100 μL of it was transferred to a 96 well plate. After adding 100 μL of luciferin-luciferase solution (TOYO Ink, Tokyo, Japan), 150 μL of the mixed solution was transferred to another 96-well plate and incubated for 10 min. After 10 min of incubation, light emission was recorded using a luminometer (Powerscan HT; Dainippon Pharmaceutical, Osaka, Japan).

Cell Culture

PC12 cell culture and MTT assay were performed in accordance with our previous work (Sasaki et al., 2013). PC12 cells (RIKEN, Tsukuba, Japan) were cultured in 75 cm^2 flasks (BD Biosciences, San Jose, CA, USA) and maintained in Dulbecco's Modified Eagle's Medium (DMEM) (Sigma-Aldrich, St. Louis, MO, USA) containing 10% heat-inactivated horse serum (Gibco, Yokohama, Japan), 5% fetal bovine serum (Sigma-Aldrich), and supplemented with 100 $U{\cdot}ml^{-1}$ penicillin and 100 $\mu g{\cdot}ml^{-1}$ streptomycin (ICN Biomedicals, Tokyo, Japan), in a water-saturated 5% CO_2 atmosphere at 37°C. For the experiments in this study, cells were used between passage 3 and passage 8.

MTT Assay for Neuroprotection

Cell viability was measured using the 3-(4,5-dimethylthiazol-2-yl)-2,5-diphenyltetrazolium bromide (MTT) assay. PC12 cells (1×10^5 $cells{\cdot}ml^{-1}$) cultured in a 96-well plate (BD Biosciences) were pretreated with 1/1,000 dilution of EEB for 10 min, followed by the addition of 200 μM corticosterone (Sigma-Aldrich, St. Louis, MO, USA) for 48 h. After sample treatment, 100 μl of culture medium and 10 μl of MTT (5 $mg{\cdot}ml^{-1}$) were added and the cells were incubated for 6 h. The MTT formazan formed was dissolved in 100 μl of 10% SDS (w/v) and the absorbance was measured using a microtiter plate reader (Powerscan HT; Dainippon Sumitomo Pharma Co. Ltd., Osaka, Japan).

Statistical Analysis

Results are expressed as mean ± standard error of the mean (SEM). Statistical analysis of the results obtained in the FST was carried out using two-way ANOVA with Ryan-einot-gabriel-welsch multiple range test. One-way ANOVA followed by Ryan-einot-gabriel-welsch multiple range test was also used. The statistical evaluation was performed using the Student's *t*-test between control and corticosterone-treatment group in *in vitro* experiment. A $P < 0.05$ was considered statistically significant.

RESULTS

EEB Reversal of Depression-Like Behavior Induced by FST

FST is a behavioral animal model that has been widely adopted for investigating depression. To determine whether EEB has antidepressant-like activity, its effect on FST-induced stress in mice was investigated. The administration of 100 mg/kg EEB for 14 consecutive days caused no mortality or significant body weight change in any animal. As shown in **Figure 1**, the immobility time in the water-administered control (FST stress) group gradually increased from day 1 to day 14 (D = day; D1, 46.5 ± 13.2 s; D2, 55.4 ± 12.0 s; D6, 68.4 ± 11.5 s; D10, 71.5 ± 7.14 s; D14, 80.3 ± 6.40 s; $P < 0.05$). However, this trend was not observed in the imipramine- and EEB-administered groups.

At day 14, the average immobility time for the EEB-administered group (33.3 ± 7.0 s) was similar to that in the imipramine-administered group (26.3 ± 10.7 s), which represented our positive control (**Figure 1**). In mice treated with imipramine, EEB induced a three-fold reduction of the average immobility time compared with that in the water-administered control mice (80.3 ± 6.40 s; $P < 0.01$).

EEB-Induced Variation of Energy Metabolism-, Dopamine Production-, and Neurogenesis-Related Gene Expression

To evaluate the molecular mechanism behind the antidepressant-like effect of EEB, we performed microarray analysis of ICR mouse cerebrum to investigate changes in gene expression. We found that the expression of eight genes was altered in the ICR mice administered EEB compared with their levels in the control group (**Table 1**). These included the short stature homeobox 2 (Shox2), paired-like homeodomain transcription factor 2 (Pitx2), teashirt zinc finger family member 1 (Tshz1), and LIM homeobox protein 9 (Lhx9) genes associated with neurogenesis ($P < 0.05$; compared with the control group). Moreover, the expression of the polyribonucleotide nucleotidyltransferase 1 (Pnpt1) gene associated with energy metabolism was upregulated, while that of the arrestin domain containing 4 (Arrdc4) gene involved in the regulation of ATP production was downregulated ($P < 0.05$; compared with the control group). In addition, the expression of two genes associated with dopamine synthesis was modulated: the arginine/serine-rich coiled-coil 1 (Rsrc1) gene was upregulated, while the protein phosphatase 1, regulatory (inhibitor) subunit 1B (Ppp1r1b) gene was downregulated ($P < 0.05$; compared with the control group). A similar pattern of alterations of expression for the genes involved in neurogenesis and dopamine synthesis was observed in the imipramine-administered group. In summary, our results show that the administration of EEB induced variation in the expression of energy metabolism-, dopamine production-, and neurogenesis-related genes.

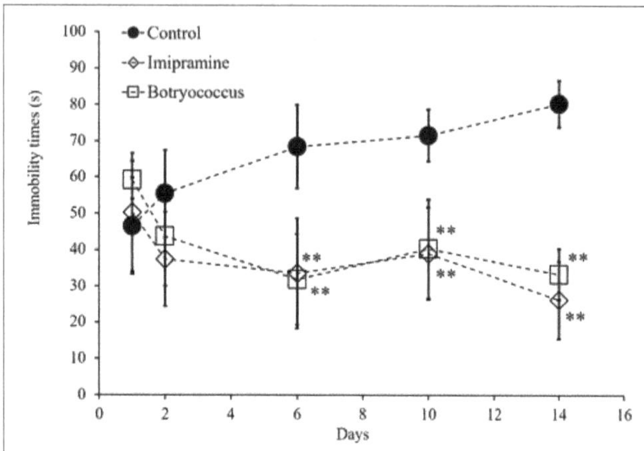

FIGURE 1 | Effects of administration of ethanol extract of *Botryococcus braunii* (EEB) on the immobility time in the forced swimming test (FST). Mice were orally administered water (control), imipramine (20 mg/kg), and EEB (100 mg/kg) daily for 14 consecutive days. FST was carried out on days 1, 2, 6, 10, and 14. The immobility time during the final 4 min of a 5-min total session was measured. FST immobility time measured for each group. Each data point expressed as the means ± SEM (n = 8) and were analyzed by two-way ANOVA followed by Ryan-einot-gabriel-welsch multiple range test, $^{**}P < 0.01$ vs. control group.

EEB-Induced Upregulation of BDNF, TH, and PC Gene Expression in ICR Mouse Cerebrum

Based on the results obtained from the microarray analysis, we investigated the mRNA expression levels of TH, PC, and BDNF in the ICR mouse cerebrum from the four experimental groups. Real-time (RT) PCR results (**Figure 2**) showed that the mRNA expression levels of TH were significantly upregulated in the EEB-administered groups (168.6 ± 21.0%, compared with the control group; $P < 0.01$; **Figure 2A**). The mRNA expression levels of PC and BDNF were also upregulated in the EEB-administered groups (PC: 142 ± 14.6% compared with the control group, $P < 0.01$; BDNF: 151.1 ± 22.4% compared with the control group, $P < 0.01$; **Figures 2B,C**). The administration of imipramine induced the overexpression of TH and BDNF, while it did not affect the mRNA level of PC (**Figure 2**).

EEB-Induced Production of ATP in ICR Mouse Cerebrum

The results obtained from the microarray analysis and RT-PCR showed that the upregulation of PC expression occurred in the EEB-administered groups, but not in the imipramine-administered mice. This indicates that EEB may increase the energy level of mice. Therefore, we determined the ATP content in the brains of the mice administered EEB. ATP is a multifunctional nucleotide referred to as the "molecular unit of currency" of intracellular energy transfer. It is also widely used as a marker of cell proliferation as it transports the chemical energy necessary for metabolic activity into the cells. The levels of ATP production in the EEB-administered mice were measured using a luciferase method. Mice administered EEB had significantly

TABLE 1 | Classification of the modulated genes and their fold change in expression in imipramine- and EEB-administered imprinting control region mice in comparison to the control, as identified by DNA microarray analysis.

Gene symbol	Gene name	Fold change (Control vs. imipramine)	Fold change (Control vs. EEB)	Molecular function	Associated phenotype
Shox2	Short stature homeobox 2	2.41**	3.09**	Plays an important role during the cerebellar neurogenesis, by maintaining the bone morphogenetic protein expression levels (Rosin et al., 2015)	Neurogenesis
Pitx2	Paired-like homeodomain transcription factor 2	1.84*	2.37*	Necessary for the normal development of the subthalamic nucleus	
Tshz1	Teashirt zinc finger family member 1	2.24**	2.02**	Maintain the expression of the prokineticin receptor 2, a G protein–coupled receptor essential for OB development and related to prokineticin signaling (Ragancokova et al., 2014)	
Lhx9	LIM homeobox protein 9	1.69**	1.39*	The typical marker genes of neurogenesis at the stage of immature neuronal cells (Ng et al., 2005).	
Pnpt1	Polyribonucleotide nucleotidyltransferase 1	1.06	2.05**	Gene encoding for PNPase, associate with Mitochondrial importation of nucleus-encoded RNAs (Kamenski et al., 2007; Tarassov et al., 2007; Duchene et al., 2009; Smirnov et al., 2011).	Energy Promotion
Arrdc4	Arrestin domain containing 4	−1.08	−1.33**	Negative regulator of glucose uptake (Patwari et al., 2009)	
Rsrc1	Arginine/serine-rich coiled-coil 1	1.63**	1.49**	Function in dopamine, glutamate, and fibroblast growth factor receptor signaling (Potkin et al., 2009)	Dopamine synthesis
Ppp1r1b	Protein phosphatase 1, regulatory (inhibitor) subunit 1B	−3.83**	−5.54**	Involved in the regulation of dopaminergic and glutaminergic signaling (Albert et al., 2002; Svenningsson et al., 2002)	

*Table values are expressed as mean ± SEM for three mice in each group. *$P < 0.05$, **$P < 0.01$ in comparison to control mice.*

upregulated levels of luminescence (152.8 ± 25.9%) compared with the control group ($P < 0.05$; **Figure 3**). In contrast, ATP levels of imipramine-administered mice were not significantly altered (**Figure 3**).

EEB-Mediated Protection against Corticosterone-Induced Cell Death

We next performed the MTT assay to investigate the viability of PC12 cells after treatment with corticosterone. Application of 200 μM corticosterone significantly decreased cell viability to 42.4 ± 4.3% compared with that of untreated cells ($P < 0.01$; **Figure 4**). However, pretreatment with a 1/1,000 dilution of EEB for 10 min reversed this corticosterone-induced cell death, resulting in a significant increase of cell viability by 34.3 ± 3.2% compared with that in the corticosterone-treated group" and revise ($P < 0.01$; **Figure 4**).

DISCUSSION

The present study was conducted to investigate the potential antidepressant-like effect of the microalga *B. braunii* and to elucidate the mechanism behind this effect. It is estimated that about 72,500 algal species have been characterized globally (Guiry, 2012). Algae produce bioactive secondary metabolites that include polyphenolic compounds, polysaccharides, steroids, fatty acids, carotenoids, mycosporine-like amino acids, halogenated compounds, polyketides, lectins, peptides, and their derivatives (Faulkner, 2001; Cardozo et al., 2007). Among the large number of biological functionalities of marine algal natural products, antioxidant, anti-inflammatory, anticancer, immunomodulatory, antidiabetic, antimicrobial, anticoagulant, tyrosinase inhibitory, and UV-protective effects have been highlighted, based on extensive studies (Blunt et al., 2015). However, there have been no reports on the antidepressant-like effect of *B. braunii*. Therefore, the discovery of novel antidepressants from these microalgae could provide new insight in the fields of biomedical and pharmaceutical research.

The FST is a standard animal model for behavioral measurement of depression. In this test, the degree to which the animal ceases to struggle and becomes relatively passively immobile is used to assess the depressive behavior. Immobility displayed in this behavioral model has been hypothesized to reflect behavioral despair, which may mimic depressive disorders in humans. Moreover, there is a significant correlation between the clinical potency of antidepressants and the potency of the same drugs in this model. Therefore, FST is usually adopted to screen or evaluate antidepressant drugs (Porsolt et al., 1978). The current study showed that the duration of immobility in

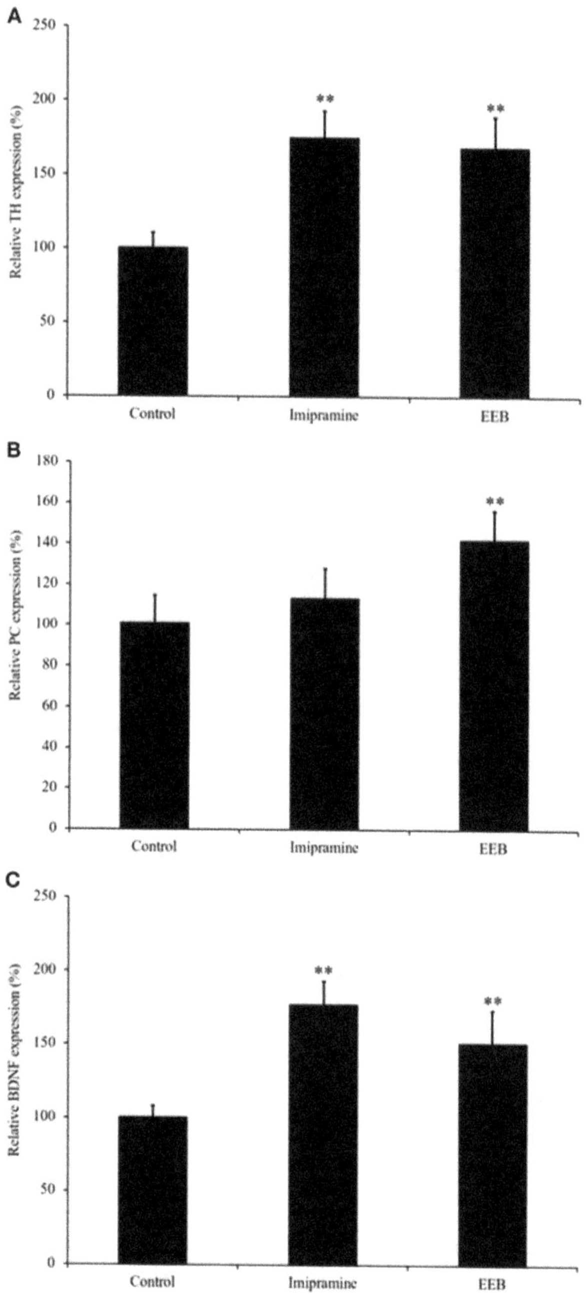

FIGURE 2 | Effect of the administration of ethanol extract of *Botryococcus braunii* (EEB) on mRNA expression of pyruvate carboxylase (PC), brain-derived neurotrophic factor (BDNF), and tyrosine hydroxylase (TH) in imprinting control region mouse cerebrum. Mice were orally administered water (control), imipramine (20 mg/kg), and EEB (100 mg/kg) daily for 14 consecutive days. Gene expression levels of TH **(A)**, PC **(B)**, and BDNF **(C)** were normalized to the GAPDH level and were expressed as the ratio of that in the control group. Values are expressed as the means ± SEM ($n = 3$ independent experiments) and were analyzed by one-way ANOVA followed by Ry8an-einot-gabriel-welsch multiple range test, $^{**}P < 0.01$ vs. control group.

the FST was significantly decreased after the administration of 100 mg/kg EEB, indicating that *B. braunii* has antidepressant effects. Furthermore, the oral administration of *B. braunii* showed a comparable effect to that of imipramine, a commercial antidepressant drug.

Microarray studies have been utilized as a useful tool to characterize depression-related biomarkers in patients as well as to further our understanding of the mechanisms underlying depression in rodent models of this disease. In this study, we identified eight genes that may be related to the pathophysiology of depressive-like behavior induced by FST-related stress. Three biological pathways (I: dopamine synthesis; II: energy metabolism; III: neurogenesis) were identified to be significantly altered in EEB-administered groups compared with their levels in the control group.

As proposed by Li et al. (2015), the monoamine hypothesis suggests that major depression might result from the dysregulation of monoaminergic neurotransmitters such as dopamine, serotonin, and norepinephrine in the central nervous system. Dopamine is the most abundant monoamine neurotransmitter in the brain, and plays a critical role in the regulation of emotions, motivation, cognition, reward circuits, and reinforcement behavior (Nieoullon and Coquerel, 2003; Wise, 2004; Perkins et al., 2008). In this study, microarray results showed that EEB induced downregulation of the Ppp1r1b gene, which encodes the dopamine- and cAMP-regulated neuronal phosphoprotein (DARPP-32). DARPP-32 is involved in the regulation of dopaminergic and glutaminergic signaling, and it has been implicated in various neurological and psychiatric disorders including schizophrenia (Albert et al., 2002) and depression (Svenningsson et al., 2002). In addition, EEB also induced overexpression of the Rscl gene, which functions in dopamine, glutamate, and fibroblast growth factor receptor signaling (Potkin et al., 2009). Moreover, we determined the mRNA expression of tyrosine hydroxylase (or tyrosine 3-monooxygenase, TH), the rate-limiting enzyme in the biosynthesis of the catecholamine neurotransmitters dopamine (DA) and norepinephrine (NE), and of adrenaline in neurons. The regulated activity of TH is thought to play a critical role in modulating the functional activity of the dopaminergic neuronal systems in the brain (Fu et al., 2006). Catecholamines, such as DA and NE, are known to play an important role in several behavioral and neurodegenerative diseases such as depression and Parkinson's disease. In our study, we demonstrated that EEB treatments increased the level of TH by 168.6 ± 21.0%, in comparison to that in vehicle-treated animals. Therefore, our results demonstrate that *B. braunii* may act as an antidepressant by enhancing catecholamine synthesis in the brain.

Energy metabolic pathways [including glycolysis/gluconeogenesis, the tricarboxylic acid (TCA) cycle, and oxidative phosphorylation] have been studied extensively in major depression disorder (Reininghaus et al., 2013). In our study, we reported the variation in the expression of Pnpt1 and Arrdc4 genes, which are involved in energy production. The Pnpt1 gene product is a polynucleotide phosphorylase (PNPase), an enzyme associated with the import of nucleus-encoded RNAs such as transfer RNA (tRNA), 5S ribosomal RNA (5S rRNA), ribonuclease P RNA (RNase P RNA), and MRP (mitochondrial RNA processing) RNAse into mitochondria. These nucleus-encoded RNAs are essential for mitochondrial DNA replication,

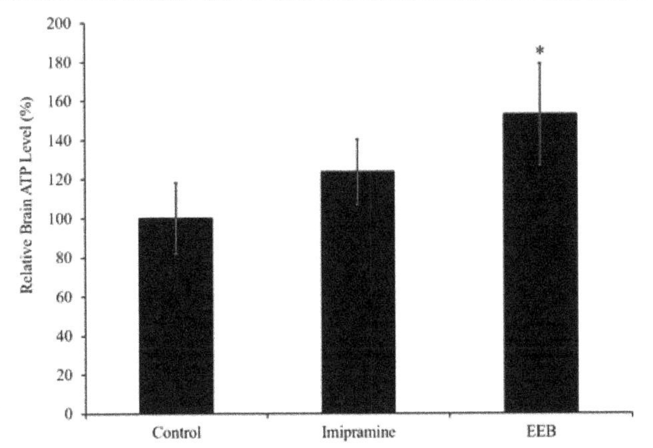

FIGURE 3 | Effects of the administration of ethanol extract of *B. braunii* (EEB) on the ATP levels in imprinting control region mouse cerebrum. Mice were orally administered water (control), imipramine (20 mg/kg), and EEB (100 mg/kg) daily for 14 consecutive days. Values are expressed as the means ± SEM ($n = 4$ independent experiments) and were analyzed by one-way ANOVA followed by Ryan-einot-gabriel-welsch multiple range test, $^{*}P < 0.05$ vs. control group.

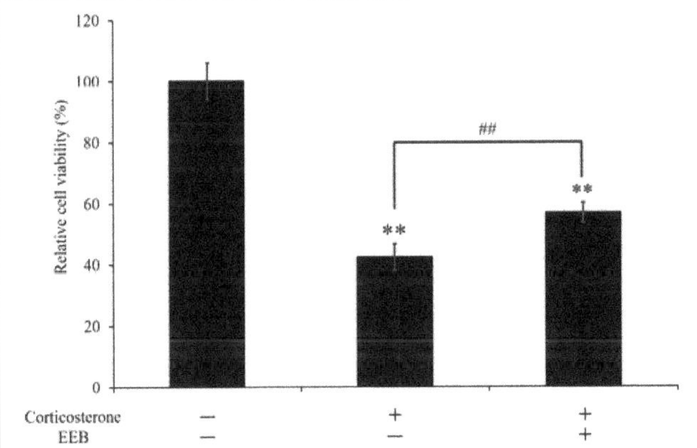

FIGURE 4 | Effect of ethanol extract of *B. braunii* (EEB) on the corticosterone-induced changes in PC12 cell viability. Values are expressed as the means ± SEM ($n = 5$ independent experiments) and were analyzed by one-way ANOVA followed by Ryan-einot-gabriel-welsch multiple range test, $^{**}P < 0.01$ vs. control cells, $^{\#\#}P < 0.01$ vs. corticosterone-treated cells.

transcription, and translation (Kamenski et al., 2007; Tarassov et al., 2007; Duchene et al., 2009; Smirnov et al., 2011). It is reported that deficiency of PNPase leads to cellular changes secondary to mitochondrial dysfunction, which include lactate accumulation, reduction in steady-state ATP levels, and reduced cell proliferation (Chen et al., 2006). The expression of Arrdc4, a negative regulator of glucose uptake (Patwari et al., 2009), was also downregulated in the cerebrum of EEB-administered ICR mice. Glucose is a fundamental nutrient, providing ATP for energy as well as carbon for biosynthesis (Vander Heiden et al., 2009). In addition, from the microarray results, we determined the gene expression of pyruvate carboxylase (PC), the rate-limiting enzyme catalyzing the ATP-dependent carboxylation of pyruvate to oxaloacetate. Our findings demonstrate that EEB may have an antidepressant-like effect by enhancing the level of energy availability. Interestingly, we demonstrated that only EEB treatments increased PC expression and ATP level in mouse cerebrum, while treatment with imipramine was ineffective on both of these parameters.

It is reported that ATP can induce an increase of BDNF expression (Klein et al., 2012). In our study, we demonstrated that EEB significantly increased BDNF gene expression in mouse brain. BDNF is essential for neurogenesis and for the rearrangement of axonal arbors in the brain (Jeanneteau et al., 2010). Furthermore, it has been shown that the exogenous application of BDNF to hippocampal neurons alleviates the neurotoxic insult induced by corticosterone (Nitta et al., 1999). In our *in vitro* experiment, we confirmed that 200 μM corticosterone induced a significant decrease in the viability of PC12 cells. However, EEB attenuated the cell death induced by corticosterone. This result indicates a close functional relationship between BDNF and glucocorticoids, and may explain the important role of BDNF in the modulation of major depressive disorder. In addition to our findings, previous publications demonstrated that the promotion of neurogenesis in mouse hippocampus could be the mechanism underlying the antidepressant-like effect of some drugs (Ito et al., 2008). Moreover, it was shown that compounds with an antidepressant-like effect in animal models of chronic unpredicted stress restored the levels of BDNF expression in hippocampal neurons and astrocytes (Jin et al., 2013).

Our results from the microarray analysis also revealed that EEB treatment induced the overexpression of a few genes related to the process of neurogenesis (Shox2, Pitx2, Tshz1, and Lhx9). Shox2 plays an important role during cerebellar neurogenesis, by maintaining the proper balance of morphogen sonic hedgehog and bone morphogenetic protein (BMP) expression levels (Rosin et al., 2015). The Pitx2 gene product is necessary for the normal development of the subthalamic nucleus and its projections to the tegmentum, as well as for the development of the projections arising in the midbrain. Pitx2 protein is expressed in postmitotic neurons of the midgestation central nervous system, including GABAergic neurons of the future thalamus and midbrain, and neurons of the subthalamic nucleus (Martin et al., 2002). Moreover, Pitx2 is required to establish functional connectivity of these terminally differentiated neurons (Martin et al., 2004). Tshz1 is expressed in the developing olfactory bulb (OB) and the dorsolateral ganglionic eminence (Caubit et al., 2005). It is reported that the major function of Tshz1 in the OB is to maintain the expression of prokineticin receptor 2, a G protein-coupled receptor essential for OB development and related to prokineticin signaling (Ragancokova et al., 2014). Prokineticin signaling is involved in several biological processes, including nociception, circadian rhythm, and neurogenesis (Ng et al., 2005; Hu et al., 2006; Li et al., 2012). Lhx9 was isolated by degenerate RT-PCR followed by mouse embryonic library screening. Lhx9 is one of the typical marker genes of neurogenesis at the stage of immature neuronal cells (Peukert et al., 2011). These results suggest that EEB treatment induced the enhancement of neurogenesis through the promotion of energy production.

The results from our study showed that *B. braunii* has an antidepressant-like effect in ICR mice with FST-induced depression. This microalga may contain proteins, carbohydrates, lipids, or bioactive molecules such as n-3 PUFA and carotenoids that exert an antidepressant-like effect. And, *B. braunii* produces carotenoids including β-carotene, lutein, violaxanthin, canthaxanthin, astaxanthin, and zeaxanthin (Ranga Rao et al., 2006, 2010). A number of reports have been published on studies in which attempts were made to elucidate the antidepressant effect of these active substances. For example, astaxanthin was shown to improve the impaired behavior in an animal model of autism, presumably by its antioxidant activity (Al-Amin et al., 2015). Additionally, n-3 PUFAs are under investigation for their possible use in the treatment and prevention of depression. An early study in rodents demonstrated that a reduction of dietary n-3 PUFA intake induced a decrease in the levels of nerve growth factor (NGF) in the hippocampus, and that NGF levels in different brain regions were affected differently by dietary n-3 PUFA deficiency and restoration (Ikemoto et al., 2000). Interestingly, meta-analysis of clinical trials using a combination of different types of n-3 PUFA, such as EPA and DHA, supplementation in patients with affective disorders and depression showed the therapeutic benefit of this combination for the amelioration of symptoms in patients affected by major depressive disorder (Grosso et al., 2014). Therefore, *B. braunii*, which is rich in n-3 PUFA and carotenoids, may be useful as a new therapeutic agent for depression. Further studies on the chemical composition of *B. braunii* will be necessary.

CONCLUSION

In summary, we report here for the first time evidence showing that *B. braunii* exerts an antidepressant-like effect in an animal model of depression. This appears to be mediated by the enhancement of energy promotion, neurogenesis, and dopamine synthesis in the brain. The observed effects of this alga showed in terms of significant differences compared with imipramine, a commercial antidepressant drug that was used as a positive control in this study, indicating a difference in the molecular mechanism underlying their antidepressant effects. These molecular mechanisms are currently not understood and will be the focus of our future research.

AUTHOR CONTRIBUTIONS

KS, MO, and HI conceived and designed the experiments; KS and MO performed the experiments; KS prepared the figures and tables; KS analyzed and interpreted the results, and wrote the paper; MD and MW provided *B. braunii*; and HI edited and revised the manuscript.

FUNDING

This study was supported by the Fukushima Algae Project.

ACKNOWLEDGMENTS

We wish to thank Hiroshi Kobayashi (ABES) for purification of the botryococcene.

We also wish to thank Shinji Kayano (Sobio Technologies Inc.), Hidenori Michikawa (Sobio Technologies Inc.), and Yuki Sakai (Sobio Technologies Inc.) for the cultivation of *B. braunii*.

REFERENCES

Al-Amin, M. M., Rahman, M. M., Khan, F. R., Zaman, F., and Mahmud Reza, H. (2015). Astaxanthin improves behavioral disorder and oxidative stress in prenatal valproic acid-induced mice model of autism. *Behav. Brain Res.* 286, 112–121. doi: 10.1016/j.bbr.2015.02.041

Albert, K. A., Hemmings, H. C. Jr., Adamo, A. I. B., Potkin, S. G., Akbarian, S., Sandman, C. A., et al. (2002). Evidence for decreased DARPP-32 in the prefrontal cortex of patients with schizophrenia. *Arch. Gen. Psychiatry* 59, 705–712. doi: 10.1001/archpsyc.59.8.705

Ben Othman, M., Han, J., El Omri, A., Ksouri, R., Neffati, M., and Isoda, H. (2013). Antistress effects of the ethanolic extract from *Cymbopogon schoenanthus* growing wild in Tunisia. *Evid. Based Complement. Alternat. Med.* 2013:737401. doi: 10.1155/2013/737401

Blunt, J. W., Copp, B. R., Keyzers, R. A., Munro, M. H. G., and Prinsep, M. R. (2015). Marine natural products. *Nat. Prod. Rep.* 32, 116–211. doi: 10.1039/C4NP00144C

Bouvier, N., Trenque, T., and Millart, H. (2003). Development of antidepressant drugs. experience and prospects. *Presse Med.* 32, 519–522.

Cardozo, K. H. M., Guaratini, T., Barros, M. P., Falcão, V. R., Tonon, A. P., Lopes, N. P., et al. (2007). Metabolites from algae with economical impact. *Comp. Biochem. Physiol. C Pharmacol. Toxicol.* 146, 60–78. doi: 10.1016/j.cbpc.2006.05.007

Caubit, X., Tiveron, M. C., Cremer, H., and Fasano, L. (2005). Expression patterns of the three teashirt-related genes define specific boundaries in the developing and postnatal mouse forebrain. *J. Comp. Neurol.* 486, 76–88. doi: 10.1002/cne.20500

Chen, H. W., Rainey, R. N., Balatoni, C. E., Dawson, D. W., Troke, J. J., Wasiak, S., et al. (2006). Mammalian polynucleotide phosphorylase is an intermembrane space RNase that maintains mitochondrial homeostasis. *Mol. Cell Biol.* 26, 8475–8487. doi: 10.1128/MCB.01002-06

Duchene, A. M., Pujol, C., and Marechal-Drouard, L. (2009). Import of tRNAs and aminoacyl-tRNA synthetases into mitochondria. *Curr. Genet.* 55, 1–18. doi: 10.1007/s00294-008-0223-9

Faulkner, D. J. (2001). Marine natural products. *Nat. Prod. Rep.* 18, 1–49. doi: 10.1039/B006897G

Fava, M. (2003). Diagnosis and definition of treatment-resistant depression. *Biol. Psychiatry* 53, 649–659. doi: 10.1016/S0006-3223(03)00231-2

Fu, A. L., Wu, S. P., Dong, Z. H., and Sun, M. J. (2006). A novel therapeutic approach to depression via supplement with tyrosine hydroxylase. *Biochem. Biophys. Res. Commun.* 351, 140–145. doi: 10.1016/j.bbrc.2006.10.013

Grosso, G., Pajak, A., Marventano, S., Castellano, S., Galvano, F., Bucolo, C., et al. (2014). Role of omega-3 fatty acids in the treatment of depressive disorders, a comprehensive meta-analysis of randomized clinical trials. *PLoS ONE* 9:e96905. doi: 10.1371/journal.pone.0096905

Guiry, M. D. (2012). How many species of algae are there? *J. Phycol.* 48, 1057–1063. doi: 10.1111/j.1529-8817.2012.01222.x

Hu, W. P., Zhang, C., Li, J. D., Luo, Z. D., Amadesi, S., Bunnett, N., et al. (2006). Impaired pain sensation in mice lacking prokineticin 2. *Mol. Pain.* 2:35. doi: 10.1186/1744-8069-2-35

Ikemoto, A., Nitta, A., Furukawa, S., Ohishi, M., Nakamura, A., Fujii, Y., et al. (2000). Dietary n-3 fatty acid deficiency decreases nerve growth factor content in rat hippocampus. *Neurosci. Lett.* 285, 99–102. doi: 10.1016/S0304-3940(00)01035-1

Isoda, H., Motojima, H., Margout, D., Neves, M., Han, J., Nakajima, M., et al. (2012). Antiallergic effect of picholine olive oil-in-water emulsions through β-hexosaminidase release inhibition and characterization of their physicochemical properties. *J. Agric. Food Chem.* 60, 7851–7858. doi: 10.1021/jf3016078

Ito, N., Yabe, T., Gamo, Y., Nagai, T., Oikawa, T., Yamada, H., et al. (2008). Rosmarinic acid from Perillae herba produces an antidepressant-like effect in mice through cell proliferation in the hippocampus. *Biol. Pharm. Bull.* 31, 1376–1380. doi: 10.1248/bpb.31.1376

Jeanneteau, F., Deinhardt, K., Miyoshi, G., Bennett, A. M., and Chao, M. V. (2010). The MAP kinase phosphatase MKP-1 regulates BDNF-induced axon branching. *Nat. Neurosci.* 13, 1373–1379. doi: 10.1038/nn.2655

Jin, X., Liu, P., Yang, F., Zhang, Y. H., and Miao, D. (2013). Rosmarinic acid ameliorates depressive-like behaviors in a rat model of CUS and Up-regulates BDNF levels in the hippocampus and hippocampal-derived astrocytes. *Neurochem. Res.* 38, 1828–1837. doi: 10.1007/s11064-013-1088-y

Kamenski, P., Kolesnikova, O., Jubenot, V., Entelis, N., Krasheninnikov, I. A., Martin, R. P., et al. (2007). Evidence for an adaptation mechanism of mitochondrial translation via tRNA import from the cytosol. *Mol. Cell.* 26, 625–637. doi: 10.1016/j.molcel.2007.04.019

Klein, K., Aeschlimann, A., Jordan, S., Gay, R., Gay, S., and Sprott, H. (2012). ATP induced brain-derived neurotrophic factor expression and release from osteoarthritis synovial fibroblasts is mediated by purinergic receptor P2X4. *PLoS ONE.* 7:e36693. doi: 10.1371/journal.pone.0036693

Li, J. D., Hu, W. P., and Zhou, Q. Y. (2012). The circadian output signals from the suprachiasmatic nuclei. *Prog. Brain Res.* 199, 119–127. doi: 10.1016/B978-0-444-59427-3.00028-9

Li, Z., He, Y., Tang, J., Zong, X., Hu, M., and Chen, X. (2015). Molecular imaging of striatal dopamine transporters in major depression - a meta-analysis. *J. Affect. Disord.* 174, 137–143. doi: 10.1016/j.jad.2014.11.045

Liu, W., Sheng, H., Xu, Y., Liu, Y., Lu, J., and Ni, X. (2013). Swimming exercise ameliorates depression-like behavior in chronically stressed rats, relevant to proinflammatory cytokines and IDO activation. *Behav. Brain Res.* 242, 110–116. doi: 10.1016/j.bbr.2012.12.041

Lu, S. H., Guo, J., Cai, C., Liang, X. B., Guan, J. H., Peng, X., et al. (2015). Effects of kaixin powder on expression of 5-HT receptor in hippocampus of depressed rats induced by CUMS. *Chin. Herb. Med.* 7, 150–154. doi: 10.1016/S1674-6384(15)60031-4

Martin, D. M., Skidmore, J. M., Fox, S. E., Gage, P. J., and Camper, S. A. (2002). Pitx2 distinguishes subtypes of terminally differentiated neurons in the developing mouse neuroepithelium. *Dev. Biol.* 252, 84–99. doi: 10.1006/dbio.2002.0835

Martin, D. M., Skidmore, J. M., Philips, S. T., Vieira, C., Gage, P. J., Condie, B. G., et al. (2004). PITX2 is required for normal development of neurons in the mouse subthalamic nucleus and midbrain. *Dev. Biol.* 267, 93–108. doi: 10.1016/j.ydbio.2003.10.035

Ng, K. L., Li, J. D., Cheng, M. Y., Leslie, F. M., Lee, A. G., and Zhou, Q. Y. (2005). Dependence of olfactory bulb neurogenesis on prokineticin 2 signaling. *Science* 308, 1923–1927. doi: 10.1126/science.1112103

Nieoullon, A., and Coquerel, A. (2003). Dopamine: a key regulator to adapt action, emotion, motivation and cognition. *Curr. Opin. Neurol.* 16(Suppl. 2), S3–S9. doi: 10.1097/00019052-200312002-00002

Nitta, A., Ohmiya, M., Sometani, A., Itoh, M., Nomoto, H., Furukawa, Y., et al. (1999). Brain-derived neurotrophic factor prevents neuronal cell death induced by corticosterone. *J. Neurosci. Res.* 57, 227–235. doi: 10.1002/(SICI)1097-4547(19990715)57:2<227::AID-JNR8>3.0.CO;2-E

Norton, T. A., Melkonian, M., and Andersen, R. A. (1996). Algal biodiversity. *Phycologia* 35, 308–326. doi: 10.2216/i0031-8884-35-4-308.1

Pangestuti, R., and Kim, S. K. (2011). Biological activities and health benefit effects of natural pigments derived from marine algae. *J. Funct. Foods* 3, 255–266. doi: 10.1016/j.jff.2011.07.001

Patwari, P., Chutkow, W. A., Cummings, K., Verstraeten, V. L. R. M., Lammerding, J., Schreiter, E. R., et al. (2009). Thioredoxin-independent regulation of metabolism by the α-arrestin proteins. *J. Biol. Chem.* 284, 24996–25003. doi: 10.1074/jbc.M109.018093

Perkins, K. A., Lerman, C., Grottenthaler, A., Ciccocioppo, M. M., Milanak, M. E., Conklin, C. A., et al. (2008). Dopamine and opioid gene variants are associated with increased smoking reward and reinforcement owing to negative mood. *Behav. Pharmacol.* 19, 641–649. doi: 10.1097/FBP.0b013e32830c367c

Peukert, D., Weber, S., Lumsden, A., and Scholpp, S. (2011). Lhx2 and Lhx9 determine neuronal differentiation and compartition in the caudal forebrain by regulating Wnt signaling. *PLoS Biol.* 9:e1001218. doi: 10.1371/journal.pbio.1001218

Porsolt, R. D., Bertin, A., and Jalfre, M. (1978). "Behavioral despair" in rats and mice, strain differences and the effects of imipramine. *Eur. J. Pharmacol.* 51, 291–294. doi: 10.1016/0014-2999(78)90414-4

Potkin, S. G., Turner, J. A., Fallon, J. A., Lakatos, A., Keator, D. B., Guffanti, G., et al. (2009). Gene discovery through imaging genetics, identification of two novel genes associated with schizophrenia. *Mol. Psychiatry* 14, 416–428. doi: 10.1038/mp.2008.127

Ragancokova, D., Rocca, E., Oonk, A. M., Schulz, H., Rohde, E., et al. (2014). TSHZ1-dependent gene regulation is essential for olfactory bulb development and olfaction. *J. Clin. Invest.* 124, 1214–1227. doi: 10.1172/JCI72466

Ranga Rao, A., Sarada, R., Baskaran, V., and Ravishankar, G. A. (2006). Antioxidant activity of *Botryococcus braunii* extract elucidated *in vitro* models. *J. Agric. Food Chem.* 54, 4593–4599. doi: 10.1021/jf060799j

Ranga Rao, A., Sarada, R., and Ravishankar, G. A. (2010). Enhancement of carotenoids in green alga-*Botryococcus braunii* in various autotrophic media under stress conditions. *Int. J. Pharm. Bio Sci.* 4, 87–92.

Reininghaus, E. Z., Reininghaus, B., Ille, R., Fitz, W., Lassnig, R. M., Ebner, C., et al. (2013). Clinical effects of electroconvulsive therapy in severe depression and concomitant changes in cerebral glucose metabolism-an exploratory study. *J. Affect. Disord.* 146, 290–294. doi: 10.1016/j.jad.2012.07.034

Rosin, J. M., McAllister, B. B., Dyck, R. H., Percival, C. J., Kurrasch, D. M., and Cobb, J. (2015). Mice lacking the transcription factor SHOX2 display impaired cerebellar development and deficits in motor coordination. *Dev. Biol.* 399, 54–67. doi: 10.1016/j.ydbio.2014.12.013

Samet, I., Villareal, M. O., Motojima, H., Han, J., Sayadi, S., and Isoda, H. (2015). Olive leaf components apigenin 7-glucoside and luteolin 7-glucoside direct human hematopoietic stem cell differentiation towards erythroid lineage. *Differentiation* 89, 146–155. doi: 10.1016/j.diff.2015.07.001

Sasaki, K., El Omri, A., Kondo, S., Han, J., and Isoda, H. (2013). *Rosmarinus officinalis* polyphenols produce anti-depressant like effect through monoaminergic and cholinergic functions modulation. *Behav. Brain Res.* 238, 86–94. doi: 10.1016/j.bbr.2012.10.010

Shahidi, F., and Janak Kamil, Y. V. A. (2001). Enzymes from fish and aquatic invertebrates and their application in the food industry. *Trends Food Sci. Technol.* 12, 435–464. doi: 10.1016/S0924-2244(02)00021-3

Shen, J. W., and Liang, Z. J. (2007). Advances in research on biological etiology of depression and the antidepressants. *Pharm Care Res.* 7, 94–99.

Smirnov, A., Entelis, N., Martin, R. P., and Tarassov, I. (2011). Biological significance of 5S rRNA import into human mitochondria, role of ribosomal protein MRP-L18. *Genes Dev.* 25, 1289–1305. doi: 10.1101/gad.624711

Svenningsson, P., Tzavara, E. T., Witkin, J. M., Fienberg, A. A., Nomikos, G. G., and Greengard, P. (2002). Involvement of striatal and extrastriatal DARPP-32 in biochemical and behavioral effects of fluoxetine (Prozac). *Proc. Natl. Acad. Sci. U.S.A.* 99, 3182–3187. doi: 10.1073/pnas.052712799

Tarassov, I., Kamenski, P., Kolesnikova, O., Karicheva, O., Martin, R. P., Krasheninnikov, I. A., et al. (2007). Import of nuclear DNA- encoded RNAs into mitochondria and mitochondrial translation. *Cell Cycle* 6, 2473–2477. doi: 10.4161/cc.6.20.4783

Vander Heiden, M. G., Cantley, L. C., and Thompson, C. B. (2009). Understanding the Warburg effect, the metabolic requirements of cell proliferation. *Science* 324, 1029–1033. doi: 10.1126/science.1160809

Wise, R. A. (2004). Dopamine, learning and motivation. *Nat. Rev. Neurosci.* 5, 483–494. doi: 10.1038/nrn1406

9

Astrocyte Activation in Locus Coeruleus is Involved in Neuropathic Pain Exacerbation Mediated by Maternal Separation and Social Isolation Stress

*Kazuo Nakamoto[1], Fuka Aizawa[1], Megumi Kinoshita[1], Yutaka Koyama[2] and Shogo Tokuyama[1]**

[1] Department of Clinical Pharmacy, School of Pharmaceutical Sciences, Kobe Gakuin University, Kobe, Japan, [2] Laboratory of Pharmacology, Faculty of Pharmacy, Osaka Ohtani University, Osaka, Japan

Correspondence:
Shogo Tokuyama
stoku@pharm.kobegakuin.ac.jp

Our previous studies demonstrated that emotional dysfunction associated with early life stress exacerbated nerve injury-induced mechanical allodynia. Sex differences were observed in several anxiety tests, but not in mechanical allodynia. To elucidate the mechanism underlying these findings, we have now investigated the involvement of astrocytes in emotional dysfunction and enhancement of nerve injury-induced mechanical allodynia in mice subjected to maternal separation combined with social isolation (MSSI) as an early life stress. We measured expression of glial fibrillary acidic protein (GFAP), an astrocyte maker, in each brain area by immunohistochemistry. GFAP expression in the locus coeruleus (LC) of female, but not of male mice, significantly increased after MSSI, corresponding to the behavioral changes at 7 and 12 weeks of age. Lipopolysaccharide (LPS)-treated astrocyte-derived supernatant was administered to local brain regions, including LC. Intra-LC injection of conditioned medium from cultured astrocytes treated with LPS increased GFAP expression, anxiety-like behavior and mechanical allodynia in both male and female mice. Furthermore, increases in anxiety-like behavior correlated with increased mechanical allodynia. These findings demonstrate that emotional dysfunction and enhanced nerve injury-induced mechanical allodynia after exposure to MSSI are mediated, at least in part, by astrocyte activation in the LC. Male but not female mice may show resistance to MSSI stress during growth.

Keywords: early life stress, astrocyte, glia, locus coeruleus, maternal separation and social isolation stress

INTRODUCTION

Pain is a complex experience that involves purely sensory aspects, such as nociceptive stimuli, as well as emotional effects and feelings of unease (Bushnell et al., 2013). While pain serves as a warning against noxious stimuli (Woolf, 2010), chronic pain severely decreases quality of life. Also, emotional states heavily influence pain (Villemure and Bushnell, 2009). The severity of psychopathology in patients with major depressive disorder was positively associated with the prevalence of pain (Kishi et al., 2015). Thus, pain is modulated by both sensory and emotional factors. We previously demonstrated that emotional states altered mechanical allodynia and behavioral responses in mice (Nishinaka et al., 2015b). Another report showed that exposure to restraint stress before induction of neuropathic pain significantly increased mechanical allodynia (Norman et al., 2010). To obviate hyperalgesic effects associated directly with a physical stressor, we chose to use the maternal separation and social interaction (MSSI) stress model, a purely psychological form of stress. The MSSI model shows long-lasting behavioral and pathophysiological impairments (Niwa et al., 2011). We previously indicated that MSSI exacerbated mechanical allodynia. Interestingly, mice showed sex differences in several anxiety tests following MSSI, while pain was observed in both sexes after MSSI (Nishinaka et al., 2015b). These findings suggested that differences in sex may influence the relationship between pain control and emotional states.

Accumulating evidence indicates that astrocytes play a crucial role in the regulation of neural function in the central nervous system (CNS). Astrocytes are the most numerous type of glial cell. (Sofroniew and Vinters, 2010) and are important regulators of neural activity. For example, they contribute to neurotransmitter uptake and the CNS vascular response to neural activity (Sattler and Rothstein, 2006; Gordon et al., 2007). Moreover, astrocytes alter neural excitability via direct release of neuromodulator molecules (Halassa et al., 2009). In fact, astrocytes can release gliotransmitters (e.g., glutamate, GABA, D-serine, ATP) in response to neuronal activity including increase in the intracellular Ca^{2+} concentration (Araque et al., 2014; Gundersen et al., 2015). Exocytotic release of gliotransmitters or channel-mediated release via Ca^{2+}-dependent Cl^- channel and volume-regulated anion channel (Kimelberg et al., 2006; Park et al., 2013) were induced by increase in the cytosolic Ca^{2+} concentration. Furthermore, gliotransmitters can also be released through Ca^{2+}-independent opening of P2X purinergic receptors (Duan et al., 2003) or connexin/pannexin such as Cx43 hemichannels (Montero and Orellana, 2015). These factors can act on receptors on the presynaptic nerve terminal, or on post-synaptic dendrites when gliotransmitters are released from astrocytes. Astrocytes also contribute to the clinical and pathological mechanisms of disease processes. In a chronic pain study, reactive transformation of astrocytes following neuropathic pain contributed to the enhancement of neuropathic pain by releasing growth factors and inflammatory mediators (Zhang et al., 2013). Further, an astrocyte specific intermediate filament is up-regulated after nerve injury (Wei et al., 2008) and matrix metalloproteinase (MMP)-2-cleaved interleukin (IL)-1β induced astrocyte activation in the later phase of neuropathic pain (Kawasaki et al., 2008). More recently, glucocorticoid regulation of ATP release from spinal astrocytes underlies diurnal exacerbation of neuropathic mechanical allodynia (Koyanagi et al., 2016). Based on these reports, it is thought that astrocytes may play a role in modulation of pain.

On the other hand, astrocytes may influence neural networks that underlie specific behaviors, including aberrant behaviors associated with stress. For example, Cui et al. (2014), showed that glial dysfunction causes depressive-like behaviors and sleep disturbance. Chronic restraint stress causes dysfunction of astrocytes (Imbe et al., 2013). Zhang et al. (2015), showed that Chronic corticosterone exposure reduces hippocampal astrocyte structural plasticity in mice. A postmortem study reported that levels of glial fibrillary acidic protein (GFAP), a marker of reactive astrocytes, decreased in multiple brain regions in mood disorder patients (Miguel-Hidalgo et al., 2000; Bowley et al., 2002; Banasr and Duman, 2008; Chocyk et al., 2011; Gittins and Harrison, 2011). Although the mechanisms underlying emotional dysfunction mediated by astrocytes are unclear, these findings suggest that astrocytic abnormalities are associated with stress. In addition, astrocytes are regulated by sex hormones (Schwarz and Bilbo, 2012), indicating that there are sex differences in astrocytic function. We hypothesized that astrocytes are involved in sex-dependent emotional dysfunction induced by MSSI.

To examine our hypothesis, we investigated the influence of MSSI on GFAP expression levels and associated nociception and emotion in neuropathic pain states. Furthermore, to evaluate the involvement of local astrocytic activation, we developed a local activation model involving microinjection of supernatant from lipopolysaccharide (LPS)-treated astrocytes.

MATERIALS AND METHODS

Animals

Pregnant ddY mice at gestational day 14 and timed-pregnant Wister rats (day 16 or 17) and were obtained from Japan SLC, Inc. (Hamamatsu, Japan). The pregnant mice and rat were housed individually under standard conditions (23–24°C, 12 h light/dark cycle with lights on from 8 a.m. to 8 p.m.) with food and water available ad libitum. The present study was conducted in accordance with the Guiding Principles for the Care and Use of Laboratory Animals adopted by the Japanese Pharmacological Society. The Ethical Committee for Animal Experimentation of Kobe Gakuin University approved all experiments (approval number A15-33; Kobe, Japan).

Maternal Separation Combined with Social Isolation Stress Paradigm

Maternal separation combined with social isolation was performed as previously described (Nishinaka et al., 2015b). Pups both MSSI and control groups were housed with dams until postnatal day 14. On postnatal day 15, the pups in the MSSI group were placed in individual isolation cages (25 cm × 15 cm × 13 cm) for 6 h/day. The isolation cage was surrounded by the black paper to shut out visualization of other. After maternal separation for 7 days, pups were kept in isolation cages until 12 weeks of age. Dams and pups assigned to the control group were reared in standard conditions without maternal separation until weaning. After weaning, the control pups were separated by sex and housed 2–4 per cage.

Elevated Plus-Maze Test

The elevated plus-maze (EPM) test was performed as previously described (Nishinaka et al., 2015b). Mice were placed on the EPM consisted of two open arms and two enclosed arms (both 25 cm length × 8 cm width) which elevated 50 cm above the floor. The illumination levels of the open and enclosed arms were similar (approximately 360 lx). The behavior was tracked for 5 min by using a web camera. The number of entries to the open arms was expressed as a percentage of enties to all arms. The time spent in the open arms was expressed as a percentage of times in the open arms. A decreased the number of entry and the time spent to the open arms indicaeted anixis-behavior (Nishinaka et al., 2015b).

Partial Sciatic Nerve Ligation (PSL)

Mice were deeply anesthetized with sodium pentobarbital (65 mg/kg), and then surgery was performed as previously described at 9 weeks of age (Seltzer et al., 1990). In brief, the sciatic nerve of the right hind limb was exposed through a small incision. Half or two-thirds of the nerve thickness was tightly ligated with a silk suture. In sham-operated mice, the sciatic nerve was exposed without ligation.

von Frey Test

Mechanical allodynia after nerve injury was measured using the von Frey test as previously described (Nishinaka et al., 2015b). Mice were placed on a 5 mm × 5 mm wire mesh grid floor for 2–3 h prior to testing. The middle of the plantar surface of each hind paw was probed with 0.4 g von Frey filaments (Neuroscience, Inc., Tokyo, Japan). The withdrawal response to probing of the hind paw was measured 10 times. The intertrial interval was >10 s. An increase in the number of withdrawals indicates the degree of pain associated with mechanical stimulation (Nishinaka et al., 2015b).

Immunoflurorescence

Immunofluorescence staining was performed as previously described (Nakamoto et al., 2015) with some modifications. Mice were deeply anesthetized with diethyl ether and perfused transcardially with phosphate-buffered saline (PBS, pH 7.4) followed by 4% paraformaldehyde in 0.1 M PBS, pH 7.4. After perfusion, brain sections were incubated in 10% sucrose at 4°C for 3 h, and were kept 20% sucrose at 4°C overnight. Sections were cut at 20 μm on a cryostat (CM1850, Leica, Microsystems GmbH, Wetzlar, Germany). The brain sections were incubated with blocking buffer (3% BSA in PBST) for 1 h at room temperature, and then incubated overnight at 4°C with a mouse monoclonal anti-GFAP antibody (MAB3402, Merck Millipore KGaA, Darmstadt, Germany; 1:1000) and chicken polyclonal anti- tyrosine hydroxylase (TH) (Abcam, Tokyo, Japan; 1:200). The slices were incubated at room temperature for 2 h in secondary antibody (goat polyclonal anti-mouse IgG conjugated with AlexaFluor 488 or 594, goat polyclonal anti-chicken IgG conjugated with AlexaFluor 594; Life Technologies, Inc., Carlsbad, CA, United States; 1:200). The positive cells were detected with a confocal fluorescence microscope (FV1000, Olympus Corporation, Tokyo, Japan) or BZ-X710 microscope (Keyence, Itasca, IL, United States). Reactive astrocytes are characterized by cellular hypertrophy, hyperplasia, immunoreactivity of increased GFAP on tissue slides. The immunoreactivity of GFAP-positive astrocytic cells were quantified with the Image J cell counter analysis tool (ImageJ; NIH, Bethesda, MD, United States) in defined area of interest on the locus coeruleus (LC). The score was blinded to sampling times and animal treatments.

Preparation of Primary Cultured Astrocytes from Rat Brain

Astrocytes were prepared from the cerebra of 1- to 2-day-old Wistar rats as described (Koyama et al., 2004). The isolated cells were seeded at 1×10^4 cells/cm^2 in 75 cm^2 culture flasks and grown in minimal essential medium supplemented with 10% fetal bovine serum. To remove small process-bearing cells (mainly oligodendrocyte progenitors and microglia from the protoplasmic cell layer), the culture flasks were shaken at 250 rpm overnight 10–14 days after seeding. The monolayer cells were trypsinized and seeded on six-well culture plates or on 15 mm glass cover slips in 24-well culture plates. At this stage, approximately 95% of the cells showed immunoreactivity for GFAP.

Lipopolysaccharide (LPS) Stimulation of Rat Astrocytes

Before treatment, astrocytes in six well-culture plates were incubated in serum-free medium for 48 h. LPS was minimally diluted using serum-free medium before treatment. After incubation in serum-free medium, the cells were treated with 1,000 ng/mL LPS for 24 h.

Microinjection of Astrocyte Supernatant

Microinjection of astrocyte culture supernatant into the LC was performed as previously described (Nakamoto et al., 2015), with some modifications. Briefly, mice were anesthetized with pentobarbital (65 mg/kg) and immobilized on a stereotaxic frame (SR-5M; NARISHIGE, Co., Ltd, Tokyo, Japan). A microsyringe with a 30-gauge stainless steel needle was inserted unilaterally into the LC (5.4 mm posterior to bregma, 0.9 mm lateral from the midline, and 4.0 mm deep) and astrocyte supernatant (0.2 μL) injected incrementally over 1 min (**Figure 3A**). The injection site in LC was confirmed using 0.5% Trypan blue in saline.

Statistical Analyses

All data are expressed as the mean ± the standard error of the mean (SEM). Significant differences were determined by a one-way analysis of variance (ANOVA) followed by Scheffe's multiple comparison tests (for comparisons between more than three groups) or Student's *t*-test (for comparisons between two groups). A *P*-value < 0.05 was considered significant.

RESULTS

MSSI Stress Induced an Increase in GFAP Protein Expression in the LC Area of Female But Not Male Mice

Immunoreactivity for GFAP was observed surrounding TH positive cells in the LC. In males, MSSI stress did not affect GFAP

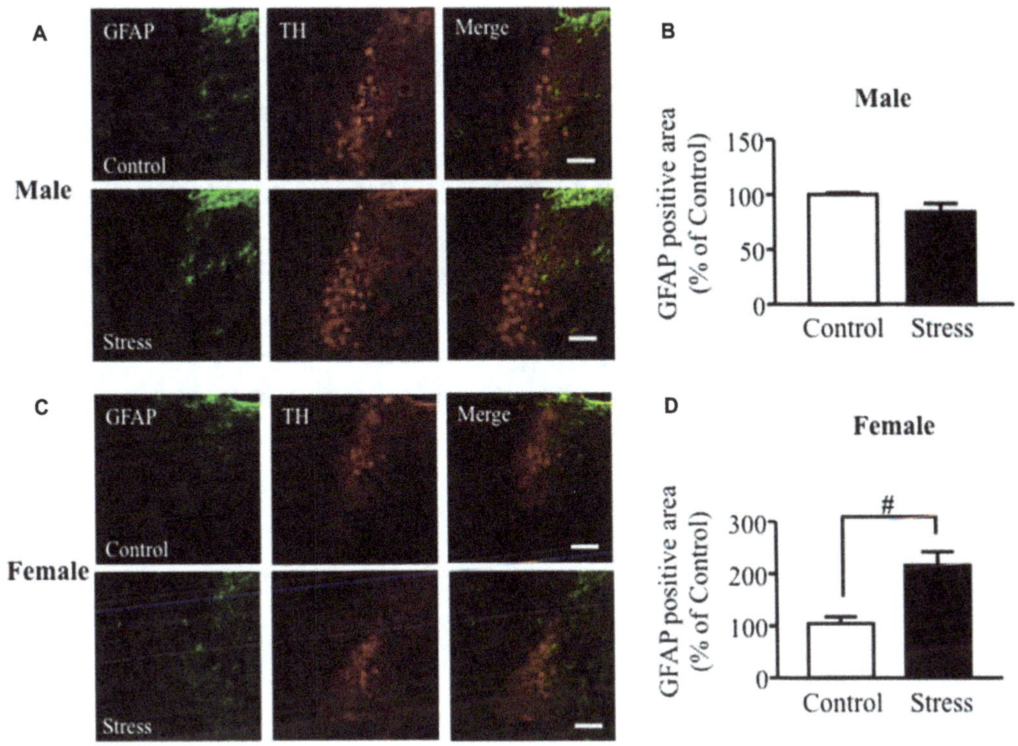

FIGURE 1 | Maternal separation combined with social isolation (MSSI) stress induced an increase in GFAP protein expression in the LC area of female but not male mice. Representative images showing immunofluorescence labeling of GFAP (green) and TH (Red) in the LC of MSSI stressed mice at 7 weeks of age, before PSL. Percentage of the GFAP positive area over the total area including LC after MSSI in **(A,B)** male mice and **(C,D)** female mice. Panel shows representative images of the GFAP positive area. Results expressed as percent of Control (mean ± SEM) from $n = 3$ male mice and $n = 3$ female mice. $^{\#}P < 0.05$, vs. Control, Student's *t*-test. Scale bar = 100 mm. LC, locus coeruleus.

expression in the LC at 7 weeks of age, before PSL (**Figures 1A,B**). In contrast, MSSI stress induced a significant increase in GFAP expression in the LC of female mice, compared to control female mice, at 7 weeks of age (**Figures 1C,D**).

The MSSI-Induced Increase in LC GFAP Expression Was Suppressed by PSL in Female Mice

At 12 weeks of age, the increased GFAP protein expression was observed in brain regions including the LC of MSSI-stressed female mice, compared to control female mice. This MSSI-induced increase in LC GFAP expression was suppressed by PSL (**Figures 2A,B**). In other region of the brain, GFAP protein expression did not change in male and female mice (Supplementary Figure 1).

LPS-Treated Astrocyte-Conditioned Medium Microinjection into the LC Induced Increased GFAP Expression in Male and Female Mice

In male and female mice, microinjection of LPS-treated astrocyte-derived supernatant into the brainstem area, including the LC, significantly increased local GFAP expression compared to non-treated control medium (**Figures 3B–E**). GFAP positive cells were observed surrounding TH positive cells in the LC (**Figure 3F**).

LPS-Treated Astrocyte-Conditioned Medium Microinjection into the LC Induced Anxiety-Like Behavior and PSL-Induced Mechanical Allodynia in Male Mice

In male mice, microinjection of LPS-treated astrocyte-derived supernatant into the brainstem area, including the LC, significantly decreased the number of open arm crossings and time spent in the open arms compared to vehicle-treated male mice (**Figures 4A,B**). In contrast, there was no difference in the number of center zone crossings between vehicle- and LPS-treated groups (**Figure 4C**). The entries into open arms (%) or the time spent in open arms (%) correlated negatively with the response time to mechanical stimuli after PSL in vehicle- or LPS-treated male mice (**Figure 4D**). At 1 week after PSL, the vehicle- and LPS-treated astrocyte-derived supernatant treated mice showed an increased number of responses to mechanical stimuli compared to vehicle- and LPS-treated injected sham injured male mice. Mice injected with LPS-treated astrocyte-derived supernatant showed a tendency toward an

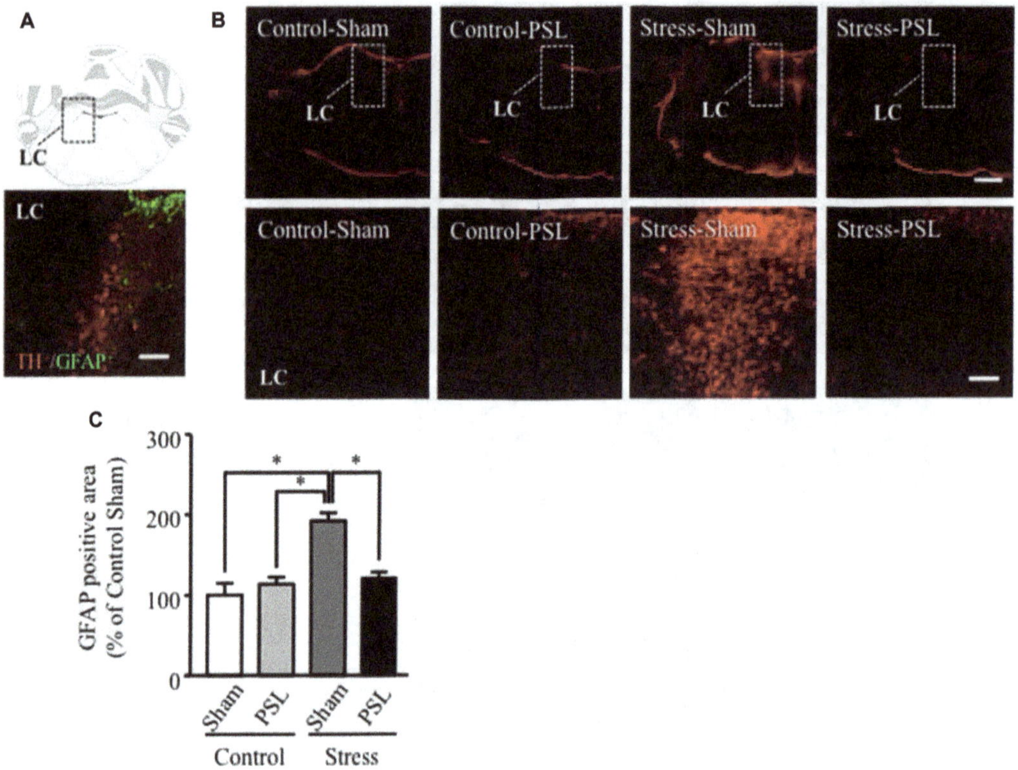

FIGURE 2 | The MSSI-induced increase in LC GFAP expression was suppressed by PSL in female mice. Representative images showing immunofluorescence labeling of GFAP (green) and TH (Red) in the LC of mice **(A)**. Percentage of the GFAP positive area over the total area including LC of MSSI stressed mice at 12 weeks of age, after PSL after PSL **(B)**. Panel shows representative images of the GFAP positive area. Results expressed as percent of Control (mean ± SEM in female mice: $n = 3$) **(C)**. *$P < 0.01$ vs. Control-Sham, vs. Control-PSL, vs. Stress-PSL, Scheffe's test. Scale bar = 100 mm. LC, locus coeruleus.

increase in the number of responses to mechanical stimuli compared to vehicle-treated injected PSL male mice. However, the number of responses against mechanical stimuli did not change between the vehicle treated group and the LPS-treated astrocyte-derived supernatant group prior to PSL (**Figure 4E**).

LPS-Treated Astrocyte-Derived Supernatant Microinjection into the LC Caused Anxiety-Like Behavior and PSL-Induced Mechanical Allodynia in Female Mice

Similar results were obtained in female mice. Female mice microinjected with LPS-treated astrocyte-derived supernatant showed a decreased number of open arm crossings and time spent in the open arms compared to vehicle-treated female mice (**Figures 5A,B**). The number of crossings in the center zone was comparable to that in vehicle-treated female mice (**Figure 5C**). The entries into open arms (%) or the time spent in open arms (%) correlated negatively with the response time to mechanical stimuli after PSL in vehicle- or LPS-treated female mice (**Figure 5D**). At 1 week after PSL, vehicle- and LPS-treated astrocyte-derived supernatant female mice showed an increased number of responses to mechanical stimuli compared to vehicle- and LPS-treated supernatant- injected female mice. Furthermore, the number of responses to mechanical stimuli showed a significant increase in LPS-treated PSL female mice compared to vehicle-treated PSL female mice. In contrast, the number of responses to mechanical stimuli before PSL was similar in both vehicle- and LPS-treated supernatant-injected female mice (**Figure 5E**).

DISCUSSION

Both the LC in the pons and the rostral ventromedial medulla (RVM) contribute to the regulation of pain and emotion (Aston-Jones et al., 1999; Yoshimura and Furue, 2006). Noradrenergic and serotonergic neurons are localized to the LC and RVM, respectively, and project to multiple higher brain areas as well as to the spinal cord. The descending pathways regulate nociceptive signaling in the spinal cord. It has been reported that chronic stress activates or suppress neuronal activity in the LC, and neuropathic pain suppress neuronal activity in the LC, which is associated with the development of anxiety-like behaviors in mice (Borges et al., 2015). Selective depletion of noradrenaline in the LC causes anxiety- and depression-like behaviors (Itoi et al., 2011). Physiological changes in glial cells of the medulla oblongata are associated with disease states and altered neuronal activity (Alvarez-Maubecin et al., 2000;

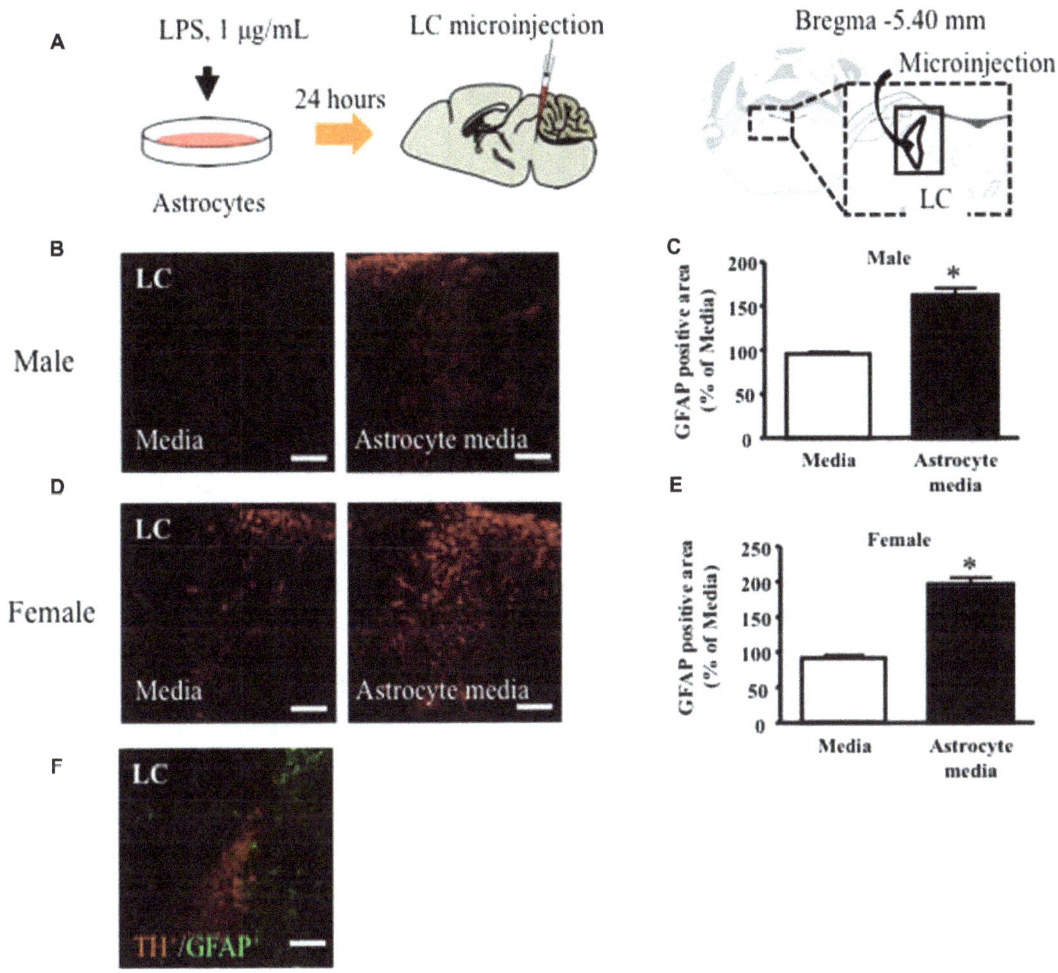

FIGURE 3 | Lipopolysaccharide (LPS)-treated astrocyte-conditioned medium microinjection into the LC increased GFAP expression in male and female mice. **(A)** Schematic diagram of the experimental protocol for microinjection into the LC. LC, locus coeruleus. Representative images showing immunofluorescence labeling of GFAP (red) in the LC of mice. **(A)** Percentage of the GFAP positive area over the total area including LC after microinjection in male **(B,C)** and female **(D,E)** mice. GFAP (Red) *$P < 0.05$, vs. Media, Student's *t*-test. Representative images showing immunofluorescence labeling of GFAP (green) and TH (Red) in the LC of mice **(F)**. Representative images of astrocytes in LC after microinjection. GFAP (Green), TH (Red). Scale bar = 100 mm.

O'Donnell et al., 2012). For example, downregulation of astrocytic gene expression was observed in the postmortem LC of major depressive disorder patients (Chandley et al., 2013). Chronic restraint stress decreased the expression of GFAP and S100β calcium-binding protein in the cytoplasm of astrocytes (Gerlai et al., 1995) in the RVM (Imbe et al., 2013), while inflammation-induced reactive astrocytes enhanced the activity of the serotonergic descending pain facilitation system, which increased nociceptive signaling in the spinal cord via the RVM (Cunha and Dias, 2009; Roberts et al., 2009). In this study, we examined the influence of MSSI on astrocytes in the LC to determine whether astrocytes were involved in the exacerbation of neuropathic pain by emotional dysfunction. We found that MSSI significantly increased GFAP expression in the LC of female but not male mice. Furthermore, we found that GFAP expression in the medulla oblongata of MSSI stressed female mice shows tendency of increase at 12 weeks age, but not male mice (Supplementary Figures 1, 2). It is well-known that up-regulation of GFAP levels is associated with functional changes in astrocytes that in turn affect neuronal function, due to changes in astrocyte-neuron signaling (Gómez-Galán et al., 2013). Therefore, these findings suggest that MSSI-induced dysfunctional astrocytes in the LC are involved in the development of abnormal emotional states and alterations of the pain modulatory system.

Our previous results demonstrated that MSSI increased anxiety-like behaviors in female but not male mice (Nishinaka et al., 2015b) and MSSI did not influence GFAP expression in the LC of male mice. However, Niwa et al. (2011) previously found that MSSI increased EPM anxiety-like behavior in both male and female C57BL/6J mice. In mice, anxiety and depression-like behaviors differ according to strain or sex (Millstein and Holmes, 2007; McDermott et al., 2015). Generally, females have increased stress sensitivity, likely due to differences in sex hormones,

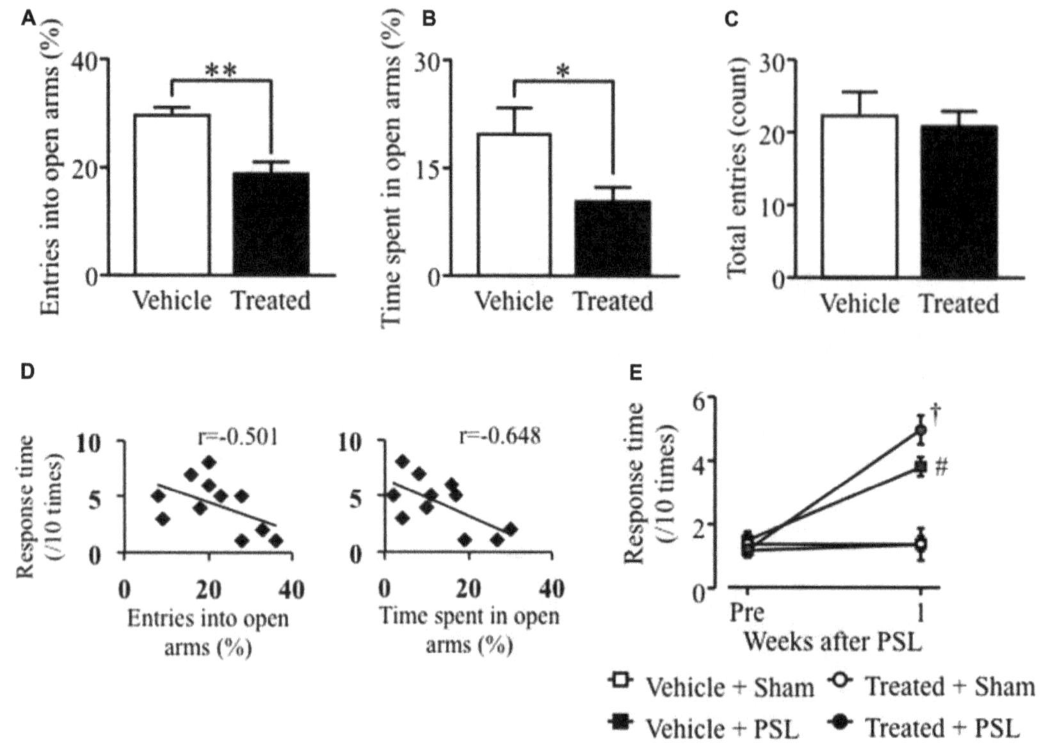

FIGURE 4 | Lipopolysaccharide-treated astrocyte-conditioned medium microinjection into the LC induced anxiety-like behavior and PSL-induced mechanical allodynia in male mice. **(A)** The number of entries into open arms (%). **(B)** Time spent in the open arms (%). **(C)** The total number of entries into the four arms. Vehicle group: $n = 8$, Treated group: $n = 9$. **(D)** Correlation between the entries into open arms (%) or the time spent in open arms (%) and mechanical stimuli after PSL in vehicle- or LPS-treated male mice. **(E)** 0.4 g filament. Vehicle-Sham group: $n = 5$, Vehicle-PSL group: $n = 6$, Treated-Sham group: $n = 5$, Treated-PSL group: $n = 11$. Data expressed as the mean ± SEM. $^{*}P < 0.05$, $^{**}P < 0.01$ vs. Vehicle, Student's t-test. $^{\#}P < 0.05$ vs. Vehicle + Sham, $^{\dagger}P < 0.05$ vs. Treated + Sham, Scheffe's test.

although the detailed mechanisms are not clear (Maeng and Milad, 2015). As show in **Figures 1, 2**, at 7 or 12 weeks age, the GFAP expression in the LC of MSSI stressed mice with or without PSL treated was different between male and female. These results indicate that MSSI-mediated emotional dysfunction and neuropathic pain exacerbation might be more sensitively induced or worked astrocyte activation in female stressed mice, but not male stressed mice. Therefore, our findings suggest that sex differences in LC astrocytic activation induced by MSSI are responsible, at least in part, for the sex differences in anxiety-like behavior and are mediated through the damaging effects of reactive astrocytes on female LC neurons.

Furthermore, to investigate the effect of acute and region-selective activation of LC astrocytes on anxiety-like or nociceptive behaviors, we microinjected the supernatant of LPS-treated astrocytes into the LC region. We found that LC astrocytes up-regulated GFAP expression and showed morphological changes, indicating that astrocytes were activated by the supernatant injection. LPS binds to toll like receptor (TLR) 4, which is expressed in astrocytes. It is thought that these signaling-induced inflammatory responses, which are mediated by the NF-κB pathway, may result in activation of astrocytes (Gorina et al., 2011; Li et al., 2016). Activated astrocytes show up-regulated GFAP protein levels and morphological changes, such as cellular hypertrophy and outgrowth of astrocytic foot processes (von Boyen et al., 2004; Pekny and Pekna, 2014). In this study, we used the LPS-treated astrocytes from rat cell culture. As shown in previous reports, co-culture systems have been used which combined rat astrocytes with mouse neurons. And also, it is reported that rat astrocytes provided optimum conditions for synaptic functioning of mouse neurons (Goudriaan et al., 2014). Further, it is reported that there was no cross-reactivity toward mouse-derived embryonic stem cells injected into rat retina (Gregory-Evans et al., 2009). In this study, microinjection of supernatant from vehicle-treated astrocytes was not affected GFAP expression in the LC area. Based on these reports, we believe that cross-reactivity which may be induced by the microinjection of supernatant from rat astrocytes into mice may have a negligible effect on GFAP protein expression.

The important point is that LC administration of supernatant derived from LPS-treated astrocytes increased anxiety-like behavior and GFAP expression in both male and female mice. These results indicate that activation of astrocytes in the LC might result in emotional dysfunction and exacerbated mechanical allodynia. However, the GFAP expression in the LC of MSSI mice with PSL was different between males and females. We previously showed that MSSI sex-dependently induced emotional dysfunction after nerve injury, which was associated with sex

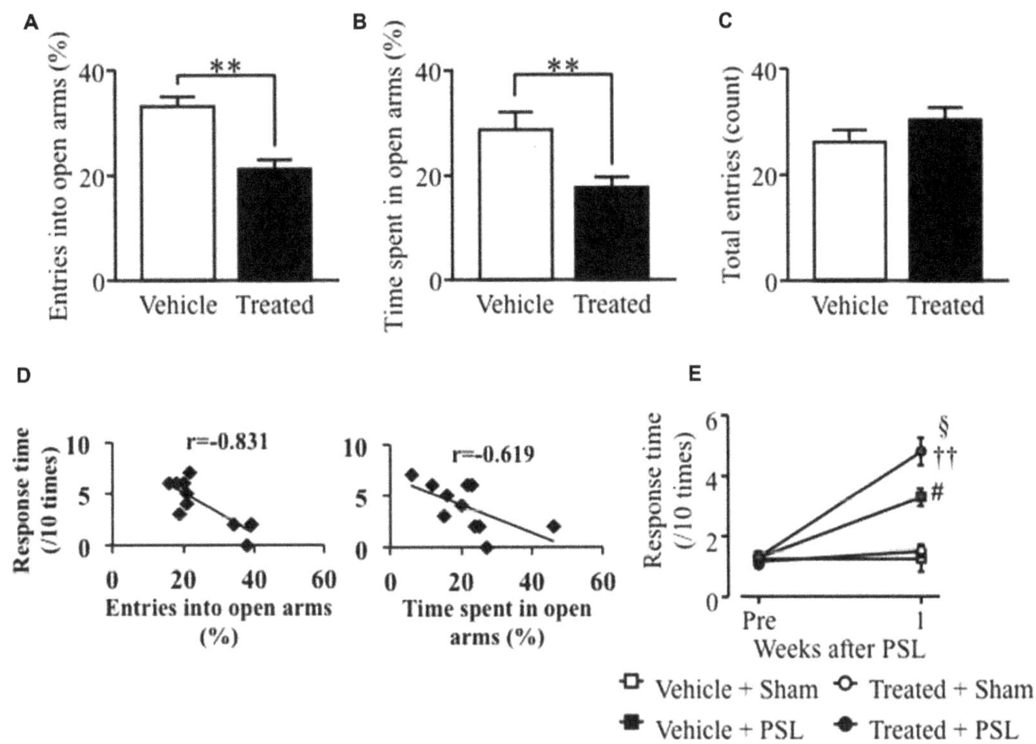

FIGURE 5 | Lipopolysaccharide-treated astrocyte-derived supernatant microinjection into the LC caused anxiety-like behavior and PSL-induced mechanical allodynia in female mice. **(A)** The number of entries into open arms (%). **(B)** Time spent in the open arms (%). **(C)** The total number of entries into the four arms. Vehicle group: $n = 8$, Treated group: $n = 11$. **(D)** Correlation between the entries into open arms (%) or the time spent in open arms (%) and mechanical stimuli after PSL in vehicle- or LPS-treated female mice. **(E)** 0.4 g filament. Vehicle-Sham group: $n = 4$, Vehicle-PSL group: $n = 7$, Treated-Sham group: $n = 6$, Treated-PSL group: $n = 10$. Data expressed as mean ± SEM. $^{**}P < 0.01$ vs. Vehicle, Student's *t*-test. $^{\#}P < 0.05$ vs. Vehicle + Sham, $^{\dagger\dagger}P < 0.01$ vs. Treated + Sham, $^{\S}P < 0.05$ vs. Treated + PSL, Scheffe's test.

differences in the stress-induced regulation of BDNF expression (Nishinaka et al., 2015a). It is thought that neuronal function in the brain of male mice is protected from early life stresses, such as MSSI, by altered expression of several stress-responsive factors, including BDNF upregulation, such that MSSI male mice might acquire resistance to stress. Our findings suggest that activation of astrocytes in the LC, caused by MSSI, might be involved in the induction of emotional dysfunction.

We also found that LC astrocytic dysfunction caused by MSSI contributes to the exacerbation of mechanical allodynia after PSL. Despite downregulation of MSSI-induced LC GFAP overexpression by PSL, MSSI enhanced nerve injury-induced mechanical allodynia. Many studies on the relationship between pain and astrocytic function have demonstrated that inflammation or nerve injury activates astrocytes in the spinal cord and supraspinal area, and that these activated cells contribute to the development and maintenance of persistent pain (Ji et al., 2013). Previous studies have also shown that anti-inflammatory drugs, such as steroids, suppress activated astrocytes (Kuypers et al., 2013; Evans et al., 2014). The MSSI-induced increase in GFAP expression was reversed to control levels by PSL, which would appear to be an improvement in the MSSI effect. From our results, it is unclear whether PSL-induced downregulation of LC GFAP expression in MSSI-stressed mice is associated with the exacerbation of nerve injury-induced mechanical allodynia. We suggest that the MSSI-induced increase in LC GFAP expression in the absence of nerve injury may induce a reduction in mechanical threshold in the presence of nerve injury. The activated astrocytes produce various neurotrophic factors, cytokines, chemokines, and free radicals, with both neuroprotective and neurotoxic effects. The balance between these factors is important for preservation of neuronal function and may act to trigger a compensatory condition against MSSI. Nerve injury may shift this balance and thereby enhance mechanical allodynia.

Furthermore, as shown in **Figures 4, 5**, we found that activation of astrocytes which induced by microinjection of astrocyte conditioned medium with LPS caused emotional dysfunction and exacerbated mechanical allodynia. On the other hand, there is no increased GFAP expression following MSSI in male mice although MSSI-mediated neuropathic pain exacerbation observed in male mice (Nishinaka et al., 2015a). This discrepancy between male and female indicates that other factors which inhibit astrocyte activation may be produced in MSSI stressed male mice, but not female stressed mice.

Further studies will be needed to clarify sex difference between astrocyte activation and pain.

CONCLUSION

We found that MSSI sex-dependently activated astrocytes in the LC, as indicated by increased GFAP expression, with increases in anxiety-like behavior. These MSSI-induced activated astrocytes in the LC may contribute to the exacerbation of neuropathic pain. Furthermore, male mice, but not female mice, might acquire resistance to MSSI-induced stress during growth. We have thus identified one possible and unexpected mechanism linking emotional state with changes in the pain control system, i.e., astroglial activation in the LC.

AUTHOR CONTRIBUTIONS

Study conception and design: KN and ST; acquisition of data: KN, MK, YK; analysis and interpretation: KN, MK and ST; drafting of the manuscript: KN and ST; critical revision of the manuscript for important intellectual content; ST, statistical analysis; KN, MK; obtained funding; KN, ST, administrative, technical, or material support; KN, MK, YK, study supervision; KN, ST. All authors read and approved the final manuscript.

ACKNOWLEDGMENTS

Part of this work was supported by Grants-in-Aid and Special Coordination Funds from the Kobe Gakuin University Joint Research (B). We thank Dr. Takashi Nishinaka for technical help in performing animal study. The authors would like to thank Enago (www.enago.jp) for the English language review.

REFERENCES

Alvarez-Maubecin, V., Garcia-Hernandez, F., Williams, J. T., and Van Bockstaele, E. J. (2000). Functional coupling between neurons and glia. *J. Neurosci.* 20, 4091–4098.

Araque, A., Carmignoto, G., Haydon, P. G., Oliet, S. H., Robitaille, R., and Volterra, A. (2014). Gliotransmitters travel in time and space. *Neuron* 81, 728–739. doi: 10.1016/j.neuron.2014.02.007

Aston-Jones, G., Rajkowski, J., and Cohen, J. (1999). Role of locus coeruleus in attention and behavioral flexibility. *Biol. Psychiatry* 46, 1309–1320. doi: 10.1016/S0006-3223(99)00140-7

Banasr, M., and Duman, R. S. (2008). Glial loss in the prefrontal cortex is sufficient to induce depressive-like behaviors. *Biol. Psychiatry* 64, 863–870. doi: 10.1016/j.biopsych.2008.06.008

Borges, G., Berrocoso, E., Mico, J. A., and Neto, F. (2015). ERK1/2: Function, signaling and implication in pain and pain-related anxio-depressive disorders. *Prog. Neuropsychopharmacol. Biol. Psychiatry* 60, 77–92. doi: 10.1016/j.pnpbp.2015.02.010

Bowley, M. P., Drevets, W. C., Ongür, D., and Price, J. L. (2002). Low glial numbers in the amygdala in major depressive disorder. *Biol. Psychiatry* 52, 404–412. doi: 10.1016/S0006-3223(02)01404-X

Bushnell, M. C., Ceko, M., and Low, L. A. (2013). Cognitive and emotional control of pain and its disruption in chronic pain. *Nat. Rev. Neurosci.* 14, 502–511. doi: 10.1038/nrn3516

Chandley, M. J., Szebeni, K., Szebeni, A., Crawford, J., Stockmeier, C. A., Turecki, G., et al. (2013). Gene expression deficits in pontine locus coeruleus astrocytes in men with major depressive disorder. *J. Psychiatry Neurosci.* 38, 276–284. doi: 10.1503/jpn.120110

Chocyk, A., Dudys, D., Przyborowska, A., Majcher, I., Maćkowiak, M., and Węzony, K. (2011). Maternal separation affects the number, proliferation and apoptosis of glia cells in the substantia nigra and ventral tegmental area of juvenile rats. *Neuroscience* 173, 1–18. doi: 10.1016/j.neuroscience.2010.11.037

Cui, W., Mizukami, H., Yanagisawa, M., Aida, T., Nomura, M., Isomura, Y., et al. (2014). Glial dysfunction in the mouse habenula causes depressive-like behaviors and sleep disturbance. *J. Neurosci.* 34, 16273–16285. doi: 10.1523/JNEUROSCI.1465-14.2014

Cunha, T. M., and Dias, Q. M. (2009). Glial modulation of pain: a step beyond. *J. Neurosci.* 29, 3340–3342. doi: 10.1523/JNEUROSCI.5938-08.2009

Duan, S., Anderson, C. M., Keung, E. C., Chen, Y., Chen, Y., and Swanson, R. A. (2003). P2X7 receptor-mediated release of excitatory amino acids from astrocytes. *J. Neurosci.* 23, 1320–1328.

Evans, M. C., Gaillard, P. J., de Boer, M., Appeldoorn, C., Dorland, R., Sibson, N. R., et al. (2014). CNS-targeted glucocorticoid reduces pathology in mouse model of amyotrophic lateral sclerosis. *Acta Neuropathol. Commun.* 2:66. doi: 10.1186/2051-5960-2-66

Gerlai, R., Wojtowicz, J. M., Marks, A., and Roder, J. (1995). Overexpression of a calcium-binding protein, S100 beta, in astrocytes alters synaptic plasticity and impairs spatial learning in transgenic mice. *Learn. Mem.* 2, 26–39. doi: 10.1101/lm.2.1.26

Gittins, R. A., and Harrison, P. J. (2011). A morphometric study of glia and neurons in the anterior cingulate cortex in mood disorder. *J. Affect. Disord.* 133, 328–332. doi: 10.1016/j.jad.2011.03.042

Gómez-Galán, M., De Bundel, D., Van Eeckhaut, A., Smolders, I., and Lindskog, M. (2013). Dysfunctional astrocytic regulation of glutamate transmission in a rat model of depression. *Mol. Psychiatry* 18, 582–594. doi: 10.1038/mp.2012.10

Gordon, G. R. J., Mulligan, S. J., and MacVicar, B. A. (2007). Astrocyte control of the cerebrovasculature. *Glia* 55, 1214–1221. doi: 10.1002/glia.20543

Gorina, R., Font-Nieves, M., Márquez-Kisinousky, L., Santalucia, T., and Planas, A. M. (2011). Astrocyte TLR4 activation induces a proinflammatory environment through the interplay between MyD88-dependent NFκB signaling, MAPK, and Jak1/Stat1 pathways. *Glia* 59, 242–255. doi: 10.1002/glia.21094

Goudriaan, A., Camargo, N., Carney, K. E., Oliet, S. H., Smit, A. B., and Verheijen, M. H. (2014). Novel cell separation method for molecular analysis of neuron-astrocyte co-cultures. *Front. Cell Neurosci.* 8:12. doi: 10.3389/fncel.2014.00012

Gregory-Evans, K., Chang, F., Hodges, M. D., and Gregory-Evans, C. Y. (2009). Ex vivo gene therapy using intravitreal injection of GDNF-secreting mouse embryonic stem cells in a rat model of retinal degeneration. *Mol. Vis.* 15, 962–973.

Gundersen, V., Storm-Mathisen, J., and Bergersen, L. H. (2015). Neuroglial transmission. *Physiol. Rev.* 95, 695–726. doi: 10.1152/physrev.00024.2014

Halassa, M. M., Fellin, T., and Haydon, P. G. (2009). Tripartite synapses: roles for astrocytic purines in the control of synaptic physiology and behavior. *Neuropharmacology* 57, 343–346. doi: 10.1016/j.neuropharm.2009.06.031

Imbe, H., Kimura, A., Donishi, T., and Kaneoke, Y. (2013). Effects of restraint stress on glial activity in the rostral ventromedial medulla. *Neuroscience* 241, 10–21. doi: 10.1016/j.neuroscience.2013.03.008

Itoi, K., Sugimoto, N., Suzuki, S., Sawada, K., Das, G., Uchida, K., et al. (2011). Targeting of locus ceruleus noradrenergic neurons expressing human interleukin-2 receptor α-subunit in transgenic mice by a recombinant immunotoxin anti-Tac(Fv)-PE38: a study for exploring noradrenergic influence upon anxiety-like and depression-like beha. *J. Neurosci.* 31, 6132–6139. doi: 10.1523/JNEUROSCI.5188-10.2011

Ji, R. R., Berta, T., and Nedergaard, M. (2013). Glia and pain: is chronic pain a gliopathy? *Pain* 154(Suppl.), S10–S28. doi: 10.1016/j.pain.2013.06.022

Kawasaki, Y., Xu, Z. Z., Wang, X., Park, J. Y., Zhuang, Z. Y., Tan, P. H., et al. (2008). Distinct roles of matrix metalloproteases in the early- and late-phase development of neuropathic pain. *Nat. Med.* 14, 331–336. doi: 10.1038/nm1723

Kimelberg, H. K., MacVicar, B. A., and Sontheimer, H. (2006). Anion channels in astrocytes: biophysics, pharmacology, and function. *Glia* 54, 747–757. doi: 10.1002/glia.20423

Kishi, T., Matsuda, Y., Mukai, T., Matsunaga, S., Yasue, I., Fujita, K., et al. (2015). A cross-sectional survey to investigate the prevalence of pain in Japanese patients with major depressive disorder and schizophrenia. *Compr. Psychiatry* 59, 91–97. doi: 10.1016/j.comppsych.2015.02.004

Koyama, Y., Yoshioka, Y., Shinde, M., Matsuda, T., and Baba, A. (2004). Focal adhesion kinase mediates endothelin-induced cyclin D3 expression in rat cultured astrocytes. *J. Neurochem.* 90, 904–912. doi: 10.1111/j.1471-4159.2004.02546.x

Koyanagi, S., Kusunose, N., Taniguchi, M., Akamine, T., Kanado, Y., Ozono, Y., et al. (2016). Glucocorticoid regulation of ATP release from spinal astrocytes underlies diurnal exacerbation of neuropathic mechanical allodynia. *Nat. Commun.* 7:13102. doi: 10.1038/ncomms13102

Kuypers, E., Jellema, R. K., Ophelders, D. R. M. G., Dudink, J., Nikiforou, M., Wolfs, T. G. A. M., et al. (2013). Effects of intra-amniotic lipopolysaccharide and maternal betamethasone on brain inflammation in fetal sheep. *PLoS ONE* 8:e81644. doi: 10.1371/journal.pone.0081644

Li, N., Zhang, X., Dong, H., Zhang, S., Sun, J., and Qian, Y. (2016). Lithium ameliorates LPS-induced astrocytes activation partly via inhibition of toll-like receptor 4 expression. *Cell Physiol. Biochem.* 38, 714–725. doi: 10.1159/000443028

Maeng, L. Y., and Milad, M. R. (2015). Sex differences in anxiety disorders: interactions between fear, stress, and gonadal hormones. *Horm. Behav.* 76, 106–117. doi: 10.1016/j.yhbeh.2015.04.002

McDermott, C. M., Liu, D., Ade, C., and Schrader, L. A. (2015). Estradiol replacement enhances fear memory formation, impairs extinction and reduces COMT expression levels in the hippocampus of ovariectomized female mice. *Neurobiol. Learn. Mem.* 118, 167–177. doi: 10.1016/j.nlm.2014.12.009

Miguel-Hidalgo, J. J., Baucom, C., Dilley, G., Overholser, J. C., Meltzer, H. Y., Stockmeier, C. A., et al. (2000). Glial fibrillary acidic protein immunoreactivity in the prefrontal cortex distinguishes younger from older adults in major depressive disorder. *Biol. Psychiatry* 48, 861–873. doi: 10.1016/S0006-3223(00)00999-9

Millstein, R. A., and Holmes, A. (2007). Effects of repeated maternal separation on anxiety- and depression-related phenotypes in different mouse strains. *Neurosci. Biobehav. Rev.* 31, 3–17. doi: 10.1016/j.neubiorev.2006.05.003

Montero, T. D., and Orellana, J. A. (2015). Hemichannels: new pathways for gliotransmitter release. *Neuroscience* 286, 45–59. doi: 10.1016/j.neuroscience.2014.11.048

Nakamoto, K., Nishinaka, T., Sato, N., Aizawa, F., Yamashita, T., Mankura, M., et al. (2015). The activation of supraspinal GPR40/FFA1 receptor signalling regulates the descending pain control system. *Br. J. Pharmacol.* 172, 1250–1262. doi: 10.1111/bph.13003

Nishinaka, T., Kinoshita, M., Nakamoto, K., and Tokuyama, S. (2015a). Sex differences in depression-like behavior after nerve injury are associated with differential changes in brain-derived neurotrophic factor levels in mice subjected to early life stress. *Neurosci. Lett.* 592, 32–36. doi: 10.1016/j.neulet.2015.02.053

Nishinaka, T., Nakamoto, K., and Tokuyama, S. (2015b). Enhancement of nerve-injury-induced thermal and mechanical hypersensitivity in adult male and female mice following early life stress. *Life Sci.* 121, 28–34. doi: 10.1016/j.lfs.2014.11.012

Niwa, M., Matsumoto, Y., Mouri, A., Ozaki, N., and Nabeshima, T. (2011). Vulnerability in early life to changes in the rearing environment plays a crucial role in the aetiopathology of psychiatric disorders. *Int. J. Neuropsychopharmacol.* 14, 459–477. doi: 10.1017/S1461145710001239

Norman, G. J., Karelina, K., Zhang, N., Walton, J. C., Morris, J. S., and Devries, A. C. (2010). Stress and IL-1beta contribute to the development of depressive-like behavior following peripheral nerve injury. *Mol. Psychiatry* 15, 404–414. doi: 10.1038/mp.2009.91

O'Donnell, J., Zeppenfeld, D., McConnell, E., Pena, S., and Nedergaard, M. (2012). Norepinephrine: a neuromodulator that boosts the function of multiple cell types to optimize CNS performance. *Neurochem. Res.* 37, 2496–2512. doi: 10.1007/s11064-012-0818-x

Park, H., Han, K. S., Oh, S. J., Jo, S., Woo, J., Yoon, B. E., et al. (2013). High glutamate permeability and distal localization of Best1 channel in CA1 hippocampal astrocyte. *Mol. Brain* 6:54. doi: 10.1186/1756-6606-6-54

Pekny, M., and Pekna, M. (2014). Astrocyte reactivity and reactive astrogliosis: costs and benefits. *Physiol. Rev.* 94, 1077–1098. doi: 10.1152/physrev.00041.2013

Roberts, J., Ossipov, M. H., and Porreca, F. (2009). Glial activation in the rostroventromedial medulla promotes descending facilitation to mediate inflammatory hypersensitivity. *Eur. J. Neurosci.* 30, 229–241. doi: 10.1111/j.1460-9568.2009.06813.x

Sattler, R., and Rothstein, J. D. (2006). Regulation and dysregulation of glutamate transporters. *Handb. Exp. Pharmacol.* 175, 277–303. doi: 10.1007/3-540-29784-7_14

Schwarz, J. M., and Bilbo, S. D. (2012). Sex, glia, and development: interactions in health and disease. *Horm. Behav.* 62, 243–253. doi: 10.1016/j.yhbeh.2012.02.018

Seltzer, Z., Dubner, R., and Shir, Y. (1990). A novel behavioral model of neuropathic pain disorders produced in rats by partial sciatic nerve injury. *Pain* 43, 205–218. doi: 10.1016/0304-3959(90)91074-S

Sofroniew, M. V., and Vinters, H. V. (2010). Astrocytes: biology and pathology. *Acta Neuropathol.* 119, 7–35. doi: 10.1007/s00401-009-0619-8

Villemure, C., and Bushnell, M. C. (2009). Mood influences supraspinal pain processing separately from attention. *J. Neurosci.* 29, 705–715. doi: 10.1523/JNEUROSCI.3822-08.2009

von Boyen, G. B., Steinkamp, M., Reinshagen, M., Schäfer, K. H., Adler, G., and Kirsch, J. (2004). Proinflammatory cytokines increase glial fibrillary acidic protein expression in enteric glia. *Gut* 53, 222–228. doi: 10.1136/gut.2003.012625

Wei, F., Guo, W., Zou, S., Ren, K., and Dubner, R. (2008). Supraspinal glial-neuronal interactions contribute to descending pain facilitation. *J. Neurosci.* 28, 10482–10495. doi: 10.1523/JNEUROSCI.3593-08.2008

Woolf, C. J. (2010). What is this thing called pain? *J. Clin. Invest.* 120, 3742–3744. doi: 10.1172/JCI45178

Yoshimura, M., and Furue, H. (2006). Mechanisms for the anti-nociceptive actions of the descending noradrenergic and serotonergic systems in the spinal cord. *J. Pharmacol. Sci.* 101, 107–117. doi: 10.1254/jphs.CRJ06008X

Zhang, H., Zhao, Y., and Wang, Z. (2015). Chronic corticosterone exposure reduces hippocampal astrocyte structural plasticity and induces hippocampal atrophy in mice. *Neurosci. Lett.* 592, 76–81. doi: 10.1016/j.neulet.2015.03.006

Zhang, Z. J., Cao, D. L., Zhang, X., Ji, R. R., and Gao, Y. J. (2013). Chemokine contribution to neuropathic pain: respective induction of CXCL1 and CXCR2 in spinal cord astrocytes and neurons. *Pain* 154, 2185–2197. doi: 10.1016/j.pain.2013.07.002

10

Non-Invasive Focused Ultrasound Stimulation can Modulate Phase-Amplitude Coupling between Neuronal Oscillations in the Rat Hippocampus

Yi Yuan[1†], Jiaqing Yan[2†], Zhitao Ma[1] and Xiaoli Li[3,4]*

[1] Institute of Electrical Engineering, Yanshan University, Qinhuangdao, China, [2] School of Electrical and Control Engineering, North China University of Technology, Beijing, China, [3] State Key Laboratory of Cognitive Neuroscience and Learning and IDG/McGovern Institute for Brain Research, Beijing Normal University, Beijing, China, [4] Center for Collaboration and Innovation in Brain and Learning Sciences, Beijing Normal University, Beijing, China

***Correspondence:**
Xiaoli Li
xiaoli@bnu.edu.cn

[†] These authors have contributed equally to this work.

Noninvasive focused ultrasound stimulation (FUS) can be used to modulate neural activity with high spatial resolution. Phase-amplitude coupling (PAC) between neuronal oscillations is tightly associated with cognitive processes, including learning, attention, and memory. In this study, we investigated the effect of FUS on PAC between neuronal oscillations and established the relationship between the PAC index and ultrasonic intensity. The rat hippocampus was stimulated using focused ultrasound at different spatial-average pulse-average ultrasonic intensities (3.9, 9.6, and 19.2 W/cm^2). The local field potentials (LFPs) in the rat hippocampus were recorded before and after FUS. Then, we analyzed PAC between neuronal oscillations using a PAC calculation algorithm. Our results showed that FUS significantly modulated PAC between the theta (4–8 Hz) and gamma (30–80 Hz) bands and between the alpha (9–13 Hz) and ripple (81–200 Hz) bands in the rat hippocampus, and PAC increased with incremental increases in ultrasonic intensity.

Keywords: focused ultrasound stimulation, neuronal oscillation, phase-amplitude coupling, hippocampus, ultrasonic intensity

INTRODUCTION

Neuronal oscillations provide a mechanism for forming cell assemblies and coordinating cell assemblies by linking the activity of multiple neurons (Wiley, 2010). Neuronal oscillations, which are the complex cognitive functions of the brain that occur from the synergistic interaction of multiple neurons, are mainly involved in cognitive processes, including feature binding, selective attention, and memory. In neuronal oscillations, the amplitude of a faster rhythm is coupled to the phase of a slower rhythm; this is termed phase-amplitude coupling (PAC) and reflects the interactions between local micro-scale and systems-level macro-scale neuronal ensembles. Therefore, PAC can be used as an index of cortical excitability and network interactions (Klausberger et al., 2003; Knight, 2007; Haider and McCormick, 2009; Voytek et al., 2010). Recent findings have shown that PAC was a mechanism for working memory capacity and the discrete nature of perception. PAC also plays an important role during sleep (Penny et al., 2008; Wang et al., 2014). In brief, PAC is a new index that reflects the dynamic interactions between neuronal oscillations.

Noninvasive focused ultrasound stimulation (FUS) of isolated turtle nerve fibers was first performed in 1929 (Newton, 1929). A previous study showed that the mechanism of FUS involves ultrasound-induced cavitation of nanometric bilayer sonophores, which can induce a complex mechanoelectrical interplay that leads to excitation, primarily through the effect of currents induced by membrane capacitance changes of neurons (Plaksin et al., 2014).Changes in neural networks induced by FUS may be caused by changes in the firing rhythm of several neurons. Low-intensity ultrasound can directly modulate neuronal activity in peripheral nerves (Mihran et al., 1990; Tyler, 2011), elicit action potentials in hippocampal slices (Tyler et al., 2008), synchronous oscillations in the intact hippocampus (Tufail et al., 2010) and stimulate the retina (Menz et al., 2013). Furthermore, it can noninvasively stimulate the intact mouse motor cortex (Tufail et al., 2010). Recently, low-intensity focused ultrasound was used to modulate visuomotor behavior in monkeys (Deffieux et al., 2013). Focused ultrasound was also applied to modulate the activity of the primary somatosensory cortex in humans (Legon et al., 2014). Tufail and Yoo et al used pulses of low-frequency (250–700 kHz) ultrasound to modulate brain function (Tufail et al., 2010; Yoo et al., 2011). Mehiæ et al. used a higher frequency (2 MHz), pulsed and focused ultrasound to stimulate the brain of lightly anesthetized mice (Mehiæ et al., 2014). Compared with transcranial direct current stimulation (tDCS) and repetitive transcranial magnetic stimulation (rTMS), FUS has a higher spatial resolution (<2 mm; Tufail et al., 2010; Bystritsky et al., 2011; Yoo et al., 2011). To date, there have been no reports on the effect of low-intensity ultrasound on PAC between neuronal oscillations. In this study, we focused exclusively on the effect of FUS on PAC between neuronal oscillations derived from the hippocampus. A thorough study of the relationship between PAC and ultrasonic intensity is necessary to evaluate the effects of FUS on neuromodulation and to provide a reference for choosing ultrasonic intensities when applying FUS. Our study investigated PAC between neuronal oscillations in the rat hippocampus induced by different ultrasonic intensities of FUS. Local field potentials (LFPs) were recorded from the rat hippocampus before and after FUS. The effects of FUS on PAC between the theta (4–8 Hz) and gamma (30–80 Hz) bands and between the alpha (9–13 Hz) and ripple (81–200 Hz) bands were analyzed using the phase-amplitude coupling index (PACI).

MATERIALS AND METHODS

Experimental Setup for FUS and Data Acquisition

The schematic of the experimental setup is shown in **Figure 1**. The pulse signals were generated by an ultrasonic transmitter and receiver card (USB-UT350T, Ultratek, USA) that drove the focused ultrasound transducer. In our study, the ultrasound transducer, with a bandwidth of 50% and focal length of 30 mm, was driven at a high frequency (2.5 MHz). The active volume of the ultrasound probe was ~625.36 mm^3 and the diameter of the ultrasound intensity focus field was ~4.5 mm. A single stimulation consisted of 4 cycle (1.6 μs) ultrasound pulses with a pulse repetition frequency of 500 Hz and a duration of 160 ms (80 repetitions). An ultrasonic sound power measuring instrument with a diameter of 9.5 mm was used to measure the average intensity of the ultrasound (YP0511F, Hangzhou, China). The spatial-average pulse-average intensities of the ultrasound were 3.9, 9.6, and 19.2 W/cm^2.

LFP signals from the hippocampus were recorded using a 16-channel microelectrode (GBMA S16, Blackrock Microsystems,

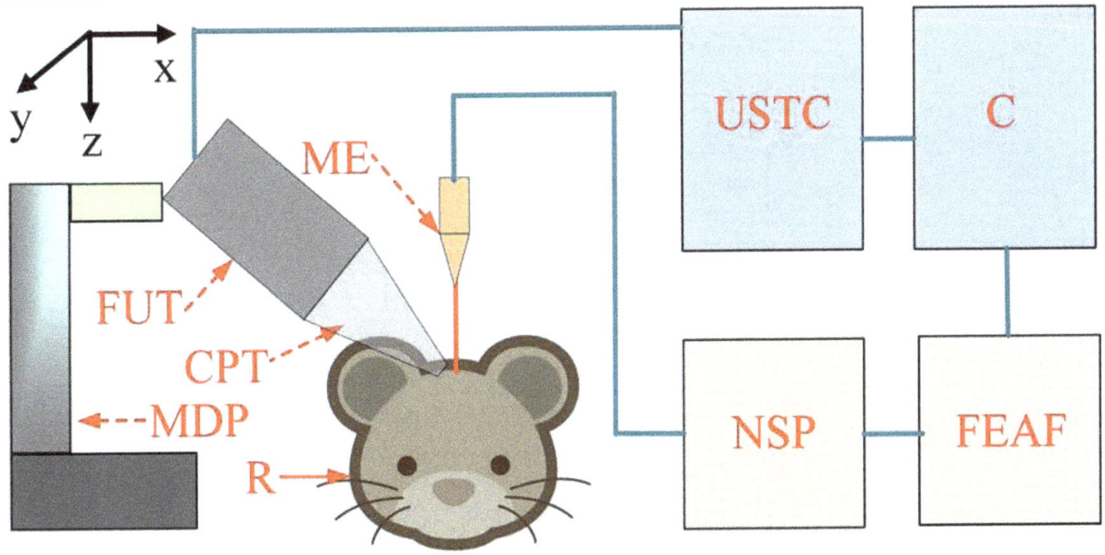

FIGURE 1 | The schematic of the experiment setup. C, computer; USTC, ultrasonic transmitter card; ME, microelectrode; FUT, focused ultrasound transducer; CPT, conic plastic tube; R, rat; MDP, manual displacement platform; NSP, neural signal processor; FEAF, front-end amplifier.

USA) and amplified using a 128-channel front-end amplifier (Cerebus, 128 channels, Blackrock Microsystems, USA). The analog signals were converted into digital signals using a 128-channel neural signal processor (Cerebus128 channels, Cyberknetics, USA), which was then transmitted to a computer for data storage and processing. The data were digitized at a sample rate of 30 kHz, and a low-pass filter with a 250 Hz cutoff frequency for the LFPs was set in the Cerebus system. A heating blanket was used to maintain normal body temperature in the rats. A cold-light source and microscope were used for surgery and a shielding net was used to prevent outside electrical interference.

Animal Surgery and Anesthesia

A total of six Sprague-Dawley rats (3-month-old males, body weights ~270 g) were used in the experiment. All procedures were carried out in accordance with the Animal Ethics and Administrative Council of Yanshan University and Hebei Province, China. Surgical anesthesia was induced with sodium pentobarbital (3%, 5 mg/100 g, i.p.). The anesthetized rats were fixed on the stereotaxic apparatus (ST-5ND-C, Stoelting Co., USA) with ear bars and a clamping device. The fur covering the rat's skull was shaved, and the skin was cleaned with a 0.9% sodium chloride physiological solution. The scalp was cut along the midline of the skull, and the subcutaneous tissue and periosteum were removed. The location of the hippocampus was determined using an atlas. A section of the skull was removed to expose the brain tissue in an area of ~0.5 × 0.5 cm. After completion of the surgical procedure, a 16-channel metal microelectrode (GBMA-S16, Blackrock Microsystems, USA) was inserted into the hippocampus. The anteroposterior (AP), mediolateral (ML), and dorsoventral (DL) coordinates of the center of the recording electrode were -5.3, 3.4, and 3 mm, respectively.

Experimental Procedure

In the ultrasound stimulation experiment, the anesthetized rats were fixed on the stereotaxic apparatus (ST-5ND-C, Stoelting Co., USA) with ear bars and a clamping device. The focused transducer was aimed at the rat hippocampus by adjusting a three-axis manual displacement platform (Zolix, China). A 27 mm plastic cone was filled with degassed ultrasound gel and used to couple the ultrasound transducer to the cortex over the hippocampus. The ultrasound transducer then transmitted an ultrasonic wave. The focused ultrasonic wave passed through the ultrasonic coupling medium and stimulated the brain tissue to induce noninvasive brain neuromodulation. The angle between the ultrasound and the recording microelectrode was ~60°.

PAC Analyses

PAC is the coupling degree index between the low-frequency phase and the high-frequency amplitude. In this study, we

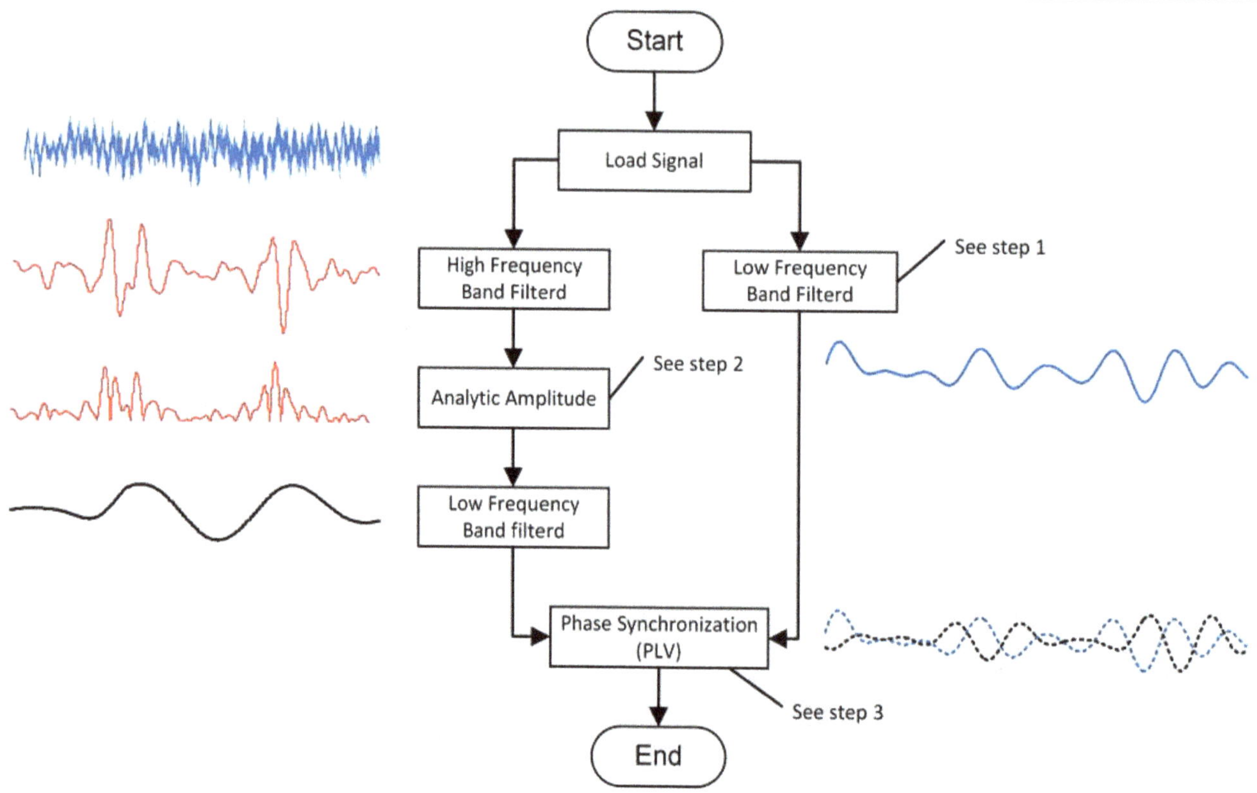

FIGURE 2 | The schematic of PAC calculation algorithm.

modified Voytek's method to calculate the PACI between the low and high frequencies (Voytek et al., 2013). The process (shown in **Figure 2**) of this calculation method included three steps.

Step 1: band-pass filter

A harmonic wavelet was used to provide an unbiased and consistent estimation of the EEG power spectrum (Kapiris et al., 2005). The harmonic wavelet was chosen instead of the more commonly used Morlet wavelet because it is orthogonal and its expression is simple. The wavelet transform passes a filter $\psi(\bullet)$over a time series $x(t)$ to obtain a finite number of filtered signals.

$$W_x(a,\tau) = \frac{1}{\sqrt{|a|}} \int x(t)\, \psi\left(\frac{t-\tau}{a}\right) dt, \quad (1)$$

where $\psi(\bullet)$ is the basic or mother wavelet function and a and τ denote the scale factor and the translation of the origin, respectively. The variable $1/a$ gives the frequency scale, and τ gives the temporal location of an event. $W_x(a,\tau)$ can be interpreted as the "energy" of x of scale a at $t=\tau$. Moreover, the harmonic wavelet function is defined as

$$\psi_{m,n}(t) = \frac{e^{jn2\pi t} - e^{jm2\pi t}}{j(n-m)\,2\pi t}, \quad (2)$$

where m and n are the real scale parameters but not necessarily integers. For the discrete time series $t=\tau$, the wavelet transform is expressed as

$$W_S(n) = \sum_{n=0}^{N-1} x_n \psi_0^* \left(\frac{n-N}{S}\right), \quad (3)$$

where * indicates the complex conjugate. By varying the wavelet scale s and translating along the localized time index k, one can construct a picture that shows both the amplitude of any feature

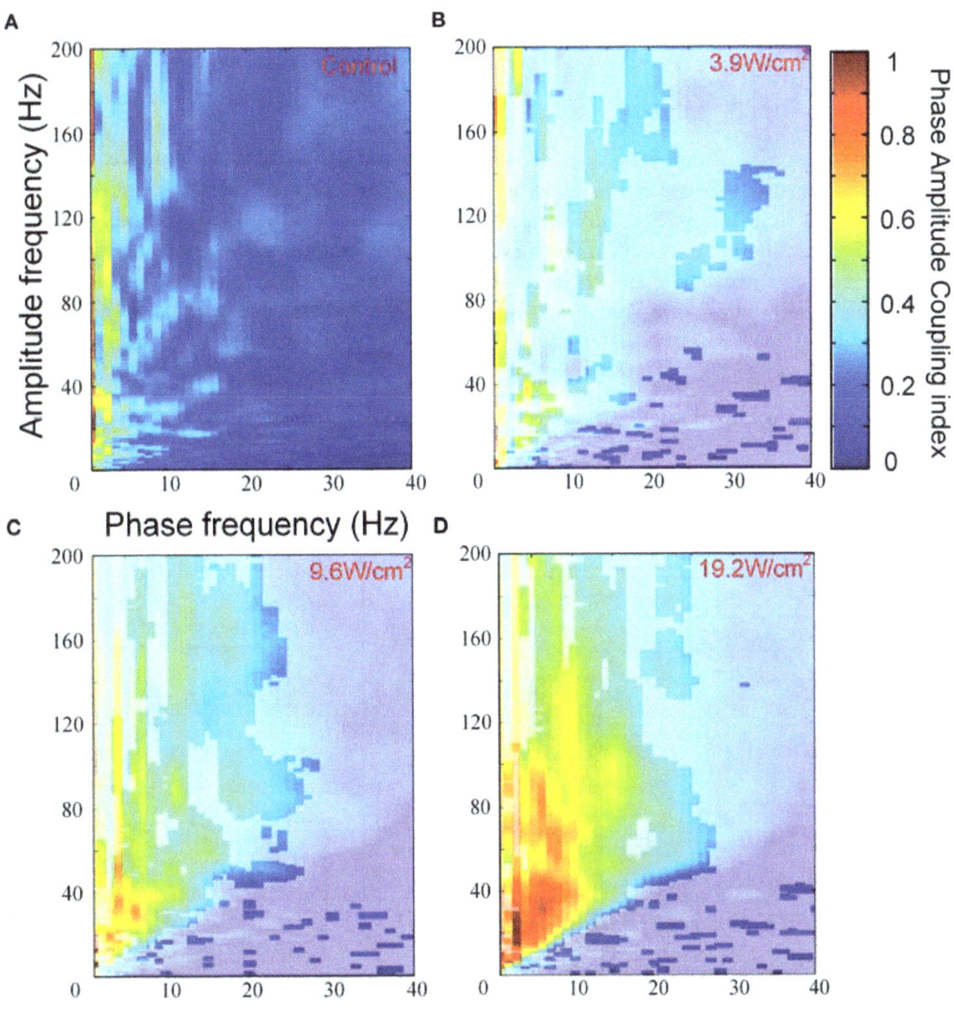

FIGURE 3 | (A) The images of the PACI as a function of the analytic phase (1–40 Hz) and the analytic amplitude (1–200 Hz) for the control ($n = 6$). **(B–D)** The images of the PACI as a function of the analytic phase (1–40 Hz) and the analytic amplitude (1–200 Hz) for the FUS with different ultrasonic intensities: **(B)** 3.9 W/cm^2, **(C)** 9.6 W/cm^2, **(D)** 19.2 W/cm^2 ($n = 6$).

vs. the scale and how this amplitude varies with time. The band pass filtered discrete sequence x_n is defined as

$$x_{filt}(f) = 2 \times real\left(W\left(f\right)\right). \tag{4}$$

Step 2: analytic amplitude

For the filtered signal x_{filt_s}, we used the absolute value to reflect the power of the signal. The power of the discrete sequencex_{filt_s} is defined as

$$P\left(s\right) = \left|x_{filt_s}\right|, \tag{5}$$

where |•| indicates the absolute value.

Step 3: phase synchronization

Phase synchronization describes the phase relationship of the two signals. In this study, we applied the Hilbert transform to estimate the phases (ϕ_l, ϕ_h) for the two signals: (i) the low-frequency oscillation and (ii) the low-frequency band-pass filtered high–frequency oscillation amplitude.

Then, the PACI between the two signals was defined by the following equation

$$PACI = \left|\frac{1}{K}\sum_{k=1}^{K-1} \exp\left(i\left(\phi_l\left[k\right] - \phi_h\left[k\right]\right)\right)\right|, \tag{6}$$

where *PACI* is the phase-locking value between the ongoing phase ϕ_l and ϕ_k, and k is the time index. PAC differences between the control and FUS at the different ultrasonic intensities were analyzed for all subjects using Kruskal-Wallis with Tukey-Kramer *post-hoc* test that is a non-parametric statistical test method.

RESULTS

We investigated PAC that was induced by FUS at different ultrasonic intensities. **Figures 3A–D** show the images of the PACI as a function of the analytic phase (1–40 Hz) and analytic amplitude (1–200 Hz) for the control and FUS at the different intensities. In **Figures 3B–D**, the area not covered by white shadows indicated that they are mean ranks significantly different from the control group (Kruskal-Wallis with Tukey-Kramer *post-hoc* test). When the ultrasonic intensity was 3.9 W/cm^2, the PACI showed that there was a significant difference between FUS and the control in a small frequency range (**Figures 3A,B**). These changes were mainly reflected in the theta, alpha and gamma frequency bands. Compared to the ultrasonic intensity (3.9 W/cm^2), the PACI in the large frequency range was significantly enhanced with an ultrasonic intensity of 9.6 W/cm^2 (**Figure 3C**). This enhancement was obvious in the theta and gamma frequency bands, the alpha and gamma frequency bands, and the ripple frequency bands. When the ultrasonic intensity was 19.2 W/cm^2 (**Figure 3D**), the PACI was further increased compared to the ultrasonic intensity of 9.6 W/cm^2. However, it is worth noting that there were no significant changes in the frequency bands. Based the comparison of the PACI between the three ultrasonic intensities and the control, we found that the change in PAC was obvious in the theta and gamma frequency bands and the alpha and ripple frequency bands. Therefore, to further analyze the effects of ultrasonic intensity on the PACI, we separately calculated the mean PACI in the theta and gamma frequency bands and the alpha and ripple frequency bands.

Furthermore, in **Figures 3A–D**, we quantitatively computed the mean PACI, which is equal to the total PACI divided by the total points. As is shown in **Figure 4A**, the mean PACI between

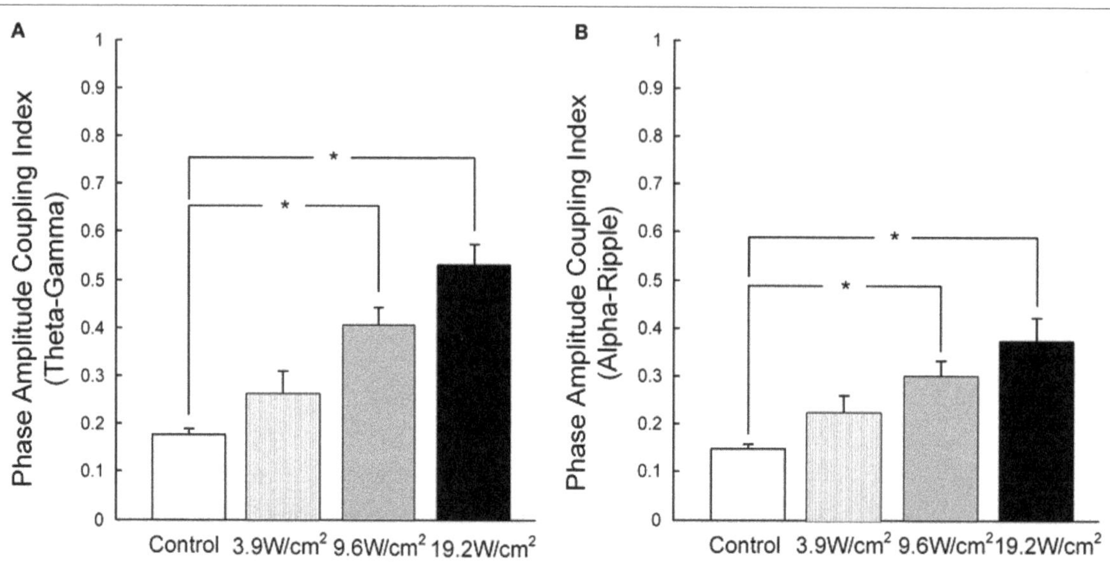

FIGURE 4 | (A) The mean PACI of theta (4–8 Hz) and gamma coupling (30–80 Hz) in the control and with ultrasonic intensities of 3.9, 9.6, and 19.2 W/cm^2 [mean ± SEM, $n = 6$, Chi-Sq (3, 20) = 16.49, *$p = 0.0009$: mean ranks mean ranks significantly different, Kruskal-Wallis with Tukey-Kramer *post-hoc* test]. **(B)** The mean PACI of alpha (9–13 Hz) and ripple coupling (81–200 Hz) in the control and with ultrasonic intensities of 3.9, 9.6, 19.2 W/cm^2 [mean ± SEM, $n = 6$, Chi-Sq (3, 20) =14.25, *$p = 0.0026$: mean ranks significantly different, Kruskal-Wallis with Tukey-Kramer *post-hoc* test].

the theta (4–8 Hz) and gamma (30–80 Hz) bands for the control and the different ultrasonic intensities (3.9, 9.6, and 19.2 W/cm^2) was 0.17 ± 0.01, 0.26 ± 0.04, 0.41 ± 0.03, and 0.53 ± 0.04, respectively [mean ± SEM, $n = 6$, Chi-Sq (3, 20) = 16.49, $^*p = 0.0009$: mean ranks significantly different, Kruskal-Wallis with Tukey-Kramer *post-hoc* test). Compared with the control, the mean PACI between the theta and gamma band increased by 1.53-, 2.41-, and 3.12-fold for the ultrasonic intensities of 3.9, 9.6, and 19.2 W/cm^2, respectively. Therefore, the mean PACI between the theta and gamma band significantly increased as the ultrasonic intensity increased. A similar result was found for the alpha (9–13 Hz)-ripple (81–200 Hz) coupling (**Figure 4B**). The mean PACI between the alpha (9–13 Hz) and ripple (81–200 Hz) bands for the control and the different ultrasonic intensities (3.9, 9.6, and 19.2 W/cm^2) was 0.15 ± 0.01, 0.22 ± 0.03, 0.30 ± 0.03, and 0.37 ± 0.05, respectively [mean ± SEM, $n = 6$, Chi-Sq (3, 20) = 14.25, $^*p = 0.0026$: mean ranks significantly different, Kruskal-Wallis with Tukey-Kramer *post-hoc* test]. Compared with the control, the mean PACI between the alpha and ripple band increased by 1.46−, 2.01−, and 2.46−fold for the ultrasonic intensities of 3.9, 9.6, and 19.2 W/cm^2, respectively. These results show that the FUS can significantly enhance the PAC index between the theta and gamma band and between the alpha and ripple band as the ultrasonic intensity increases.

DISCUSSION

In our previous work (Yuan et al., 2015), we used focused ultrasound with different parameters to stimulate the rat hippocampus. We recorded LFPs evoked by FUS in the rat hippocampus. The mean absolute power of the LFPs was calculated using the Welch algorithm at the delta, theta, alpha, beta and gamma frequency bands. The experimental results demonstrate that the mean absolute power of the LFPs at the different frequency bands increases as the ultrasound power increases. However, we did not pay particular attention to the effect of the ultrasonic parameters on PAC of LFP signals. Subsequently, we found that ultrasonic power can influence PAC of the LFP between the low and high-frequency bands, specifically, in the theta and gamma frequency bands and the alpha and ripple frequency bands.

Previous studies have shown that PAC is associated with brain functions. For example, human memory strength can be predicted by theta-frequency phase-locking of singles (Rutishauser et al., 2010). Therefore, investigating the relationship between PAC and FUS is important. We calculated the mean PACI between the alpha and ripple band and between the theta and gamma band at different ultrasonic intensities (3.9, 9.6, and 19.2 W/cm^2). Our results indicated that the PACI between the theta and gamma band and between the alpha and ripple band were closely connected with the ultrasonic intensity. We can alter the amplitude characteristics of the high-frequency LFPs by modulating the phase characteristics of the low-frequency LFPs by adjusting the ultrasonic intensity. Cognitive abilities (such as memory storage, retrieval, etc.) are closely related to PAC (Mann and Mody, 2010); therefore, we can modulate cognitive abilities by altering ultrasonic intensity. PAC can also optimize ultrasonic intensity by modulating brain oscillations during the application of FUS to treat neurological diseases.

In our study, we analyzed PAC in the rat hippocampus using three ultrasonic intensities (3.9, 9.6, and 19.2 W/cm^2). To obtain a more accurate understanding of the functional relationship between PAC and different ultrasonic intensities, we plan to stimulate the rat hippocampus with additional ultrasound intensities in future studies. The range of acoustic parameters can affect neural activity. A previous study showed that the success of ultrasound stimulation increases as a function of both the acoustic intensity and acoustic duration (King et al., 2013). Perhaps other ultrasonic parameters, including the center frequency, stimulus frequency, duration and number of cycles, can also affect PAC in the hippocampus. In this study, we only quantitatively analyzed the effect of different ultrasonic intensities of FUS on PAC in the rat hippocampus. In future studies, we will evaluate the effect of the other ultrasonic parameters mentioned above on PAC in the hippocampus.

Because ultrasound at high intensities or during long exposures can burn and damage tissues, it is very important to control the ultrasonic intensity when FUS is applied to modulate brain activity. In this study, the maximum ultrasonic intensity was 19.2 W/cm^2, which was not only below the maximum recommended limit for diagnostic imaging applications (190 W/cm^2) but was also below the 23.87 W/cm^2 that was used to modulate the activity in the primary somatosensory cortex in humans (Nyborg, 2001). Therefore, the ultrasonic dose in our experiment is safe. Studies have shown that neuromodulation using TMS is based on the motor threshold (Awiszus, 2003). However, TMS cannot modulate brain activity due to the weak intensity of the magnetic field. This study demonstrates that PAC between neuronal oscillations in the rat hippocampus can be altered using different ultrasonic intensities, which may support the use of PAC between neuronal oscillations to select the appropriate ultrasound intensity for FUS.

In summary, PAC between neuronal oscillations in the rat hippocampus can be altered by FUS, and the PACI increased as the ultrasonic intensity increased. To our knowledge, this is the first study of its kind to demonstrate the effect of FUS with different ultrasonic intensities on PAC between neuronal oscillations.

AUTHOR CONTRIBUTIONS

YY and XL designed and coordinated the study, YY, JY, and ZM carried out experiment and data process, and drafted the manuscript. All authors gave final approval for publication.

ACKNOWLEDGMENTS

This research was supported by National Natural Science Foundation of China (61503321, 61273063), Natural science foundation of Hebei Province (F2014203161).

REFERENCES

Awiszus, F. (2003). TMS and threshold hunting. *Suppl. Clin. Neurophysiol.* 56, 13–23. doi: 10.1016/S1567-424X(09)70205-3

Bystritsky, A., Korb, A. S., Douglas, P. K., Cohen, M. S., Melega, W. P., Mulgaonkar, A. P., et al. (2011). A review of low-intensity focused ultrasound pulsation. *Brain Stimul.* 4, 125–136. doi: 10.1016/j.brs.2011.03.007

Deffieux, T., Younan, Y., Wattiez, N., Tanter, M., Pouget, P., and Aubry, J.-F. (2013). Low-intensity focused ultrasound modulates monkey visuomotor behavior. *Curr. Biol.* 23, 2430–2433. doi: 10.1016/j.cub.2013.10.029

Kapiris, P. G., Polygiannakis, J., Li, X. L., Yao, X., and Eftaxias, K. A. (2005). Similarities in precursory features in seismic shocks and epileptic seizures. *Europhys. Lett.* 69, 657–663. doi: 10.1209/epl/i2004-10383-2

Klausberger, T., Magill, P., Márton, L. F., Roberts, J. D., Cobden, P. M., Buzsáki, G., et al. (2003). Brainstate- and cell-type-specific firing of hippocampal interneurons *in vivo*. *Nature* 421, 844–848. doi: 10.1038/nature01374

King, R. L., Brown, J., Newsome, W. T., and Pauly, K. B. (2013). Effective parameters for ultrasound-induced *in vivo* neurostimulation. *Ultrasound Med. Biol.* 393, 312–331. doi: 10.1016/j.ultrasmedbio.2012.09.009

Knight, R. T. (2007). Neural networks debunk phrenology. *Science* 316, 1578–1579. doi: 10.1126/science.1144677

Haider, B., and McCormick, D. (2009). Rapid neocortical dynamics: cellular and network mechanisms. *Neuron* 62, 171–189. doi: 10.1016/j.neuron.2009.04.008

Legon, W., Sato, T. F., Opitz, A., Mueller, J., Barbour, A., Williams, A., et al. (2014). Transcranial focused ultrasound modulates the activity of primary somatosensory cortex in humans. *Nat. Neurosci.* 17, 322–329. doi: 10.1038/nn.3620

Mann, E. O., and Mody, I. (2010). Control of hippocampal gamma oscillation frequency by tonic inhibition and excitation of interneurons. *Nat. Neurosci.* 13, 205–213. doi: 10.1038/nn.2464

Mehiæ, E., Xu, J. M., Caler, C. J., Coulson, N. K., Moritz, C. T., and Mourad, P. D. (2014). Increased anatomical specificity of neuromodulation via modulated focused ultrasound. *PLoS ONE* 9:e86939. doi: 10.1371/journal.pone.0086939

Menz, M. D., Oralkan, Ö., Khuri-Yakub, P. T., and Baccus, S. A. (2013). Precise neural stimulation in the retina using focused ultrasound. *J. Neurosci.* 33, 4550–4560. doi: 10.1523/jneurosci.3521-12.2013

Mihran, R. T., Barnes, F. S., and Wachtel, H. (1990). Temporally-specific modification of myelinated axon excitability *in vitro* following a single ultrasound pulse. *Ultrasound Med. Biol.* 16, 297–309. doi: 10.1016/0301-5629(90)90008-Z

Newton, H. E. (1929). The effect of high frequency sound waves on heart muscle and other irritable tissues. *Am. J. Physiol.* 9, 1284–1290.

Nyborg, W. L. (2001). Biological effects of ultrasound: development of safety guidelines. Part II: general review. *Ultrasound Med. Biol.* 27, 301–333. doi: 10.1016/S0301-5629(00)00333-1

Penny, W. D., Duzel, E., Miller, K. J., and Ojemann, J. G. (2008). Testing for nested oscillation. *J. Neurosci. Methods* 174, 50–61. doi: 10.1016/j.jneumeth.2008.06.035

Plaksin, M., Shoham, S., and Kimmel, E. (2014). Intramembrane cavitation as a predictive bio-piezoelectric mechanism for ultrasonic brain stimulation. *Phys. Rev. X* 4:011004. doi: 10.1103/PhysRevX.4.011004

Rutishauser, U., Ross, I. B., Mamelak, A. N., and Schuman, E. M. (2010). Human memory strength is predicted by theta-frequency phase-locking of single neurons. *Nature* 464, 903–907. doi: 10.1038/nature08860

Tufail, Y., Matyushov, A., Baldwin, N., Tauchmann, M. L., Georges, J., Yoshihiro, A., et al. (2010). Transcranial pulsed ultrasound stimulates intact brain circuits. *Neuron* 66, 681–694. doi: 10.1016/j.neuron.2010.05.008

Tyler, W. J. (2011). Noninvasive neuromodulation with ultrasound? A continuum mechanics hypothesis. *Neuroscientist* 17, 25–36. doi: 10.1177/10738584093 48066

Tyler, W. J., Tufail, Y., Finsterwald, M., Tauchmann, M. L., Olson, E. J., and Majestic, C. (2008). Remote excitation of neuronal circuits using low intensity, low-frequency ultrasound. *PLoS ONE* 3:3511. doi: 10.1371/journal.pone.0003511

Voytek, B., Canolty, R. T., Shestyuk, A., Crone, N. E., Parvizi, J., and Knight, R. T. (2010). Shifts in gamma phase-amplitude coupling frequency from theta to alpha over posterior cortex during visual tasks. *Front. Hum. Neurosci.* 4:191. doi: 10.3389/fnhum.2010.00191

Voytek, B., D'Esposito, M., Crone, N., and Knight, R. T. (2013). A method for event-related phase/amplitude coupling. *Neuroimage* 64, 416–424. doi: 10.1016/j.neuroimage.2012.09.023

Wang, J., Gao, D. Q., Li, D., Desroches, A. S., Liu, L., and Li, X. L. (2014). Theta-gamma coupling reflects the interaction of bottom-up and top-down processes in speech perception in children. *Neuroimage* 102, 637–645. doi: 10.1016/j.neuroimage.2014.08.030

Wiley, B. G. (2010). Neural syntax: cell assemblies, synapsembles, and readers. *Neuron* 68, 362–385. doi: 10.1016/j.neuron.2010.09.023

Yoo, S.-S., Bystritsky, A., Lee, J.-H., Zhang, Y. Z., Fischer, K., Min, Y.-K., et al. (2011). Focused ultrasound modulates region-specific brain activity. *Neuroimage* 56, 1267–1275. doi: 10.1016/j.neuroimage.2011.02.058

Yuan, Y., Lu, C. B., and Li, X. L. (2015). Effect of focused ultrasound stimulation at different ultrasonic power levels on the local field potential power spectrum. *Chin. Phys. B* 24:088704. doi: 10.1088/1674-1056/24/8/088704

11

Deep Brain Stimulation Improves the Symptoms and Sensory Signs of Persistent Central Neuropathic Pain from Spinal Cord Injury

*Walter J. Jermakowicz[1,2], Ian D. Hentall[1,2,3], Jonathan R. Jagid[1,3], Corneliu C. Luca[3,4], James Adcock[1,3], Alberto Martinez-Arizala[1,2,3,4] and Eva Widerström-Noga[1,2,3]**

[1]The Miami Project to Cure Paralysis, Miller School of Medicine, University of Miami, Miami, FL, USA, [2]Department of Neurological Surgery, Miller School of Medicine, University of Miami, Miami, FL, USA, [3]Research Service, Bruce W. Carter Department of Veterans Affairs Medical Center, Miami, FL, USA, [4]Department of Neurology, Miller School of Medicine, University of Miami, Miami, FL, USA

Correspondence:
Eva Widerström-Noga
ewiderstrom-noga@med.miami.edu

Central neuropathic pain (CNP) is a significant problem after spinal cord injury (SCI). Pharmacological and non-pharmacological approaches may reduce the severity, but relief is rarely substantial. While deep brain stimulation (DBS) has been used to treat various chronic pain types, the technique has rarely been used to attenuate CNP after SCI. Here we present the case of a 54-year-old female with incomplete paraplegia who had severe CNP in the lower limbs and buttock areas since her injury 30 years prior. She was treated with bilateral DBS of the midbrain periaqueductal gray (PAG). The effects of this stimulation on CNP characteristics, severity and pain-related sensory function were evaluated using the International SCI Pain Basic Data Set (ISCIPBDS), Neuropathic Pain Symptom Inventory (NPSI), Multidimensional Pain Inventory and Quantitative Sensory Testing before and periodically after initiation of DBS. After starting DBS treatment, weekly CNP severity ratings rapidly decreased from severe to minimal, paralleled by a substantial reduction in size of the painful area, reduced pain impact and reversal of pain-related neurological abnormalities, i.e., dynamic-mechanical and cold allodynia. She discontinued pain medication on study week 24. The improvement has been consistent. The present study expands on previous findings by providing in-depth assessments of symptoms and signs associated with CNP. The results of this study suggest that activation of endogenous pain inhibitory systems linked to the PAG can eliminate CNP in some people with SCI. More research is needed to better-select appropriate candidates for this type of therapy. We discuss the implications of these findings for understanding the brainstem's control of chronic pain and for future progress in using analgesic DBS in the central gray.

Keywords: neuromodulation, low-frequency stimulation, periaqueductal gray, pain severity, evoked pain, chronic pain

INTRODUCTION

Persistent neuropathic pain is a common and serious consequence of spinal cord injury (SCI) that is especially refractory to both pharmacological and non-pharmacological treatments (Siddall et al., 2003; Vranken, 2009; Finnerup et al., 2014). Electrical stimulation of specific brain structures with the purpose of relieving chronic pain has been used for a long time but the reported efficacy for central neuropathic pain (CNP) is relatively low and difficult to predict. For certain patients, effects of stimulation on CNP may be tremendous (Boccard et al., 2013; Pereira and Aziz, 2014). Nevertheless, because deep brain stimulation (DBS) is an invasive procedure, its use for SCI pain is rare and currently restricted to severe cases refractory to non-invasive therapies. In order to be accepted as a therapy for chronic pain, success rates need to improve. This will require, *inter alia*, a better understanding of CNP mechanisms along with improved patient selection.

The present article describes an almost complete reversal of CNP (which had been present since injury 30 years ago) and associated sensory dysfunction paralleled by a reduction in psychosocial impact in a 54-year-old female with SCI-related CNP who underwent DBS of the periaqueductal gray (PAG). The optimization of stimulation parameters and the time-course of daily changes in general pain intensity over a 42-week period were previously reported for this subject and one other with SCI-related chronic pain (Hentall et al., 2016). Here we provide a more detailed analysis specifically focusing on the CNP below the level of injury evaluating a broader set of pain characteristics, somatosensory function and psychosocial impact conducted at intervals over a 52-week period. We also conducted an exit interview to obtain her personal perspectives on her pain and treatments. The "Discussion" Section contains a brief review of possible mechanisms underlying successful amelioration of CNP by DBS and the prospects for improving treatment efficacy.

BACKGROUND

Clinical History

The subject was a 54-year-old female veteran with an incomplete SCI (T11 level) due to electrocution 30 years ago. Examination according to the International Standards for Neurological Classification of SCI classified her injury as AIS-B (sensory but no motor function preserved).

The patient's worst pain problem was chronic below-level CNP in both lower extremities, with onset shortly after her initial injury. The average weekly pain level for this specific pain preceding the baseline measurement was 8 of 10 on a numerical rating scale (NRS). CNP was daily and constant, and most intense during the night and therefore significantly interfering with sleep. She reported severe "electric" and moderate "stabbing" pain, moderate to severe evoked pain in response to brushing, severe evoked pain to cold stimuli and moderate tingling and pins and needles in the painful area. She was taking a daily dose of 75 mg pregabalin for the pain but had previously tried a wide range of pharmacological options (including opiates and higher doses of pregabalin) and she said: "Medication? I don't like medication. I don't like the way it makes me feel. I don't like the side effects. It . . . They all leave me feeling stupid and foggy and disoriented and . . . So, that's why I wouldn't take them until I absolutely just couldn't . . ."

Pain and Sensory Assessments

Pain was evaluated with respect to location, classification, intensity, temporal pattern and pain interference using the International SCI Pain Basic Dataset (ISCIPBDS; Widerström-Noga et al., 2014). Neuropathic pain symptom severity was evaluated with the Neuropathic Pain Symptom Inventory (NPSI; Bouhassira et al., 2004), and psychosocial impact with the Multidimensional Pain Inventory-SCI version (Widerström-Noga et al., 2006). Sensory function was assessed below the level of injury in the neuropathic pain area with the TSA-II Neurosensory Analyzer (Medoc Ltd., Ramat Yishai, Israel), either via a thermode or a vibratory pin applied to the painful area below the level of injury. Thresholds for cool detection, warm detection, cold pain, hot pain and vibration detection were determined using the method of limits (reaction-time inclusive). We also evaluated thermal allodynia using thermorollers (Somedic, Sweden), and mechanical allodynia using a soft brush and Semmes-Weinstein monofilaments (10 g, #5.07). Further details regarding all QST procedures can be found in a previous publication (Widerström-Noga et al., 2016). Baseline pain testing was performed twice in the subject (1 and 5 weeks before the first surgery) and baseline results were averaged. For a study timeline see **Figure 1**.

DBS Surgery

The work was performed under an Investigative Device Exemption of the U.S. Food and Drug Administration (IDE G120202), and Clinical Trials.gov (NCT02006433).

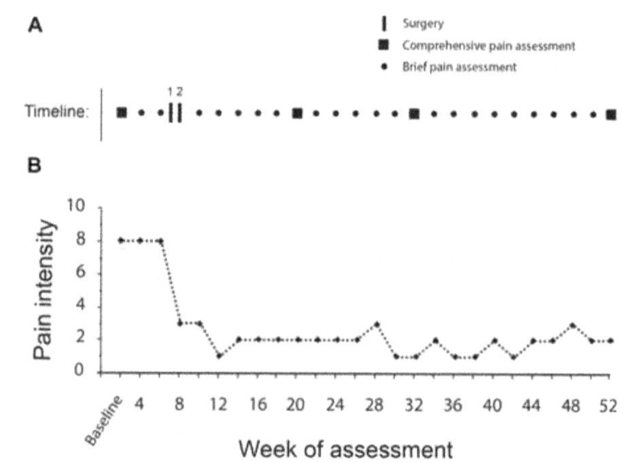

FIGURE 1 | (A) Timeline of study. The subject underwent a comprehensive pain assessment (entire battery of pain tests) on week 2, prior to the two surgical procedures performed on weeks 6 and 7. This was followed by biweekly brief pain assessments (average pain intensity ratings past 7 days by patient in clinic) and periodic repeat comprehensive assessments postoperatively (weeks 20, 32 and 52). **(B)** Average pain intensity ratings past 7 days through duration of the study. Immediately following activation of the device the subject noticed a profound reduction of her central neuropathic pain (CNP).

All study procedures were approved by the University of Miami Institutional Review Board (IRB) with written consent from the subject in accordance with the Declaration of Helsinki.

Two surgeries were performed 1 week apart: (1) bilateral implantation of electrode leads (Medtronic3387S-40) in the anterolateral PAG with the subject awake; and (2) connection of both leads to extension cables under general anesthesia and tunneling to a generator (Activa PC Neurostimulator 37601, Medtronic). Stimulation was briefly tested during the first surgery, eliciting an emotional response in the subject due to near-complete relief of her long-standing symptoms. For more details see Hentall et al. (2016).

RESULTS

The subject reported a rapid and profound improvement in her CNP, from severe to minimal intensity, when the DBS device was activated on the day after the second surgery. Her DBS stimulation settings were adjusted in periodic office visits (monthly, later every 2 months). In addition, the stimulator was programmed with several blinded choices of parameters (frequency or voltage) for selection at home (Hentall et al., 2016). Among salient findings reported previously, she preferred a very low mean pulse rate (0.67 Hz) and the pain level took several days to shift to a new steady state when the blinded stimulation setting was changed. The blinded choice of settings (ineffective 0.1 V vs. effective 4.5 V) also allowed exclusion of potentially powerful placebo effects.

Figure 1B shows a time-line of the subject's average weekly CNP intensity following her DBS procedure. Whereas she typically reported a pain intensity of 7–8 at baseline, following the procedure her median reported CNP intensity was 2 and remained so the length of the study. The subject also noted a significant decrease in the size of the painful area (**Figure 2**). Pain medication was discontinued by the 17th postoperative week.

The rapid reduction in overall neuropathic pain symptom severity after initiation of DBS was maintained over the course of the study (**Figure 3A**). Evoked pain was reduced to a minimal level. Paresthesia/dysesthesia (pins and needles and tingling) in the painful area also decreased to a significantly lower level.

Before surgery, the subject exhibited both dynamic mechanical allodynia evoked by very weak vibratory stimuli and static mechanical allodynia in the painful area in response to punctuate stimuli applied with the von Frey filament (100 g). Cold allodynia was evoked within a normally non-noxious range, between 22.9°C and 25.2°C. After onset of DBS treatment, however, there were no signs of allodynia in the painful area, consistent with the reduction in pain symptoms. Vibratory stimuli at the threshold level for perception and the punctuate stimulus applied with the large von Frey filament (300 g; 6.65) did not evoke pain after DBS was initiated. Cool and warm detection thresholds were in the normal range (**Figure 3B**). Although she initially perceived pain at the maximal temperature (50°C), both cold and hot stimuli within the default minimum/maximum temperatures of 0°C and 50°C did not evoke a pain sensation at follow-up.

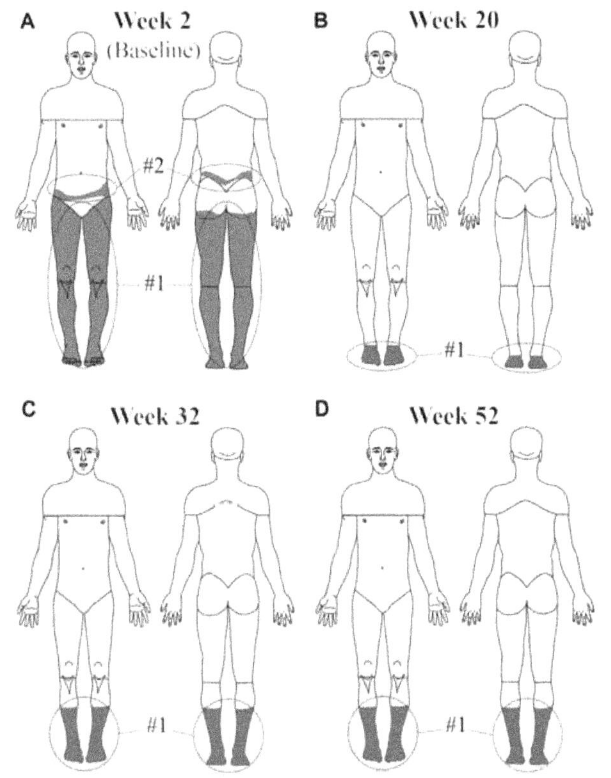

FIGURE 2 | The area of neuropathic pain was greatly reduced in the subject with activation of the device. Whereas before surgery **(A)** her pain was located at the anterior and posterior aspects of both legs and the superior buttocks, by the 20th week after surgery **(B)** pain was only perceived below the ankles. By the 32nd postoperative week **(C)** the pain extended back up to her mid-calf region of both legs and remained unchanged the remainder of the study **(D)**.

Though formal neurocognitive evaluation was not performed, the Beck depression inventory (BDI), MPI-SCI subscales, perceived life control and affective distress did not indicate any negative effects of the DBS (**Supplementary Figure S1**). The BDI scores are not shown because the subject never scored above "1" (including the baseline assessments). Indeed, placement of the PAG DBS device had a tremendous positive impact on the quality of life of the subject. During a qualitative interview after the surgery she stated "It's a whole new world. I'm learning my body all over again. It's life-changing. It still brings tears to my eyes". The DBS device has remained activated with consistent efficacy reported by the patient since implantation over 2 years ago.

DISCUSSION

Electrical stimulation of the PAG significantly reduced the intensity and distribution of CNP-related symptoms and associated abnormal sensory signs (i.e., mechanical and thermal allodynia) in our subject and, consequently, had a profound effect on her quality of life. The consistent beneficial effects on multiple aspects of CNP over the entire study period and the blinded choice of settings controlling for potential placebo

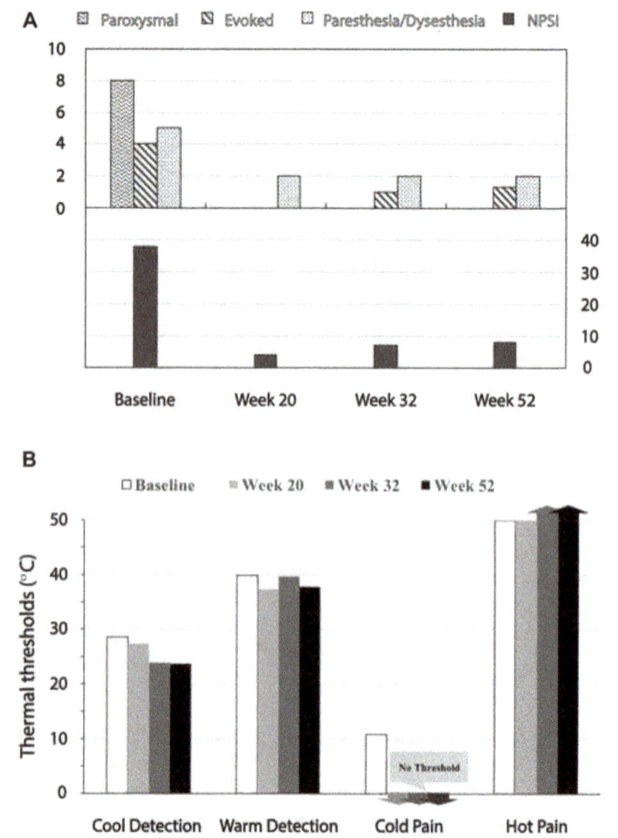

FIGURE 3 | Reduction of Neuropathic Pain Symptom Inventory (NPSI) and QST test scores with device activation. (A) The top graph shows paroxysmal, evoked and paresthesia/dysesthesia scores, all of which were reduced to minimal levels with stimulation. The bottom graph shows the reduction in the NPSI sum score. **(B)** Effects on QST measures. Whereas the subject had significant allodynia before surgery in response to cold and warm, these stimuli within the default minimum/maximum temperatures (0°C and 50°C, respectively) did not evoke pain sensations in follow-up.

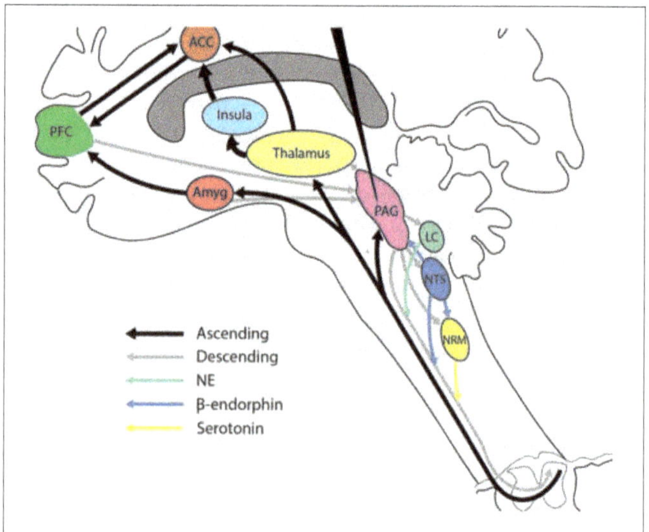

FIGURE 4 | Illustration showing the central role of the periaqueductal gray (PAG) in the modulation of various descending pain systems. Various neurotransmitter systems have been implicated in the treatment of central pain. The PAG has strong ascending and descending connections with each of these systems and is thus in a strong position to modulate CNP. Conventions for the arrows are shown at the bottom left of the figure. ACC, anterior cingulate cortex; Amyg, amygdala; PFC, prefrontal cortex; LC, locus coeruleus; NRM, nucleus raphe magnus; NTS, nucleus tractus solitarius.

effects (Hentall et al., 2016) supports the validity of this case report. Despite 30 years of limited pain relief with various pharmacological treatments she had near-complete relief of her CNP with activation of the DBS device. Such profound and long-lasting improvements in people with CNP pain are rarely reported with conservative measures or other surgical options (Vranken, 2009; Cardenas et al., 2013; Gao et al., 2016).

DBS for Neuropathic Pain

DBS has been used for the treatment of various types of pain since the 1970s, following advances in implantable stimulation devices and the influence of Melzack and Wall's (1965) gate theory. Most evidence available supports the PAG as a useful stimulation target (Pereira and Aziz, 2014). In addition to ascending somatosensory projections, the PAG receives significant inputs from the prefrontal cortex (PFC) and amygdala and then projects to nucleus raphe magnus (NRM) and locus coeruleus (LC) in the midbrain and dorsal horn neurons in the spinal cord (Van Bockstaele et al., 1991; Li et al., 2016). Recent case series on DBS for chronic neuropathic pain, which have utilized superior targeting methods compared to earlier studies and multi-day trials with an externalized electrode prior to final implantation, suggest clinically-relevant improvements of pain symptoms in 67%–83% of patients with heterogeneous types of pain (Boccard et al., 2013). Gray et al. (2014) showed that beyond improving pain symptoms, DBS may also improve mood, anxiety and quality of life. However, very few studies have examined the pain reducing ability of DBS in people with CNP. The acceptance of this therapy in the U.S. has been hindered by the variability of outcomes. Even in cases where patients respond favorably to a several day trial with an externalized stimulator prior to permanent implantation, roughly a quarter of those patients do not experience benefit 1 year after surgery (Boccard et al., 2013).

The recent renewal of interest in DBS for chronic pain has arisen from various factors: (1) improved safety of DBS in general; (2) success with other indications for DBS; (3) advances in imaging and targeting methods; and (4) renewed recognition by the public and health administrators of the detrimental effects of prolonged opioid medication (Schofferman et al., 2014). For patients with CNP of whose etiological or pathological classification is known to make it particularly refractory to typical treatment interventions, particularly if they have failed to respond to conservative measures over many years, DBS may offer benefits. The challenge is to determine which pain phenotypes and patients are most likely to respond. This is an especially hard problem in populations with CNP stemming from CNS injuries, in which multiple pain mechanisms are likely to operate simultaneously (Carlton et al., 2009; Hari et al., 2009; Zeilig et al., 2012; Finnerup et al., 2014).

Possible Mechanisms of DBS for CNP

Spontaneous and evoked excitability within the somatosensory system is normally well-controlled by ascending and descending pain pathways (Basbaum and Fields, 1984; Vranken, 2009). CNP after spinal injury may arise as a consequence of the amplification of signals in residual sensory neurons by spinal and supraspinal processes, such as astrocytic and microglial activation, ultimately influencing various neurotransmitter systems, local connectivity and cytokines (Scholz and Woolf, 2007; Zeilig et al., 2012; Finnerup et al., 2014; Robinson et al., 2016).

The raphe nuclei and their associated modulatory neurotransmitter, serotonin, have long been implicated as important factors influencing pain. However, although selective serotonin reuptake inhibitors are among the most prescribed medications for CNP, little efficacy has been shown in clinical pain trials (Vranken, 2009; Urtikova et al., 2012). While initial behavioral experiments suggested an anti-nociceptive role for serotonin, the link between the neurotransmitter and pain is now viewed as more complex and serotonin may have both pro- and anti-nociceptive properties, depending on the location and mechanism of release (central from raphe vs. peripheral from mast cells) and the serotonergic receptors involved (Urtikova et al., 2012; Bobinski et al., 2015).

The NRM is the largest CNS source of spinal cord serotonin and the PAG is its major input (Van Bockstaele et al., 1991). Serotonergic neurons in the raphe are responsive to inflammatory molecules and markers of CNS injury (Vanegas and Schaible, 2004; Bobinski et al., 2015). It was shown that stimulation of the NRM acutely increases levels of spinal cord PKA, cAMP and CREB, signaling molecules with important roles in development, repair and long-term potentiation. Interestingly, these beneficial effects were elicited at quite low stimulation frequencies (4–8 Hz), not the high frequencies (typically 50–150 Hz) used for nearly all other indications of DBS (Hentall et al., 2006; Carballosa-Gonzalez et al., 2014). This is relevant because while high-frequency DBS is thought to functionally inhibit its target, low-frequency stimulation is considered stimulatory and, in the present case, should lead to activation of PAG and NRM and the release of modulatory neurotransmitters in the spinal cord (Hentall and Gonzalez, 2012).

Norepinephrine (NE) has also been implicated in the modulation of pain (Hickey et al., 2014; Li et al., 2016). NE reuptake inhibitors or combinations of NE and 5-HT reuptake inhibitors are common therapies for CNP and are recommended first-line treatments for patients with SCI (Guy et al., 2016). Also, the $\alpha 2$ receptor agonist clonidine is used to treat the withdrawal effects of opioids (Siddall et al., 2000). Recent optogenetic studies have shown that focal activation of the LC, whose major inputs are from the PFC, amygdala, PAG and dorsal noradrenergic bundle, may be either pro- or anti-nociceptive, suggestive of different neuron subgroups within the LC (Hickey et al., 2014). Consistent with this, recently Li et al. (2016), used a canine adenoviral vector expressing channelrhodopsin2 to target ponto-spinal NE neurons, and found a subset of ventral LC neurons with spinal projections that is likely involved in the regulation of nociception. Interestingly, this subgroup of LC neurons had lower average firing rate than other noradrenergic neurons of the LC.

DBS of the PAG could also relieve pain via neurons that secrete β-endorphin (Siddall et al., 2000; Schofferman et al., 2014). β-endorphin is derived from the prohormone pro-opiomelanocortin (POMC). Cerritelli et al. (2016) recently identified a subset of 100–200 POMC neurons in the nucleus tractus solitarius (NTS) that, when optogenetically stimulated, led to significant analgesic effects, that were blocked by administration of naloxone, an opioid receptor antagonist. Thus several highly interconnected pathways may be involved in modulating ascending pain information and are accessible by DBS in the PAG. For a schematic overview see **Figure 4.**

Prospects for Improved Rates of Success

DBS of brainstem targets can be considered for ameliorating severe CNP that is refractory to pharmacological treatment. The best evidence for any pharmacological treatment of CNP after SCI is for the anticonvulsant pregabalin (Guy et al., 2016). However, the treatment responses to pregabalin for CNP are not consistent. Indeed, a large recent randomized trial showed the numbers needed to treat for >30% pain reduction was about 7 (Cardenas et al., 2013). Long-term opioid therapy has already proven to be a poor long-term option (Schofferman et al., 2014). When available, non-invasive brain stimulation methods, such as repetitive transcranial magnetic stimulation, are preferrable over DBS. However, their efficacy is yet to be proven in heterogeneous pain conditions and they are currently not recommended treatment approaches for patients with CNP related to SCI (Gao et al., 2016; Guy et al., 2016).

If DBS is to become an accepted therapy for CNP, its efficacy and consistency need to be improved. Anecdotally patients may experience outstanding results, but many are left to a greater or lesser extent with the original debilitating pain (Coffey, 2001; Boccard et al., 2013; Pereira and Aziz, 2014). It is thus important to identify predictors of long-term efficacy and understand mechanisms of tolerance. Comprehensive evaluation of neuropathic pain symptoms including severity, location and temporal pattern, and quantitative pain assessments, such as used in this study, may help in this task, along with novel brain imaging techniques. Thus, better defined pain phenotypes based on comprehensive pain assessment protocols may lead to more reliable selection of patients amenable to this therapy. Better knowledge of responsive pain phenotypes in this notoriously difficult patient population is also important for comparing treatments, especially because novel therapies continue to emerge, such as minimally invasive ablative techniques (Tiwari et al., 2014).

AUTHOR CONTRIBUTIONS

WJJ performed the majority of work on preparing the manuscript, figures and integrating other authors' comments.

JA conducted pain assessments and helped prepare the pain data and figures. IDH prepared the application for the clinical trial and helped prepare the manuscript. JRJ, AM-A and CCL performed the surgical and neurological procedures and revised the final versions of the manuscript. EW-N helped prepare the manuscript and oversee and summarize all pain assessments.

SUPPLEMENTARY MATERIAL

FIGURE S1 | Assessment of psychosocial impact and subjective distress experienced by the patient before and after surgery. Comparison of MPI—spinal cord injury (SCI) subscales, Life Control and Affective Distress, suggest the patient did not develop new cognitive or affective impairments following the surgery. Each assessment was performed by the same assessor. More details about the MPI-SCI may be found at Widerström-Noga et al. (2006).

REFERENCES

Basbaum, A. I., and Fields, H. L. (1984). Endogenous pain control systems: brainstem spinal pathways and endorphin circuitry. *Annu. Rev. Neurosci.* 7, 309–338. doi: 10.1146/annurev.neuro.7.1.309

Bobinski, F., Ferreira, T. A., Córdova, M. M., Dombrowski, P. A., da Cunha, C., Santo, C. C., et al. (2015). Role of brainstem serotonin in analgesia produced by low-intensity exercise on neuropathic pain after sciatic nerve injury in mice. *Pain* 156, 2595–2606. doi: 10.1097/j.pain.0000000000000372

Boccard, S. G., Pereira, E. A., Moir, L., Aziz, T. Z., and Green, A. L. (2013). Long-term outcomes of deep brain stimulation for neuropathic pain. *Neurosurgery* 72, 221–230; discussion 231. doi: 10.1227/NEU.0b013e31827b97d6

Bouhassira, D., Attal, N., Fermanian, J., Alchaar, H., Gautron, M., Masquelier, E., et al. (2004). Development and validation of the neuropathic pain symptom inventory. *Pain* 108, 248–257. doi: 10.1016/j.pain.2003.12.024

Carballosa-Gonzalez, M. M., Vitores, A., and Hentall, I. D. (2014). Hindbrain raphe stimulation boosts cyclic adenosine monophosphate and signaling proteins in the injured spinal cord. *Brain Res.* 1543, 165–172. doi: 10.1016/j.brainres.2013.11.013

Cardenas, D. D., Nieshoff, E. C., Suda, K., Goto, S., Sanin, L., and Knapp, L. E. (2013). A randomized trial of pregabalin in patients with neuropathic pain due to spinal cord injury. *Neurology* 80, 533–539. doi: 10.1212/WNL.0b013e318281546b

Carlton, S. M., Du, J., Tan, H. Y., Nesic, O., Hargett, G. L., Bopp, A. C., et al. (2009). Peripheral and central sensitization in remote spinal cord regions contribute to central neuropathic pain after spinal cord injury. *Pain* 147, 265–276. doi: 10.1016/j.pain.2009.09.030

Cerritelli, S., Hirschberg, S., Hill, R., Balthasar, N., and Pickering, A. E. (2016). Activation of brainstem pro-opiomelanocortin neurons produces opioidergic analgesia, bradycardia and bradypnoea. *PLoS One* 11:e0153187. doi: 10.1371/journal.pone.0153187

Coffey, R. J. (2001). Deep brain stimulation for chronic pain: results of two multicenter trials and a structured review. *Pain Med.* 2, 183–192. doi: 10.1046/j.1526-4637.2001.01029.x

Finnerup, N. B., Norrbrink, C., Trok, K., Piehl, F., Johannesen, I. L., Sørensen, J. C., et al. (2014). Phenotypes and predictors of pain following traumatic spinal cord injury: a prospective study. *J. Pain* 15, 40–48. doi: 10.1016/j.jpain.2013.09.008

Gao, F., Chu, H., Li, L., Yang, M., Du, L., Chen, L., et al. (2016). Repetitive transcranial magnetic stimulation for pain after spinal cord injury: a systematic review and meta-analysis. *J. Neurosurg. Sci.* [Epub ahead of print].

Gray, A. M., Pounds-Cornish, E., Eccles, F. J., Aziz, T. Z., Green, A. L., and Scott, R. B. (2014). Deep brain stimulation as a treatment for neuropathic pain: a longitudinal study addressing neuropsychological outcomes. *J. Pain* 15, 283–292. doi: 10.1016/j.jpain.2013.11.003

Guy, S. D., Mehta, S., Casalino, A., Côté, I., Kras-Dupuis, A., Moulin, D. E., et al. (2016). The CanPain SCI clinical practice guidelines for rehabilitation management of neuropathic pain after spinal cord: recommendations for treatment. *Spinal Cord* 54, S14–S23. doi: 10.1038/sc.2016.90

Hari, A. R., Wydenkeller, S., Dokladal, P., and Halder, P. (2009). Enhanced recovery of human spinothalamic function is associated with central neuropathic pain after SCI. *Exp. Neurol.* 216, 428–430. doi: 10.1016/j.expneurol.2008.12.018

Hentall, I. D., and Gonzalez, M. M. C. (2012). Promotion of recovery from thoracic spinal cord contusion in rats by stimulation of medullary raphe or its midbrain input. *Neurorehabil. Neural Repair* 26, 374–384. doi: 10.1177/1545968311425178

Hentall, I. D., Luca, C. C., Widerstrom-Noga, E., Vitores, A., Fisher, L. D., Martinez-Arizala, A., et al. (2016). The midbrain central gray best suppresses chronic pain with electrical stimulation at very low pulse rates in two human cases. *Brain Res.* 1632, 119–126. doi: 10.1016/j.brainres.2015.12.021

Hentall, I. D., Pinzon, A., and Noga, B. R. (2006). Spatial and temporal patterns of serotonin release in the rat's lumbar spinal cord following electrical stimulation of the nucleus raphe magnus. *Neuroscience* 142, 893–903. doi: 10.1016/j.neuroscience.2006.06.038

Hickey, L., Li, Y., Fyson, S. J., Watson, T. C., Perrins, R., Hewinson, J., et al. (2014). Optoactivation of locus ceruleus neurons evokes bidirectional changes in thermal nociception in rats. *J. Neurosci.* 34, 4148–4160. doi: 10.1523/JNEUROSCI.4835-13.2014

Li, Y., Hickey, L., Perrins, R., Werlen, E., Patel, A. A., Hirschberg, S., et al. (2016). Retrograde optogenetic characterization of the pontospinal module of the locus coeruleus with a canine adenoviral vector. *Brain Res.* 1641, 274–290. doi: 10.1016/j.brainres.2016.02.023

Melzack, R., and Wall, P. D. (1965). Pain mechanisms: a new theory. *Science* 150, 971–979. doi: 10.1126/science.150.3699.971

Pereira, E. A., and Aziz, T. Z. (2014). Neuropathic pain and deep brain stimulation. *Neurotherapeutics* 11, 496–507. doi: 10.1007/s13311-014-0278-x

Robinson, C., Apgar, C., and Shapiro, L. A. (2016). Astrocyte hypertrophy contributes to aberrant neurogenesis after traumatic brain injury. *Neural Plast.* 2016:1347987. doi: 10.1155/2016/1347987

Schofferman, J., Fishman, S. M., Harden, R. N., and Kirschner, K. L. (2014). Did we reach too far? The opioid epidemic and chronic pain. *PM R* 6, 78–84. doi: 10.1016/j.pmrj.2013.12.003

Scholz, J., and Woolf, C. J. (2007). The neuropathic pain triad: neurons, immune cells and glia. *Nat. Neurosci.* 10, 1361–1368. doi: 10.1038/nn1992

Siddall, P. J., McClelland, J. M., Rutkowski, S. B., and Cousins, M. J. (2003). A longitudinal study of the prevalence and characteristics of pain in the first 5 years following spinal cord injury. *Pain* 103, 249–257. doi: 10.1016/s0304-3959(02)00452-9

Siddall, P. J., Molloy, A. R., Walker, S., Mather, L. E., Rutkowski, S. B., and Cousins, M. J. (2000). The efficacy of intrathecal morphine and clonidine in the treatment of pain after spinal cord injury. *Anesth. Analg.* 91, 1493–1498. doi: 10.1097/00000539-200012000-00037

Tiwari, P., Danish, S., and Madabhushi, A. (2014). Identifying MRI markers to evaluate early treatment related changes post laser ablation for cancer pain management. *Proc. SPIE Int. Soc. Opt. Eng.* 9036:90362L. doi: 10.1117/12.2043729

Urtikova, N., Berson, N., Van Steenwinckel, J., Doly, S., Truchetto, J., Maroteaux, L., et al. (2012). Antinociceptive effect of peripheral serotonin

5-HT_{2B} receptor activation on neuropathic pain. *Pain* 153, 1320–1331. doi: 10.1016/j.pain.2012.03.024

Van Bockstaele, E. J., Aston-Jones, G., Pieribone, V. A., Ennis, M., and Shipley, M. T. (1991). Subregions of the periaqueductal gray topographically innervate the rostral ventral medulla in the rat. *J. Comp. Neurol.* 309, 305–327. doi: 10.1002/cne.903090303

Vanegas, H., and Schaible, H. G. (2004). Descending control of persistent pain: inhibitory or facilitory? *Brain Res. Rev.* 46, 295–309. doi: 10.1016/j.brainresrev.2004.07.004

Vranken, J. H. (2009). Mechanisms and treatment of neuropathic pain. *Cent. Nerv. Syst. Agents Med. Chem.* 9, 71–78. doi: 10.2174/187152409787601932

Widerström-Noga, E., Biering-Sørensen, F., Bryce, T. N., Cardenas, D. D., Finnerup, N. B., Jensen, M. P., et al. (2014). The international spinal cord injury pain basic data set (version 2.0). *Spinal Cord* 52, 282–286. doi: 10.1038/sc.2014.4

Widerström-Noga, E. G., Cruz-Almeida, Y., Martinez-Arizala, A., and Turk, D. C. (2006). Internal consistency, stability and validity of the spinal cord injury version of the multidimensional pain inventory. *Arch. Phys. Med. Rehabil.* 87, 516–523. doi: 10.1016/j.apmr.2005.12.036

Widerström-Noga, E., Felix, E. R., Adcock, J. P., Escalona, M., and Tibbett, J. (2016). Multidimensional neuropathic pain phenotypes after spinal cord injury. *J. Neurotrauma* 33, 482–492. doi: 10.1089/neu.2015.4040

Zeilig, G., Enosh, S., Rubin-Asher, D., Lehr, B., and Defrin, R. (2012). The nature and course of sensory changes following spinal cord injury: predictive properties and implications on the mechanism of central pain. *Brain* 135, 418–430. doi: 10.1093/brain/awr270

12

Frontal Connectivity in EEG Gamma (30–45 Hz) Respond to Spinal Cord Stimulation in Minimally Conscious State Patients

Yang Bai[1], *Xiaoyu Xia*[2], *Zhenhu Liang*[1], *Yong Wang*[1], *Yi Yang*[2], *Jianghong He*[2]* and *Xiaoli Li*[3,4]*

[1] *Institute of Electrical Engineering, Yanshan University, Qinhuangdao, China,* [2] *Department of Neurosurgery, PLA General Hospital, Beijing, China,* [3] *State Key Laboratory of Cognitive Neuroscience and Learning, Beijing Normal University, Beijing, China,* [4] *IDG/McGovern Institute for Brain Research, Beijing Normal University, Beijing, China*

Correspondence:
Jianghong He
he_jianghong@sina.cn
Xiaoli Li
xiaoli@bnu.edu.cn

Spinal cord stimulation (SCS) has become a valuable brain-intervention technique used to rehabilitate patients with disorders of consciousness (DOC). To explore how the SCS affects the cerebral cortex and what possible electrophysiological mechanism of SCS effects on the cortex, the present study investigated the functional connectivity and network properties during SCS in minimally conscious state (MCS) patients. MCS patients received both SCS and sham sessions. Functional connectivity of the phase lock value (PLV) in the gamma band (30–45 Hz) was investigated at the pre-, on- and post-SCS stages. In addition, to evaluate global network properties, complex network parameters, including average path length, cluster coefficient and small-world, were measured. When SCS was turned on, significantly decreased connectivity was noted in the local scale of the frontal-frontal region and in the large scales of the frontal-parietal and frontal-occipital regions. The global network showed fewer small-world properties, average path lengths increased and cluster coefficients decreased. When SCS was turned off, the large-scale connectivity and global network returned to its pre-SCS level, but the local scale of frontal-frontal connectivity remained significantly lower than its pre-SCS level. Sham sessions produced no significant changes in either functional connectivity or network. The findings directly showed that SCS could effectively intervene cortical gamma activity, and the intervention included immediate global effects (large scale connectivity and network alteration only occurred in stimulation period) and long-lasting local effects (local scale connectivity alteration persist beyond stimulation period). Moreover, considering the mechanism and propagation of gamma activity, it indicates that the frontal cortex plays a crucial role in the SCS effects on the cerebral cortex.

Keywords: spinal cord stimulation, EEG, minimally conscious state, gamma, functional connectivity

INTRODUCTION

Despite considerable research, there is currently no effective standardized treatment for patients with disorders of consciousness (DOC). However, in recent years, spinal cord stimulation (SCS) has become a valuable brain-intervention technique for rehabilitating DOC patients because it is a less-invasive, simpler surgical procedure than deep-brain stimulation (Georgiopoulos et al., 2010;

Mattogno et al., 2017). Studies have shown its efficacy in modulating the brains of DOC patients (Yamamoto et al., 2012, 2013, 2017), but the underlying mechanism of its effects on the cerebral cortex is still unclear.

Electrophysiological studies investigating the effects of SCS on DOC patients are limited. Studies using pain-related P250 amplitude have shown that SCS may indirectly stimulate the frontal cortex, which is part of the awareness and attention network (Yampolsky et al., 2012; Yamamoto et al., 2013). In a previous study, we reported that SCS modulated frontal delta and gamma activity in patients in a minimally conscious state (MCS) (Bai et al., 2017), showing that SCS modulated the brain functions of MCS patients and providing EEG evidence supporting the potential mechanism for doing so: stimulating the reticular formation and further affecting the frontal cortical region through the formation-thalamus-cortex network. However, further research is needed to provide detailed evidence about the pathway by which SCS affects the cerebral cortices of DOC patients.

Gamma oscillatory activity is thought to be a fundamental mechanism that integrates neural networks within and across brain structures, facilitates coherent sensory registration and mediates cognitive functions (Kaiser and Lutzenberger, 2005; Herrmann et al., 2010; Roye et al., 2010). This activity may represent a coding operator for brain functions and inter-area communications (Basar, 2013). Gamma connectivity has been implicated relevant in subjective consciousness (Llinas et al., 1998; Singer, 1998), and gamma coherence has been shown to be a fundamental prerequisite in the aware process and the potential to participate cognitive processes (Naro et al., 2016). In addition, gamma connectivity has been identified as an important awareness-level marker in DOC patients (Cavinato et al., 2015; Naro et al., 2016). In MCS and vegetative state (VS) patients, significant differences have been demonstrated in the responses of short-range parietal and long-range fronto-parietal gamma coherences to simple sensory stimulus modalities (Cavinato et al., 2015). Our previous study found that SCS, particularly at 70 Hz, significantly changed gamma activity, increasing its relative power and decreasing both coherence and global synchronization. Therefore, considering gamma activity's critical role in cognitive and brain function, gamma activity alteration induced by SCS may increase understanding of the possible physiological basis for the effects of SCS.

Functional connectivity and corresponding network parameters have been identified as valuable characteristic to assess the brain states of DOC patients (Kotchoubey et al., 2013; Chennu et al., 2014; Monti et al., 2015). Functional connectivity measures the relationships among the activities measured in various regions of interest in the brain. Analysing complex networks based on graph theory has enabled the application of new methods useful to investigating both local and global properties of functional connectivity in the brain (Bullmore and Sporns, 2009). Combination of functional connectivity and network properties play a prominent role in analysing, describing and understanding human brain function (Stam and Reijneveld, 2007). Therefore, the present study focused on assessing the functional connectivity and network characteristics of gamma activity. Given that SCS at a frequency of 70 Hz proved to significantly change gamma activity, 70 Hz was chosen as the frequency parameter of stimulation during sessions that included EEG recording at the pre-, on- and post-SCS stages. We hypothesized that the relationships among various brain regions would identify the pathway responsible for the SCS effects.

EXPERIMENTAL PROCEDURES

Patients

As reported in our previous study, 16 MCS patients, aged 19–65, who had received SCS implants were enrolled in a multiple-session stimulation study. All participants were at least 3 weeks post-surgery and had stable clinical states. During the study, 5 participants dropped out due to infection and other clinical factors. **Table 1** shows the clinical features of the 11 participants who completed the entire study. The consciousness state of each patient was assessed using the JFK Coma Recovery Scale-Revised (JFK CRS-R) (Giacino et al., 2004). Any treatment or drugs that could modify cortical excitability were excluded. Written informed consent to participate in the study was obtained from the patient's caregivers, and the study was approved by the ethics committee of PLA Army General Hospital.

Stimulation Protocol

The participants received both sessions that included real stimulation and sham stimulations, with at least 2 days' washout between sessions. Stimulation was delivered by a pulse generator (Prime Advanced, Medtronic Inc., Minneapolis, MN, USA) that delivered electric pulses with a 3-V amplitude and a 210-μs pulse width. The pulse generator was implanted under the anterior chest wall. And the pulse generator was connected to stimulation electrodes through Touhy needle. The needle was implanted into the midline epidural space at the cervical-thoracic junction. And the stimulation electrodes were inserted into the epidural space of the cervical vertebrae, and placed at the C2–C4 levels. The stimulation was caused by periodic occurrence of voltage

TABLE 1 | Participants' demographic characteristics.

Patient	Etiology	Post-injury (months)	CRS-R
Patient 1	Hemorrhage	18	8
Patient 2	Hemorrhage	12	10
Patient 3	Hemorrhage	11	7
Patient 4	Hemorrhage	11	7
Patient 5	Anoxia	4	10
Patient 6	Hemorrhage	3	9
Patient 7	Hemorrhage	4	7
Patient 8	Anoxia	3	7
Patient 9	Infarction	4	7
Patient 10	Anoxia	8	7
Patient 11	Anoxia	28	9

CRS-R, Coma recovery scale-revised.

difference between two electrodes. The stimulation parameters could be setup by a wireless controller *in vitro*. In this study, the stimulation frequency parameter was set at 70 Hz and delivered for 20 min consecutively. Sham stimulations were conducted with the stimulator turned off.

EEG Recordings and Pre-processing

Resting state EEG was recorded for 10 min before stimulation, for 20 min during the real or sham stimulation and for 10 min immediately after the stimulation. EEGs were recorded using 32 channels (BrainAmp 64 MRplus, Brain Products, Germany) and Ag/AgCl pin electrodes having a sampling rate of 1 kHz. The skin/electrode impedance was maintained below 5 kΩ. During the experiments, participants were behaviorally awake (eyes open, EO), and if they showed signs of sleepiness (prolonged eye closure, EC), either the JFK CRS-R arousal-facilitation protocol was applied or the experiment was suspended.

EEG pre-processing was conducted using EEGLAB software version 12.0.2.5b, running on a MATLAB environment (Version 2013b, MathWorks Inc.; Natick, MA, USA). The 50-Hz power signal was removed by a notch filter. The EEG signal was band filtered between 1 and 45 Hz. The Independent Component Analysis (ICA) was used to identify and remove artifact-relevant components, including eye movements and muscle activation. The EEG data were divided into epochs of 10 s with overlaps of 50%. The selected artifact-free epochs were average referenced.

EEG Analysis

Phase Locking Value (PLV)

Connectivity between pairwise channels in the gamma band (30–45 Hz) was computed using phase synchronization, which is briefly described as follows. For each epoch EEG signal, the instantaneous phases $\varphi_x(t)$ and $\varphi_y(t)$ of the pairwise channel were evaluated based on the Hilbert transform. Then, the phase difference was defined by

$$\Delta\phi_{xy}(t) = \varphi_x(t) - \varphi_y(t). \quad (1)$$

Several indices based on the phase difference within a short term can be used to indicate the phase synchronization between two series (Rosenblum et al., 2001). The present study applied PLV based on the circular variance of the phase difference, yielding

$$PLV_{xy} = \frac{1}{N}\left|\sum_{t=1}^{N} e^{j\Delta\varphi_{xy}(t)}\right|. \quad (2)$$

This measure of PLV varied between 0 and 1, and the computation involved no parameter choices. Therefore, the synchrony can be described by a phase-synchronization matrix C with each element of PLV_{xy}.

Graph Theoretical Analysis

Graph theoretical analysis was performed on the phase synchronization matrices. The nodes in the graph were defined as the electrodes and the links as the measure of the phase synchronization between the nodes. Weighted graphs were created using synchronization matrix C with each element of PLV_{xy}.

Graphs can be characterized using various measures, two of the most fundamental of which are the clustering coefficient, which denotes the likelihood that neighbors of a vertex will also be connected to each other, and the average path length, which indicates the average number of edges of the shortest path between pairs of vertices. Stam et al. (2009) provided full definitions for calculating the clustering index (C_w) and the path length (L_w) to analyse weighted networks. To calculate the clustering index from weighted networks, the weights between the node i and the other nodes j should be symmetrical ($\omega_{ij} = \omega_{ji}$), and $0 \le \omega_{ij} \le 1$, as proposed by Onnela et al. (2005). Indeed, both conditions are readily fulfilled when using PLV values as the weight definition. Then, the weighted clustering index of vertex i is defined as

$$C_i = \frac{\sum_{k\neq i}\sum_{l\neq i, l\neq k} \omega_{ik}\omega_{il}\omega_{kl}}{\sum_{k\neq i}\sum_{l\neq i, l\neq k} \omega_{ik}\omega_{il}}. \quad (3)$$

Note that all sums terms with $k = i$, $l = i$ or $k = l$ are skipped. The mean clustering of the total network is defined as

$$C_w = \frac{1}{N}\sum_{i=1}^{N} C_i \quad (4)$$

Then, the length of a weighted path between two vertices is defined as the sum of the lengths of the edges of this path. The shortest path L_{ij} between two vertices i and j is the path between i and j with the shortest length. The averaged path length of the entire network is computed as

$$L_w = \frac{1}{(1/N(N-1))\sum_{i=1}^{N}\sum_{j\neq i}^{N}(1/L_{ij})} \quad (5)$$

In this formula, the harmonic mean is used to handle disconnected edges resulting in infinite path lengths (i.e., $1/\infty \to 0$) (Newman, 2003). Then, the small-world parameter can be calculated as $S = \frac{C_w}{L_w}$.

To obtain measures that are independent of network size, the mean edge weight and the mean path length were compared to the mean of 50 random networks. The C_w^s and L_w^s denote weighted clustering coefficient and path length, respectively, averaged over an ensemble of 50 random, surrogate networks that were derived from the original network by randomly reshuffling the edge weights. Then, the final index was obtained from $\widehat{C}_w = C_w/C_w^s$ and $\widehat{L}_w = L_w/L_w^s$. Finally, the small-world parameter was denoted as $S = \frac{\widehat{C}_w}{\widehat{L}_w}$.

RESULTS

Functional connectivity was measured using the PLV between each set of pairwise EEG channels. Then, interest regions were defined as follows: frontal (Fp1, Fp2, Fz, F3, and F4), central (Cz, C3, and C4), parietal (Pz, P3, and P4) and occipital (Oz, O3, and O4). **Figure 1** shows the functional connectivity of electrodes in the regions of interest and the overall brain in gamma band. Comparison of on-SCS and pre-SCS shows a

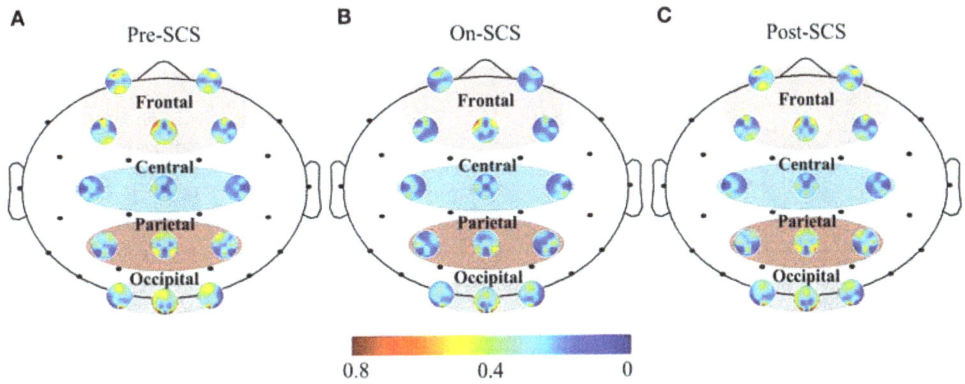

FIGURE 1 | Functional connectivity of electrodes in regions of interest and overall brain in gamma band. **(A)** Average functional connectivity of the electrodes with overall brain pre-SCS. **(B)** Average functional connectivity of the electrodes with overall brain on-SCS. **(C)** Average functional connectivity of the electrodes with others post-SCS. Each colored circle shows the connectivity between the identified electrode and other electrodes. The regions of interest are the frontal, central, parietal and occipital. Colors indicate the average strength of connectivity.

distinct decrease of connectivity among the frontal, frontal-parietal and frontal-occipital regions. After the SCS was turned off, connectivity of frontal-frontal, frontal-parietal and frontal-occipital were markedly returned.

SCS induced connectivity changes were found in frontal-frontal, frontal-parietal, and frontal-occipital (**Figure 2A**). To investigate the changes at different stages, we compared the average connectivity between pairwise stages using paired *t*-tests: On-SCS vs. Pre-SCS, Post-SCS vs. On-SCS and Post-SCS vs. Pre-SCS (**Figure 2B**). Bonferroni correction was performed after multiple comparisons. When SCS was turned on (On-SCS vs. Pre-SCS), significant decreases of connectivity were found in frontal-frontal ($p < 0.001$), frontal-parietal ($p < 0.001$) and frontal-occipital ($p = 0.011$). When SCS was turned off, all the connectivity rebounded but only with significance in the frontal-parietal ($p < 0.001$). But when post-SCS compared with pre-SCS, significance was only found within frontal-frontal connectivity ($p < 0.001$). As **Table 2** shows, in sham sessions, in all three stages, the average connectivity showed no significant changes.

Then, pairwise comparisons of each connectivity were performed using paired *t*-tests, and correction of the false discovery rate was performed after multiple comparisons (q-value $= 0.05$). Top panel of **Figure 2C** shows the significantly altered connecitities in comparison of pairwise stages. Then, we defined the electrodes which were included in at least three significantly changed connectivities as critical electrodes (bottom panel of **Figure 2C**). The location of the significantly altered connectivity and critical eletrodes was generally consistent with the average connectivity findings. When SCS was turned on or turned off, the significantly altered connectivity and critical electrodes were both located mostly in the frontal and parietal regions. And after SCS stimulation, the locations of the significantly decreased connectivity and the critical electrodes were found in frontal regions.

In order to explore the effects of SCS on the global cerebral cortex, graph theoretical based network parameters were calculated using the connectivity matrix in the gamma band at three stages: path length, cluster coefficient and small-world. Comparisons between pairwise stages were performed using paired *t*-tests with Bonferroni corrections. **Figure 3** shows the boxplot of the parameters at each stage. Significant increases of average path length ($p = 0.004$) and decreases of cluster coefficient ($p = 0.040$) were found during SCS stimulation period. The global network showed less small-world property. And the network perturbation company with the stimulation. When SCS was turned off, the network parameters rebound to the baseline level. In sham sessions, the various stages produced no significant alterations of the network parameters.

DISCUSSION

SCS has been demonstrated as a valuable brain-intervention technique for rehabilitating DOC patients (Georgiopoulos et al., 2010; Mattogno et al., 2017; Yamamoto et al., 2017). But there was still few studies investigating the potential mechanism. In a previous study (Bai et al., 2017), we reported that SCS at a frequency of 70 Hz could effectively modulate MCS patients' frontal gamma activities by increasing the relative power and decreasing the coherence and global synchronization. In order to further explore the effects of SCS with 70 Hz on interventing gamma activity, the present study measured functional connectivity and network properties in the gamma band at different SCS stages. By this way, we aim to investigate how the SCS effects on the cortex and what the potential pathway participate SCS modulation on the cerebral. Comparing with pre-SCS, SCS turning on induced significant decreases in functional connectivity in local scale of frontal-frontal and large scale of frontal-parietal and frontal-occipital regions. When SCS was turned off, the large scale connectivity and global network features returned to the pre-SCS level. But the local scale of frontal-frontal connectivity stays lower than pre-SCS. The findings directly show that, SCS turning on effectively modulate the gamma activity. The interventaion includes immediate global

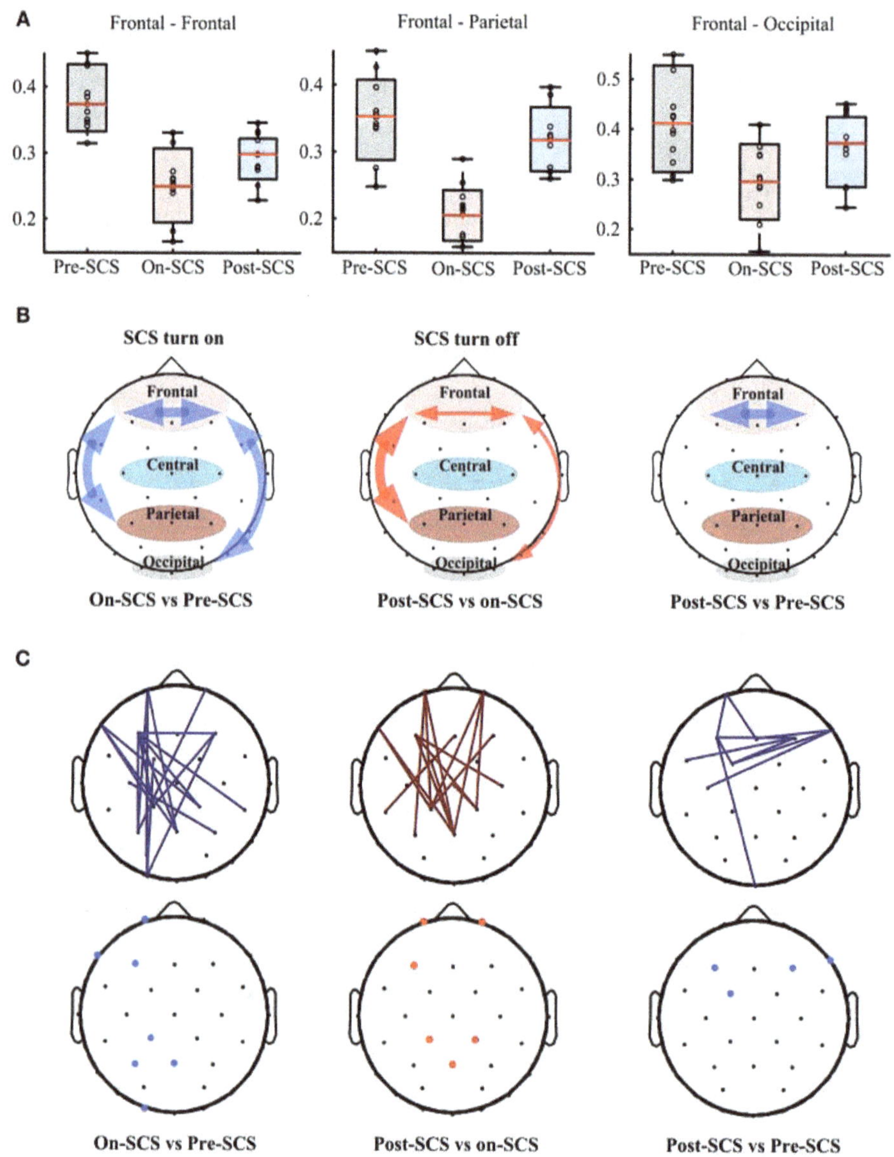

FIGURE 2 | (A) Functional connectivity in patients' gamma bands at pre-, on- and post-SCS. **(B)** Compasions of patients' average frontal-frontal, frontal-parietal and frontal-occipital connectivity using paired *t*-test. Heavy red arrows mean significant increases, thin red arrows mean increase without significance, and blue arrows mean significant decreases. **(C)** Top panel shows significantly altered connectivities and bottom panel shows critical electrodes compared between pairwise stages. Red lines mean significantly increased connectivity, and blue lines mean significant decreased connectivity. Red dots mean critical electrodes included in significantly increased connectivities, and blue dots mean critical electrodes included in significantly decreased connectivities.

TABLE 2 | Gamma band functional connectivity and network parameters (mean ± standard deviation) pre-SCS, on-SCS and post-SCS in sham sessions.

	Pre-SCS	On-SCS	Post-SCS
Frontal-Frontal	0.374 ± 0.047	0.380 ± 0.042	0.357 ± 0.031
Frontal-Parietal	0.341 ± 0.052	0.358 ± 0.070	0.332 ± 0.060
Frontal-Occipital	0.399 ± 0.076	0.389 ± 0.076	0.386 ± 0.073
Average path length	0.189 ± 0.020	0.186 ± 0.018	0.190 ± 0.013
Cluster coefficient	5.664 ± 0.396	5.584 ± 0.458	5.627 ± 0.048
Small-World	31.26 ± 5.448	31.24 ± 6.784	31.29 ± 3.806

effects (large scale connectivity and network property), and local effects (local scale connectivity) which last beyond period of the stimulation. The global and local effects imply that regions of frontal, parietal and occipital were the direct targets of SCS. But, potential after-effects of local or global effects of SCS on consciousness rehabilitation should be further explored in long-term clinical assessment.

These results provide further evidence supporting the critical role of the frontal cortex in the SCS effects. All significantly altered connectivity was relevant to the frontal region, no matter whether it was in global or local effects. When SCS was turned off,

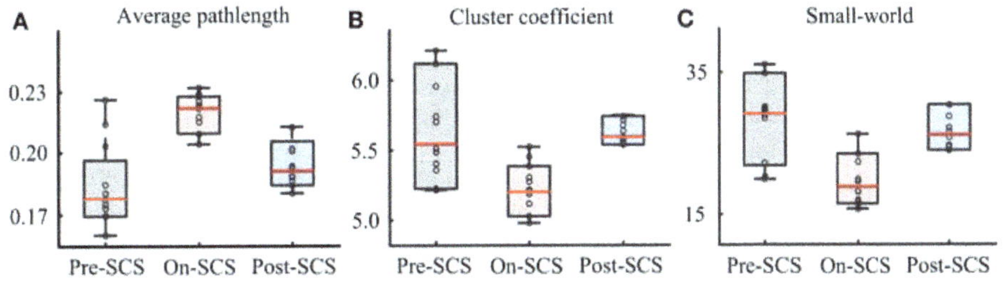

FIGURE 3 | Network parameters in gamma bands at pre-SCS, on-SCS and post-SCS. **(A)** Average path length. **(B)** Cluster coefficients. **(C)** Small-world.

connectivity of the frontal-parietal and frontal-occipital returned to pre-SCS levels, but frontal-frontal connectivity in post-SCS remained lower than pre-SCS. These decreases in the frontal regions were consistent with the coherence results from our previous study (Bai et al., 2017). Evidence demonstrating the role of the frontal cortex in SCS has also been provided by other studies using pain-related P250 amplitude. These studies demonstrated the capability of SCS to directly affect the frontal cortex (Yampolsky et al., 2012; Yamamoto et al., 2013). Therefore, the intervention global effects occurring in the parietal and occipital cortices may be induced by their interaction with frontal cortex, and the interaction could be represented in gamma connectivity.

Considering the crucial role of gamma activity in brain function, the gamma alteration induced by SCS stimulation may imply brain modulation in DOC patients. Gamma activity can be measured in a wide range of cortical and subcortical structures (Basar and Bullock, 1992). One important potential mechanism considered existing a subcortical pacemaker (thalamus) that drove the cortex at a frequency in the gamma band (Llinas et al., 1998). Then, the gamma activity measured in the cortex was propagated by thalamo-cortical connections (Steriade et al., 1996; Llinas et al., 2005), meaning that the intra-laminar thalamic nuclei might drive large areas of the cortex using gamma oscillations (Llinas and Ribary, 1993). Therefore, these global changes in connectivity and network in the gamma activity suggest the capability of SCS to modulate the gamma pacemaker: thalamus. The altered thalamus interrupts the established model of gamma "command" activity in the cortex, thus causing fewer small-world network features, including increasing average path length and decreasing cluster coefficient, in the cortex. When combined with the results of our previous research, those of the present study suggest that gamma activity detected in the cortex, especially the frontal cortex, may be a significant biomarker for evaluating the effects of SCS.

The results of the present study provide EEG evidence demonstrating the anatomical pathway by which SCS modulates the brain: the thalamus-cortex connection. This is consistent with the indications that the SCS mechanism may be that it enhances the specific firing of the cerebral cortex by exerting a direct effect on the reticular formation-thalamus pathway. In addition, the crucial role of the frontal region in altering connectivity along with SCS stimulation prompts us to propose the frontal cortex as a relay station in the SCS modulation pathway. SCS affects the cerebral cortex by first modulating the frontal cortex and then propagating to other regions via frontal cortex connectivity. Coincidentally, this pathway has been included in a meso-circuit model that attempts to explain DOC after brain injuries (Schiff, 2010). In this explanation, the connections between the thalamus, frontal cortex and parietal/occipital/temporal cortices are crucial to maintaining the consciousness-related network (Giacino et al., 2014). The significant changes in connectivity in the gamma that are induced by SCS being turned on and off are closely related to the three important nodes (thalamus, frontal cortex and parietal/occipital cortices) in this circuit-level pathway. Therefore, we propose that the effects of SCS on consciousness may benefit from interfering with the circuit-level network.

CONCLUSIONS

The present study investigated connectivity and network characteristics in the gamma band at pre-, on- and post-SCS using an SCS frequency of 70 Hz. Significantly frontal related connectivity alterations and network parameters changes were found in gamma band. The findings indicated that SCS could effectively affect the cerebral cortex and the intervention includes immediate global effects (large scale connectivity of frontal-parietal and frontal-occipital, and network alteration) and long-lasting local effects (local connectivity of frontal-frontal). Considering the mechanism of gamma generation and propagation, we suggest that the frontal cortex plays the crucial role in pathway of the stimulation: the SCS alters the frontal cortex by using the thalamus-cortex connection, and then the global brain are modulated via connectivity with the frontal cortex. In addition, the pathway may be the anatomical basis by which the SCS modulates the brain. Since the thalamus, frontal cortex and parietal/occipital cortex play crucial roles in the consciousness-related network, the effects of SCS on consciousness may benefit from interfering with the circuit-level network.

ETHICS STATEMENT

This study was carried out in accordance with the recommendations of the ethics committee of PLA Army

General Hospital with written informed consent from all subjects. All subjects gave written informed consent in accordance with the Declaration of Helsinki. The protocol was approved by the ethics committee of PLA Army General Hospital.

AUTHOR CONTRIBUTIONS

YB had full access to all the data in the study and takes responsibility for the integrity of the data and the accuracy of the data analysis. Study concept and design: YB and XX. Acquisition, analysis, or interpretation of data: YB and XX. Drafting of the manuscript: YB. Critical revision of the manuscript for important intellectual content: All authors. Statistical analysis: YB. Obtained funding: JH and XL. Administrative, technical, or material support: YW. Study supervision: JH and XL.

FUNDING

This work was supported by the National Natural Science Foundation of China (grant numbers 61273063, 81230023); the Beijing Municipal Science and Technology Commission (grant number Z141107002514111); the Innovation Cultivation Fund of the PLA Army General Hospital (grant number 2015-LC-09); The commercialization of research fund supported by Beijing Municipal Commission of Education.

ACKNOWLEDGMENTS

The authors are grateful for the assistance of all persons and volunteers whose participation was essential for the successful completion of this study.

REFERENCES

Bai, Y., Xia, X., Li, X., Wang, Y., Yang, Y., Liu, Y., et al. (2017). Spinal cord stimulation modulates frontal delta and gamma in patients of minimally consciousness state. *Neuroscience* 346, 247–254. doi: 10.1016/j.neuroscience.2017.01.036

Basar, E. (2013). A review of gamma oscillations in healthy subjects and in cognitive impairment. *Int. J. Psychophysiol.* 90, 99–117. doi: 10.1016/j.ijpsycho.2013.07.005

Basar, E., and Bullock, T. H. (1992). *Induced Rhythms in the Brain.* Boston, MA: Springer. doi: 10.1007/978-1-4757-1281-0

Bullmore, E., and Sporns, O. (2009). Complex brain networks: graph theoretical analysis of structural and functional systems. *Nat. Rev. Neurosci.* 10, 186–198. doi: 10.1038/nrn2575

Cavinato, M., Genna, C., Manganotti, P., Formaggio, E., Storti, S. F., Campostrini, S., et al. (2015). Coherence and consciousness: study of fronto-parietal gamma synchrony in patients with disorders of consciousness. *Brain Topogr.* 28, 570–579. doi: 10.1007/s10548-014-0383-5

Chennu, S., Finoia, P., Kamau, E., Allanson, J., Williams, G. B., Monti, M. M., et al. (2014). Spectral signatures of reorganised brain networks in disorders of consciousness. *PLoS Comput. Biol.* 10:e1003887. doi: 10.1371/journal.pcbi.1003887

Georgiopoulos, M., Katsakiori, P., Kefalopoulou, Z., Ellul, J., Chroni, E., and Constantoyannis, C. (2010). Vegetative state and minimally conscious state: a review of the therapeutic interventions. *Stereotact. Funct. Neurosurg.* 88, 199–207. doi: 10.1159/000314354

Giacino, J. T., Fins, J. J., Laureys, S., and Schiff, N. D. (2014). Disorders of consciousness after acquired brain injury: the state of the science. *Nat. Rev. Neurol.* 10, 99–114. doi: 10.1038/nrneurol.2013.279

Giacino, J. T., Kalmar, K., and Whyte, J. (2004). The JFK Coma Recovery Scale-Revised: measurement characteristics and diagnostic utility. *Arch. Phys. Med. Rehabil.* 85, 2020–2029. doi: 10.1016/j.apmr.2004.02.033

Herrmann, C. S., Frund, I., and Lenz, D. (2010). Human gamma-band activity: a review on cognitive and behavioral correlates and network models. *Neurosci. Biobehav. Rev.* 34, 981–992. doi: 10.1016/j.neubiorev.2009.09.001

Kaiser, J., and Lutzenberger, W. (2005). Cortical oscillatory activity and the dynamics of auditory memory processing. *Rev. Neurosci.* 16, 239–254. doi: 10.1515/REVNEURO.2005.16.3.239

Kotchoubey, B., Merz, S., Lang, S., Markl, A., Muller, F., Yu, T., et al. (2013). Global functional connectivity reveals highly significant differences between the vegetative and the minimally conscious state. *J. Neurol.* 260, 975–983. doi: 10.1007/s00415-012-6734-9

Llinas, R., and Ribary, U. (1993). Coherent 40-Hz oscillation characterizes dream state in humans. *Proc. Natl. Acad. Sci. U.S.A.* 90, 2078–2081. doi: 10.1073/pnas.90.5.2078

Llinas, R., Ribary, U., Contreras, D., and Pedroarena, C. (1998). The neuronal basis for consciousness. *Philos. Trans. R. Soc. Lond. B Biol. Sci.* 353, 1841–1849. doi: 10.1098/rstb.1998.0336

Llinas, R., Urbano, F. J., Leznik, E., Ramirez, R. R., and van Marle, H. J. (2005). Rhythmic and dysrhythmic thalamocortical dynamics: GABA systems and the edge effect. *Trends Neurosci.* 28, 325–333. doi: 10.1016/j.tins.2005.04.006

Mattogno, P. P., Barbagallo, G., Iacopino, G., Pappalardo, G., LA Rocca, G., Signorelli, F., et al. (2017). Recovery from chronic diseases of consciousness: state of the art in neuromodulation for persistent vegetative state and minimally conscious state. *Acta Neurochir. Suppl.* 124, 19–25. doi: 10.1007/978-3-319-39546-3_4

Monti, M. M., Rosenberg, M., Finoia, P., Kamau, E., Pickard, J. D., and Owen, A. M. (2015). Thalamo-frontal connectivity mediates top-down cognitive functions in disorders of consciousness. *Neurology* 84, 167–173. doi: 10.1212/WNL.0000000000001123

Naro, A., Russo, M., Leo, A., Cannavo, A., Manuli, A., Bramanti, A., et al. (2016). Cortical connectivity modulation induced by cerebellar oscillatory transcranial direct current stimulation in patients with chronic disorders of consciousness: a marker of covert cognition? *Clin. Neurophysiol.* 127, 1845–1854. doi: 10.1016/j.clinph.2015.12.010

Newman, M. E. (2003). Properties of highly clustered networks. *Phys. Rev. E Stat. Nonlin. Soft Matter Phys.* 68(2 Pt 2):026121. doi: 10.1103/PhysRevE.68.026121

Onnela, J. P., Saramaki, J., Kertesz, J., and Kaski, K. (2005). Intensity and coherence of motifs in weighted complex networks. *Phys. Rev. E Stat. Nonlin. Soft Matter Phys.* 71(6 Pt 2):065103. doi: 10.1103/PhysRevE.71.065103

Rosenblum, M., Pikovsky, A., Kurths, J., Schäfer, C., and Tass, P. A. (2001). Phase synchronization: from theory to data analysis. *Handb. Biol. Phys.* 4, 279–321. doi: 10.1016/S1383-8121(01)80012-9

Roye, A., Schroger, E., Jacobsen, T., and Gruber, T. (2010). Is my mobile ringing? Evidence for rapid processing of a personally significant sound in humans. *J. Neurosci.* 30, 7310–7313. doi: 10.1523/JNEUROSCI.1113-10.2010

Schiff, N. D. (2010). Recovery of consciousness after brain injury: a mesocircuit hypothesis. *Trends Neurosci.* 33, 1–9. doi: 10.1016/j.tins.2009.11.002

Singer, W. (1998). Consciousness and the structure of neuronal representations. *Philos. Trans. R. Soc. Lond. B Biol. Sci.* 353, 1829–1840. doi: 10.1098/rstb.1998.0335

Stam, C. J., de Haan, W., Daffertshofer, A., Jones, B. F., Manshanden, I., van Cappellen van Walsum, A. M., et al. (2009). Graph theoretical analysis of magnetoencephalographic functional connectivity in Alzheimer's disease. *Brain* 132(Pt 1), 213–224. doi: 10.1093/brain/awn262

Stam, C. J., and Reijneveld, J. C. (2007). Graph theoretical analysis of complex networks in the brain. *Nonlin. Biomed. Phys.* 1:3. doi: 10.1186/1753-4631-1-3

Steriade, M., Contreras, D., Amzica, F., and Timofeev, I. (1996). Synchronization of fast (30–40 Hz) spontaneous oscillations in intrathalamic and thalamocortical networks. *J. Neurosci.* 16, 2788–2808.

Yamamoto, T., Katayama, Y., Obuchi, T., Kobayashi, K., Oshima, H., and Fukaya, C. (2012). Spinal cord stimulation for treatment of patients in the minimally conscious state. *Neurol. Med. Chir.* 52, 475–481. doi: 10.2176/nmc.52.475

Yamamoto, T., Katayama, Y., Obuchi, T., Kobayashi, K., Oshima, H., and Fukaya, C. (2013). Deep brain stimulation and spinal cord stimulation for vegetative state and minimally conscious state. *Neurosurgery* 80, S30 e31–39. doi: 10.1016/j.wneu.2012.04.010

Yamamoto, T., Watanabe, M., Obuchi, T., Kobayashi, K., Oshima, H., Fukaya, C., et al. (2017). Spinal cord stimulation for vegetative state and minimally conscious state: changes in consciousness level and motor function. *Acta Neurochir. Suppl.* 124, 37–42. doi: 10.1007/978-3-319-39546-3_6

Yampolsky, C., Hem, S., and Bendersky, D. (2012). Dorsal column stimulator applications. *Surg. Neurol. Int.* 3, S275–S289. doi: 10.4103/2152-7806.103019

13

Influence of Brain Stem on Axial and Hindlimb Spinal Locomotor Rhythm Generating Circuits of the Neonatal Mouse

Céline Jean-Xavier[†] *and Marie-Claude Perreault*[*]

Department of Physiology, Emory University School of Medicine, Atlanta, GA, United States

***Correspondence:**
Marie-Claude Perreault
m-c.perreault@emory.edu

[†]Present Address:
Céline Jean-Xavier,
Department of Comparative Biology and Experimental Medicine, Faculty of Veterinary Medicine, Hotchkiss Brain Institute, University of Calgary, Calgary, AB, Canada

The trunk plays a pivotal role in limbed locomotion. Yet, little is known about how the brain stem controls trunk activity during walking. In this study, we assessed the spatiotemporal activity patterns of axial and hindlimb motoneurons (MNs) during drug-induced fictive locomotor-like activity (LLA) in an isolated brain stem-spinal cord preparation of the neonatal mouse. We also evaluated the extent to which these activity patterns are affected by removal of brain stem. Recordings were made in the segments T7, L2, and L5 using calcium imaging from individual axial MNs in the medial motor column (MMC) and hindlimb MNs in lateral motor column (LMC). The MN activities were analyzed during both the rhythmic and the tonic components of LLA, the tonic component being used as a readout of generalized increase in excitability in spinal locomotor networks. The most salient effect of brain stem removal was an increase in locomotor rhythm frequency and a concomitant reduction in burst durations in both MMC and LMC MNs. The lack of effect on the tonic component of LLA indicated specificity of action during the rhythmic component. Cooling-induced silencing of the brain stem reproduced the increase in rhythm frequency and accompanying decrease in burst durations in L2 MMC and LMC, suggesting a dependency on brain stem neuron activity. The work supports the idea that the brain stem locomotor circuits are operational already at birth and further suggests an important role in modulating trunk activity. The brain stem may influence the axial and hindlimb spinal locomotor rhythm generating circuits by extending their range of operation. This may represent a critical step of locomotor development when learning how to walk in different conditions and environments is a major endeavor.

Keywords: motor command, subcortical, reticulospinal, vestibulospinal, CPG, trunk-hindlimb coordination

INTRODUCTION

Locomotion in mammals is efficient when both trunk and hindlimbs are appropriately controlled (Carlson et al., 1979; Thorstensson et al., 1982; Gramsbergen, 1998; Jamon, 2006; Schilling, 2011). Evidence indicates that both the brainstem and the spinal cord participate in the control of trunk and hindlimb activity during locomotion (Musienko et al., 2014). However, little is known about the respective contribution of these two control systems.

Our understanding of the circuits controlling locomotor activity in trunk muscles relies heavily on studies in vertebrates that either have no legs or only simple forms of hindlimbs, including lamprey (Grillner, 2006; Ryczko et al., 2010), xenopus (Combes et al., 2004; Beyeler et al., 2008; Roberts et al., 2012), leech (Kristan et al., 2005), zebrafish (Thorsen, 2004; Bagnall and McLean, 2014; Kishore et al., 2014; Grillner and Manira, 2015), and amphibian tetrapods (Cabelguen et al., 2014; Ryczko et al., 2015). Recent work in rodents suggests that some of the basic mechanisms that underlie control of trunk in limbless vertebrates are retained in limbed mammals (Falgairolle et al., 2013; Beliez et al., 2015; Hinckley et al., 2015). However, the more complex mechanisms that have developed along with the specialization that came with the morphological evolution of the hindlimbs (Beyeler et al., 2008; Le Gal et al., 2016) have yet to be studied.

The present study in a brain stem-spinal cord preparation of the neonatal mouse was designed to examine the contribution of the brain stem to trunk and hindlimb motoneurons (MNs) activities during drug-induced fictive locomotor-like activity (LLA; Kudo and Yamada, 1987; Smith and Feldman, 1987; Jiang et al., 1999; Bonnot et al., 2002). We used calcium imaging to record locomotor activity from individual MNs in T7, L2, or L5 segments and compare recordings from MNs in the medial and lateral motor column (MMC and LMC) before and after removal of the brain stem. This approach enables before/after comparison in the same preparation, making for a more robust interpretation of the results.

The findings suggest an early influence of the brain stem directed to the axial and hindlimb spinal locomotor rhythm generating circuits. This early influence may be critical when animals learn how to walk in different conditions and environment. Preliminary results have been published previously in abstract form (Jean-Xavier and Perreault, 2013).

MATERIALS AND METHODS

Animals

Experiments were performed on neonatal [post-natal day (P) 0–2] ICR/Ha mice ($n = 36$). All animal protocols followed US National Institutes of Health guidelines and were approved by Emory University Institutional Animal Care and Use Committee.

In Vitro Brain Stem-Spinal Cord Preparation

Under deep isoflurane (4%) anesthesia, animals were decerebrated by transecting the brain rostral to the superior colliculus and eviscerated. Preparations were then placed in a dissection chamber filled with ice cold oxygenated (95% O_2/5% CO_2) glycerol-based dissecting solution containing (in mM): glycerol 250, KCl 2, D-glucose 11, $CaCl_2$ 0.15, $MgSO_4$ 2, NaH_2PO_4 1.2, HEPES 5 and $NaHCO_3$ 25 (pH of 7.4). After a craniotomy and a laminectomy, the brain stem-spinal cords, with the dorsal and ventral roots attached, were gently dissected out. Brain stem-spinal cords were then transferred to a Sylgard-coated recording chamber where they were positioned ventral side up. The recording chamber was partitioned into a brain stem and a spinal cord compartments using a plastic wall sealed with petroleum jelly at cervical segment C1-C2. Room temperature (RT; 23°C) oxygenated artificial cerebrospinal fluid (aCSF) containing (in mM): NaCl 128, KCl 3, D-glucose 11, $CaCl_2$ 2.5, $MgSO_4$ 1, NaH_2PO_4 1.2, HEPES 5 and $NaHCO_3$ 25, was pumped into each compartment. The tightness of the seal was verified by adding phenol red to one of the compartment.

Loading of Motoneurons with Fluorescent Calcium Indicator

Spinal segments were identified by counting the ventral roots using as a starting point the C1 ventral root and/or the L5 ventral root which is last large diameter root of the lumbar enlargement. Motoneurons (MNs) in the thoracic segment T7 and lumbar segments L2 and L5 were loaded with Calcium Green 1-conjugated dextran amine (CaGDA; 3000 MW; Molecular Probes, for indicator kinetics (see Zhao et al., 1996; Kreitzer et al., 2000; Putney, 2006) by applying reconstituted CaGDA crystals (Glover, 1995) to the cut end of the corresponding ventral roots. Labeling via retrograde axonal transport continued in the dark at RT for at least 3 h.

Drug-Induced Fictive Locomotor-Like Activity (LLA)

LLA was induced by applying a neurochemical cocktail composed of N-Methyl-D-aspartate (5 μM NMDA), 5-hydroxytryptamine hydrochloride (10 μM 5-HT) and dopamine hydrochloride (50 μM DA) dissolved in aCSF. The locomotor cocktail was applied specifically to the spinal cord compartment (recycling flow rate of 15 ml/min). All neurochemicals were purchased from Sigma Aldrich and kept as frozen (−30°C) stock (10–100 mM).

Removal of the Brain Stem

The brain stem was removed by complete transection of the spinal cord at the level of C1 segment using superfine Vannas scissors (WPI, USA). To avoid transecting during states of high excitability, neurochemicals were washed out for ≥20 min prior to transection. The locomotor cocktail solution was re-applied to the isolated spinal cord only after a post-transection recovery period of ≥20 min.

Reversible Cooling of the Brain Stem

In a subset of experiments, the excitability of the brain stem was reduced using cooling. For these experiments, temperature probes (Yellow Spring Instruments, YSI-402) were placed in each bath compartment. Prior to cooling, the brain stem compartment was set to an initial temperature of 28°C using warm aCSF. The brain stem was then cooled down to 18°C using ice-cold aCSF. After cooling, but before final removal of the brain stem, the brain stem compartment was rewarmed to 28°C. The spinal cord compartment was kept at RT at all times. Isothermal values were reached in 5 min.

Calcium Imaging

Drug-induced LLA is usually monitored using electrical recording from ventral roots which contain mixed axonal populations (axons from axial and limb MNs and sympathetic preganglionic neurons). Here, we used calcium imaging, which enable us to resolve activity in individual MNs identified as axial MNs of the medial motor column (MMC) or limb MNs of the lateral motor column (LMC) based on their mediolateral locations (Lev-Tov and O'Donovan, 1995; O'Donovan et al., 2008; Szokol and Perreault, 2009; Hinckley et al., 2015). Individual CaGDA-labeled MNs were visualized through the ventral white matter up to about 100 μm under the surface (Szokol and Perreault, 2009) using a 40x water immersion objective (LUMPLFLN 40X, 0.8 NA, Olympus USA) of an epi-fluorescence microscope (BX51, Olympus, USA) equipped with a 100 W halogen lamp driven by a DC power supply (PAN35-20A, Kikusui Electronics Corporation, Japan) and excitation and emission filters (BP 450–490 nm and LP 515 nm, respectively). Fluorescence images were captured using a sCMOS camera (PCO.edge, PCO, Canada) mounted on a video zoom adapter set at 0.5x. Image (16 bit) streams (480 frames) were stored at 4 frames/s (binning 2×2, gain 1) using the acquisition software Metamorph (v7.7, Universal Imaging Corporation, Molecular Devices, USA). All recording sessions (controls and trials) lasted 120 s.

Data Analysis

Using the acquisition and image analysis software Metamorph, circular regions of interest (ROIs) were positioned over the soma of individual MNs so as to cover as much of the field of view as possible. The selection of the MN somata was made according to labeling intensity and availability in the same focus plane. Fluorescence intensity within each ROI averaged over all pixels. These data were converted to text files and exported to pClamp (Clampfit 10.4, Molecular Devices, USA) where they were expressed as waveforms or changes in fluorescence over time for further analysis. Changes in fluorescence were measured and reported as percent changes from an average baseline level F0 [ΔF/F or (F–F0)/F0]. For the recordings that contained the onset of LLA (see "Tonic component" section below), F0 was measured prior to the arrival of the neurochemicals in the bath and thus estimated well the true baseline calcium level ("rest" period in absence of neurochemicals). For the recordings that contained only rhythmic activity (see "Rhythmic component" section below), F0 was measured as the minimum inter-burst fluorescence and thus likely overestimated the true baseline calcium level.

Locomotor-Like Activity (LLA)

Tonic component

An initial, slowly rising, tonic plateau of activity often preceded rhythmic LLA. Its onset was detected using a threshold function (Clampfit 10.4, Molecular Devices, USA) set to average baseline fluorescence + 4SD (horizontal dotted lines in **Figure 1B**) whereas its magnitude was quantified as the average plateau fluorescence (measured once the plateau had stabilized) minus the average baseline fluorescence. The baseline fluorescence and the plateau fluorescence were average over a 5 s-period.

Rhythmic component

Although cyclic changes in fluorescence were often observed within 3 min of neurochemicals application, we only analyzed recordings obtained ≥20 min (stable rhythm).

Frequency of occurrence of double-peak bursts in MMC MNs. Double-peak bursts were defined as bursts with a transient dip in fluorescence (>30% decrease from the highest peak value and duration of at least 1 s) about midway through their crest (**Figure 3A**). The proportion of double-peak bursts was assessed by compiling their numbers during 2 min- recording sessions (2–5 MMC MNs per experiment).

Rhythm frequency and burst durations. The onset and offset of the locomotor bursts in individual MNs were detected using a threshold function (single channel search function in Clampfit 10.4) set at 30% of the peak value (Tazerart et al., 2007). Times between consecutive onsets were used to determine the duration of each locomotor cycle and assess rhythm frequency whereas times between onsets and offsets were used to calculate burst durations.

Temporal relationships and coupling strengths. Temporal relationships and coupling strengths between pairs of MNs were determined for MNs of the same motor column (intra-columnar) and MNs of different motor columns (inter-columnar). For these analyses, we used "Spinalcore," a program for signal processing and analyses in frequency/time domain of stationary and non-stationary time series (Mor and Lev-Tov, 2007). Briefly, the calcium signal from each individual MN was decomposed in the frequency domain over the time course of the recordings using a continuous Morlet wavelet transform (10 octaves per scale). Then, using coherent cross-power wavelet transform (CXWT, spectrograms in **Figure 6A**), we determined if two individual signals had 1) common bands of high-power frequencies and 2) a phase relationship that was consistent over time. The degree of consistency of the phase relationship (coupling strength or coherence) ranged from zero to one for highly coherent signals. The high-power frequencies band of interest in the CXWT was selected (white rectangle in spectrograms of **Figure 6A**) and used to extract rhythm frequency, phase differences and coupling strengths (coherence) between pairs of MNs. Rhythm frequencies and coupling strengths were presented as bar graphs and phase differences as circular plots.

Statistics

Data are reported as mean±SEM, unless indicated otherwise. Tests of significance were performed on the grand averages across preparations and included: the paired *t*-test, unpaired *t*-test and one-way ANOVA followed by Holm-Sidak *post-hoc* multiple comparison. When the assumption of normality was violated, we instead used the Fisher's exact-test, Wilcoxon matched-paired test, Mann-Whitney test and Kruskal-Wallis test followed by Dunn's multiple comparison. These tests were performed using GraphPad Prism 6 (San Diego, CA, USA). To test mean phase differences, we performed Watson–Williams *F*-test using Oriana (Kovach Computing Services, Pentraeth, UK). Significance level was set at $p < 0.05$.

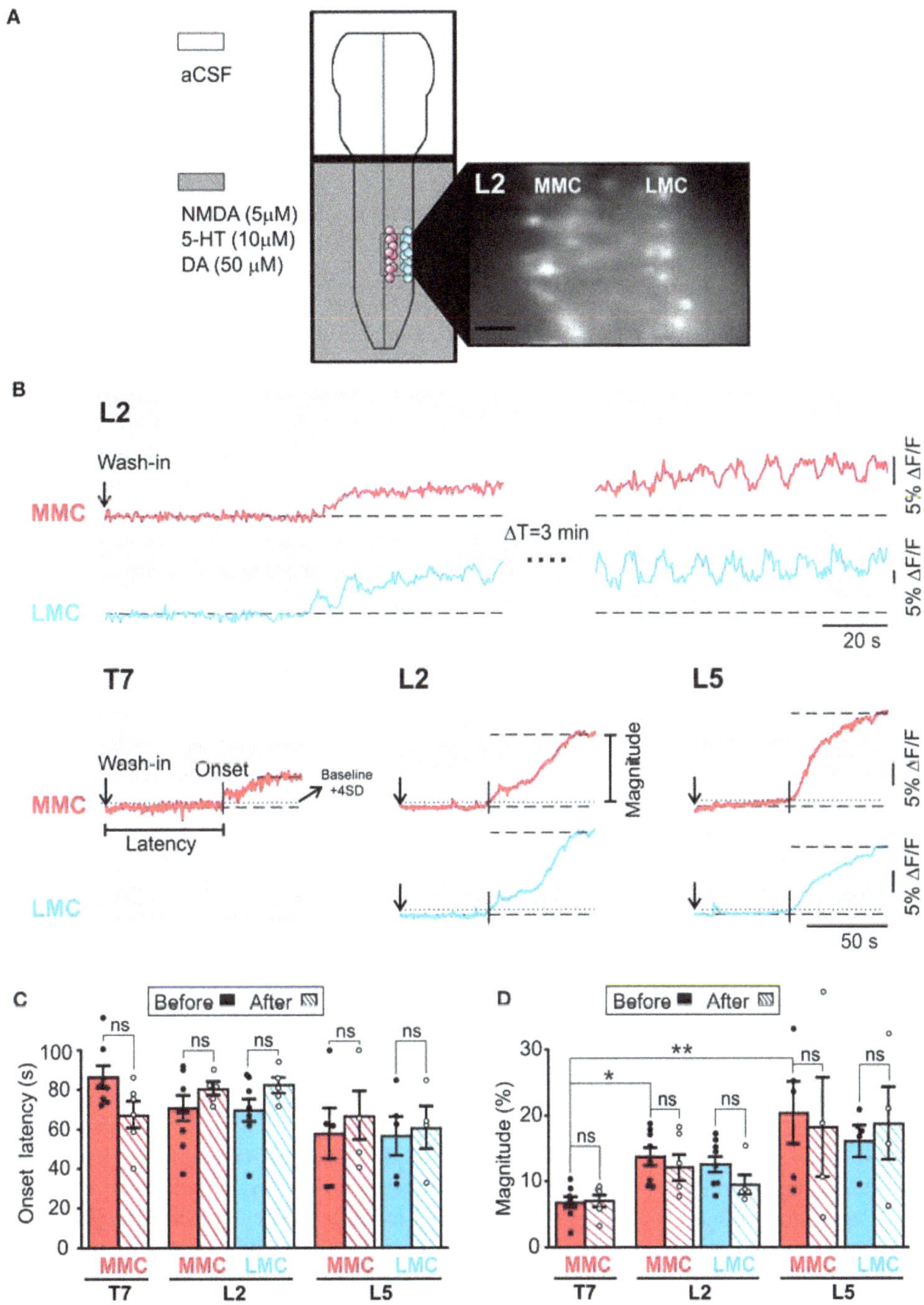

FIGURE 1 | An initial period of tonic activity accompanies rhythmic activity both in MMC and in LMC MNs. **(A)** Schematic representation of the experimental arrangement. The recording chamber was partitioned in two compartments with a plastic bridge sealed with petroleum jelly. The brain stem compartment (top) was superfused with aCSF while the spinal cord compartment (bottom) was superfused with aCSF plus NMDA (5 μM), 5HT (10 μM), and DA (50 μM). The presence of the neurochemicals is indicated by the gray shading. MNs in the MMC (red circles) and LMC (blue circles) were loaded with fluorescent calcium indicator CaGDA (see Methods). Inset: Photomicrograph of CaGDA loaded MMC and LMC MNs in L2. Scale bar is 25 μm. **(B)** Top: Changes in fluorescence following the arrival of the neurochemicals to the spinal cord compartment in a single MMC MN (red waveform) and LMC MN (blue waveform). The recording bouts on the left show the slow building up of the tonic component of LLA in each MNs. The recording bouts on the right, which were acquired 3 min later, show the same tonic component as it reaches maximal magnitude (plateau). Bottom: Population responses (large ROI covering the entirety of the motor columns) showing the tonic component of LLA in MMC MNs of T7, L2, and L5 segments and LMC MNs of L2 and L5 segment. Vertical arrows: Time of application of neurochemicals. Vertical bars: Onset latency. Horizontal dashed line: Mean baseline fluorescence. Horizontal dotted line: Mean baseline fluorescence +4 SD. **(C)** Bar graph showing the mean onset latency of the tonic component in T7, L2, and L5 MNs before (solid bars) and after (hatched bars) removal of the brain stem. Each bar is a grand average across all experiments (individual points). Mean onset latencies of tonic activity were similar before and after removal of the brain stem (Wilcoxon matched-pairs test, T7 MMC^{before} vs.

(Continued)

FIGURE 1 | MMC^{after} $p = 0.22$; L2 MMC^{before} vs. MMC^{after} $p = 0.31$; L5 MMC^{before} vs. MMC^{after} $p = 0.25$; L2 LMC^{before} vs. LMC^{after} $p = 0.31$; L5 LMC^{before} vs. LMC^{after} $p > 0.99$). **(D)** Bar graph showing the magnitude of the tonic component in T7, L2, and L5 MNs before (solid bars) and after (hatched bars) removal of the brain stem. Each bar is a grand average across all experiments (individual points). The mean magnitudes of tonic component were similar before and after removal of the brain stem (Wilcoxon matched-pairs test, T7 MMC^{before} vs. MMC^{after} $p = 0.84$; L2 MMC^{before} vs. MMC^{after} $p = 0.88$; L5 MMC^{before} vs. MMC^{after} $p > 0.99$; L2 LMC^{before} vs. LMC^{after} $p > 0.99$; L5 LMC^{before} vs. LMC^{after} $p > 0.99$). $^{*}p < 0.05$, $^{**}p < 0.01$.

RESULTS

We analyzed optical recordings from more than 4000 individual MNs in the T7, L2, and L5 segments during drug-induced LLA. To achieve single-cell resolution each segment was investigated in different preparations. Below, sample sizes "*n*" refer to the number of animals.

Initial Tonic Activity

An initial period of tonic activity preceding rhythmic activity has been reported during drug-induced LLA in the isolated spinal cord of the neonatal rat (Kjaerulff and Kiehn, 1996; Beliez et al., 2015) and during MLR-evoked fictive locomotion in adult the decerebrate cat and rat (Perreault et al., 1999; MacDonell et al., 2015). However, this tonic activity has not been described in the mouse. Here, we measured tonic activity in individual MNs in T7, L2, and L5 segments (5–10 MNs per motor column) and show that tonic activity develops both in MMC and in LMC MNs (**Figure 1**, $n = 21$). In both MN groups, tonic activity appeared within less than 2 min and increased until it reached a plateau (**Figure 1B**). Few minutes after that, rhythmic activity started. Occasionally, tonic and rhythmic activity would appear concomitantly (LMC trace in **Figure 1B**). On average, the magnitude of the tonic activity in MMC MNs was significantly smaller in T7 than that in L2 and L5 (**Figure 1D**, Kruskal-Wallis test followed by Dunn's multiple comparison, T7 vs. L2, $p = 0.02$; T7 vs. L5, $p = 0.01$), suggesting an inter-segmental difference between thoracic and lumbar segments. However, in the absence of dependable measure for difference in excitability between preparations, this suggestion must remain tentative.

Pairwise comparisons before and after removal of the brain stem ($n = 15$) revealed no significant differences in mean onset latency or magnitude (compare solid and hatched bars in **Figures 1C,D**, see figure legend for *p*-values). Since the presence of the brain stem did not appear to change the inherent capability of the spinal cord to generate tonic activity, we suggest that initial tonic activity during drug-induced LLA is organized largely by neural networks in the spinal cord.

Rhythmic Locomotor-Like Activity

Rhythmic activity was analyzed in T7, L2, and L5 segments ($n = 10$ animals per segment) before and after removal of the brain stem. Measurements were performed on individual MNs (10 MNs per motor column) and included rhythm frequency, burst durations, phase relationships and strengths of coupling between MNs. Data presented below include the first measurements of rhythmic locomotor activity in MMC MNs of the brain stem-spinal cord of the neonatal mouse.

Rhythm frequency and burst duration

The rhythm frequencies and burst durations were assessed in all three segments and, when eligible, in both MMC and LMC MNs (**Figure 2**). Analyses were performed on both combined (**Figure 2C**) and individual segments/columns (**Figures 2D,E**).

Before removal of the brain stem, the average frequencies ranged between 0.11 and 0.31 Hz without significant difference in average frequencies between the segments (one-way ANOVA test followed by a Holm-Sidak multiple comparison, all $p > 0.17$). Removal of the brain stem increased the average rhythm frequency (solid circles in **Figure 2C**, paired *t*-test, $p = 0.0008$). When motor columns were analyzed separately, L2 showed that the increase in frequency occurred both in MMC and LMC (**Figure 2D**, solid vs. hatched bars, see figure legend for *p*-values).

We then tested whether the increase in locomotor frequency might have arisen from a reduction in locomotor burst durations. Prior to removal of the brain stem, the average burst durations ranged between 3.3 and 4.5 s without significant difference in average burst duration between segments (One-way ANOVA test followed by a Holm-Sidak multiple comparison, all $p > 0.85$). When motor columns were analyzed separately, L2 showed significantly longer burst durations in MMC than LMC MNs (paired *t*-test, $p = 0.04$). Removal of the brain stem reduced the average burst duration (solid triangles in **Figure 2C**, paired *t*-test, $p = 0.0007$). Again, when motor columns were analyzed separately, L2 showed that the reduction in burst duration occurred both in MMC and LMC (**Figure 2E**, solid vs. hatched bars, see figure 1 egend for *p*-values). Thus, it is likely that the increase in rhythm frequency after removal of the brainstem arose from a reduction in locomotor burst durations in both MMC and LMC MNs.

Additionally, removal of the brain stem eliminated the difference in L2 burst duration between MMC and LMC MNs seen in the brain stem-attached preparation (paired *t*-test, $p = 0.10$). This observation prompted us to look more closely at the shape of the bursts in MMC MNs. We observed that some of the bursts in MMC MNs displayed double-peak, similar to those reported previously in the L3–L5 segments of the isolated spinal cord (O'Donovan et al., 2008). Therefore, we wanted to test whether regulation of double-peak bursts by the brain stem could contribute to the reduction in burst duration in L2 MMC MNs. We compared the proportion of double-peak bursts during 2 min-recording sessions before and after removal of the brain stem ($n = 7$, **Figure 3**). Comparisons were made for L2 and T7 segments. Before removal of the brain stem, we observed double-peak bursts in MMC MNs (asterisks in **Figure 3A**, see also MMC traces in **Figure 2**) in both L2 and T7, albeit at a lower proportion in T7 (54% in L2 vs. 21% in T7, **Figure 3B**, solid bars). After removal of the brain

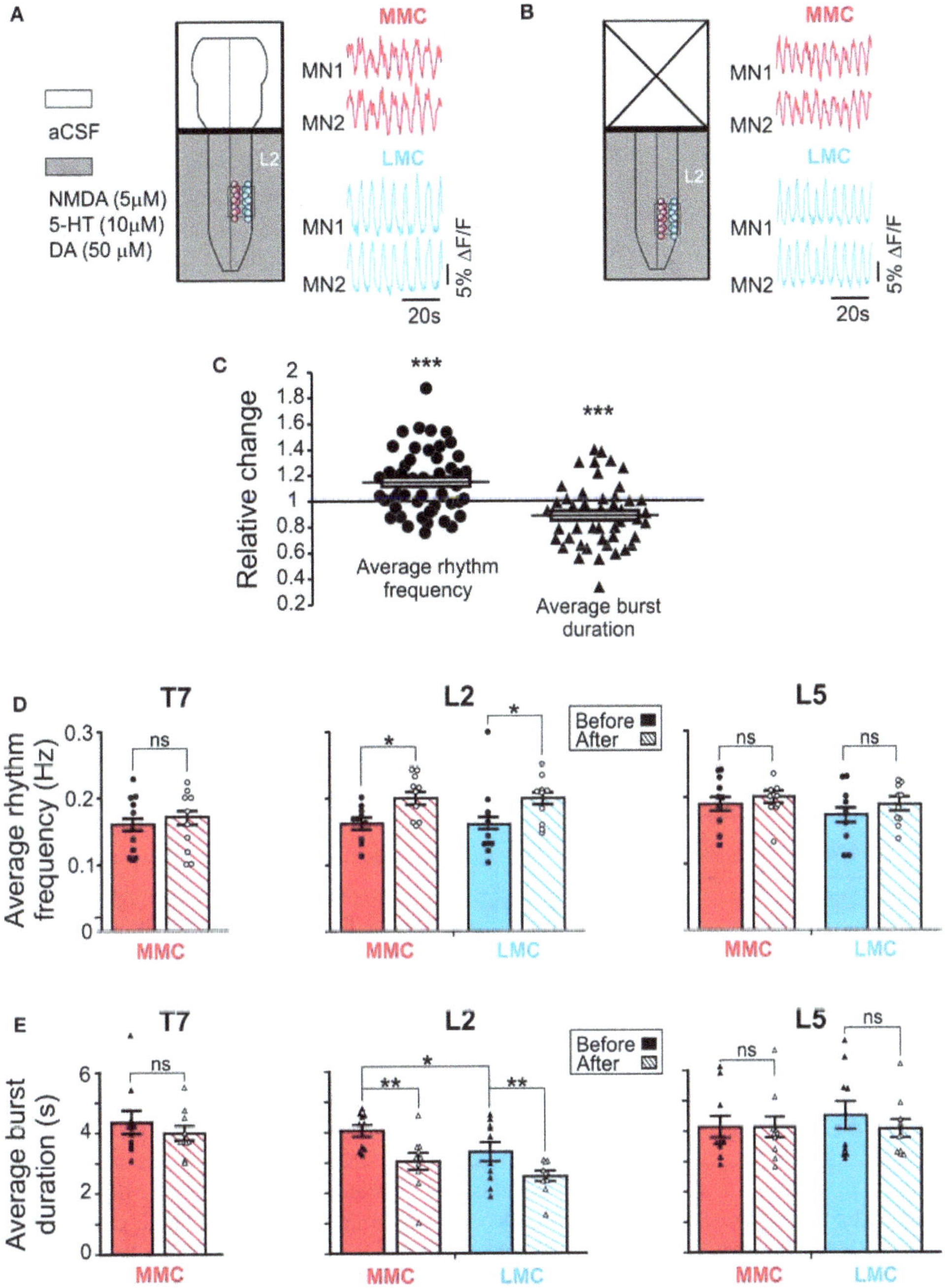

FIGURE 2 | Regulation of the locomotor rhythm frequency and burst durations by the brain stem. Schematic representations of the experimental arrangement before **(A)** and after **(B)** removal of the brain stem shown together with corresponding set of waveforms displaying changes in fluorescence in two L2 MMC MNs (red) and two L2 LMC (blue) MNs (for other details, see **Figure 1A**). The same four MNs are shown in the two panels. **(C)** Pooled data from 50 motor columns (10 motor columns in T7, 20 motor columns in L2 and in L5) showing relative change in average rhythm frequency (solid circles) and burst duration (solid triangles) after removal of the brain stem. **(D,E)** Bar graphs showing the average rhythm frequency and average burst duration in MMC (red) and LMC MNs (blue) in the individual segments before and after removal of the brain stem (solid and hatched bars, respectively). Each bar is a grand average across all experiments. The increase in rhythm frequency after removal of the brainstem was statistically significant in L2 (paired *t*-test, L2 MMC^{before} vs. MMC^{after} $p = 0.003$; L2 LMC^{before} vs. LMC^{after} $p= 0.048$; T7 MMC^{before} vs. MMC^{after} $p=0.79$; L5 MMC^{before} vs. MMC^{after} $p =0.86$; L5 LMC^{before} vs. LMC^{after} $p =0.26$). Removal of the brain stem also significantly reduced the average burst durations in L2 (paired *t*-test, L2 MMC^{before} vs. MMC^{after} $p = 0.003$; L2 LMC^{before} vs. LMC^{after} $p = 0.004$; T7 MMC^{before} vs. MMC^{after} $p = 0.26$; L5 MMC^{before} vs. MMC^{after} $p = 0.97$; L5 LMC^{before} vs. LMC^{after} $p = 0.34$). $^{*}p < 0.05$, $^{**}p < 0.01$, $^{***}p < 0.001$.

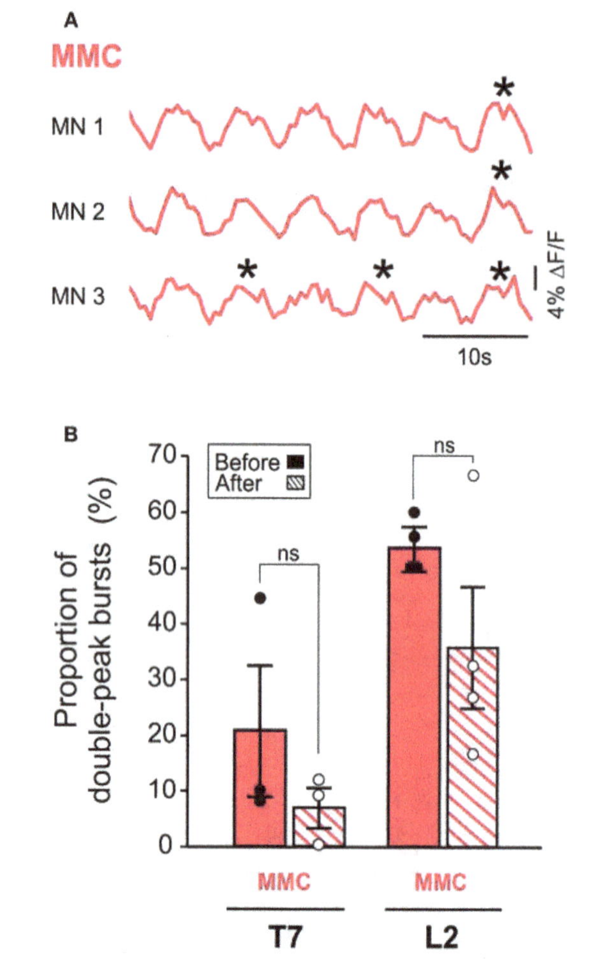

FIGURE 3 | MMC MNs display double-peak bursts during LLA. **(A)** Changes in fluorescence in three individual MNs in the left MMC (top) and right MMC (bottom). *Asterisks* indicate double-peak bursts (see Methods). **(B)** Bar graphs showing the mean frequency of occurrence of double-peak bursts in MMC MNs of T7 and L2 before (solid bars) and after (hatched bars) removal of the brain stem. Each bar is a grand average across all experiments (individual points).

stem (**Figure 3B**, hatched bars), the proportion of double-peak bursts in L2 decreased to 36%. However, the decrease was not statistically significant (Fisher's exact test, $p = 0.07$) nor was it specific to L2 (decrease to 7% in T7, Fisher's exact test, $p = 0.11$).

Altogether, these findings suggest that the brain stem contributes to the regulation of the rhythm frequency and burst duration of both MMC and LMC MNs during drug-induced LLA. When columns were analyzed separately, the threshold for significance was reached in L2 but not in T7 or L5. This is likely because MNs in this segment display tighter temporal relationships (see Supplemental Figure 1 and section below). We also observed a reduced incidence of double-peak bursts in L2 MMC MNs after removal of the brain stem but this does not appear to contribute to the reduction in locomotor burst durations in these MNs.

Phase relationships and coupling strengths between MNs of the same motor column

We then sought to determine the temporal relationships and strengths of coupling between MNs within individual motor columns. Several pair of MNs were analyzed within each motor column. Each pair consisted of a reference MN and another, randomly selected, MN within the motor column. The reference MN was selected based on its rostral most location in the field of view. All intra-columnar phase relationships (mean phase vector) and coupling strengths (mean coherence) analyzed in T7, L2, and L5 are shown in **Figure 4**.

Before removal of the brain stem (**Figure 4A**), all the mean phase vectors were close to 0°, suggesting that MN pairs discharged synchronously. However, the mean vector length "rvec" was lower in T7 MMC compared to L2 or L5 MMC, indicating a more widespread distribution of phase differences. As shown in the circular plot of T7, this widespread distribution was not the result of a uniform distribution of phase differences around the circle (Watson's U^2-test, $p < 0.01$), but rather a clustering of phase differences into two groups separated by 180°; one large cluster of MN pairs discharging synchronously and a smaller cluster of MN pairs discharging out-of-phase. Removal of the brain stem did not significantly alter the mean phase vectors in any of the segment (**Figure 4B**, see figure legend for p-values).

The mean coherences between MN pairs ranged between 0.75 and 0.96 and were significantly higher between MNs of L2 motor columns than between MNs of the T7 and L5 motor columns (**Figure 4C**, filled bars, see figure legend for p-values). The lower coherence between T7 MMC MNs T7 may be attributable to the presence of less well-correlated MN pairs (dots close to the thick, black outline circle in circular plots). This is consistent with the recent finding of Beliez et al. (2015) who reported a substantial number of non-locomotor-driven MNs in this segment. Removal of the brain stem did not significantly alter the mean coherences (**Figure 4C**, hatched bars; see figure legend for p-values).

Altogether, these data indicate that MNs within L2 and L5 motor columns discharge in phase with each other during drug-induced LLA in the brain stem-spinal cord preparation. In T7 motor columns, many MNs discharge in phase while a substantial number discharge out-of-phase. We also found that the temporal relationships between MNs were tightest in L2, a finding that is compatible with a higher potential for rhythmogenesis (see Discussion). Removal of the brain stem, despite its clear effect on the locomotor frequency and burst durations, did not significantly affect intra-columnar phase relationships or coupling strengths between MNs.

Phase relationships and coupling strengths between MNs of different motor columns

We next examined the temporal relationships and strengths of coupling between MNs in different motor columns. Inter-columnar relationships were determined between MNs of the left and right MMCs in L2 and between MNs in the MMC and LMC in both L2 and L5. All inter-columnar phase relationships

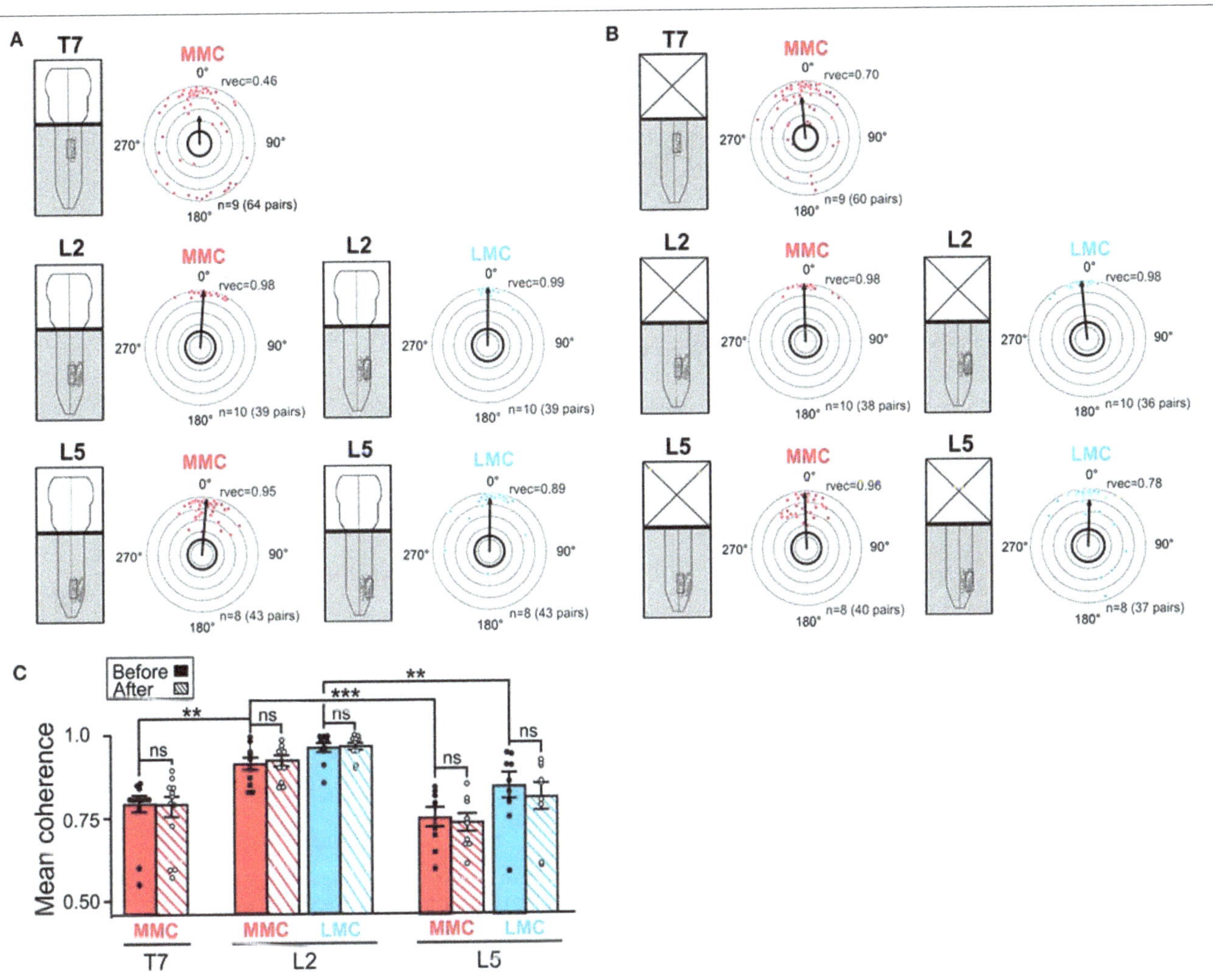

FIGURE 4 | Temporal relationships and coupling strengths (coherence) between MNs of the same motor column before and after removal of the brain stem. **(A,B)** Intra-columnar phase relationships between pairs of MNs in T7 MMC (top), L2 MMC and LMC (middle) and L5 MMC and LMC (bottom) before and after removal of the brain stem, respectively. Phase relationships between MN pairs are shown as phase differences in circular plots. Individual dots represent individual MN pairs (red=>MMC, blue=>LMC). The direction of the vectors (arrows) indicates mean phase difference (0° =>synchronous, 180° difference=>alternating) whereas the length of the vectors (rvec) indicates the extent to which the phase differences are clustered around the mean on a scale from 0.0 (origin) to 1.0 (outermost gray circle). The circle with thick black outline indicates the $p < 0.05$ level of statistical significance as determined by the Rayleigh test. Number of experiments and number MN pairs analyzed indicated at the bottom of each circular plots. The lower average vector length "rvec" in T7 indicates a more widespread distribution of phase differences between MNs in this segment than in L2 or L5. Phase differences were clustered in two groups around 0 and 180°. The changes in mean phase vectors after removal of the brainstem were not statistically significantly (Watson–Williams F-test, T7 MMC^{before} vs. MMC^{after} $F = 0.83$, $p = 0.38$; L2 MMC^{before} vs. MMC^{after} $F = 2.25$, $p = 0.15$; L2 LMC^{before} vs. LMC^{after} $F = 2.53$, $p = 0.13$; L5 MMC^{before} vs. MMC^{after} $F = 1.28$, $p = 0.28$; L5 LMC^{before} vs. LMC^{after} $F = 1.28$, $p = 0.63$). **(C)** Bar graph showing the mean coherence before (solid bars) and after (hatched bars) removal of the brain stem. The coupling between MNs was significantly tighter in L2 than in T7 or L5 both before and after removal of the brain stem (Kruskal-Wallis test followed by a Dunn's multiple comparison, L2 MMC^{before} vs. T7 MMC^{before} $p = 0.007$; L2 MMC^{before} vs. L5 MMC^{before} $p = 0.0004$; L2 LMC^{before} vs. L5 LMC^{before} $p = 0.001$; L5 MMC^{before} vs. T7 MMC^{before} $p > 0.99$; Wilcoxon matched paired test, T7 MMC^{before} vs. MMC^{after} $p = 0.82$; L2 MMC^{before} vs. MMC^{after} $p = 0.56$; L2 LMC^{before} vs. LMC^{after} $p > 0.99$; L5 MMC^{before} vs. MMC^{after} $p = 0.73$; L5 LMC^{before} vs. LMC^{after} $p = 0.57$). $^{**}p < 0.01$, $^{***}p < 0.001$.

(mean phase vector) and coupling strengths (mean coherence) are shown in **Figure 5**.

Before removal of the brain stem (**Figure 5A**), the mean phase vector between left and right L2 MMC MNs was around 180°, indicating left/right alternation between axial MNs. In contrast, the mean phase vector between MMC and LMC MNs on the same side of L2 was close to 0°, indicating synchronous activation. In L5, the mean phase vector between MMC and LMC MNs was close to 90°, differing significantly from the mean phase vector in L2 (Watson–Williams F-test, $F = 9.462$, $p = 0.007$). The mean vector length in L5 was also smaller than in L2, indicating a more widespread distribution of phase differences. However, the distribution was not uniform (Watson's U^2-test, $p < 0.01$) and close inspection of the L5 circular plots revealed a clustering of phase differences into at least two groups; one group where MMC and LMC MNs discharged mostly in-phase (quadrant 0–90°)

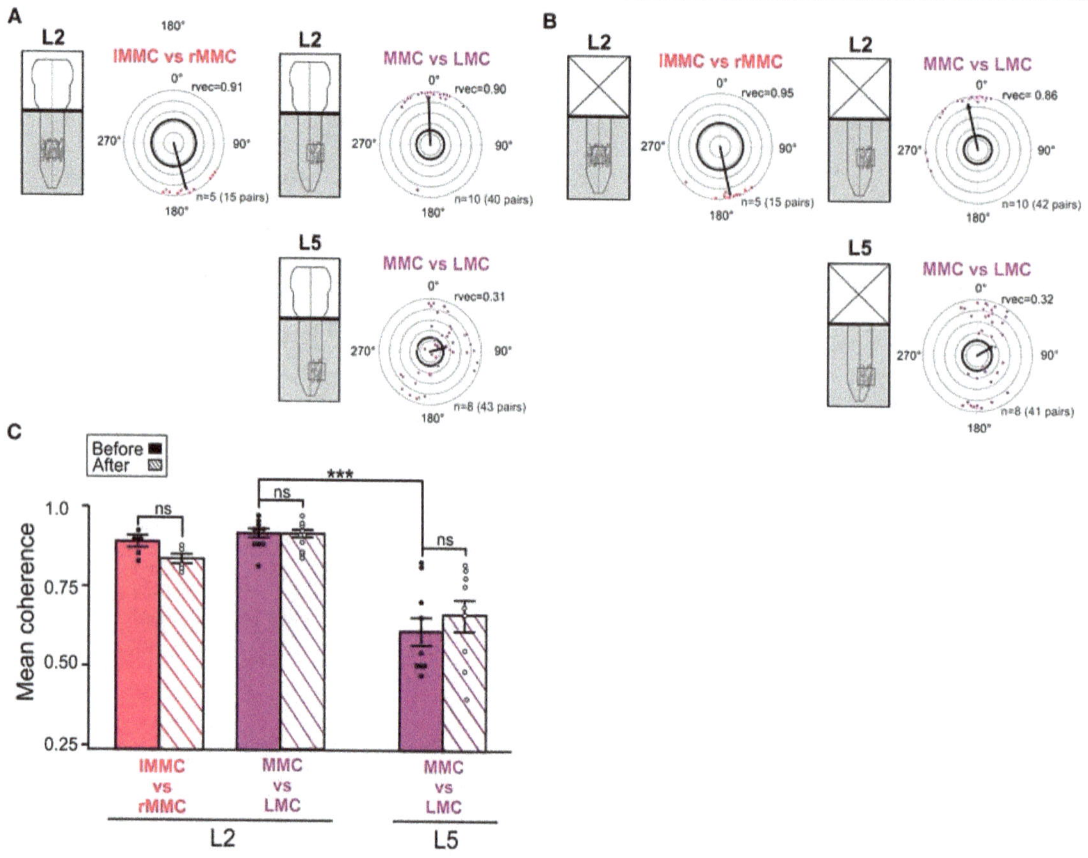

FIGURE 5 | Temporal relationships and coupling strengths between MNs of different motor columns before and after removal of the brain stem. **(A,B)** Inter-columnar phase relationships between pairs of MNs in left and right MMC in L2, MMC and LMC in L2, and MMC and LMC in L5 before and after removal of the brain stem. Phase relationships between MMCs are shown in red and phase relationships between MMC and LMCs are shown in purple. Removal of the brain stem did not significantly change the mean phase differences between MNs (Watson–Williams F-test, L2 lMMC/rMMC^{before} vs. lMMC/rMMC^{after} $F = 0.03$, $p = 0.87$; L2 MMC/LMC^{before} vs. MMC/LMC^{after} $F = 0.60$, $p = 0.45$; L5 MMC/LMC^{before} vs. MMC/LMC^{after} $F = 0.21$, $p = 0.65$). **(C)** Bar graph showing mean coherence before (solid bars) and after (hatched bars) removal of the brain stem. The strengths of the coupling between MNs was not significantly affected by removal of the brain stem (Wilcoxon matched-pairs test, L2 lMMC/rMMC^{before} vs. lMMC/rMMC^{after} $p = 0.19$; Kruskal-Wallis test followed by a Dunn's multiple comparison, L2 MMC/LMC^{before} vs. L2 MMC/LMC^{after} $p > 0.99$; L5 MMC/LMC^{before} vs. L5 MMC/LMC^{after} $p > 0.99$). ***$p < 0.001$. For other details, see **Figure 4**.

and another one group where MMC and LMC MNs discharged out-of-phase (around 180°).

In addition, several MMC/LMC pairs were less, or not, correlated (dots close or within the thick black outline circle). Removal of the brain stem did not significantly change the mean phase vectors between left and right L2 MMC MNs or between MMC and LMC MNs in L2 and L5 (**Figure 5B**, see figure legend for p-values).

The coherence between MMC and LMC MNs was found to be significantly lower in L5 than in L2 (MMC vs. LMC solid bars in **Figure 5C**, Kruskal-Wallis test followed by a Dunn's multiple comparison, $p = 0.0005$), suggesting a much more labile coupling between MMC and LMC MNs in L5 than in L2. This might be attributable to the presence of some poorly correlated MNs in the MMC (see previous section) rather than in the LMC. Removal of the brain stem did not significantly change the coherence between MMC and LMC MNs either in L2 or L5 (**Figure 5C**, hatched bars see figure legend for p-values).

Altogether, these findings demonstrate left/right alternation between L2 MMC MNs, synchrony between L2 MMC and LMC MNs, and combinations of synchrony and alternation between L5 MMC and LMC MNs during drug-induced LLA in the brain stem-spinal cord preparation. As intra-columnar relationships, inter-columnar relationships were not significantly affect by removal of the brain stem, suggesting that during drug-induced LLA these relationships are organized largely by the spinal networks.

Effect of Reversible Cooling of the Brain Stem on L2 Rhythm Frequency

To investigate whether activity in brain stem neurons contributed to the increase in L2 rhythm frequency observed after removal of the brain stem, we cooled down the brain stem to 18°C ($n = 4$). At this temperature, activity in neuronal somata is blocked and transmission along axons is greatly reduced (Brooks, 1983).

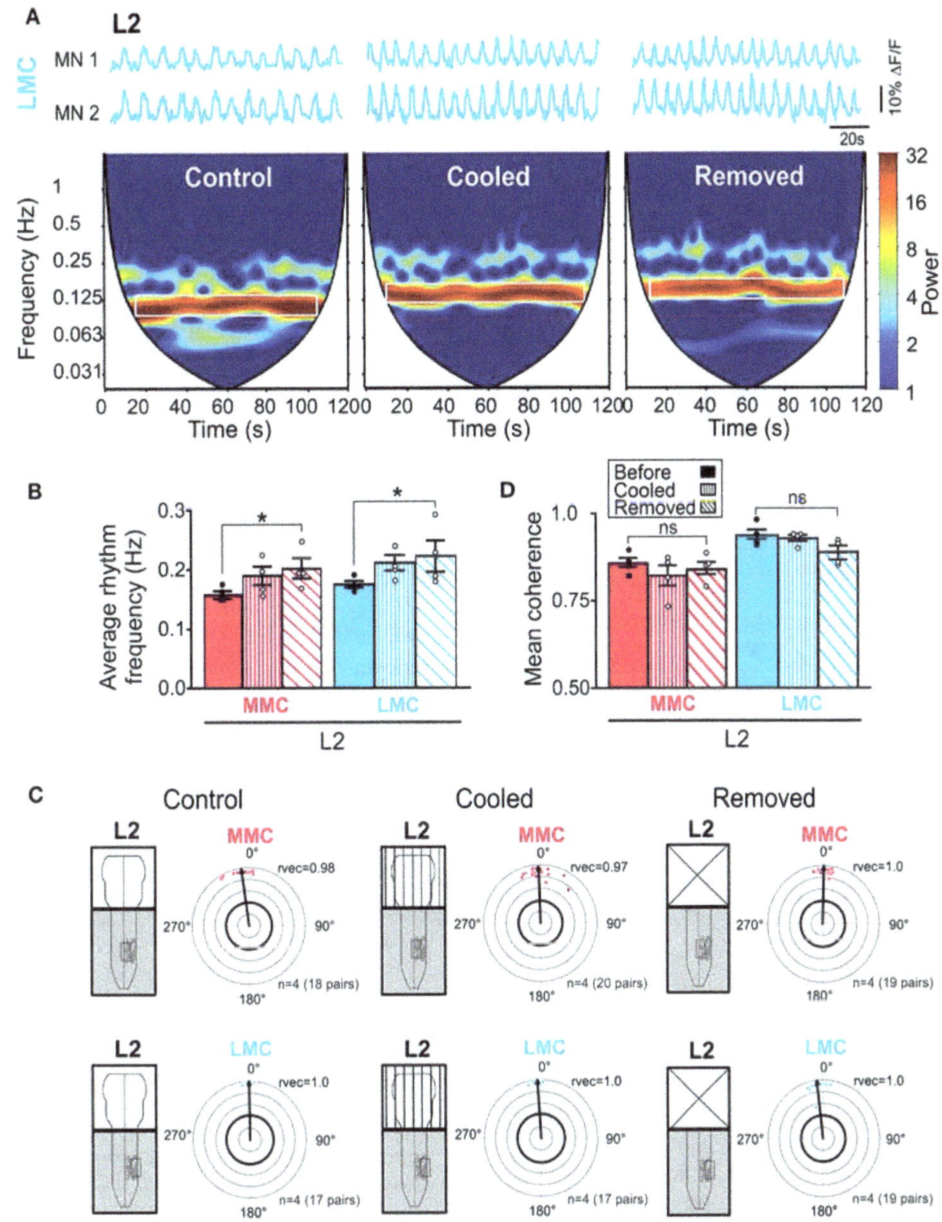

FIGURE 6 | Reduced brain stem activity also increases locomotor rhythm frequency. **(A)** Three sets of waveforms showing changes in fluorescence in two L2 LMC MNs before and during cooling of the brain stem and after removal of the brain stem. Each set of waveforms is shown with corresponding coherent cross-wavelet transform (CXWT) spectrogram (see Methods). The band of high-power (red) frequencies is marked with a white rectangle indicates a significantly coherence between the two signals in the neighborhood of the locomotor rhythm frequency. The two bottom white regions on either side of the V-shaped "cone of influence" indicate spectra regions not analyzed due to edge effects (Mor and Lev-Tov, 2007). **(B)** Bar graphs showing the average rhythm frequency in each motor column before (solid bars) and during cooling (vertically hatched bars) of the brain stem, and after removal of the brain stem (obliquely hatched bars). The increase after cooling was not as large as the increase after complete removal of the brain stem but it was observed in all experiments in both MMC and LMC MNs (Friedman test followed by Dunn's multiple *post-hoc* comparison, $MMC^{control}$ vs. MMC^{cooled} $p = 0.23$ $MMC^{control}$ vs. $MMC^{removed}$ $p = 0.04$; MMC^{cooled} vs. $MMC^{removed}$ $p > 0.99$; $LMC^{control}$ vs. LMC^{cooled} $p = 0.23$; $LMC^{control}$ vs. $LMC^{removed}$ $p = 0.04$; LMC^{cooled} vs. $LMC^{removed}$ $p > 0.99$). **(C)** Circular plots showing the effect of cooling and removing the brain stem on the intra-columnar phase differences (Watson–Williams *F*-test, $MMC^{control}$ vs. MMC^{cooled} $F = 0.69$, $p = 0.46$; $MMC^{control}$ vs. $MMC^{removed}$ $F = 2.23$, $p = 0.19$; MMC^{cooled} vs. $MMC^{removed}$ $F = 0.18$, $p = 0.68$; $LMC^{control}$ vs. LMC^{cooled} $F = 2.28$, $p = 0.18$; $LMC^{control}$ vs. $LMC^{removed}$ $F = 5.56$, $p = 0.06$ LMC^{cooled} vs. $LMC^{removed}$ $F = 1.07$, $p = 0.34$). **(D)** Bar graphs showing the effect of cooling and removal the brain stem on the intra-columnar coupling strengths (Friedman test followed by a Dunn's multiple comparison, $MMC^{control}$ vs. MMC^{cooled} $p = 0.47$; $MMC^{control}$ vs. $MMC^{removed}$ $p > 0.99$; MMC^{cooled} vs. $MMC^{removed}$ $p > 0.99$; $LMC^{control}$ vs. LMC^{cooled} $p > 0.99$; $LMC^{control}$ vs. $LMC^{removed}$ $p = 0.23$; LMC^{cooled} vs. $LMC^{removed}$ $p = 0.47$). $^*p < 0.05$.

Cooling of the brain stem increased the locomotor rhythm frequency (**Figure 6A**), an effect that was reversible. In the spectrograms of **Figure 6A**, the increase is shown as a shift of the high-power frequencies band (white rectangle) toward higher frequencies. The increase was not as large as the increase observed after complete removal of the brain stem but it was observed in all experiments both in MMC and LMC MNs (**Figure 6B**, see figure legend for *p*-values). We also analyzed intra-columnar phase relationships and strengths of coupling during cooling and, as shown in **Figures 6C,D**, the effects of cooling on these parameters were indistinguishable from the effects observed after removal of the brain stem (see figure legend for *p*-values).

These results demonstrate a similar effect of cooling and removal of the brain stem on the locomotor rhythm and support a contribution from brain stem descending neurons.

DISCUSSION

General Findings

In this study, we characterized for the first time the activities of trunk (MMC) and hindlimb (LMC) MNs during drug-induced fictive locomotion in the brain stem-spinal cord preparation of the neonatal mouse. We found that (1) trunk and hindlimb MNs display a preparatory period of tonic activity prior to rhythmic activity, (2) trunk MNs in T7 burst either in-phase or out-of-phase during rhythmic activity whereas trunk MNs in L2 or L5 burst in-phase, and (3) most trunk MNs in L2 burst in-phase with hindlimb MNs whereas in L5, several trunk MNs also burst out-of-phase with hindlimb MNs. Removal of the brain stem significantly increased the locomotor rhythm frequency with concomitant shortening in locomotor bursts. When individual segments were considered separately, the effects of removing the brain stem were significant in L2 but not T7 or L5. One interpretation of this result is that, in neonatal mouse, the brain stem targets its influence specifically on the thoracolumbar segments that have the highest potential for generating rhythmic locomotor activity (Ho and O'Donovan, 1993; Cazalets et al., 1995; Kjaerulff and Kiehn, 1996; Cowley et al., 2009; Hägglund et al., 2013).

Our work adds to a previous study in neonatal decerebrate mice in which an increase in locomotor rhythm frequency after removal of the brainstem was observed in L2 MNs (Gordon and Whelan, 2008). Both the recording method and the method used to induce fictive locomotion in this study differed from the methods used in the present study, suggesting that the increase in L2 locomotor rhythm frequency after removal of the brainstem is a robust phenomenon. In the adult decerebrate mice, spinalization also produces an increase in locomotor frequency (Meehan et al., 2012).

Candidate Subcortical Descending Systems

The increase in locomotor rhythm frequency after brainstem removal may be attributable to the loss of inputs from one or more brainstem descending systems. Prime candidates are the reticulospinal and the vestibulospinal systems (Grillner, 1981; Armstrong, 1988; Jordan, 1991; Zaporozhets et al., 2004; Jordan et al., 2008; Hägglund et al., 2010; Bretzner and Brownstone, 2013; Perreault and Glover, 2013).

Both the reticulospinal system and the lateral vestibulospinal system have the functional connectivity that would allow control over MMC and LMC MNs in the newborn mouse (Szokol et al., 2008; Szokol and Perreault, 2009; Kasumacic et al., 2010; Sivertsen et al., 2014). Although there is currently no available data on the discharge pattern of the reticulo- or vestibulospinal neurons during locomotor activity in the decerebrated mouse, earlier studies in adult decerebrate lampreys, guinea pigs, and cats indicate that the majority of these neurons discharge rhythmically during fictive locomotion (Kasicki et al., 1989; Bussières and Dubuc, 1992; Marlinsky, 1992; Perreault et al., 1993). Electrical or optogenetic stimulation to increase the ongoing locomotor discharge of reticulo- or vestibulospinal neurons in decerebrated preparations can lead to a prolongation of the locomotor cycle (Russell and Zajac, 1979; Vinay and Grillner, 1993; Perreault et al., 1994; Leblond and Gossard, 1997; Bouvier et al., 2015). Hence, loss of reticulo- and/or vestibulo-spinal inputs after spinal cord transection would be consistent with a decrease in locomotor cycle.

Monoaminergic descending systems such as the coerulospinal and raphespinal systems could also participate. The discharge pattern of monoaminergic descending neurons during locomotor activity has not been investigated in decerebrate neonatal mouse but available evidence from experiments in adult cats suggests that a majority of raphespinal neurons are tonically active during locomotion (Veasey et al., 1995; Noga et al., 2017). Serotonin prolongs locomotor cycle and axial MN burst durations in adult decerebrate lampreys (Buchanan, 2011). Conversely, serotoninergic receptor antagonists reduce the locomotor burst and cycle duration in limb MNs in decerebrate rats (Cabaj et al., 2017). Thus, loss of tonic raphespinal input after spinal transection would also be consistent with a decrease in locomotor cycle. However, a more precise assessment of the relative contribution of the different supraspinal neuronal groups must await a future characterization of their locomotor discharge patterns in the mouse.

Tonic Activity, Double-Peak Bursts in Axial MNs and Trunk-Hindlimb Coordination

We report tonic and rhythmic LLA in axial MNs of T7, L2, and L5 segment. The tonic activity in axial MNs have similar spatiotemporal characteristics as the tonic activity in hindlimb MNs, a finding that is consistent with the idea that tonic activity in MNs act as a constant background for rhythmic activity (Kjaerulff and Kiehn, 1996). Tonic activity was not affected by removal of the brain stem, suggesting that it is produced by neuronal networks located in the spinal cord. We speculate that these spinal networks may play an important role in production of the postural responses that accompany locomotor movement by setting the level of excitability of the spinal neurons that form the locomotor rhythm generator.

We report single locomotor burst and double-peak locomotor bursts in axial MNs. The functional significance of the double-peak bursts is unclear but *double-bursts* in trunk muscles in various adult mammalian species has been associated with a multifunctional role in mobilization and stabilization of the trunk and pelvis, a requirement for movement of the limbs during walking (Carlson et al., 1979; English, 1980; Thorstensson et al., 1982; Zomlefer et al., 1984; Ritter et al., 2001; Wada and Kanda, 2004; Wada et al., 2006; de Sèze et al., 2008; Ceccato et al., 2009; Schilling and Carrier, 2010). Double-peak locomotor bursts tend to be less common after removal of the brainstem. Interestingly, double-bursts in adult trunk muscles are also less frequent after spinal transection unless animals are provided with neurochemicals, training, or sensory afferent input activation (Koehler et al., 1984; Zomlefer et al., 1984; Barbeau and Rossignol, 1987). Future experiments on the development of double-peak bursts are required to determine if more parallels exist between double-peak bursts in neonates and double-bursts in adults, and ultimately inform about the possibility that double-peak bursts lead to the expression of full-fledge double-bursts in adults.

Our findings on the temporal dynamic of the locomotor activities between axial and hindlimb MNs add to previous single-cell resolution work in the isolated lumbar spinal cord and confirm a more complex coupling between axial and hindlimb MNs in the L5 (O'Donovan et al., 2008; Hinckley et al., 2015). Removal of the brain stem does not significantly affect inter-columnar phase relationships either in L2 or in L5, suggesting that trunk-hindlimb coordination in neonates greatly relies on propriospinal mechanisms. These mechanisms may include segmental as well as inter-segmental mechanisms (Falgairolle and Cazalets, 2007). Finally, in addition to their role in trunk-hindlimb coordination, thoracolumbar MNs innervating abdominal and pelvic musculature (Schrøder, 1980; Canon et al., 1991; Giraudin et al., 2008) may also assist respiratory exhalation during rhythmic motor activity (Iscoe, 1998; Hodges et al., 2007). Compatible with such a role, thoracolumbar MNs innervating abdominal muscles have recently been shown to display LLA during drug-induced fictive locomotion both before and after silencing of the brain stem (Le Gal et al., 2016).

CONCLUSION

In the current study, we have assessed the influence of the brain stem on locomotor activity in axial and hindlimb spinal networks in newborn mammals. The study reveals an influence on the timing of the locomotor activity not only in hindlimb but also in axial motor pools. This influence on the axial and hindlimb spinal locomotor rhythm generating circuits may extend the range of frequencies over which these circuits operate. Having this ability early during development may be critical when learning how to walk is a major undertaking.

AUTHOR CONTRIBUTIONS

Funding acquisition: M-CP; Conceptualization: M-CP and CJ-X; Supervision: M-CP; Methodology: CJ-X and M-CP; Experiments: CJ-X; Analyses: CJ-X and M-CP; Interpretation: M-CP and CJ-X; Writing of original draft: M-CP; Editing and approval of final version approval: M-CP and CJ-X.

ACKNOWLEDGMENTS

Ms. Renee Shaw for technical support, Drs Yoav Mor and Aharon Lev-Tov providing the SpinalCore software, and Dr. Morten Raastad for constructive comments on an earlier draft of this manuscript. This research was supported by the International Foundation for Research on Paraplegia (IRP), the Craig H. Neilsen Foundation and the National Institutes of Health (NIH) grant R01 NS085387.

REFERENCES

Armstrong, D. M. (1988). The supraspinal control of mammalian locomotion. *J. Physiol.* 405, 1–37. doi: 10.1113/jphysiol.1988.sp017319

Bagnall, M. W., and McLean, D. L. (2014). Modular organization of axial microcircuits in zebrafish. *Science* 343, 197–200. doi: 10.1126/science.1245629

Barbeau, H., and Rossignol, S. (1987). Recovery of locomotion after chronic spinalization in the adult cat. *Brain Res.* 412, 84–95. doi: 10.1016/0006-8993(87)91442-9

Beliez, L., Barrière, G., Bertrand, S. S., and Cazalets, J.-R. (2015). Origin of thoracic spinal network activity during locomotor-like activity in the neonatal rat. *J. Neurosci.* 35, 6117–6130. doi: 10.1523/JNEUROSCI.4145-14.2015

Beyeler, A., Métais, C., Combes, D., Simmers, J., and Le Ray, D. (2008). Metamorphosis-induced changes in the coupling of spinal thoraco-lumbar motor outputs during swimming in *Xenopus laevis*. *J. Neurophysiol.* 100, 1372–1383. doi: 10.1152/jn.00023.2008

Bonnot, A., Whelan, P. J., Mentis, G. Z., and O'Donovan, M. J. (2002). Locomotor-like activity generated by the neonatal mouse spinal cord. *Brain Res. Rev.* 40, 141–151. doi: 10.1016/S0165-0173(02)00197-2

Bouvier, J., Caggiano, V., Leiras, R., Caldeira, V., Bellardita, C., Balueva, K., et al. (2015). Descending command neurons in the brainstem that halt locomotion. *Cell* 163, 1191–1203. doi: 10.1016/j.cell.2015.10.074

Bretzner, F., and Brownstone, R. M. (2013). Lhx3-Chx10 Reticulospinal neurons in locomotor circuits. *J. Neurosci.* 33, 14681–14692. doi: 10.1523/JNEUROSCI.5231-12.2013

Brooks, V. B. (1983). Study of brain function by local, reversible cooling. *Rev. Physiol. Biochem. Pharmacol.* 95, 1–109. doi: 10.1007/BFb0034097

Buchanan, J. T. (2011). Flexibility in the patterning and control of axial locomotor networks in lamprey. *Integr. Comp. Biol.* 51, 869–878. doi: 10.1093/icb/icr077

Bussières, N., and Dubuc, R. (1992). Phasic modulation of vestibulospinal neuron activity during fictive locomotion in lampreys. *Brain Res.* 575, 174–179. doi: 10.1016/0006-8993(92)90441-B

Cabaj, A. M., Majczynski, H., Couto, E., Gardiner, P. F., Stecina, K., Sławinska, U., et al. (2017). Serotonin controls initiation of locomotion and afferent modulation of coordination via 5-HT 7 receptors in adult rats: 5-HT 7 receptors in locomotor control. *J. Physiol.* 595, 301–320. doi: 10.1113/JP272271

Cabelguen, J.-M., Charrier, V., and Mathou, A. (2014). Modular functional organisation of the axial locomotor system in salamanders. *Zoology* 117, 57–63. doi: 10.1016/j.zool.2013.10.002

Canon, E., Reznik, M., and Timmermans, L. M. (1991). Morphometry of sacral neurons innervating the pelvic muscles. Experimental study. *Acta Urol. Belg.* 59, 1–16.

Carlson, H., Halbertsma, J., and Zomlefer, M. (1979). Control of the trunk during walking in the cat. *Acta Physiol. Scand.* 105, 251–253. doi: 10.1111/j.1748-1716.1979.tb06338.x

Cazalets, J.-R., Borde, M., and Clarac, F. (1995). Localization and organization of the central pattern generator for hindlimb locomotion in newborn rat. *J. Neurosci.* 15, 4943–4951.

Ceccato, J.-C., de Sèze, M., Azevedo, C., and Cazalets, J.-R. (2009). Comparison of trunk activity during gait initiation and walking in humans. *PLoS ONE* 4:e8193. doi: 10.1371/journal.pone.0008193

Combes, D., Merrywest, S. D., Simmers, J., and Sillar, K. T. (2004). Developmental segregation of spinal networks driving axial- and hindlimb-based locomotion in metamorphosing *Xenopus laevis*. *J. Physiol.* 559, 17–24. doi: 10.1113/jphysiol.2004.069542

Cowley, K. C., Zaporozhets, E., Joundi, R. A., and Schmidt, B. J. (2009). Contribution of commissural projections to bulbospinal activation of locomotion in the *in vitro* neonatal rat spinal cord. *J. Neurophysiol.* 101, 1171–1178. doi: 10.1152/jn.91212.2008

de Sèze, M., Falgairolle, M., Viel, S., Assaiante, C., and Cazalets, J.-R. (2008). Sequential activation of axial muscles during different forms of rhythmic behavior in man. *Exp. Brain Res.* 185, 237–247. doi: 10.1007/s00221-007-1146-2

English, A. W. (1980). The functions of the lumbar spine during stepping in the cat. *J. Morphol.* 165, 55–66. doi: 10.1002/jmor.1051650106

Falgairolle, M., Ceccato, J.-C., de Seze, M., Herbin, M., and Cazalets, J.-R. (2013). Metachronal propagation of motor activity. *Front. Biosci.* 18, 820–837. doi: 10.2741/4146

Falgairolle, M., and Cazalets, J.-R. (2007). Metachronal coupling between spinal neuronal networks during locomotor activity in newborn rat: synchronization between neuronal networks. *J. Physiol.* 580, 87–102. doi: 10.1113/jphysiol.2006.115709

Giraudin, A., Cabirol-Pol, M.-J., Simmers, J., and Morin, D. (2008). Intercostal and abdominal respiratory motoneurons in the neonatal rat spinal cord: spatiotemporal organization and responses to limb afferent stimulation. *J. Neurophysiol.* 99, 2626–2640. doi: 10.1152/jn.01298.2007

Glover, J. C. (1995). Retrograde and anterograde axonal tracing with fluorescent dextrans in the embryonic nervous system. *Neurosci. Protoc.* 30, 1–13.

Gordon, I. T., and Whelan, P. J. (2008). Brainstem modulation of locomotion in the neonatal mouse spinal cord: descending control of locomotion in the developing mouse. *J. Physiol.* 586, 2487–2497. doi: 10.1113/jphysiol.2007.148320

Gramsbergen, A. (1998). Posture and locomotion in the rat: independent or interdependent development? *Neurosci. Biobehav. Rev.* 22, 547–553. doi: 10.1016/S0149-7634(97)00043-2

Grillner, S. (1981). "Control of locomotion in bipeds, tetrapods, and fish," in *Comprehensive Physiology*, Vol. II, ed R. Terjung (Hoboken, NJ: John Wiley & Sons, Inc.), 1179–1236.

Grillner, S. (2006). Biological pattern generation: the cellular and computational logic of networks in motion. *Neuron* 52, 751–766. doi: 10.1016/j.neuron.2006.11.008

Grillner, S., and Manira, A. E. (2015). The intrinsic operation of the networks that make us locomote. *Curr. Opin. Neurobiol.* 31, 244–249. doi: 10.1016/j.conb.2015.01.003

Hägglund, M., Borgius, L., Dougherty, K. J., and Kiehn, O. (2010). Activation of groups of excitatory neurons in the mammalian spinal cord or hindbrain evokes locomotion. *Nat. Neurosci.* 13, 246–252. doi: 10.1038/nn.2482

Hägglund, M., Dougherty, K. J., Borgius, L., Itohara, S., Iwasato, T., and Kiehn, O. (2013). Optogenetic dissection reveals multiple rhythmogenic modules underlying locomotion. *Proc. Natl. Acad. Sci. U.S.A.* 110, 11589–11594. doi: 10.1073/pnas.1304365110

Hinckley, C. A., Alaynick, W. A., Gallarda, B. W., Hayashi, M., Hilde, K. L., Driscoll, S. P., et al. (2015). Spinal locomotor circuits develop using hierarchical rules based on motorneuron position and identity. *Neuron* 87, 1008–1021. doi: 10.1016/j.neuron.2015.08.005

Ho, S., and O'Donovan, M. J. (1993). Regionalization and intersegmental coordination of rhythm-generating networks in the spinal cord of the chick embryo. *J. Neurosci.* 13, 1354–1371.

Hodges, P. W., Sapsford, R., and Pengel, L. H. M. (2007). Postural and respiratory functions of the pelvic floor muscles. *Neurourol. Urodyn.* 26, 362–371. doi: 10.1002/nau.20232

Iscoe, S. (1998). Control of abdominal muscles. *Prog. Neurobiol.* 56, 433–506. doi: 10.1016/S0301-0082(98)00046-X

Jamon, M. (2006). The early development of motor control in neonate rat. *Comptes Rendus Palevol* 5, 657–666. doi: 10.1016/j.crpv.2005.11.018

Jean-Xavier, C., and Perreault, M.-C. (2013). "Brainstem control of trunk and hindlimb motoneurons during fictive locomotion in the neonatal mouse," in *Neuroscience Meeting Planner, Society for Neuroscience*. Online Program No 560.08 (San Diego, CA).

Jiang, Z., Carlin, K. P., and Brownstone, R. M. (1999). An *in vitro* functionally mature mouse spinal cord preparation for the study of spinal motor networks. *Brain Res.* 816, 493–499. doi: 10.1016/S0006-8993(98)01199-8

Jordan, L. M. (1991). "Brainstem and spinal cord mechanisms for the initiation of locomotion", in *Neurobiological Basis of Human Locomotion*, eds M. Shimamura, S. Grillner, and V. R. Edgerton (Tokyo: Japan Scientific Societies), 3–20.

Jordan, L. M., Liu, J., Hedlund, P. B., Akay, T., and Pearson, K. G. (2008). Descending command systems for the initiation of locomotion in mammals. *Brain Res. Rev.* 57, 183–191. doi: 10.1016/j.brainresrev.2007.07.019

Kasicki, S., Grillner, S., Ohta, Y., Dubuc, R., and Brodin, L. (1989). Phasic modulation of reticulospinal neurones during fictive locomotion and other types of spinal motor activity in lamprey. *Brain Res.* 484, 203–216. doi: 10.1016/0006-8993(89)90363-6

Kasumacic, N., Glover, J. C., and Perreault, M.-C. (2010). Segmental patterns of vestibular-mediated synaptic inputs to axial and limb motoneurons in the neonatal mouse assessed by optical recording: imaging vestibulospinal inputs to spinal motoneurons. *J. Physiol.* 588, 4905–4925. doi: 10.1113/jphysiol.2010.195644

Kishore, S., Bagnall, M. W., and McLean, D. L. (2014). Systematic shifts in the balance of excitation and inhibition coordinate the activity of axial motor pools at different speeds of locomotion. *J. Neurosci.* 34, 14046–14054. doi: 10.1523/JNEUROSCI.0514-14.2014

Kjaerulff, O., and Kiehn, O. (1996). Distribution of networks generating and coordinating locomotor activity in the neonatal rat spinal cord *in vitro*: a lesion study. *J. Neurosci.* 16, 5777–5794.

Koehler, W. J., Schomburg, E. D., and Steffens, H. (1984). Phasic modulation of trunk muscle efferents during fictive spinal locomotion in cats. *J. Physiol.* 353, 187–197. doi: 10.1113/jphysiol.1984.sp015331

Kreitzer, A. C., Gee, K. R., Archer, E. A., and Regehr, W. G. (2000). Monitoring presynaptic calcium dynamics in projection fibers by *in vivo* loading of a novel calcium indicator. *Neuron* 27, 25–32. doi: 10.1016/S0896-6273(00)00006-4

Kristan, W. B., Calabrese, R. L., and Friesen, W. O. (2005). Neuronal control of leech behavior. *Prog. Neurobiol.* 76, 279–327. doi: 10.1016/j.pneurobio.2005.09.004

Kudo, N., and Yamada, T. (1987). N-methyl-D,L-aspartate-induced locomotor activity in a spinal cord-hindlimb muscles preparation of the newborn rat studied *in vitro*. *Neurosci. Lett.* 75, 43–48. doi: 10.1016/0304-3940(87)90072-3

Leblond, H., and Gossard, J.-P. (1997). Supraspinal and segmental signals can be transmitted through separate spinal cord pathways to enhance locomotor activity in extensor muscles in the cat. *Exp. Brain Res.* 114, 188–192. doi: 10.1007/PL00005619

Le Gal, J.-P., Juvin, L., Cardoit, L., and Morin, D. (2016). Bimodal respiratory-locomotor neurons in the neonatal rat spinal cord. *J. Neurosci.* 36, 926–937. doi: 10.1523/JNEUROSCI.1825-15.2016

Lev-Tov, A., and O'Donovan, M. J. (1995). Calcium imaging of motoneuron activity in the en-bloc spinal cord preparation of the neonatal rat. *J. Neurophysiol.* 74, 1324–1334. doi: 10.1152/jn.1995.74.3.1324

MacDonell, C. W., Power, K. E., Chopek, J. W., Gardiner, K. R., and Gardiner, P. F. (2015). Extensor motoneurone properties are altered immediately before and during fictive locomotion in the adult decerebrate rat: motoneurone properties during fictive locomotion. *J. Physiol.* 593, 2327–2342. doi: 10.1113/JP270239

Marlinsky, V. V. (1992). Activity of lateral vestibular nucleus neurons during locomotion in the decerebrate guinea pig. *Exp. Brain Res.* 90, 583–588. doi: 10.1007/BF00230942

Meehan, C. F., Grondahl, L., Nielsen, J. B., and Hultborn, H. (2012). Fictive locomotion in the adult decerebrate and spinal mouse *in vivo*: fictive locomotion in the decerebrate mouse. *J. Physiol.* 590, 289–300. doi: 10.1113/jphysiol.2011.214643

Mor, Y., and Lev-Tov, A. (2007). Analysis of rhythmic patterns produced by spinal neural networks. *J. Neurophysiol.* 98, 2807–2817. doi: 10.1152/jn.00740.2007

Musienko, P. E., Deliagina, T. G., Gerasimenko, Y. P., Orlovsky, G. N., and Zelenin, P. V. (2014). Limb and trunk mechanisms for balance control during locomotion in quadrupeds. *J. Neurosci.* 34, 5704–5716. doi: 10.1523/JNEUROSCI.4663-13.2014

Noga, B. R., Turkson, R. P., Xie, S., Taberner, A., Pinzon, A., and Hentall, I. D. (2017). Monoamine release in the cat lumbar spinal cord during fictive locomotion evoked by the mesencephalic locomotor region. *Front. Neural Circuits* 11:59. doi: 10.3389/fncir.2017.00059

O'Donovan, M. J., Bonnot, A., Mentis, G. Z., Arai, Y., Chub, N., Shneider, N. A., et al. (2008). Imaging the spatiotemporal organization of neural activity in the developing spinal cord. *Dev. Neurobiol.* 68, 788–803. doi: 10.1002/dneu.20620

Perreault, M. C., Drew, T., and Rossignol, S. (1993). Activity of medullary reticulospinal neurons during fictive locomotion. *J. Neurophysiol.* 69, 2232–2247. doi: 10.1152/jn.1993.69.6.2232

Perreault, M.-C., and Glover, J. C. (2013). Glutamatergic reticulospinal neurons in the mouse: developmental origins, axon projections, and functional connectivity: glutamatergic reticulospinal neurons in the mouse. *Ann. N.Y. Acad. Sci.* 1279, 80–89. doi: 10.1111/nyas.12054

Perreault, M. C., Rossignol, S., and Drew, T. (1994). Microstimulation of the medullary reticular formation during fictive locomotion. *J. Neurophysiol.* 71, 229–245. doi: 10.1152/jn.1994.71.1.229

Perreault, M.-C., Shefchyk, S. J., Jimenez, I., and McCrea, D. A. (1999). Depression of muscle and cutaneous afferent-evoked monosynaptic field potentials during fictive locomotion in the cat. *J. Physiol.* 521, 691–703. doi: 10.1111/j.1469-7793.1999.00691.x

Putney, J. W. (ed.). (2006). *Calcium Signaling, 2nd Edn.* Boca Raton, FL: CRC/Taylor & Francis.

Ritter, D. A., Nassar, P. N., Fife, M., and Carrier, D. R. (2001). Epaxial muscle function in trotting dogs. *J. Exp. Biol.* 204, 3053–3064.

Roberts, A., Li, W.-C., and Soffe, S. R. (2012). A functional scaffold of CNS neurons for the vertebrates: the developing *Xenopus laevis* spinal cord. *Dev. Neurobiol.* 72, 575–584. doi: 10.1002/dneu.20889

Russell, D. F., and Zajac, F. E. (1979). Effects of stimulating Deiters' nucleus and medial longitudinal fasciculus on the timing of the fictive locomotor rhythm induced in cats by DOPA. *Brain Res.* 177, 588–592. doi: 10.1016/0006-8993(79)90478-5

Ryczko, D., Dubuc, R., and Cabelguen, J.-M. (2010). Rhythmogenesis in axial locomotor networks: an interspecies comparison. *Prog. Brain Res.* 187, 189–211. doi: 10.1016/B978-0-444-53613-6.00013-7

Ryczko, D., Knüsel, J., Crespi, A., Lamarque, S., Mathou, A., Ijspeert, A. J., et al. (2015). Flexibility of the axial central pattern generator network for locomotion in the salamander. *J. Neurophysiol.* 113, 1921–1940. doi: 10.1152/jn.00894.2014

Schilling, N. (2011). Evolution of the axial system in craniates: morphology and function of the perivertebral musculature. *Front. Zool.* 8:4. doi: 10.1186/1742-9994-8-4

Schilling, N., and Carrier, D. R. (2010). Function of the epaxial muscles in walking, trotting and galloping dogs: implications for the evolution of epaxial muscle function in tetrapods. *J. Exp. Biol.* 213, 1490–1502. doi: 10.1242/jeb.039487

Schrøder, H. D. (1980). Organization of the motoneurons innervating the pelvic muscles of the male rat. *J. Comp. Neurol.* 192, 567–587. doi: 10.1002/cne.901920313

Sivertsen, M. S., Glover, J. C., and Perreault, M.-C. (2014). Organization of pontine reticulospinal inputs to motoneurons controlling axial and limb muscles in the neonatal mouse. *J. Neurophysiol.* 112, 1628–1643. doi: 10.1152/jn.00820.2013

Smith, J. C., and Feldman, J. L. (1987). *In vitro* brainstem-spinal cord preparations for study of motor systems for mammalian respiration and locomotion. *J. Neurosci. Methods* 21, 321–333. doi: 10.1016/0165-0270(87)90126-9

Szokol, K., Glover, J. C., and Perreault, M.-C. (2008). Differential origin of reticulospinal drive to motoneurons innervating trunk and hindlimb muscles in the mouse revealed by optical recording: imaging reticulospinal inputs to lumbar spinal cord. *J. Physiol.* 586, 5259–5276. doi: 10.1113/jphysiol.2008.158105

Szokol, K., and Perreault, M.-C. (2009). Imaging synaptically mediated responses produced by brainstem inputs onto identified spinal neurons in the neonatal mouse. *J. Neurosci. Methods* 180, 1–8. doi: 10.1016/j.jneumeth.2009.01.018

Tazerart, S., Viemari, J.-C., Darbon, P., Vinay, L., and Brocard, F. (2007). Contribution of persistent sodium current to locomotor pattern generation in neonatal rats. *J. Neurophysiol.* 98, 613–628. doi: 10.1152/jn.00316.2007

Thorsen, D. H. (2004). Swimming of larval zebrafish: fin-axis coordination and implications for function and neural control. *J. Exp. Biol.* 207, 4175–4183. doi: 10.1242/jeb.01285

Thorstensson, A., Carlson, H., Zomlefer, M. R., and Nilsson, J. (1982). Lumbar back muscle activity in relation to trunk movements during locomotion in man. *Acta Physiol. Scand.* 116, 13–20. doi: 10.1111/j.1748-1716.1982.tb10593.x

Veasey, S. C., Fornal, C. A., Metzler, C. W., and Jacobs, B. L. (1995). Response of serotonergic caudal raphe neurons in relation to specific motor activities in freely moving cats. *J. Neurosci.* 15, 5346–5359.

Vinay, L., and Grillner, S. (1993). The spino-reticulo-spinal loop can slow down the NMDA-activated spinal locomotor network in lamprey. *Neuroreport* 4, 609–612. doi: 10.1097/00001756-199306000-00001

Wada, N., Akatani, J., Miyajima, N., Shimojo, K., and Kanda, K. (2006). The role of vertebral column muscles in level versus upslope treadmill walking—an electromyographic and kinematic study. *Brain Res.* 1090, 99–109. doi: 10.1016/j.brainres.2006.01.132

Wada, N., and Kanda, K. (2004). Trunk movements and EMG activity in the cat: level versus upslope walking. *Prog. Brain Res.* 143, 175–181. doi: 10.1016/S0079-6123(03)43017-3

Zaporozhets, E., Cowley, K. C., and Schmidt, B. J. (2004). A reliable technique for the induction of locomotor-like activity in the *in vitro* neonatal rat spinal cord using brainstem electrical stimulation. *J. Neurosci. Methods* 139, 33–41. doi: 10.1016/j.jneumeth.2004.04.009

Zhao, M., Hollingworth, S., and Baylor, S. M. (1996). Properties of tri- and tetracarboxylate Ca2+ indicators in frog skeletal muscle fibers. *Biophys. J.* 70, 896–916. doi: 10.1016/S0006-3495(96)79633-9

Zomlefer, M. R., Provencher, J., Blanchette, G., and Rossignol, S. (1984). Electromyographic study of lumbar back muscles during locomotion in acute high decerebrate and in low spinal cats. *Brain Res.* 290, 249–260. doi: 10.1016/0006-8993(84)90942-9

14

Histamine Increases Neuronal Excitability and Sensitivity of the Lateral Vestibular Nucleus and Promotes Motor Behaviors via HCN Channel Coupled to H2 Receptor

Bin Li[1†], Xiao-Yang Zhang[1†], Ai-Hong Yang[1,2], Xiao-Chun Peng[1], Zhang-Peng Chen[1], Jia-Yuan Zhou[1], Ying-Shing Chan[3], Jian-Jun Wang[1] and Jing-Ning Zhu[1*]*

[1]State Key Laboratory of Pharmaceutical Biotechnology and Department of Biological Science and Technology, School of Life Sciences, Nanjing University, Nanjing, China, [2]Department of Medicine, Huaibei Vocational and Technical College, Huaibei, China, [3]Department of Physiology, LKS Faculty of Medicine, The University of Hong Kong, Hong Kong, Hong Kong

***Correspondence:**
Jian-Jun Wang
jjwang@nju.edu.cn
Jing-Ning Zhu
jnzhu@nju.edu.cn

Histamine and histamine receptors in the central nervous system actively participate in the modulation of motor control. In clinic, histamine-related agents have traditionally been used to treat vestibular disorders. Immunohistochemical studies have revealed a distribution of histaminergic afferents in the brainstem vestibular nuclei, including the lateral vestibular nucleus (LVN), which is critical for adjustment of muscle tone and vestibular reflexes. However, the mechanisms underlying the effect of histamine on LVN neurons and the role of histamine and histaminergic afferents in the LVN in motor control are still largely unknown. Here, we show that histamine, in cellular and molecular levels, elicits the LVN neurons of rats an excitatory response, which is co-mediated by the hyperpolarization-activated cyclic nucleotide-gated (HCN) channels and K^+ channels linked to H2 receptors. Blockage of HCN channels coupled to H2 receptors decreases LVN neuronal sensitivity and changes their dynamic properties. Furthermore, in behavioral level, microinjection of histamine into bilateral LVNs significantly promotes motor performances of rats on both accelerating rota-rod and balance beam. This promotion is mimicked by selective H2 receptor agonist dimaprit, and blocked by selective H2 receptor antagonist ranitidine. More importantly, blockage of HCN channels to suppress endogenous histaminergic inputs in the LVN considerably attenuates motor balance and coordination, indicating a promotion role of hypothalamo-vestibular histaminergic circuit in motor control. All these results demonstrate that histamine H2 receptors and their coupled HCN channels mediate the histamine-induced increase in excitability and sensitivity of LVN neurons and contribute to the histaminergic improvement of the LVN-related motor behaviors. The findings suggest that histamine and the histaminergic afferents may directly modulate LVN neurons and play a critical role in the central vestibular-mediated motor reflexes and behaviors.

Keywords: histamine, histamine H2 receptor, HCN channel, lateral vestibular nucleus, motor control

INTRODUCTION

Histamine, restrictedly synthesized in the tuberomammillary nucleus neurons in the hypothalamus, plays important roles in many brain functions, including feeding, sleep/wakefulness and cardiovascular control (Passani et al., 2007; Haas et al., 2008; Panula and Nuutinen, 2013). Recently, role of histamine in somatic motor control has attracted an increasing attention (Li et al., 2014). Patients with motor disease, such as Parkinson's disease and vestibular disorders, show significant alternation in the central histaminergic system (Lacour, 2013; Shan et al., 2015). And histamine-related agents have been widely used to treat vestibular disorders in clinic (Haas et al., 2008; Tiligada et al., 2011), although the underlying mechanisms are still not entirely clear.

The role of central histaminergic system on motor behaviors is complex. The histidine decarboxylase (the histamine synthesizing enzyme) knockout mice exhibit a reduced locomotor and exploratory activity (Dere et al., 2004), whereas intracerebroventricular injection of histamine induces a transient increase followed by a decrease in locomotor activity in rats (Onodera et al., 1994). These complex effects of histamine on motor activity are mediated by different histamine receptors in various central motor structures. H1R-deficient mice display altered ambulatory activity and reduced exploratory behavior in a new environment (Inoue et al., 1996). The reduced locomotion is also observed in H3R-deficient mice (Toyota et al., 2002). Moreover, by means of pharmacological manipulation combining behavioral tests, our previous studies have demonstrated that histamine remarkably promotes motor balance and coordination on accelerating rota-rod and balance beam via activation of H2 receptors in the rat cerebellar fastigial and interposed nuclei (Song et al., 2006; He et al., 2012; Zhang et al., 2016).

The vestibular nuclei in the brainstem are important motor structures in the central nervous system and responsible for control of muscle tone, posture and body balance. In the vestibular nuclei, the lateral vestibular nucleus (LVN), one of the targets of cerebellar outputs, is implicated in the regulation of muscle tone and postural control during ongoing movements (Wilson and Peterson, 1978; Molina-Negro et al., 1980). Interestingly, neuroanatomical and immunostaining studies have showed a moderately dense histaminergic afferents in the central vestibular nuclei in various mammals, including guinea pig, rat and cat (Schwartz et al., 1991; Steinbusch, 1991; Tighilet and Lacour, 1996). Molecular, autoradiographic and pharmacological studies have also demonstrated that the LVN is endowed with H2 and/or H3 receptors in guinea pigs (Yabe et al., 1993; Vizuete et al., 1997). Our previous electrophysiological study have further reported that histamine post-synaptically depolarizes the LVN neurons via activating H2 receptors in rats (Zhang et al., 2008). However, the role of histamine H2 receptor and its mediated histaminergic modulation in the LVN-mediated motor control remains largely unknown.

Therefore, in this study, by whole-cell patch clamp recordings in brainstem slices and behavioral tests *in vivo*, we examined the ionic mechanisms underlying the histamine H2 receptor-mediated excitatory effect of histamine on LVN neurons, and particularly, the role of histamine and histaminergic afferent inputs in the LVN-mediated motor control. The results demonstrate that the histamine-elicited excitation on the LVN neurons is mediated by histamine H2 receptor and its downstream hyperpolarization-activated cyclic nucleotide-gated (HCN) channels as well as K^+ channels. The activation of HCN channels coupled to H2 receptors increase excitability and sensitivity of LVN neurons, and improves the LVN-mediated motor behaviors.

MATERIALS AND METHODS

Animals

Sprague-Dawley rats were individually housed under controlled environment conditions (22 ± 2°C; 60 ± 5% humidity; and 12-h light/dark cycle with lights on at 8:00 a.m. daily). The animals had free access to standard laboratory chow and water. All animal experiments, approved by the Experimental Animal Care and Use Committee of Nanjing University, were conducted in accordance with U.S. National Institutes of Health Guide for the Care and Use of Laboratory Animals (NIH Publication 85–23, revised 2011) and were reported in accordance with the ARRIVE guidelines (Kilkenny et al., 2010). All efforts were made to minimize the number of animals used.

Whole-Cell Patch-Clamp Recordings on Brain Slices

Under sodium pentobarbital (40 mg/kg) anesthesia, 51 Sprague-Dawley rats of either sex aged 10–16 days were used for these experiments, since the central histaminergic system in rats usually reach adult level by 2 weeks after birth (Haas et al., 2008). Coronal slices (300 μm thick) of brainstem containing the LVN were prepared with a vibroslicer (VT 1200 S, Leica Microsystems, Wetzlar, Germany), according to the rat brain atlas of Paxinos and Watson (2007). The slices were then incubated in oxygenated (95% O_2/5% CO_2) artificial cerebrospinal fluid (ACSF: 124 mM NaCl, 2.5 mM KCl, 1.25 mM NaH_2PO_4, 1.3 mM $MgSO_4$, 26 mM $NaHCO_3$, 2 mM $CaCl_2$ and 10 mM D-glucose) at 35 ± 0.5°C for at least 1 h and then maintained at room temperature. During recording sessions, the slices were transferred to a submerged chamber and continuously perfused with oxygenated ACSF at a rate of 2 mL/min at room temperature.

Whole-cell patch-clamp recordings were performed as our previous report (Zhang et al., 2008, 2011, 2013, 2016; Yu et al., 2016). Briefly, recording pipettes (3–5 MΩ) were filled with an internal solution (140 mM K-methylsulfate, 7 mM KCl, 2 mM $MgCl_2$, 10 mM HEPES, 0.1 mM EGTA, 4 mM Na_2ATP, 0.4 mM GTP-Tris, adjusted to pH 7.25 with 1 M KOH). Patch-clamp recordings were acquired with an Axopatch-200B amplifier (Axon Instruments, Foster City, CA, USA) and the signals were fed into a computer through a Digidata-1550 interface (Axon Instruments) for data capture and analysis (pClamp 10.4, Axon Instruments). Under voltage-clamp mode, the membrane potential of recorded neurons was held at −60 mV. In slow-ramp test, a voltage command ranged from −60 to −120 mV with dV/dt = −10 mV/s was employed (Zhang et al., 2011, 2013; Yu et al., 2016). Furthermore, under current-clamp mode, depolarizing voltage sag, the hallmark of HCN channel activation, was triggered by hyperpolarizing current steps (70–150 pA, 1 s) and evaluated by subtracting the peak voltage amplitude from the steady-state voltage. Moreover, in current-clamp recording, a depolarizing ramp-like current, consisting a 600 ms ramp (from −150 pA to 150 pA, slope of 0.5 nA/s) followed by a long plateau of current (150 pA, 4400 ms), was injected to evaluate the sensitivity and dynamic properties of LVN neurons (Ris et al., 2001; Uno et al., 2003; Zhang et al., 2011).

Immunofluorescence

The experimental procedures for immunostaining followed our previous reports (Zhang et al., 2011, 2013, 2016; Li et al., 2016). Rat (weighing 230–250 g) were deeply anesthetized with sodium pentobarbital and perfused transcardially with 100 ml of normal saline, followed by 450–500 ml of 4% paraformaldehyde in 0.1 M phosphate buffer. Subsequently, the brain was removed, trimmed and postfixed in the same fixative for 12 h at 4°C, and then cryoprotected in 30% sucrose for 48 h. Coronal brainstem sections (25 μm thick) containing the LVN were prepared with a freezing microtome (CM 3050S, Leica Microsystems). The sections were rinsed with PBS containing 0.1% Triton X-100 (PBST), and then incubated in 10% normal bovine serum in PBST for 30 min. Sections were incubated with a goat anti-H2 receptor polyclonal antibody (1:200; Everest Biotech, Oxfordshire, UK) overnight at 4°C. After wash in PBS, the sections were incubated with the Alexa 488-conjugated donkey anti-goat (1:2000; Invitrogen, Carlsbad, CA, USA) for 2 h at room temperature in the dark. The slides were washed and mounted in Fluoromount-G mounting medium (Southern Biotech, Birmingham, AL, USA). Negative controls were treated with incubations replacing the primary anti-serum with control immunoglobulins and/or omitting the primary antiserum. Images were acquired with a confocal laser scanning microscope (FV1000; Olympus) and recorded with FV10-ASW 3.1 Viewer Software (Olympus).

Stereotactic Implantation of Microinjection Cannulae

Male rats (230–250 g) were anesthetized with sodium pentobarbital (40 mg/kg) intraperitoneally, and then mounted on a stereotaxic frame (1404, David Kopf Instruments, Tujunga, CA, USA) for stereotactic brain surgery under aseptic conditions. A heating pad was used to maintain rectal temperature at 36–38°C. Briefly, two stainless-steel guide tubes (length 8 mm, o.d. 0.8 mm, i.d. 0.5 mm) for the microinjection cannulae were implanted into bilateral LVNs of each rat. The lower ends of the guide tubes were positioned 2.0 mm above the LVN (A −10.5 to 10.8, L 2.2 and H 6.5). After surgery, animals were caged individually and allowed to recover for at least 3 days.

Microinjection in the LVN

For microinjection in the LVNs, two injection cannulae (length 10 mm, o.d. 0.5 mm, i.d. 0.3 mm) were inserted to protrude 2 mm beyond the tip of the guide tube. The lower ends of the injection cannulae were just above bilateral LVNs to minimize lesioning the nuclei. Histamine (5 mM; Tocris, Bristol, UK), dimaprit (10 mM), ranitidine (10 mM; Tocris), ZD7288 (1 mM, 3 mM and 10 mM; Tocris) and saline (0.9% NaCl) were microinjected with Hamilton syringes (1 μl each side, lasting 2 min). The effective extent of the drug diffusion in the present study was restricted in the LVNs according to the estimate by extracellular electrophysiological recording units 0.5–2.0 mm away from the injection site in our previous reports (Song et al., 2006; Zhang et al., 2011).

Behavioral Tests

Animals used in behavioral tests were divided into eight groups: (1) microinjected with saline; (2) microinjected with 5 mM histamine; (3) microinjected with 10 mM dimaprit; (4) microinjected with 10 mM ranitidine; (5) microinjected with 1 mM ZD7288; (6) microinjected with 3 mM ZD7288; (7) microinjected with 10 mM ZD7288; and (8) microinjected with 10 mM dimaprit and 3 mM ZD7288. In order to achieve a stable motor performance, each animal was trained daily for at least 10 trials for 3–5 consecutive days. All training/tests started at 10:00 a.m. each day, and motor performances on accelerating rota-rod and balance beam of each animal were tested before, 0 h, 4 h and 24 h after microinjections.

We used accelerating rota-rod test to assess vestibular-related motor balance and coordination (Song et al., 2006; Zhang et al., 2011, 2014; He et al., 2012). Animals were placed on the rota-rod (Ugo Basile, Varese, Italy) and habituated to low rotation (4 rpm) for 30 s first. Then the rod was evenly accelerated up to 40 rpm during 360 s, and the latency for each rat to fall from the rotating rod was recorded. In the test, each rat was subjected three trials, with a resting interval of 3 min to reduce fatigue and stress.

We also employed balance beam test to evaluate vestibular motor function (Song et al., 2006; Zhang et al., 2011, 2014; He et al., 2012). The balance beam (2.5 cm in diameter) was 190 cm in length. A bright plastic platform (7 cm × 4 cm) was placed at one end of the rod as the start, and a darkened box (15 cm × 15 cm × 8 cm) was set at the opposite end as a goal nest for motivating rat to traverse the beam. The beam was suspended 90 cm above a cushion, which protected the fallen animals from injury, and 50 cm from a wall. The time that each rat spent to cross the beam was recorded. The test consisted of five consecutive trials with a 90 s resting interval.

Histological Identification

To verify the position of microinjection, each rat for behavioral tests was anesthetized with an overdose of sodium pentobarbital at the end of tests. Two insulated stainless steel wires (o.d. 0.4 mm) with 0.2 mm exposed tip were inserted (10 mm) into the brainstem under guidance of guide tubes for depositing iron at the injection site by DC current (10 μA, 20 s). The brain was then removed and fixed with 4% paraformaldehyde containing 1% potassium ferrocyanide. A week later, frozen serial coronal sections (80 μm thick) were prepared, and the dark blue dots indicating injection sites were identified according to the rat brain atlas (Paxinos and Watson, 2007). Data from rats in which the injection sites were deviated from the LVN were excluded from further analysis.

Statistical Analysis

All data were analyzed with Origin 7.5 (MicroCal Software) and presented as mean ± S.E.M. The Student's *t* test, one-way and repeated measures two-way analysis of variance (ANOVA) was performed for statistical analysis. Newman-Keuls *post hoc* testing was employed to further determine the differences between group means. The values of $P < 0.05$ were considered as statistically significant.

RESULTS

Histamine Excites LVN Neurons via the Activation of H2 Receptors

In the present study, we recorded a total of 67 LVN neurons with the input resistance higher than 150 MΩ. Of the 67 LVN neurons recorded, 42 showed spontaneous firing (mean firing rate = 6.9 ± 0.4 spikes/s) and the remaining 25 were silent at rest. The result was in agreement with the previous reports that 30–50% LVN neurons are silent (Lai and Chan, 2001; Sun et al., 2002; Uno et al., 2003; Zhang et al., 2008, 2011). All the neurons we patched have a diameter >35 μm, indicating they were giant LVN Deiters' (projection) neurons. In addition, there was no morphological difference between the spontaneous firing and silent LVN neurons (**Figures 1A1,B1**). In voltage clamp recordings, brief bath application (1 min) of 30 μm histamine increased the discharge rate of five spontaneous firing neurons in the LVN (**Figure 1A2**) from 5.8 ± 0.9 spikes/s to 7.6 ± 1.7 spikes/s ($P < 0.01$). On the other hand, 30 μM histamine evoked a strong depolarization on five silent LVN neurons, which was even sufficient to bring up the neurons firing (**Figure 1B2**). The results indicate that histamine elicits a significant excitatory response on both types of LVN neurons (**Figures 1A2,B2**).

Postsynaptic H2 receptors have been reported in our previous study to mediate the histamine-induced excitation on LVN neurons (Zhang et al., 2008). Here, we used ranitidine, a selective antagonist for histamine H2 receptor, to examine whether the receptor mechanisms on these two types of LVN neurons are the same. As shown in **Figures 1A2,B2**, bath application of ranitidine (3 μM) totally blocked the histamine-elicited excitation on both spontaneous firing and silent LVN neurons. In addition, dimaprit (30, 100, 300 μM), a highly selective agonist for histamine H2 receptors, induced an inward current (21.5 ± 2.6, 40.6 ± 4.5, 48.3 ± 5.2 pA, respectively) on LVN neurons in a concentration-dependent manner ($n = 6$, **Figures 1C,D**). Fitting the concentration-response curve from six LVN neurons yielded an EC_{50} value for dimaprit (10–300 μM) of 48.5 μM (**Figure 1D**). Notably, the inward current induced by dimaprit (10–300 μM) was totally blocked by 3 μM ranitidine (**Figures 1C,D**). Moreover, ranitidine (0.3–3 μM) concentration-dependently blocked the 100 μM dimaprit-induced inward current on LVN neurons (**Figure 1E**). The inward current elicited by dimaprit decreased remarkably from 44.3 ± 5.6 pA to 31.5 ± 2.3 ($n = 5$, $P < 0.05$), 14.5 ± 1.0 ($n = 5$, $P < 0.001$) and 2.7 ± 0.3 pA ($n = 5$, $P < 0.001$) by application of 0.3, 1 and 3 μM ranitidine (**Figure 1F**), respectively. Furthermore, the immunostaining result revealed that histamine H2 receptors were distributed in the LVN neurons in rats (**Figures 1G1–G4**), confirming our electrophysiological data. All these results demonstrate that histamine depolarizes and excites both types of LVN neurons by activation of H2 receptors.

Activation of Histamine H2 Receptor in the LVN Significantly Promotes Motor Behaviors

Since the LVN holds a key position in the vestibulospinal reflexes and posture control, we microinjected saline, histamine (5 mM), dimaprit (10 mM) and ranitidine (10 mM) into bilateral LVNs to determine the effect of activation of histamine H2 receptor on motor behaviors. The average score of 40 rats of all tested groups for the accelerating rota-rod tests was 152.78 ± 4.32 s, and no significant difference was found among the groups before microinjections ($F_{(3,36)} = 0.03$, $P = 0.992$; **Figure 2A**). A two-way ANOVA with repeated measures showed a significant effect of time ($F_{(3,108)} = 136.95$, $P < 0.01$), treatment ($F_{(3,36)} = 1.615$, $P = 0.203$) and time × treatment interaction ($F_{(9,108)} = 22.927$, $P < 0.01$) among these groups. Furthermore, Newman-Keuls *post hoc* test revealed that the endurance time of the histamine group ($n = 10$) on the rota-rod at 0 h after microinjection significantly increased compared with that of the saline group ($n = 10$; $P < 0.01$, **Figure 2A**), and such effect recovered hours later (**Figure 2A**). Activation of histamine H2 receptors in LVN by microinjection of dimaprit ($n = 10$) mimicked the histamine-induced improvement in motor performances at 0 h after injection ($P < 0.05$, **Figure 2A**). And blockage of histamine H2 receptors in the LVNs by ranitidine ($n = 10$) remarkably shortened the endurance time of rats on the rotating rod at 4 h ($P < 0.05$, **Figure 2A**) and 24 h ($P < 0.05$, **Figure 2A**) after injection.

In the balance beam test, the mean score of 40 rats of all groups on the beam was 4.46 ± 0.06 s, and there was no significant difference among the groups before injections ($F_{(3,36)} = 0.142$, $P = 0.934$; **Figure 2B**). A two-way ANOVA with repeated measures revealed a significant effect of time ($F_{(3,108)} = 151.091$, $P < 0.01$), treatment ($F_{(3,36)} = 7.626$, $P < 0.01$) and time × treatment interaction ($F_{(9,108)} = 36.534$, $P < 0.01$) among these groups. Furthermore, Newman-Keuls *post hoc* test indicated that microinjection of histamine ($n = 10$) into the LVNs significantly shortened the time that traversing the balance beam at 0 h after injection compared with the saline group ($n = 10$; $P < 0.01$, **Figure 2B**), and such effect recovered hours later (**Figure 2B**). Notably, at 0 h after injection, the spending time of the dimaprit group ($n = 10$) was significantly shorter than that of the saline group ($P < 0.01$, **Figure 2B**), whereas the time

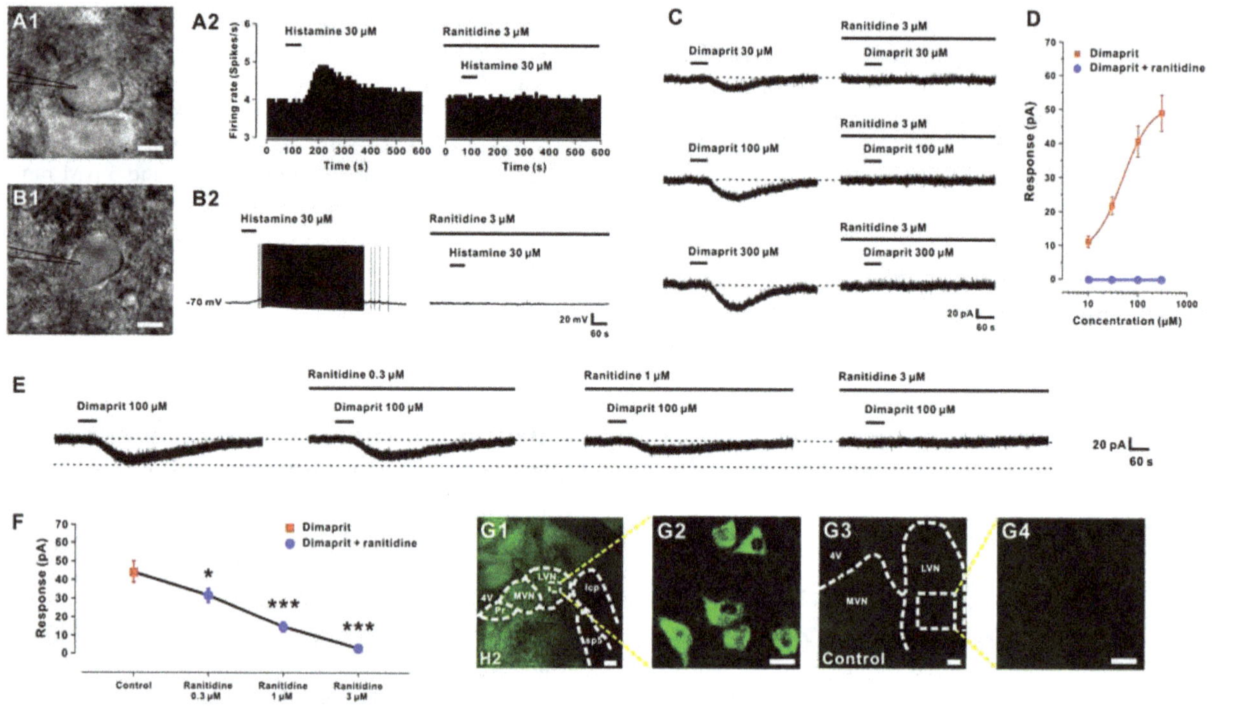

FIGURE 1 | Histamine excites LVN neurons by activation of H2 receptors. (A1,B1) Infrared differential interference contrast images of spontaneous firing and silent LVN neurons captured before whole-cell patch clamp recordings. **(A2,B2)** Histamine elicited a significant excitatory response on both spontaneous firing and silent LVN neurons. Bath application of ranitidine, a selective H2 receptor antagonist, totally blocked the histamine-elicited excitation on both types of recorded LVN neurons. **(C)** Dimaprit, a highly selective agonist for histamine H2 receptors, induced an inward current on a recorded LVN neuron in a concentration-dependent manner. And ranitidine totally blocked the inward current induced by dimaprit of all tested concentrations. **(D)** Concentration-response curves for dimaprit on recorded LVN neurons in the absence and presence of dimaprit. **(E)** Ranitidine (0.3–3 μm) concentration-dependently blocked the 100 μm dimaprit-induced inward current on a LVN neuron. **(F)** Group data of five tested LVN neurons. **(G1–G4)** Immunostaining result showed that histamine H2 receptors are present in the rat LVN neurons. Scale bars: **(A1,B1)**, 20 μm; **(G1)**, 250 μm; **(G2)**, 25 μm; **(G3)**, 150 μm; **(G4)**, 25 μm. Data shown are means ± SEM; *$P < 0.05$, ***$P < 0.001$. 4V, 4th ventricle; MVN, medial vestibular nucleus; LVN, lateral vestibular nucleus; Pr, prepositus nucleus; icp, inferior cerebellar peduncle; sp5, spinal trigeminal tract.

traversing the beam of the ranitidine group ($n = 10$) markedly prolonged at 4 h, even 24 h after injection compared with that of the saline group ($P < 0.01$, **Figure 2B**). These results indicate that activation of histamine H2 receptors in the LVNs promotes animal's motor balance and coordination.

HCN Channels and K$^+$ Channels Are Involved in the Histamine-Induced Excitation on LVN Neurons

To clarify the ionic mechanisms underlying the excitation of LVN neurons elicited by H2 receptor activation, a slow-ramp command test was employed to assess the dynamic features of dimaprit-induced current. As shown in **Figures 3A1,A2**, two types of the I-V curves induced by dimaprit were observed, indicating that more than one ionic mechanism may be underlying the depolarization induced by the activation of H2 receptors on LVN neurons. Notably, the I-V curves of 18.2% (2/11) recorded LVN neurons intersected at −110 mV (**Figure 3A2**), which means the dimaprit-elicited inward current reverses near the calculated E_K of −108 mV, suggesting an involvement of K$^+$ channels. Moreover, Ba^{2+}, a blocker of K$^+$ channels (McCormick and Williamson, 1991), was applied to examine the dynamic properties of the dimaprit-induced current excluding the component of potassium. As shown in **Figure 3B**, only one change in the I-V curves was observed after blocking K$^+$ current. Subtracting the control from the current recorded during dimaprit application yielded a difference current representing the dimaprit-induced current excluding the K$^+$ component (the insert panel in **Figure 3B**). The difference current showed a significant feature of hyperpolarization activation, which is in line with the characteristics of the current of HCN channels. Since depolarizing voltage sag induced by hyperpolarizing current steps was one of the hallmarks of HCN channel activation (Pape, 1996), we further observed the effect of dimaprit on voltage sag on LVN neurons and found that the sag was remarkably increased by dimaprit (from 11.8 ± 1.6 mV to 14.6 ± 1.9 mV, $n = 6$, $P < 0.01$; **Figures 3C,D**). Furthermore, after blockage of HCN channels with ZD7288 (10 μM), a selective blocker for HCN channels, the HCN channel activation-induced sag vanished and the increase of voltage sag elicited by dimaprit was totally blocked (**Figures 3C,D**). The results, together with the dynamic properties of hyperpolarization activation observed in slow-ramp command test after excluding the component of K$^+$, strongly suggests that HCN channels participate in the mediation of excitation of LVN neurons induced by the activation of

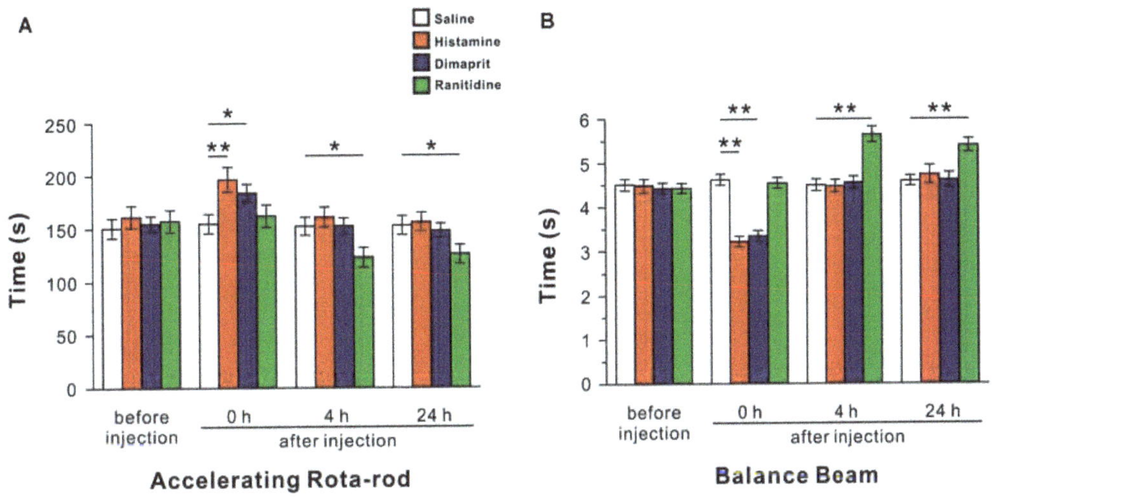

FIGURE 2 | Activation of histamine H2 receptors in the LVN promotes rat motor balance and coordination. The endurance time on an accelerating rota-rod **(A)** and the duration of passage through the balance beam **(B)** of rats treated by bilateral microinjection of saline, histamine, dimaprit, ranitidine. Data shown are means ± SEM; $^*P < 0.05$, $^{**}P < 0.01$.

H2 receptors. On the other hand, the dimaprit induced I-V curve changes were also detected in the presence of ZD7288 in the slow-ramp command test (**Figure 3E**). As shown in the insert panel of **Figure 3E**, the dimaprit-induced current excluding the component of HCN channel current reverted near the calculated E_K. Although the residual K^+ current was quite small, the data indicate a co-mediation of K^+ and HCN channels in the dimaprit-induced excitation on LVN neurons. In addition, we found that separate application of $BaCl_2$ or ZD7288 partially inhibited the dimaprit-elicited inward current (50.2 ± 5.8 pA, $n = 11$) to 31.3 ± 5.7 pA ($n = 6$, $P < 0.05$, **Figures 3F,H**) and 16.1 ± 4.7 pA ($n = 5$, $P < 0.01$, **Figures 3G,H**), respectively, whereas combined application of $BaCl_2$ and ZD7288 totally blocked the current induced by dimaprit ($n = 10$, $P < 0.001$, **Figures 3F–H**). Similarly, as shown in **Figures 3I K**, the histamine-induced inward current (67.4 ± 8.2 pA, $n = 11$) on LVN neurons was also partly blocked by separate application of $BaCl_2$ or ZD7288 to 46.0 ± 9.3 pA ($n = 6$, $P < 0.05$) or 18.8 ± 3.6 pA ($n = 5$, $P < 0.001$), respectively, and totally blocked by combined application of $BaCl_2$ and ZD7288 ($n = 9$, $P < 0.001$). All these results strongly suggest that a dual ionic mechanism, involving both the activation of HCN channels and the closure of K^+ channels, may mediate the excitatory effect of activation of H2 receptors on LVN neurons.

Activation of HCN Channels Coupled to H2 Receptors Increases Sensitivities of LVN Neurons and Changes their Dynamic Properties

Intriguingly, besides increasing the excitability, the activation of H2 receptors also enhanced the sensitivity of the LVN neurons to the stimulation of a depolarizing ramp-like current (**Figures 4A1,A2**), which consists of a 600 ms ramp (from −150 pA to 150 pA, slope of 0.5 nA/s) followed by a long plateau of current (150 pA, 4400 ms; Ris et al., 2001; Uno et al., 2003; Zhang et al., 2011). On five LVN neurons, dimaprit (100 μM) significantly increased the rate of increase in the instantaneous neuronal firing rate (from 100.0 ± 5.1% to 135.2 ± 6.9%, $n = 5$, $P < 0.001$; **Figure 4B**). However, in the presence of ZD7288 (1, 3 and 10 μM), as illustrated in **Figure 4B**, the enhancement in the rate of increase in the instantaneous firing rate induced by dimaprit (100 μM) was blocked in a concentration dependent manner. The normalized enhancement in the rate of increase in the instantaneous firing rate was decreased significantly from 35.2 ± 6.9% to 21.4 ± 4.2% ($n = 5$, $P < 0.05$), 10.0 ± 5.4% ($n = 5$, $P < 0.05$) and 2.6 ± 8.9% ($n = 5$, $P < 0.001$), respectively (**Figure 4B**). The results indicate that the increment in sensitivity of LVN neurons induced by the activation of histamine H2 receptors is mediated by HCN channels.

We also measured the difference between the instantaneous firing rate reached at the end of the ramp and the stable discharge rate at the end of the plateau, i.e., the overshoot (**Figure 4A2**). This parameter reflects the nonlinear, dynamic properties of neurons. We found that dimaprit (100 μM) effectively increased the overshoot of the LVN neurons from 100.0 ± 8.1% to 179.6 ± 12.5% ($n = 5$, $P < 0.001$; **Figure 4C**), and ZD7288 (1, 3 and 10 μM) concentration-dependently blocked the dimaprit-induced increment in overshoot from 79.6 ± 12.5% to 48.6 ± 13.2% ($n = 5$, $P < 0.05$), 20.5 ± 16.1% ($n = 5$, $P < 0.05$) and 8.9 ± 14.8% ($n = 5$, $P < 0.001$), respectively (**Figure 4C**). Therefore, the activation of HCN channels coupled to H2 receptors not only increases sensitivity of LVN neurons, but also changes their dynamic properties.

Besides activation of HCN channels, closure of K^+ channels is the other ionic mechanism underlying the activation of H2 receptors on LVN neurons. Thus, the dimaprit-induced

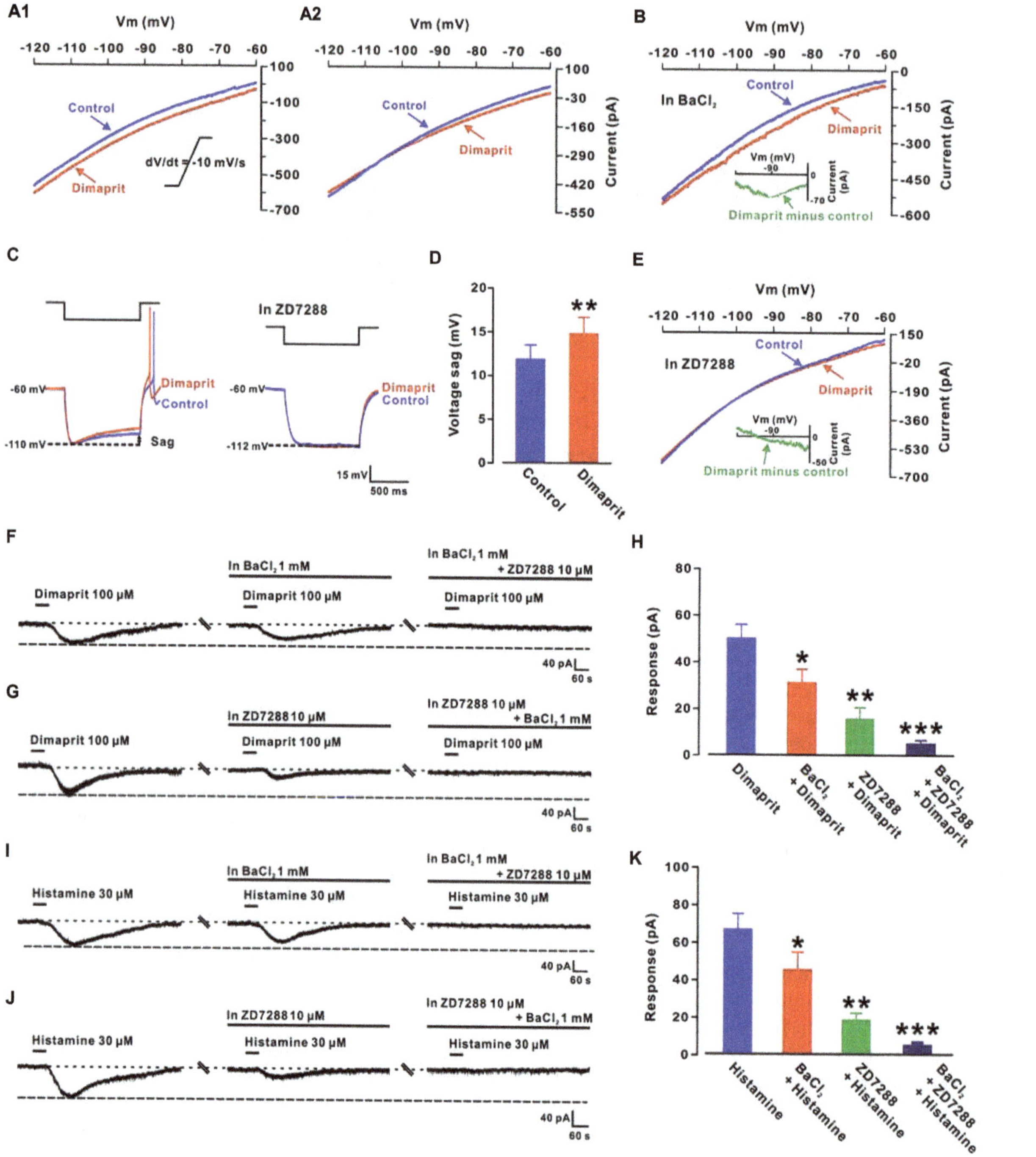

FIGURE 3 | Hyperpolarization-activated cyclic nucleotide-gated (HCN) channels and K^+ channels co-mediate the excitation induced by activation of H2 receptors on LVN neurons. (A1,A2) Two types of dimaprit-induced changes of I-V curves on LVN neurons (n = 9 and 2, respectively) responding to a slow-ramp command (dV/dt = −10 mV/s). The diversity of the dimaprit-induced changes in I-V relationships suggests that more than one ionic basis is involved in histamine H2 receptor-mediated inward current on LVN neurons. The intersection of I-V curves at calculated E_K of −108 mV **(A2)** on 18.2% (2/11) of neurons indicates an involvement of K^+ channels in the H2 receptor-mediated LVN neuronal excitation. **(B)** In the ACSF containing Ba^{2+}, a blocker of K^+ channels, the dimaprit-induced changes of I-V curves and the current excluding K^+ component in slow-ramp command tests. Note that in the presence of Ba^{2+}, the dimaprit-induced current (the inset) showed a significant feature of hyperpolarization activation, which is consistent with the characteristics of current of HCN channels. **(C)** Inward rectification (sag) triggered by hyperpolarizing current steps on an LVN neuron was increased by dimaprit (the left panel). ZD7288, a highly selective HCN channel antagonist, totally blocked the increase in the sag induced by dimaprit (the right panel). **(D)** Group data of the tested LVN neurons. **(E)** In the slow-ramp command test, in the presence of ZD7288 to exclude the component of HCN channel current, the dimaprit-induced residual current (the inset) was very small and reverted near the calculated E_K. **(F)** $BaCl_2$ partly blocked the dimaprit-elicited inward current, and combined application of $BaCl_2$ and ZD7288 totally blocked the current.

(Continued)

FIGURE 3 | Continued
(G) The dimaprit-induced inward current was also partly blocked by ZD7288, and totally blocked by combined application of ZD7288 and $BaCl_2$. **(H)** Group data of the tested LVN neurons. **(I,J)** Histamine-induced inward current was partly/totally blocked by separate/combined application of ZD7288 and $BaCl_2$. **(K)** Group data of the tested LVN neurons. Data shown are means ± SEM; $^{*}P < 0.05$, $^{**}P < 0.01$, $^{***}P < 0.001$.

changes in sensitivities of LVN neurons and their dynamic properties were also measured in the presence of $BaCl_2$. However, we found that $BaCl_2$ (1 mM) blocked neither the dimaprit-induced enhancement in the rate of increase in the instantaneous firing rate (from 30.4 ± 6.3% to 32.6 ± 5.5%, $n = 5$, $P = 0.64$, **Figure 4D**), nor the increment in overshoot (from 66.9 ± 20.2% to 60.1 ± 23.1%, $n = 5$, $P = 0.48$, **Figure 4E**). Therefore, it is HCN channels, but not K^+ channels coupled to H2 receptors, that contribute to the modulation on sensitivity and dynamic properties of LVN neurons by the activation of H2 receptors. We speculate that HCN channels may actively participate in the LVN-mediated motor behaviors.

Blockage of HCN Channels Coupled to H2 Receptors in the LVN Attenuates Motor Balance and Coordination

Given that the effects of HCN channels' activation on both sensitivity and dynamic properties of LVN neurons *in vitro*, ZD7288 (1 mM, 3 mM and 10 mM), or dimaprit together with ZD7288, was microinjected into bilateral LVNs to examine the role of HCN channels in the histamine H2 receptor-mediated promotion in motor behaviors on accelerating rota-rod and balance beam. For the accelerating rota-rod test, no significant difference among the groups before injections was observed ($F_{(3,36)} = 0.19$, $P = 0.904$; **Figure 5A**). A significant effect of time ($F_{(3,108)} = 90.146$, $P < 0.01$), treatment ($F_{(3,36)} = 8.291$, $P < 0.01$) and time × treatment interaction ($F_{(9,108)} = 34.988$, $P < 0.01$) among these groups was revealed by two-way ANOVA with repeated measures. Furthermore, *post hoc* test showed that microinjection of 3 or 10 mM ZD7288 ($n = 10$) into the LVNs remarkably decreased the endurance time of rats on the rotating rod at 0 h and 4 h after injection compared with the rats microinjected with saline ($n = 10$; $P < 0.01$, $P < 0.05$, **Figure 5A**), and such effect recovered hours later (**Figure 5A**). For the balance beam test, no significant difference was found among the groups before injections ($F_{(3,36)} = 0.497$, $P = 0.687$; **Figure 5B**). And a significant effect of time ($F_{(3,108)} = 92.131$, $P < 0.01$), treatment ($F_{(3,36)} = 45.458$, $P < 0.01$) and time × treatment interaction ($F_{(9,108)} = 42.286$, $P < 0.01$) among these groups was determined. Furthermore, *post hoc* test revealed that microinjection of 3 or 10 mM ZD7288 ($n = 10$) into the LVNs concentration-dependently lengthened the spent traversing time of rats on the beam at 0 h and 4 h after injection compared with the saline group ($n = 10$; **Figure 5B**), and such effect recovered hours later (**Figure 5B**). These results indicate that blockage of HCN channels coupled to histamine H2 receptors attenuates motor balance and coordination on the rota-rod and balance beam.

Moreover, the decrement of motor performance in both accelerating rota-rod (**Figure 5C**) and balance beam (**Figure 5D**) tests increased with the increase of the concentration of ZD7288. Also, it is noteworthy that the improvement of motor performances on rota-rod and balance beam induced by activation of H2 receptors by dimaprit was remarkably blocked by ZD7288 ($P < 0.01$, respectively; **Figures 5E,F**). All these results strongly suggest that HCN channels coupled to H2 receptors mediate improvement in motor balance and coordination of histaminergic inputs.

DISCUSSION

Although the central histaminergic system solely originates from the tuberomammillary nucleus of the hypothalamus, it participates in the regulation of various basic physiological functions (Haas et al., 2008). Brain histamine depletion or knockout of histamine receptor reduced animals' locomotor activity and exploratory behavior (Onodera et al., 1994; Inoue et al., 1996; Toyota et al., 2002), indicating the central histaminergic system may also hold a critical position in somatic motor functions. Yet, the functional role of histaminergic system in various motor structures and the underlying mechanism is still little known. Here, in the present study, we report that histamine H2 receptor and its coupled HCN channel mediate the histamine-induced enhancement of LVN neuronal excitability and sensitivity. Via activation of histamine H2 receptors and the downstream HCN channels, histaminergic inputs promote the LVN-mediated motor behaviors.

Electrophysiological and Behavioral Effects of Histamine in the LVN

Immunohistochemical studies have demonstrated that the histaminergic neurons in the tuberomammillary nucleus of the hypothalamus project directly to the vestibular nuclei in brainstem (Schwartz et al., 1991; Steinbusch, 1991; Tighilet and Lacour, 1996). As an essential part of the central histaminergic system, these histaminergic innervations on the vestibular nuclear complex, especially their physiological functions, have received increasing attention. Intriguingly, histamine exerts a uniformly excitatory effect on all four vestibular sub-nuclei (Wang and Dutia, 1995; Zhang et al., 2008, 2013; Peng et al., 2013; Zhuang et al., 2013; Yu et al., 2016). However, the receptor mechanisms underlying the histamine-induced excitation on these sub-nuclei are various (Wang and Dutia, 1995; Zhang et al., 2008, 2013; Peng et al., 2013; Zhuang et al., 2013; Yu et al., 2016). Histamine H1 and H2 receptors co-mediate the excitatory effect of histamine on neurons in the superior and inferior vestibular nuclei (Peng et al., 2013; Zhuang et al., 2013; Yu et al., 2016), whereas histamine H1, H2 and H3 receptors are all involved in the complex modulation of histamine on medial vestibular nucleus (MVN) neuron (Wang and Dutia,

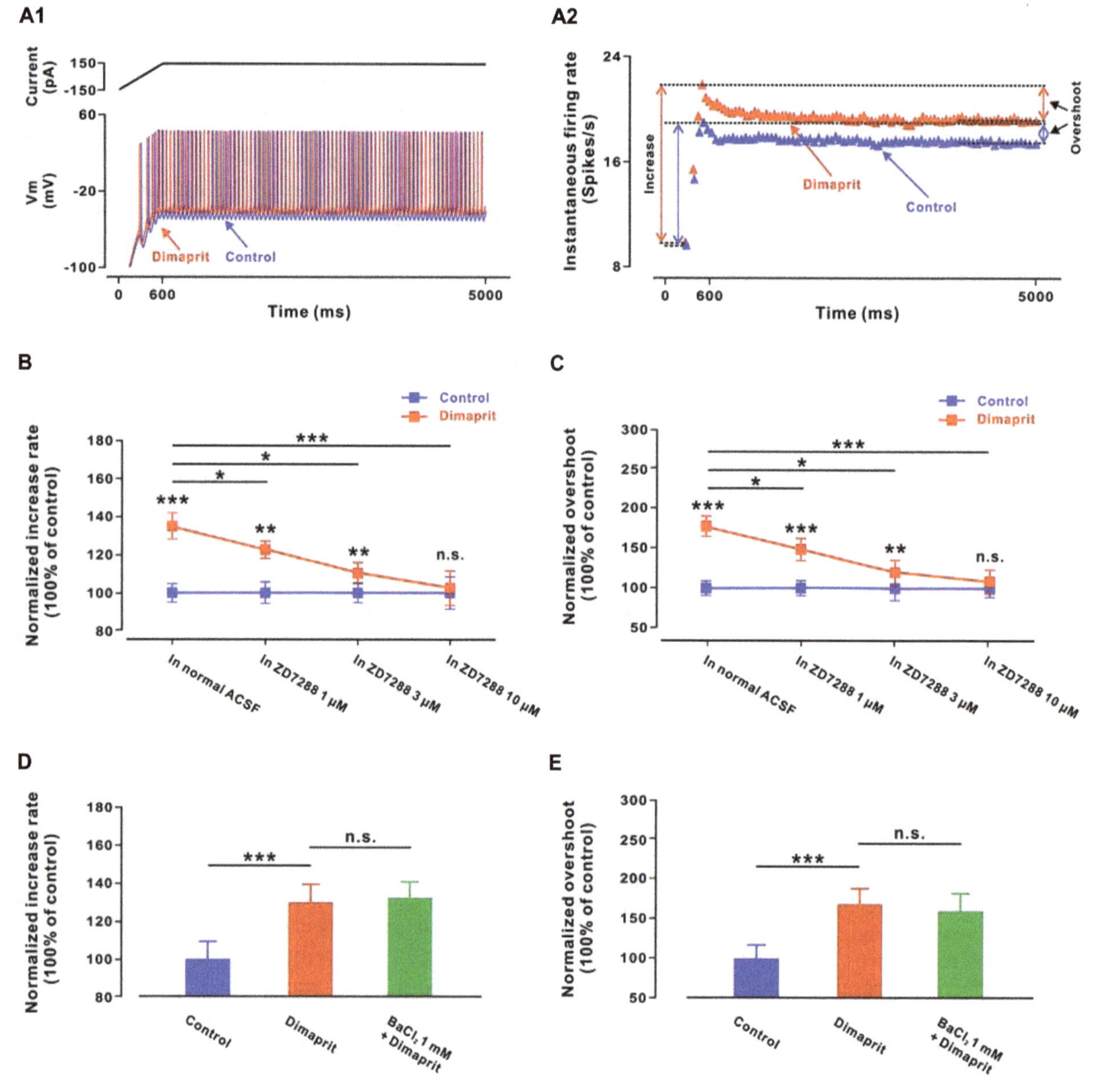

FIGURE 4 | Activation of HCN channels coupled to H2 receptors increases sensitivity of LVN neurons and change their dynamic properties. **(A1)** A ramp-like current was given from a hyperpolarized level of −150 pA for 600 ms to reach +150 pA, with the final steady-state value of +150 pA lasting 4400 ms. Firing response of a LVN neuron to the ramp-like current stimulation in the absence and presence of dimaprit. **(A2)** Instantaneous firing rates of the same LVN neuron to the ramp-like current in the absence and presence of dimaprit showed that H2 receptor activation remarkably raised both the rate of increase of the instantaneous firing rate (spikes/s/nA) and the overshooting response. **(B)** The normalized enhancement in the rate of increase in the instantaneous firing rate was concentration-dependently blocked by ZD7288 (1, 3 and 10 μM), indicating that the dimaprit-induced increment in sensitivity of LVN neurons was mediated by the activation of HCN channels coupled to H2 receptors. **(C)** ZD7288 (1, 3 and 10 μM) concentration-dependently blocked the dimaprit-induced overshoot increment, suggesting that the activation of HCN channels coupled to H2 receptors also contributed to the changes of dynamic properties of LVN neurons. **(D,E)** $BaCl_2$ (1 mM) did not block the dimaprit-induced enhancement in the rate of increase in the instantaneous firing rate and increment in overshoot on five LVN neurons. Data shown are means ± SEM; **P* < 0.05, ***P* < 0.01 and ****P* < 0.001 and n.s. indicates non-significant.

1995; Bergquist and Dutia, 2006; Zhang et al., 2013). In this study, we found that histamine elicited a significant excitatory response on LVN neurons both having spontaneous firing and being silent. These histamine-elicited excitations were totally blocked by ranitidine (selective histamine H2 receptor antagonist) and mimicked by dimaprit (highly selective agonist for histamine H2 receptors), suggesting that only histamine H2 receptors mediate the excitatory effect of histamine on LVN neurons.

Among the four vestibular sub-nuclei, the LVN receives inputs from the semicircular canals and the utricle, and projects into the lateral vestibulo-spinal tract to ipsilaterally innervate

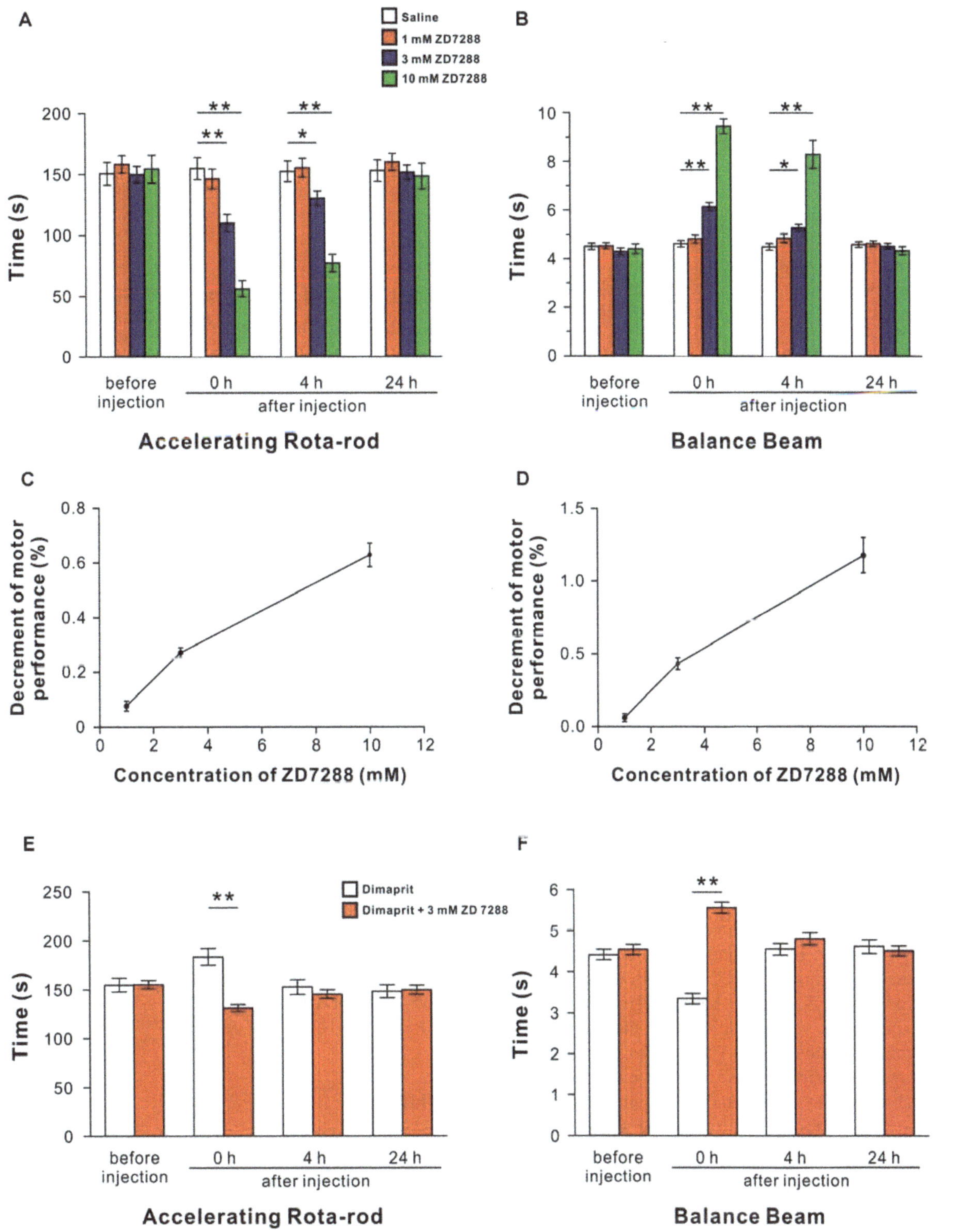

FIGURE 5 | Blockage of HCN channels coupled to H2 receptors in the LVN attenuates spontaneous and the dimaprit-induced promotion on motor balance and coordination. (A,B) The endurance time on an accelerating rota-rod and the duration of passage through the balance beam of rats treated by bilateral microinjection of saline, 1 mM ZD7288, 3 mM ZD7288 or 10 mM ZD7288. **(C,D)** The decrement of motor performance in accelerating rota-rod and balance beam tests increased with the increase of the concentration of ZD7288. **(E,F)** The endurance time on an accelerating rota-rod and the duration of passage through the balance beam of rats treated by bilateral microinjection of dimaprit or dimaprit together with 3 mM ZD7288. Data shown are means ± SEM; $^{*}P < 0.05$, $^{**}P < 0.01$.

the ventral horn of the spinal cord (Carleton and Carpenter, 1983; Sarkisian, 2000). Through facilitating the activity of spinal motoneurons innervating gravity-opposing muscles of the limb, the LVN is actively involved in the vestibule-spinal reflex and postural control. Thus, it is naturally speculated that the excitatory modulation of histamine on LVN neurons via H2 receptors may enhance the output of LVN, excite the neurons of their targets, and influence motor behaviors. In the present study, our results demonstrate that microinjection of histamine into the LVN significantly promotes motor performances on accelerating rota-rod and balance beam. Activation of histamine H2 receptors mimics the histamine-induced promotion in motor performances, whereas blockage of H2 receptors to block endogenous histaminergic inputs into the LVN attenuates motor behaviors. These results suggest that histamine H2 receptors contribute to the improvement of histaminergic inputs in the LVN-mediated motor behaviors. Interestingly, our previous studies found that histamine promoted motor balance and coordination via the activation of H2 receptors in the fastigial nucleus (He et al., 2012) and interpositus nucleus (Song et al., 2006) of the cerebellum. Therefore, histamine H2 receptors may hold a critical position in central histaminergic modulation on motor control.

Ionic Mechanisms Coupled to Histamine H2 Receptor in the LVN

Several types of ionic channels/exchangers have been reported to be linked to histamine receptors and modulate the excitability of central vestibular nuclear neurons (Ris et al., 2001; Zhang et al., 2013, 2016; Yu et al., 2016). Here, we find that both the HCN channels and K^+ channels are involved in the excitation of LVN neurons induced by the activation of histamine H2 receptors. In these dual ionic mechanisms, HCN channels seem to play a major contribution, whereas K^+ component may account for only a small one. Since HCN channels are critical "pacemaker channels" of neurons (Pape, 1996) and K^+ channels are responsible for setting membrane potential, histamine released from the hypothalamus will help to accelerate membrane depolarization and the generation of LVN neuronal activity via opening of HCN channels and closure of K^+ channels. Notably, in this study, we find that HCN channels, but not K^+ channels coupled to H2 receptors, are responsible for the histamine-induced enhancement of sensitivities of LVN neurons and modulation of their dynamic properties. This may be owing to the fact that HCN channels play an essential role in not only governing neuronal excitability but also controlling the way that neurons respond to input. Thus, by activation of HCN channels coupled to H2 receptors, histaminergic inputs may enhance the sensitivity and responsiveness of LVN neuronal circuitry to periphery vestibular inputs and consequently modulate LVN-mediated motor behaviors.

Dysfunction of HCN channels is usually associated with pathological conditions, such as epilepsy, age-related working memory decline and neuropathic pain (Lewis and Chetkovich, 2011; He et al., 2014). In the present study, by means of pharmacological manipulation to block HCN channels in the LVN, we find that rat motor performances on the rota-rod and balance beam remarkably decline (**Figures 5A–D**) and the improvement of motor performances induced by activation of histamine H2 receptors is significantly abolished (**Figures 5E,F**). These results, together with our previous findings that blockage of HCN channels in the cerebellar nuclei attenuates motor performances (Zhang et al., 2016), suggest that HCN channels coupled to histamine H2 receptors may mediate the modulation of the central histaminergic system on motor behaviors and play an important role in somatic motor control.

Functional Significance of Histaminergic Innervation on the LVN

Besides histaminergic innervation, the LVN also receives excitatory orexinergic inputs from the hypothalamus (Zhang et al., 2011). Unlike the critical role of orexinergic modulation in motor challenge (Zhang et al., 2011), excitatory histaminergic inputs on the LVN may be responsible for routine execution of normal function of the central vestibular nuclear circuitry. The functional difference in aspect of LVN's motor control between the histaminergic and orexinergic systems may depend on different functional roles of the origins of these two systems. In conclusion, the present study shows that the histamine-elicited excitation on the LVN neurons is mediated by postsynaptic histamine H2 receptor and its downstream HCN channels and K^+ channels. The activation of HCN channels coupled to H2 receptors increases sensitivity of LVN neurons, and improves the LVN-mediated motor behaviors. Based on these results, we suggest that via histamine H2 receptors and the downstream HCN channels, the excitatory histaminergic inputs may modulate both excitability and sensitivity of the LVN neurons and are actively involved in the central vestibular postural and motor control.

AUTHOR CONTRIBUTIONS

BL and X-YZ performed experiments, analyzed data, and prepared figures and drafts. A-HY, X-CP, Z-PC and J-YZ performed some experiments. Y-SC discussed the research. J-NZ and J-JW designed research and wrote the article.

FUNDING

This work was supported by the National Natural Science Foundation of China (grants 31330033, 91332124, 31471112, 31500848, 81671107, 31600834, J1210026 and NSFC/RGC Joint Research Scheme 31461163001); the Ministry of Education, China (SRFDP/RGC ERG grant 20130091140003, and Fundamental Research Fund for the Central Universities 20620140542 and 020814380048); the Natural Science Foundation of Jiangsu Province, China (grant BK20140599); and the China Postdoctoral Sciences Foundation (grant 2013T60520).

REFERENCES

Bergquist, F., and Dutia, M. B. (2006). Central histaminergic modulation of vestibular function–a review. *Sheng Li Xue Bao* 58, 293–304.

Carleton, S. C., and Carpenter, M. B. (1983). Afferent and efferent connections of the medial, inferior and lateral vestibular nuclei in the cat and monkey. *Brain Res.* 278, 29–51. doi: 10.1016/0006-8993(83)90223-8

Dere, E., De Souza-Silva, M. A., Spieler, R. E., Lin, J. S., Ohtsu, H., Haas, H. L., et al. (2004). Changes in motoric, exploratory and emotional behaviours and neuronal acetylcholine content and 5-HT turnover in histidine decarboxylase-KO mice. *Eur. J. Neurosci.* 20, 1051–1058. doi: 10.1111/j.1460-9568.2004.03546.x

Haas, H. L., Sergeeva, O. A., and Selbach, O. (2008). Histamine in the nervous system. *Physiol. Rev.* 88, 1183–1241. doi: 10.1152/physrev.00043.2007

He, C., Chen, F., Li, B., and Hu, Z. (2014). Neurophysiology of HCN channels: from cellular functions to multiple regulations. *Prog. Neurobiol.* 112, 1–23. doi: 10.1016/j.pneurobio.2013.10.001

He, Y. C., Wu, G. Y., Li, D., Tang, B., Li, B., Ding, Y., et al. (2012). Histamine promotes rat motor performances by activation of H_2 receptors in the cerebellar fastigial nucleus. *Behav. Brain Res.* 228, 44–52. doi: 10.1016/j.bbr.2011.11.029

Inoue, I., Yanai, K., Kitamura, D., Taniuchi, I., Kobayashi, T., Niimura, K., et al. (1996). Impaired locomotor activity and exploratory behavior in mice lacking histamine H1 receptors. *Proc. Natl. Acad. Sci. U S A* 93, 13316–13320. doi: 10.1073/pnas.93.23.13316

Kilkenny, C., Browne, W. J., Cuthill, I. C., Emerson, M., and Altman, D. G. (2010). Improving bioscience research reporting: the ARRIVE guidelines for reporting animal research. *PLoS Biol.* 8:e1000412. doi: 10.1371/journal.pbio.1000412

Lacour, M. (2013). Betahistine treatment in managing vertigo and improving vestibular compensation: clarification. *J. Vestib. Res.* 23, 139–151. doi: 10.3233/VES-130496

Lai, C. H., and Chan, Y. S. (2001). Spontaneous discharge and response characteristics of central otolith neurons of rats during postnatal development. *Neuroscience* 103, 275–288. doi: 10.1016/s0306-4522(00)00539-x

Lewis, A. S., and Chetkovich, D. M. (2011). HCN channels in behavior and neurological disease: too hyper or not active enough? *Mol. Cell. Neurosci.* 46, 357–367. doi: 10.1016/j.mcn.2010.11.007

Li, B., Zhu, J. N., and Wang, J. J. (2014). Histaminergic afferent system in the cerebellum: structure and function. *Cerebellum Ataxias* 1:5. doi: 10.1186/2053-8871-1-5

Li, B., Zhuang, Q. X., Gao, H. R., Wang, J. J., and Zhu, J. N. (2016). Medial cerebellar nucleus projects to feeding-related neurons in the ventromedial hypothalamic nucleus in rats. *Brain Struct. Funct.* doi: 10.1007/s00429-016-1257-2 [Epub ahead of print].

McCormick, D. A., and Williamson, A. (1991). Modulation of neuronal firing mode in cat and guinea-pig lgnd by histamine: possible cellular mechanisms of histaminergic control of Arousal. *J. Neurosci.* 11, 3188–3199.

Molina-Negro, P., Bertrand, R. A., Martin, E., and Gioani, Y. (1980). The role of the vestibular system in relation to muscle tone and postural reflexes in man. *Acta Otolaryngol.* 89, 524–533. doi: 10.3109/00016488009127170

Onodera, K., Yamatodani, A., Watanabe, T., and Wada, H. (1994). Neuropharmacology of the histaminergic neuron system in the brain and its relationship with behavioral-disorders. *Prog. Neurobiol.* 42, 685–702. doi: 10.1016/0301-0082(94)90017-5

Panula, P., and Nuutinen, S. (2013). The histaminergic network in the brain: basic organization and role in disease. *Nat. Rev. Neurosci.* 14, 472–487. doi: 10.1038/nrn3526

Pape, H. C. (1996). Queer current and pacemaker: the hyperpolarization-activated cation current in neurons. *Annu. Rev. Physiol.* 58, 299–327. doi: 10.1146/annurev.physiol.58.1.299

Passani, M. B., Giannoni, P., Bucherelli, C., Baldi, E., and Blandina, P. (2007). Histamine in the brain: beyond sleep and memory. *Biochem. Pharmacol.* 73, 1113–1122. doi: 10.1016/j.bcp.2006.12.002

Paxinos, G., and Watson, C. (2007). *The Rat Brain in Stereotaxic Coordinates.* San Diego, CA: Academic Press.

Peng, S. Y., Zhuang, Q. X., He, Y. C., Zhu, J. N., and Wang, J. J. (2013). Histamine excites neurons of the inferior vestibular nucleus in rats by activation of H1 and H2 receptors. *Neurosci. Lett.* 541, 87–92. doi: 10.1016/j.neulet.2013.02.040

Ris, L., Capron, B., Vibert, N., Vidal, P. P., and Godaux, E. (2001). Modification of the pacemaker activity of vestibular neurons in brainstem slices during vestibular compensation in the guinea pig. *Eur. J. Neurosci.* 13, 2234–2240. doi: 10.1046/j.0953-816x.2001.01603.x

Sarkisian, V. H. (2000). Input-output relations of Deiters, lateral vestibulospinal neurons with different structures of the brain. *Arch. Ital. Biol.* 138, 295–353.

Schwartz, J. C., Arrang, J. M., Garbarg, M., Pollard, H., and Ruat, M. (1991). Histaminergic transmission in the mammalian brain. *Physiol. Rev.* 71, 1–51.

Shan, L., Dauvilliers, Y., and Siegel, J. M. (2015). Interactions of the histamine and hypocretin systems in CNS disorders. *Nat. Rev. Neurol.* 11, 401–413. doi: 10.1038/nrneurol.2015.99

Song, Y. N., Li, H. Z., Zhu, J. N., Guo, C. L., and Wang, J. J. (2006). Histamine improves rat rota-rod and balance beam performances through H_2 receptors in the cerebellar interpositus nucleus. *Neuroscience* 140, 33–43. doi: 10.1016/j.neuroscience.2006.01.045

Steinbusch, H. W. M. (1991). Distribution of histaminergic neurons and fibers in rat brain. Comparison with noradrenergic and serotonergic innervation of the vestibular system. *Acta Otolaryngol. Suppl.* 479, 12–23. doi: 10.3109/00016489109121144

Sun, Y. Z., Waller, H. J., Godfrey, D. A., and Rubin, A. M. (2002). Spontaneous activity in rat vestibular nuclei in brain slices and effects of acetylcholine agonists and antagonists. *Brain Res.* 934, 58–68. doi: 10.1016/s0006-8993(02)02361-2

Tighilet, B., and Lacour, M. (1996). Distribution of histaminergic axonal fibres in the vestibular nuclei of the cat. *Neuroreport* 7, 873–878. doi: 10.1097/00001756-199603220-00008

Tiligada, E., Kyriakidis, K., Chazot, P. L., and Passani, M. B. (2011). Histamine pharmacology and new CNS drug targets. *CNS Neurosci. Ther.* 17, 620–628. doi: 10.1111/j.1755-5949.2010.00212.x

Toyota, H., Dugovic, C., Koehl, M., Laposky, A. D., Weber, C., Ngo, K., et al. (2002). Behavioral characterization of mice lacking histamine H_3 receptors. *Mol. Pharmacol.* 62, 389–397. doi: 10.1124/mol.62.2.389

Uno, A., Idoux, E., Beraneck, M., Vidal, P. P., Moore, L. E., Wilson, V. J., et al. (2003). Static and dynamic membrane properties of lateral vestibular nucleus neurons in guinea pig brain stem slices. *J. Neurophysiol.* 90, 1689–1703. doi: 10.1152/jn.00201.2003

Vizuete, M. L., Traiffort, E., Bouthenet, M. L., Ruat, M., Souil, E., Tardivel-Lacombe, J., et al. (1997). Detailed mapping of the histamine H_2 receptor and its gene transcripts in guinea-pig brain. *Neuroscience* 80, 321–343. doi: 10.1016/s0306-4522(97)00010-9

Wang, J. J., and Dutia, M. B. (1995). Effects of histamine and betahistine on rat medial vestibular nucleus neurones: possible mechanism of action of anti-histaminergic drugs in vertigo and motion sickness. *Exp. Brain Res.* 105, 18–24. doi: 10.1007/bf00242178

Wilson, V. J., and Peterson, B. W. (1978). Peripheral and central substrates of vestibulospinal reflexes. *Physiol. Rev.* 58, 80–105.

Yabe, T., de Waele, C., Serafin, M., Vibert, N., Arrang, J. M., Muhlethaler, M., et al. (1993). Medial vestibular nucleus in the guinea-pig: histaminergic receptors. II. An *in vivo* study. *Exp. Brain Res.* 93, 249–258. doi: 10.1007/bf00228391

Yu, L., Zhang, X. Y., Cao, S. L., Peng, S. Y., Ji, D. Y., Zhu, J. N., et al. (2016). Na^+-Ca^{2+} exchanger, leak K^+ channel and hyperpolarization-activated cyclic nucleotide-gated channel comediate the histamine-induced excitation on rat inferior vestibular nucleus neurons. *CNS Neurosci. Ther.* 22, 184–193. doi: 10.1111/cns.12451

Zhang, J., Han, X.-H., Li, H.-Z., Zhu, J.-N., and Wang, J.-J. (2008). Histamine excites rat lateral vestibular nuclear neurons through activation of post-synaptic H2 receptors. *Neurosci. Lett.* 448, 15–19. doi: 10.1016/j.neulet.2008.10.027

Zhang, J., Li, B., Yu, L., He, Y. C., Li, H. Z., Zhu, J. N., et al. (2011). A role for orexin in central vestibular motor control. *Neuron* 69, 793–804. doi: 10.1016/j.neuron.2011.01.026

Zhang, X. Y., Yu, L., Zhuang, Q. X., Peng, S. Y., Zhu, J. N., and Wang, J. J. (2013). Postsynaptic mechanisms underlying the excitatory action of histamine on medial vestibular nucleus neurons in rats. *Br. J. Pharmacol.* 170, 156–169. doi: 10.1111/bph.12256

Zhang, C.-Z., Zhuang, Q.-X., He, Y.-C., Li, G.-Y., Zhu, J.-N., and Wang, J.-J. (2014). 5-HT_{2A} receptor-mediated excitation on cerebellar fastigial nucleus neurons and promotion of motor behaviors in rats. *Pflugers Arch.-Eur. J. Physiol.* 466, 1259–1271. doi: 10.1007/s00424-013-1378-x

Zhang, J., Zhuang, Q. X., Li, B., Wu, G. Y., Yung, W. H., Zhu, J. N., et al. (2016). Selective modulation of histaminergic inputs on projection neurons of cerebellum rapidly promotes motor coordination via HCN channels. *Mol. Neurobiol.* 53, 1386–1401. doi: 10.1007/s12035-015-9096-3

Zhuang, Q.-X., Wu, Y.-H., Wu, G.-Y., Zhu, J.-N., and Wang, J.-J. (2013). Histamine excites rat superior vestibular nuclear neurons via postsynaptic H_1 and H_2 receptors *in vitro*. *Neurosignals* 21, 174–183. doi: 10.1159/000341980

15

LFP Oscillations in the Mesencephalic Locomotor Region during Voluntary Locomotion

Brian R. Noga[1], Francisco J. Sanchez[1], Luz M. Villamil[1], Christopher O'Toole[1], Stefan Kasicki[2], Maciej Olszewski[2], Anna M. Cabaj[2], Henryk Majczyński[2], Urszula Sławińska[2] and Larry M. Jordan[3]*

[1]The Miami Project to Cure Paralysis, Department of Neurological Surgery, University of Miami Miller School of Medicine, Miami, FL, United States, [2]Department of Neurophysiology, Nencki Institute of Experimental Biology, Warsaw, Poland, [3]Department of Physiology, Spinal Cord Research Centre, University of Manitoba, Winnipeg, MB, Canada

***Correspondence:**
Brian R. Noga
bnoga@miami.edu

Oscillatory rhythms in local field potentials (LFPs) are thought to coherently bind cooperating neuronal ensembles to produce behaviors, including locomotion. LFPs recorded from sites that trigger locomotion have been used as a basis for identification of appropriate targets for deep brain stimulation (DBS) to enhance locomotor recovery in patients with gait disorders. Theta band activity (6–12 Hz) is associated with locomotor activity in locomotion-inducing sites in the hypothalamus and in the hippocampus, but the LFPs that occur in the functionally defined mesencephalic locomotor region (MLR) during locomotion have not been determined. Here we record the oscillatory activity during treadmill locomotion in MLR sites effective for inducing locomotion with electrical stimulation in rats. The results show the presence of oscillatory theta rhythms in the LFPs recorded from the most effective MLR stimulus sites (at threshold <60 μA). Theta activity increased at the onset of locomotion, and its power was correlated with the speed of locomotion. In animals with higher thresholds (>60 μA), the correlation between locomotor speed and theta LFP oscillations was less robust. Changes in the gamma band (previously recorded *in vitro* in the pedunculopontine nucleus (PPN), thought to be a part of the MLR) were relatively small. Controlled locomotion was best achieved at 10–20 Hz frequencies of MLR stimulation. Our results indicate that theta and not delta or gamma band oscillation is a suitable biomarker for identifying the functional MLR sites.

Keywords: deep brain stimulation, mesencephalic locomotor region, local field potentials, locomotion, spinal cord injury

INTRODUCTION

Several areas of the brain have been shown to elicit locomotion when stimulated, including areas of the diencephalon and mesencephalon (Grillner et al., 1997; Jordan and Sławińska, 2014; Kiehn, 2016; Takakusaki et al., 2016). Deep brain stimulation (DBS) of the mesencephalic locomotor region (MLR), a coordination center for activation and control of spinal locomotor generator neurons, is increasingly under consideration as a potential treatment strategy for improving locomotion in Parkinson's disease (PD; freezing of gait, or FOG) and following spinal cord injury (SCI). The MLR was originally described in the cat by Shik et al. (1966), and was considered to be co-extensive with the cuneiform nucleus (CnF). This conclusion has been confirmed by many researchers in subsequent years, and this evidence has been extensively reviewed

(Mori et al., 1989, 1992; Whelan, 1996; Grillner et al., 1997; Jordan, 1998; Ryczko and Dubuc, 2013; Jordan and Sławińska, 2014). The pedunculopontine nucleus (PPN) is considered a component of the MLR, a suggestion advanced by Garcia-Rill et al. (1986, 1987, 2011). They pointed out that the PPN is defined by the presence of cholinergic neurons, and gait defects, especially in PD, have been proposed to be due to pathological changes in the cholinergic neurons in the PPN. As a result, attempts to localize the areas suitable for DBS for improving locomotion by stimulating the MLR area have focused on the PPN, but increasingly it has been recognized that the CnF and associated structures may be more appropriate targets (Mazzone et al., 2005; Stefani et al., 2007; Piallat et al., 2009; Shimamoto et al., 2010; Alam et al., 2011; Hamani et al., 2011; Thevathasan et al., 2012).

Local field potentials (LFPs) can serve as biomarkers for movement disorders and for improved electrode targeting for DBS (Thompson et al., 2014), and the increasing emphasis on MLR DBS for restoring gait in human subjects necessitates the demonstration of LFPs recorded from effective MLR sites. Surprisingly, no study has been carried out on LFPs recorded in the functionally defined MLR under controlled conditions in an animal model. Locomotor activity was initially associated with theta oscillations (6–12 Hz) in hippocampal LFP (Kramis et al., 1975), and this rhythm was subsequently shown to be prominent in hypothalamic locomotor regions that were functionally identified as locomotion-inducing sites (Sławińska and Kasicki, 1995, 1998). Similar LFP activity might be expected of other locomotor areas of the brain, because theta oscillatory rhythms in LFPs are thought to coherently bind cooperating neuronal ensembles to produce behaviors, including locomotion (Bland and Oddie, 2001). However, LFPs have never been recorded during spontaneous locomotion from MLR sites functionally defined by stimulation to evoke locomotion in the same animal, although these sites are clearly a component of the ensemble of brain areas controlling locomotion.

Gamma band activity has been proposed to be a characteristic feature of the PPN (Garcia-Rill et al., 2015), and the intrinsic properties of PPN neurons recorded *in vitro* (Simon et al., 2010; Garcia-Rill et al., 2011, 2015) have led to the suggestion that their discharge in the gamma range of frequencies "...explains the requirement to stimulate this region at 40–60 Hz to optimally induce locomotion" (Garcia-Rill et al., 2015). However, clinical studies using DBS have indicated that lower frequencies of stimulation are more effective (Ferraye et al., 2010; Nosko et al., 2015). Optogenetic activation of the MLR at frequencies lower than 40 Hz has recently been shown to reliably induce locomotion in mice (Lee et al., 2014). Moreover, Ferraye et al. (2010) concluded that "The best effects were seen in the patients with active contacts located slightly posterior to the pedunculopontine nucleus, in the cuneiform and subcuneiform nuclei..." Microelectrode recordings have suggested that neurons that modulate firing in response to imagined gait actually tend to be located in the subcuneiform region dorsal to the PPN (Piallat et al., 2009). Thevathasan et al. (2012) showed in patients with Parkinsonism that alpha power (frequency range equivalent to our theta in rats) was maximal in the caudal PPN region, and they demonstrated a correlation between alpha oscillations and improved gait performance. This caudal "pedunculopontine region" corresponds to the cuneiform and subcuneiform nuclei in humans (Ferraye et al., 2010; Alam et al., 2011). Thus there is increasing evidence that the emphasis on the PPN as the most effective site for DBS to improve locomotion may not be warranted (Alam et al., 2011), and there is increasing evidence for the CnF involvement in human studies instead. We undertook a study focusing on the CnF area of the MLR in the rat model to determine the LFP signature of this area in recordings from confirmed DBS sites for eliciting locomotion.

Takakusaki et al. (2005, 2016) and Takakusaki (2008, 2013) have demonstrated that the CnF is effective for eliciting locomotion in decerebrate cats, while the PPN controls muscle tone and stimulation in this region may actually suppress locomotion. Other workers have challenged the importance of the PPN as a component of the MLR since PPN lesions do not alter locomotor capability (Winn, 2006; Hernández-Chan et al., 2011; MacLaren et al., 2014; Gut and Winn, 2015, 2016). Moreover, neurons activated during locomotion (indicated by the presence of the activity-dependent marker Fos) are found in the CnF and other nearby areas, including the deep mesencephalic nucleus (DpMe; Jordan, 1998; Vianna et al., 2003; Heise and Mitrofanis, 2006), but not in the PPN. PPN cholinergic neurons of the MLR have been implicated in the initiation of locomotion (reviewed in Ryczko and Dubuc, 2013). However, activation of the cholinergic component of the PPN using a chemogenetic approach induced only subtle effects on locomotion in freely moving, control rats (Pienaar et al., 2015). Takakusaki et al. (2016) have shown that the effective MLR sites are not co-extensive with the cholinergic PPN neurons in cats. A recent optogenetic study in the mouse has also cast doubt on the importance of cholinergic neurons within the PPN for the initiation of locomotion from a standstill (Roseberry et al., 2016). Rather, they have demonstrated that cholinergic neurons may play a role in the modulation of ongoing locomotion. Furthermore, they found that within the MLR the glutamatergic subpopulation encodes locomotor state and speed and is necessary and sufficient for locomotion. Taken together, these studies increase the importance of determining the LFP signature of effective MLR sites, especially those in the CnF region.

In this study, we specifically targeted the CnF region to provide the first analysis of LFPs recorded from this portion of the functionally defined MLR in intact, freely moving rats and to determine the LFP signature and the most effective stimulus parameters of these effective MLR sites. We then used recordings from these sites to test the hypothesis that the theta rhythm that is a characteristic of locomotion in other structures such as the hippocampus and the hypothalamic locomotor areas (Sławińska and Kasicki, 1995, 1998) is also prominent in the MLR during voluntary locomotion in these animals, consistent with the suggestion that the theta rhythm might bind cooperating neuronal ensembles to produce locomotion. Here we focus primarily on the theta LFP oscillations, but we also subject other frequency bands to similar analysis. We also show that the same LFP features that are prominent in intact animals persist after incomplete SCI, and suggest that they might be used as a biomarker of effective sites for electrode placements for DBS.

MATERIALS AND METHODS

Experiments were performed on 28 adult female Sprague-Dawley rats (240–350 g) following their acclimation to housing, handling and treadmill locomotor assessment. Rats were housed separately. Animals were exposed to a 12-h light/dark cycle and had free access to food and water. The number of animals used, and their pain and distress were minimized. Experimental procedures were approved by the University of Miami IACUC committee in accordance with NIH guidelines (National Institutes of Health Publications, No. 80-23; revised 1996). Experiments in Poland were carried out with the approval of the First Ethics Committee for Animal Experimentation according to the principles of experimental conditions and laboratory animal care of the European Union and the Polish Law on Protection of Animals Used for Experiments.

MLR-DBS and EMG Electrode Implantation

Parylene-insulated, tungsten microelectrodes, (A-M Systems Inc., Carlsborg, WA, USA; 127 μm diameter, 12 degree tip taper, adjusted to 0.07–0.4 MΩ) were stereotaxically implanted into the region of the MLR under isoflurane anesthesia (Milner and Mogenson, 1988). After exposing the cranium with a short skin incision, a small ~1 mm diameter hole was drilled through the left side of the skull above the stereotaxic target (~0.7–1.2 mm anterior to the interaural line, 2.0 mm lateral to the midline). Small, stainless steel, self-tapping screws served to anchor the electrode base to the skull. A titanium screw was inserted into the parietal bone immediately opposite the electrode insertion point to serve as an attachment for the return lead (anode). The microelectrode assembly was lowered using a micromanipulator aiming for a site ~6.2 mm DV (Paxinos and Watson, 1998). The base of the microelectrode assembly was then rigidly fixed to the skull and to the screws using dental cement (Stoelting, Wood Dale, IL, USA). The wound was closed by sutures around the implant. Pin connectors projecting vertically from the electrode assembly allowed electrical connection to the voltage and/or current stimulators and to preamplifiers for recording of LFPs (see below).

For the electromyography (EMG) recordings, bipolar electrodes were implanted bilaterally in the soleus (Sol) muscle (extensor, active during the stance phase of the step cycle) and the tibialis anterior (TA) muscle (flexor, active during the swing phase of the step cycle). The electrodes were made of Teflon-coated stainless steel wire (0.24 mm in diameter; AS633, CoonerWire Co., Chatsworth, CA, USA). The tips of the electrodes with 1–1.5 mm of the insulation removed were pulled through a cutaneous incision on the back of the animal, and each of the hook electrode was inserted into the appropriate muscle and secured by a suture (Sławińska et al., 2000). The distance between the electrode tips was 1–2 mm. The connector with the other ends of the wires fixed to it, covered with dental cement (Spofa Dental, Prague, Czech Republic) and silicone (3140 RTV, Dow Corning, Midland, MI, USA), was secured to the back of the animal.

Locomotor Threshold Determination

The current or voltage threshold for locomotor induction (minimum strength to elicit locomotor activity) was determined for all animals by stimulating awake rats in an open field. The MLR was stimulated (cathodal stimulation) during behavioral testing after recovery from surgery (~1 week) and several weeks after that in some animals to determine stability and effect of long-term implantation. Thresholds were also tested in animals subject to SCIs. Thresholds for locomotor induction were carefully tested over the stimulation range: frequency 10–70 Hz (10, 20, 50 and 70 Hz), and pulse duration 0.2, 0.5, 1.0 and 2.0 ms (Milner and Mogenson, 1988; Coles et al., 1989). During any session, a stimulation frequency was chosen and threshold strengths determined for each pulse width. Thresholds were determined in current mode (1–350 μA), but voltage assessments (typically less than 7 V) were made in some animals. Thresholds were determined by gradually increasing the strength of stimulation until locomotor movements ensued. Locomotor responses to sudden stimulation at strengths above threshold were also examined in most animals. Locomotor responses were visually classified by three experienced independent observers (FJS, CO and BRN). *Slow speed* (walk) or *Fast speed* (trot or gallop; Gillis and Biewener, 2001) was determined based on two (or more) identical observer ratings. Then, in random order, another stimulation frequency was chosen and the process was repeated. Between each pulse width test, animals were allowed to rest for approximately 30–60 s.

LFP Recording

For the chronic LFP recordings in freely moving rats the same electrodes as for MLR-DBS stimulation were used. MLR field potential recordings were made at 2000× gain, 1–300 Hz band pass filtering, with typically a 60 Hz notch filter and sampled at 1–2 kHz for later analysis. Connection to the pre-amplifier was made via wires 60–90 cm in length attached to the pin connectors on the electrode assembly with the indifferent wire connected to the titanium screw placed in the parietal bone. Animals were placed on an adjustable speed treadmill belt enclosed by a transparent plexiglass box, with automated ventilation (Treadmill Simplex II, Columbus Instruments, Columbus, OH, USA). Animals were previously trained to voluntarily walk on the treadmill and did not receive any electrical shocks for motivation. Video of each session was recorded using a 60 Hz frame rate (3-D PeakMotus Motion Measurement System). Field potentials were recorded for 30 s periods at rest and at each treadmill speed (10, 15, 20 m/min). The order varied depending on how cooperative the animals were during the different recording sessions. In most cases, animals started from rest and the belt speed was increased incrementally to each designated speed and then the belt was turned off. In other cases, recordings commenced once stable locomotion at higher speeds was attained and then the belt speed was decreased to other speeds and then stopped. Field potentials were also recorded following SCI in some animals (up to 17 weeks). For voluntary locomotion on a treadmill in these animals, speeds were dependent upon the severity of the injury.

Spinal Cord Injuries

Mid-thoracic contusion injuries were made using the New York University Impactor device (Gruner, 1992) under isoflurane anesthesia (2% in O_2) and sterile technique. A dorsal laminectomy was performed on the T8 vertebra to expose the dura over the T9 spinal segment. The adjacent vertebrae were clamped to stabilize and support the column during impact. Mild, moderate and severe contusion injuries were made by dropping a 10-g rod onto the exposed spinal cord from a height of 6.25, 12.5 or 25 mm, respectively. The impact height and velocity errors were below 6%, within acceptable parameters to ensure consistency. Average compression distances of 1.283 ± 0.182, 1.653 ± 0.201 and 2.01 ± 0.187 mm for mild, moderate and severe injuries, respectively, were also in close agreement with previously published data (Basso et al., 1996). The muscles were sutured in layers and the skin was closed with stainless-steel surgical clips. Rats were allowed to recover in a temperature controlled environment and were provided with accessible water and food. Gentamicin (2–3 mg/kg; APP Pharmaceuticals, Lake Zurich, IL, USA) and buprenorphine (0.1 mg/kg; Buprenex Inj.; Reckitt Benckiser Pharmaceuticals Inc., Richmond, VA, USA) were administered after surgery for 7 and 3 days, respectively. Lactated Ringers solution was administered BID SC for 7 days (5 ml/injection). The bladder was expressed twice daily until each animal regained continence. Animals were monitored daily for skin and weight changes. Animals were removed from the study if any post-operative complications could not be successfully treated (e.g., excessive weight loss, infections and pain behaviors including self-mutilation such as autonomy or excessive grooming leading to ulceration).

Immunohistochemistry

Under anesthesia, an electrolytic lesion was made at each stimulation site by passing a small (1 mA), brief (2–5 s) DC current through the DBS electrode. Animals were perfused intracardially with paraformaldehyde and their brains removed for histological reconstruction. The tissue surrounding the stimulation site was processed for paraffin and cut into 15 μm coronal sections. Sections were de-paraffinized and the immunohistochemical procedures optimized using a primary antibody dilution series. For the pre-adsorption control, tissue sections were incubated only with normal donkey serum (NDS: 10%; in 0.1 M phosphate buffered saline or PBS) then in 0.3% Triton X-100 in 0.1 M PBS after blocking endogenous peroxidase with 3% H_2O_2 at room temperature. Immunoreactivity was totally absent after omission of the primary antibodies. To examine glial scar formation around the stimulation electrode and to aid in the identification of the electrode tip within the tissue, sections were stained with an antibody to glial fibrillary acidic protein (GFAP). Sections were incubated in 1:500 rabbit polyclonal anti-GFAP (Millipore AB5804) overnight (0.1 M PBS with 0.3% Triton X-100 + 5% NDS), washed in 0.1 M PBS 0.3% Triton X-100 and then incubated in secondary donkey anti-rabbit Alexa 594 (1:200; A21207, Molecular Probes) in 0.1 M PBS with 0.3% Triton X-100 + 5% NDS. Selected sections (each in a series of 10) were then counterstained and coverslipped with either Vectashield Hard-set dry mounting media (H-1500) with 4′,6′-diamidino-2-phenylindole dilactate (DAPI) a fluorescent DNA counterstain or with Cresyl Violet to confirm anatomical localization of the electrode position and anatomical regions of the brain according to Paxinos and Watson (1998). Digital epi-fluorescent images were captured on a Zeiss 200M Axiovert microscope at 5× magnification.

Data Analysis and Statistics

For statistical analysis of LFP activity, 15 of the tested animals were selected on the basis of a consistent and complete sequence of behavior and the absence of noise/movement artifact. The data files (digitized at 2 kHz, band-pass filtered between 1 Hz and 300 Hz) were converted to Spike2 (CED, UK) format. The spectrograms and power spectra were analyzed using built-in functions of Spike2. Movement artifacts in the LFP channels were manually removed before analysis, under visual inspection. For spectrograms a window of 2048 points was used; the calibration of the y axis was adjusted to the dynamics of the data and is shown on the plots. Power spectra were calculated using an FFT algorithm (Hanning window, bins/channel 2048, width of bin 0.488 Hz). The total power for the delta (0–4 Hz), low (4–6 Hz) and high (6–12 Hz) theta, beta (12–28 Hz), low (28–55 Hz) and high (65–100 Hz) gamma frequency bands and the power and frequency for the peak in the power spectra of delta and theta bands related to various locomotor speeds or resting conditions for each trial were imported to Prism 6 (GraphPad Software, Inc., La Jolla, CA, USA). The D'Agostino test was performed before statistical tests to verify that the data followed a Gaussian distribution (normality test). We chose to separate the theta band into low and high components because the theta band recorded in the hippocampus (Kramis et al., 1975) was separated into Type 1 (corresponding to our high theta and linked to locomotion) and Type II (corresponding to our low theta and associated with sleeping and immobility). Comparison of thresholds effective for inducing locomotion was performed with unpaired t-test. Other analyses were performed with two-way Repeated Measures ANOVA (RM ANOVA). The Holm-Sidak's test was used for multiple comparisons. The minimum significance was set at $p = 0.05$. Linear regression analysis was performed using Prism 6 (GraphPad Software, Inc.). The speed was taken as an independent x-variable, while the parameters describing power and frequencies were taken as y-variable (see "Results" Section). The regression coefficient and the significance of slope were calculated for each analysis.

RESULTS

Evoked Locomotion in Freely-Moving Animals

The efficacy of MLR stimulation was examined in freely moving animals within 1 week of implantation. **Figure 1A** shows an example of EMG recordings during electrically induced locomotor behavior of a rat in an open field. A stimulus applied in the MLR at a strength just above threshold (28 μA) induced increased attention indicated by an orienting reaction, looking around and then forward quadrupedal locomotion commencing around 3.5 s after the onset of the stimulation, leading to regular locomotion. This pattern of activity is similar to that observed in freely moving cats with the stimulating electrode implanted in the cuneiform nucleus (Mori et al., 1989).

Figure 1B presents EMGs and LFPs from the same effective site within the MLR during voluntary locomotion of the same rat along a runway. The animal's movement was detected with photocells positioned at intervals along the runway. MLR LFPs recorded prior to, during and after voluntary locomotor activity on a runway showed dramatic changes during the transition from rest to walking. During recording from the effective MLR site we observed irregular LFP activity during resting. Transition to the locomotor activity detected with EMG was associated with clearly enhanced theta rhythm (6–12 Hz; **Figures 1B**, **4B**). This change in LFPs was observed in all animals where the recording site was within an effective MLR stimulus site (**Figures 3A–C**). In **Figure 1B** we also present examples of activity in other filtered bands (delta, low and high theta, beta, low and high gamma). Changes related to locomotor activity were also observed in delta and low theta bands, but they did not persist throughout the locomotor trial, and the delta band activity could also be observed at rest. See below for more detailed analysis.

Stimulation Parameters for Evoked Locomotion in an Open Field

Stimulation of the MLR evoked locomotor responses ranging from slow walking to fast locomotor behavior and jumping depending upon the stimulus parameters. Stimulation strength was slowly increased during testing for locomotor threshold values. At each of the tested stimulation parameters (frequency or pulse width), when strength of stimulation approached threshold value, animals would typically orient themselves and lean forward slightly before initiating locomotion. This response could last many seconds, becoming shorter with an increase in the rate at which the stimulation strength was increased. The delay to the onset of the locomotor response was much shorter (and could be within a second) when stimulation strengths at the onset of stimulation were above threshold and the locomotor response could be abrupt (galloping with or without jumping), often resembling escape behavior.

Locomotor threshold tests over a range of frequencies (10–70 Hz) and pulse widths (0.2–2 ms) were conducted in 21 uninjured animals at ~1 week of implantation (**Figure 2**). Walking could be most readily produced at 10 or 20 Hz. Stimulation at and above threshold strength at these frequencies produced well-graded locomotor responses evolving from slow walking to galloping. Transition from slow to fast locomotion typically occurred over a range of stimulus strengths (10–20 μA), thus demonstrating good controllability. At 50 or 70 Hz stimulation frequencies the first locomotor response produced at threshold strength was predominantly fast locomotion. Increasing the strength of stimulation above threshold could induce galloping and jumping responses and typically with only slight changes in strength of stimulation (2–5 μA). Tests in SCI animals (n = 3) showed a similar frequency dependence of the locomotor response as uninjured animals at threshold stimulation strengths (**Figure 2B**). Thus, a "controlled" rate of locomotion was difficult to establish at the highest tested frequencies, in contrast to 20 Hz, which produced the best controllable, graded locomotor response.

High vs. Low Locomotor Threshold Sites

Since the most consistent controllable locomotion was obtained at a frequency of 20 Hz with pulse width of 0.5–1 ms (**Figure 2B**), we determined the threshold strengths at approximately 1 week after implantation using 1 ms pulses at 20 Hz and grouped the animals into those with either high or low threshold responses. We defined low threshold (LowTh) sites as those producing locomotion with currents of ≤60 μA and those above 60 μA were defined as high threshold (HighTh).

Locations of all electrode stimulation sites (n = 28) were plotted on three coronal planes centered on Bregma −8.00, −7.04 and −6.30 mm (interaural 1.00–2.70 mm; taken from the atlas of Paxinos and Watson, 1998). High and low current locomotor threshold groups differed in location within the midbrain (**Figures 3A–C**). Low threshold sites were found in the CnF and the DpMe more anteriorly. High threshold sites were observed surrounding these areas dorsally, medially and ventrally.

GFAP staining was observed along each electrode tract and especially at the tip. This is illustrated in **Figure 3D** taken from an animal with a 5 month implant. GFAP staining typically did not extend into surrounding tissue for more than 50 or 60 μm even after prolonged implantation. To determine whether prolonged implantation of the electrode and increased glial scar formation (He and Bellamkonda, 2008) would affect locomotor thresholds (at 20 Hz, 1 ms pulse duration), we re-tested thresholds in 19 animals at various times (9–116 days) following the initial threshold assessment. Using current controlled stimulation, eight animals showed increased current thresholds, while nine showed decreased thresholds and two were unchanged. Overall, current thresholds were not significantly different (p = 0.342; paired samples t-test) with time from implantation, indicating that the small deposition of GFAP around the electrode tip did not interfere with electrode stimulation efficacy.

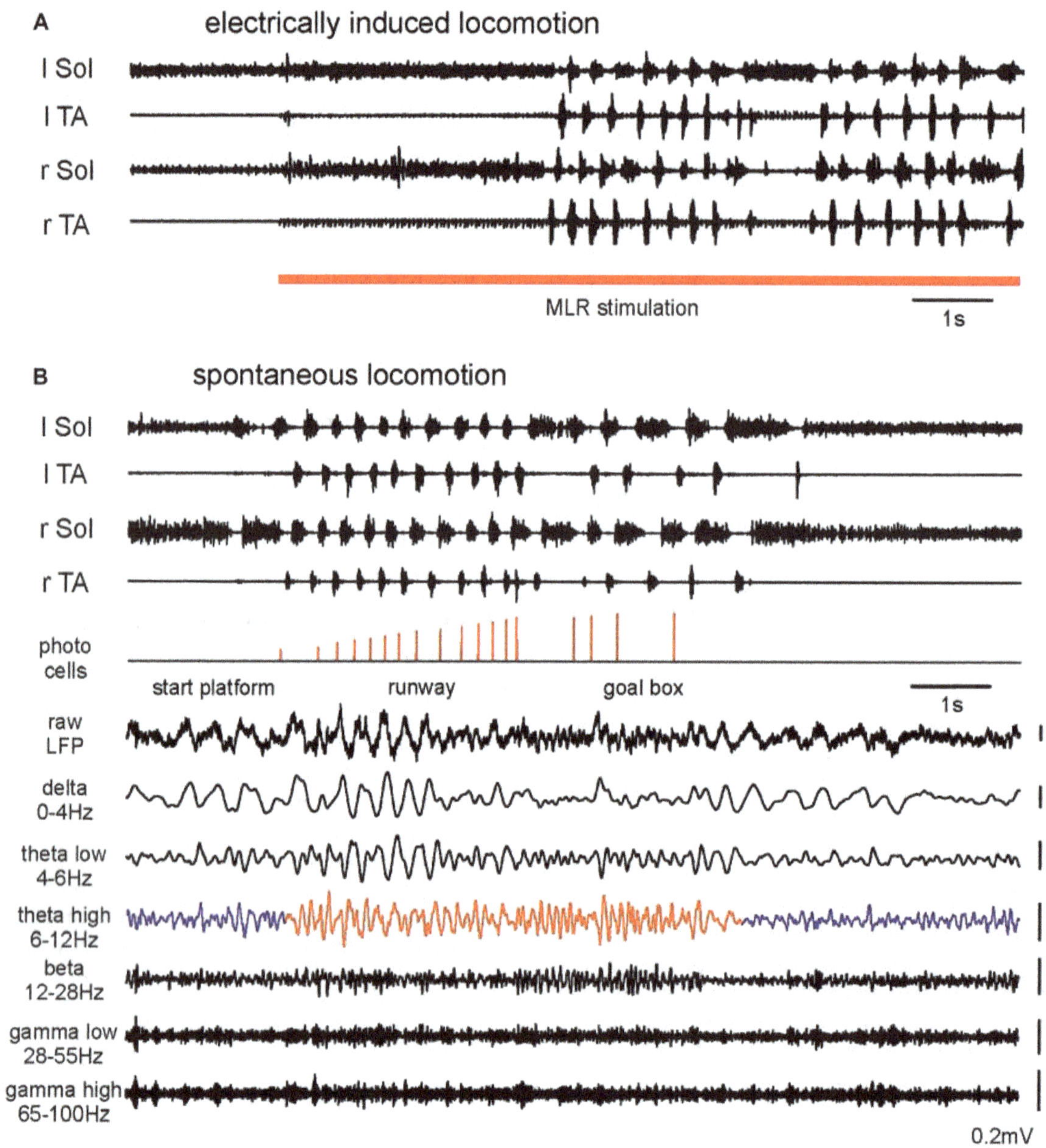

FIGURE 1 | Hindlimb muscle electromyography (EMG) and mesencephalic locomotor region (MLR) LFP activity during transition from resting to walking: (A) A rat with motor activity induced by right MLR electrical stimulation (28 μA, 20 Hz, 0.5 ms pulse duration). **(B)** The same rat walking spontaneously along a 2 m runway. Photocells events with increasing pulse amplitudes show progression along the runway. The bottom traces show simultaneously occurring raw LFP recorded from the right MLR and successive activity in filtered frequency bands. Abbreviations: Sol, Soleus muscle; TA, Tibialis Anterior muscle; r, right; l, left; LFP, local field potential.

LFP Recorded from MLR-DBS Sites during Treadmill Locomotion

The chronic LFP recordings in freely moving rats were obtained using electrodes that were implanted for DBS. Analysis of LFPs was done for periods before and during forced locomotion at various speeds (10, 15 and 20 m/min) of the treadmill belt. Examples of the LFPs (filtered within the theta range, 6–12 Hz) recorded from a HighTh and a LowTh site in rats during transition from resting to walking are shown in **Figures 4A1,B1** (bottom). In contrast to rats of the HighTh group, in all rats of the LowTh group, a regular theta rhythm was present from the start to the end of locomotion. Before locomotion started, short lasting episodes of regular activity in the LFP with a peak frequency of about 6–7 Hz were recorded (spectrogram in **Figure 4B2**—left). Interrupting these were short episodes of rhythmic LFP activity with a peak frequency below 7 Hz that were usually related to exploratory behavior of the rat in the treadmill cage. When the rat started to walk a clear peak of rhythmic theta activity (7–9 Hz) appeared in the spectrogram. A comparison of the power spectra calculated for the LFP recorded during resting and locomotion shows that the different experimental conditions differ in both frequency and amplitude of the peak in the power spectra of the theta band (see example in **Figures 4A2,B2**). There was also a change in the peak in the power spectra of the delta band (0–4 Hz; see analysis below and **Figure 7**). The data presented on the logarithmic scale show no peak in LFP power in the higher frequency bands (**Figures 4A3,B3**).

We performed an analysis comparing the frequency of the peak of theta rhythm and its power between the LowTh and HighTh groups. We selected eight LowTh and seven HighTh cases for statistical analysis based on the fact that they were all subjected to the protocol for LFP recordings at rest and at all defined treadmill speeds (10, 15 and 20 m/min). Average threshold currents for these LowTh and HighTh sites were 32.8 $\pm$ 3.2 and 151.5 $\pm$ 38.3 μA and were significantly different (*t*-test, $p \leq 0.001$). Statistical analysis (two-way RM ANOVA) showed a significant increase in frequency of the peak of theta rhythm over the resting condition at all speeds of locomotion in both groups of animals ($F_{(3,39)} = 16.34, p < 0.0001$; **Figure 5A**). Interestingly, within each experimental condition (rest or locomotion) the differences of the frequency of the theta oscillations between the LowTh and HighTh groups were not significant.

Analysis of the peak power of the theta rhythm (**Figure 5B**) showed significant differences between resting and locomotion at 15 m/min and 20 m/min, and between 10 m/min and 20 m/min in the LowTh group only ($F_{(3,39)} = 5.075$, $p < 0.005$). In the HighTh group we found no significant differences between any of the experimental conditions. Thus, it is clear that the theta rhythm was present both during rest and locomotion and the frequency of the theta rhythm was not different, but the peak power of the theta rhythm differentiated the LowTh and HighTh groups. It is noteworthy that the peak power of the theta oscillations was significantly different (Sidak's test, $p = 0.0066$) when comparing LowTh and HighTh rats during locomotion at the highest speed (20 m/min; **Figure 5B**). In summary, our results show that both the frequency and peak power of the theta rhythm change depending on the locomotor speed of animals in the LowTh group, while in the HighTh group only the frequency of the peak of the theta rhythm changes.

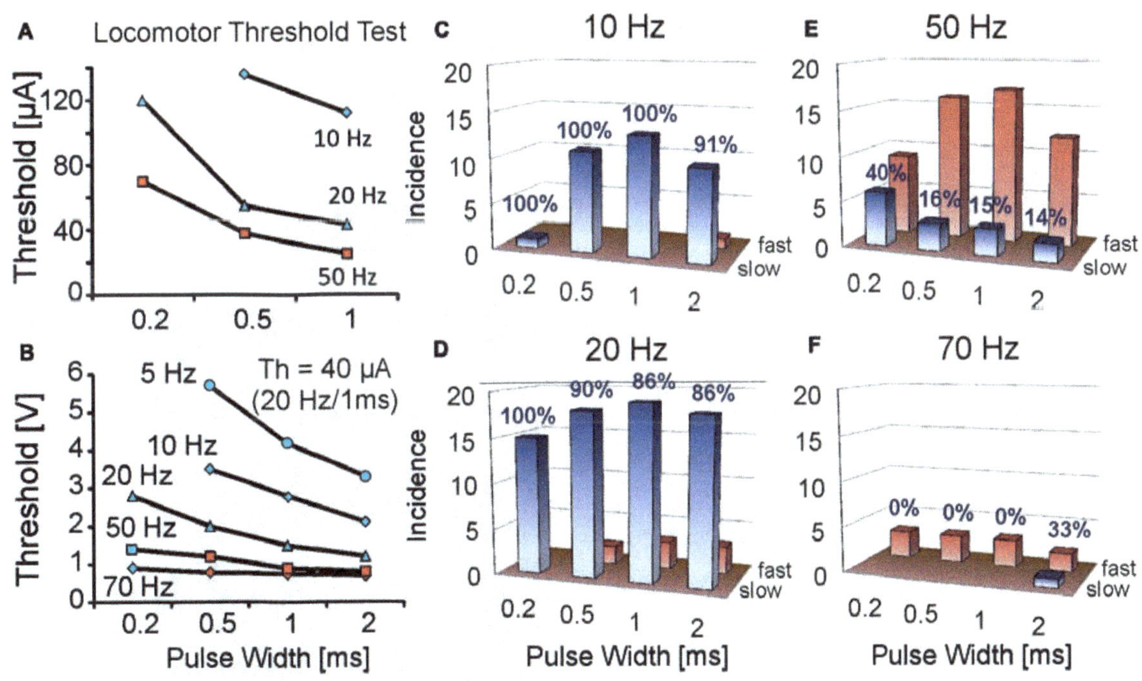

FIGURE 2 | Rate of locomotion at threshold strengths for initiating locomotion varies with different stimulation frequencies and pulse widths. Locomotor threshold parameter tests for single MLR stimulation sites were conducted at various stimulus frequencies and pulse widths. **(A,B)** Thresholds plotted relative to pulse width and frequency for two animals; one intact **(A)** and one with mid-thoracic moderate contusion injury **(B)**. Current threshold (Th) for the spinal cord injury (SCI) animal at 20 Hz, 1 ms duration was 40 μA. Note that greater strengths of stimulation were required with lower frequencies and shorter pulse widths. Initial locomotor responses vary according to frequency and pulse width of stimulation: stimulation frequencies of 20 Hz typically produce slow locomotion at threshold (blue symbols) in contrast to higher stimulation frequencies which typically initiate fast locomotion at threshold (red symbols). **(C–F)** Incidence of slow or fast locomotion at threshold strengths for initiating locomotion for different stimulation frequencies and pulse widths in uninjured animals 1 week after electrode implant. Note higher incidence of slow locomotion (percentage indicated) at low stimulation frequencies (10 and 20 Hz) vs. high frequencies (50 and 70 Hz). The number of trials is indicated on the ordinate (1 trial per animal). Red bars indicate the incidence of fast locomotion, while the blue bars indicate the incidence of slow locomotion. Only one data point per animal is included for each frequency and pulse width test combination. A similar response was observed during threshold tests in the SCI animal **(B)**.

This shows that theta oscillations are associated with sites that are most effective for eliciting locomotion. In line with this result is a conclusion presented by Thevathasan et al. (2012) who found that in PD patients the best outcome of DBS was achieved at the level of maximal alpha activity in the caudal PPN region.

Next, we analyzed the differences in power of delta, theta, beta and gamma bands between the LowTh and HighTh groups for the different experimental conditions (**Figure 6**). For the theta band we analyzed two sub-bands: low (4–6 Hz) and high (6–12 Hz) theta; for gamma we analyzed low (28–55 Hz) and high (65–100 Hz) sub-bands.

For the LowTh group a two-way RM ANOVA did not show significant differences between experimental conditions for the delta band ($F_{(3,39)} = 2.739$, $p = 0.056$). *Post hoc* Sidak's multiple comparison tests showed that power was significantly different between resting and locomotion at 15 m/min and between 10 m/min and 20 m/min locomotion (**Figure 6A**). There were no significant differences between the different behavioral states in the HighTh group. Moreover, the difference between LowTh

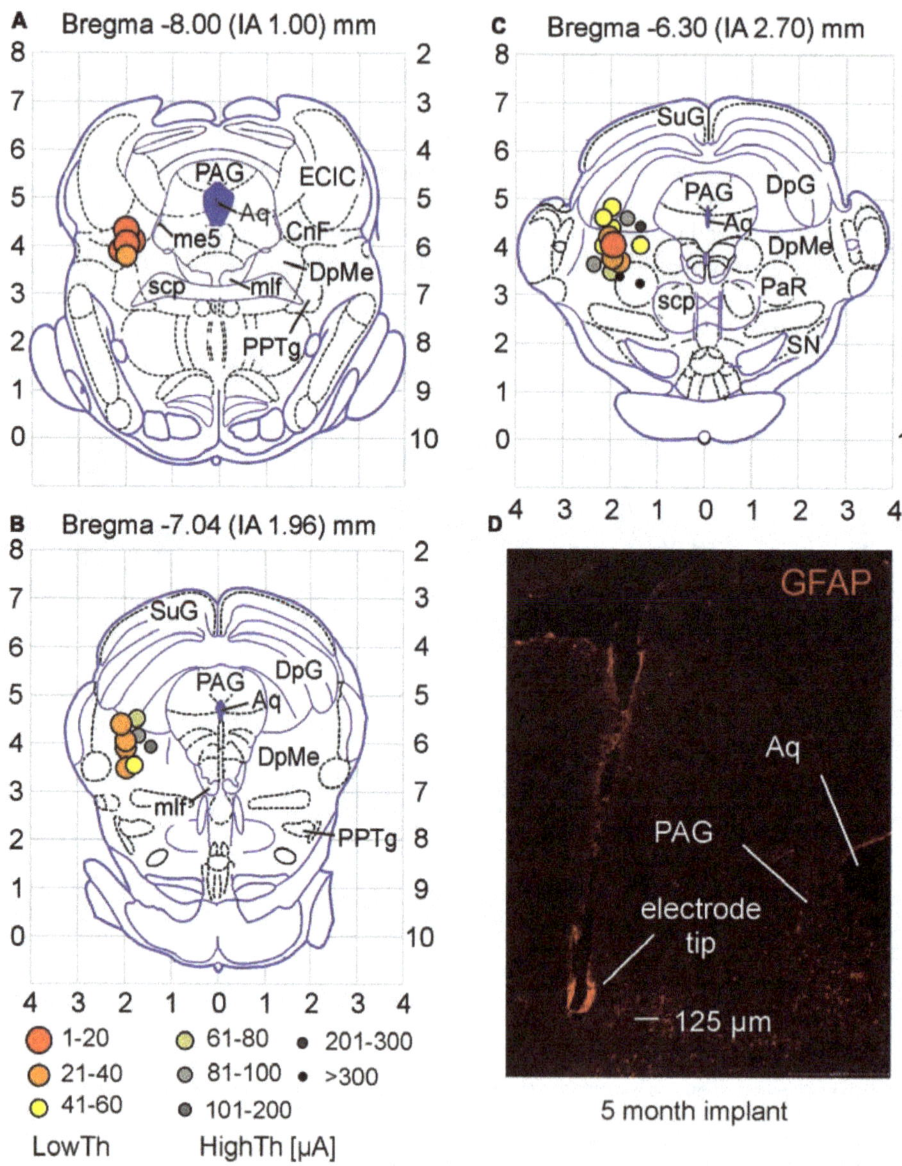

FIGURE 3 | Stimulation sites for high and low current locomotor threshold groups differ in location. (A–C) Low threshold sites were found in the CnF and DpMe of midbrain. High threshold sites were observed surrounding these areas. Current thresholds for each site are defined by symbols in **(B)**. **(D)** Example of electrode tip site in the brain tissue (coronal section). Note the minor tissue response to the electrode as observed with GFAP staining. Abbreviations as per Paxinos and Watson (1998). Aq, aqueduct; CnF, cuneiform n.; DpG, deep gray layer of superior colliculus; DpMe, deep mesencephalic n.; ECIC, external cortex of inferior colliculus; me5, mesencephalic n. of 5th nerve; mlf, medial longitudinal fasciculus; PAG, periaqueductal gray; PaR, pararubral n.; PPTg, pedunculopontine tegmental n.; scp, superior cerebellar peduncle; SN, substantia nigra; SuG, superficial gray layer of superior colliculus.

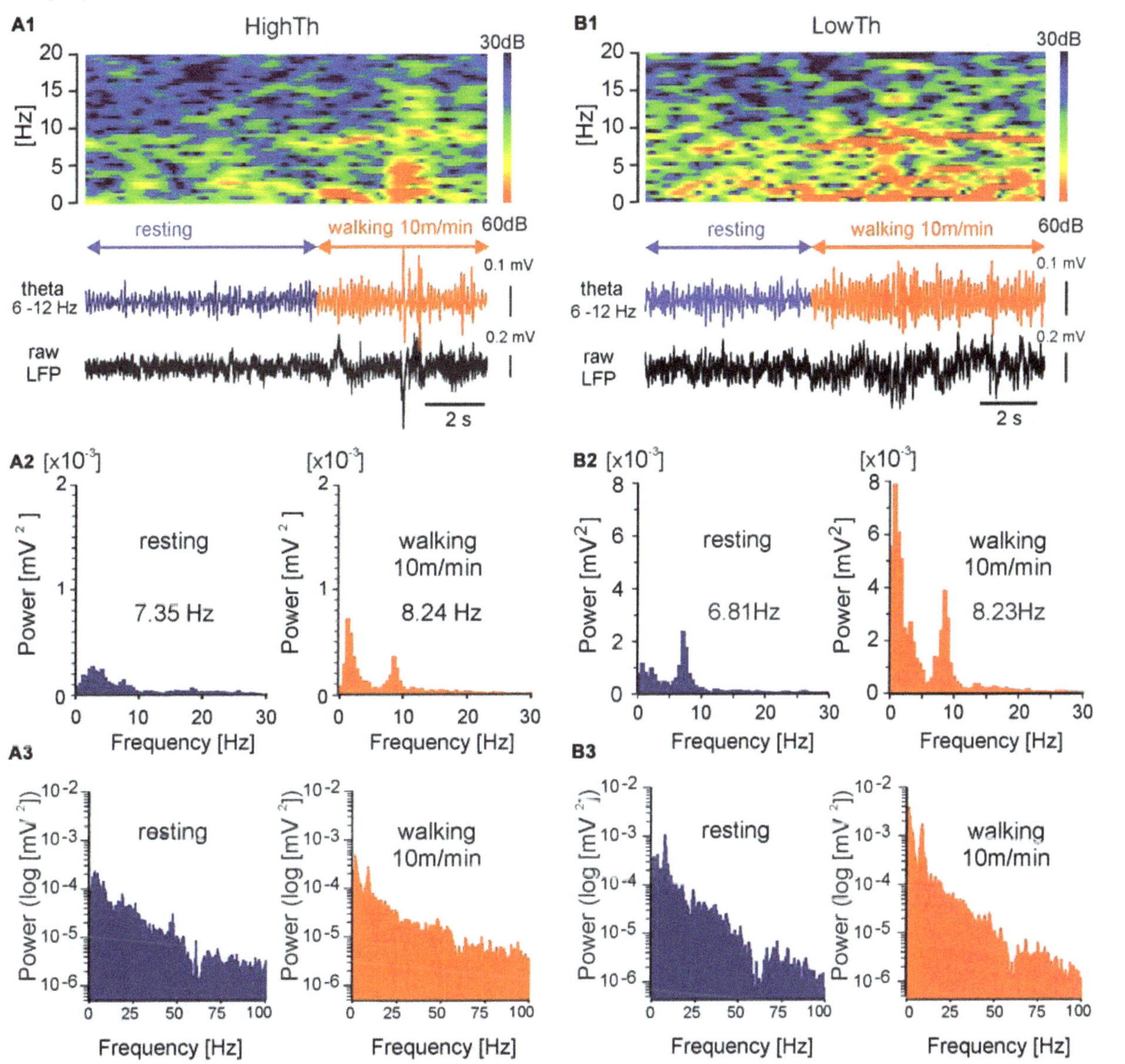

FIGURE 4 | MLR LFP activity during transition from resting to walking in freely moving rat. LFPs recorded during locomotion from LowTh sites show a larger increase in the power of delta and theta bands in comparison to the HighTh sites. Top in **(A1)** frequency spectrogram (frequencies between 0 Hz and 20 Hz) plotted vs. time of LFP recorded from a HighTh site; bottom in **(A1)** LFP, filtered 6–12 Hz and raw, recorded from a HighTh site; **(A2)** histograms of power spectra in linear scale for corresponding data segments; **(A3)** histograms of power spectra in logarithmic scale for corresponding data segments; Top in **(B1)** frequency spectrogram (frequencies between 0 Hz and 20 Hz) plotted vs. time; bottom in **(B1)** LFP, filtered 6–12 Hz and raw, recorded from LowTh site; **(B2)** histograms of power spectra for corresponding data segments. **(B3)** histograms of power spectra in logarithmic scale for corresponding data segments.

and HighTh groups for locomotion at 20 m/min was significant (**Figure 6A**).

For the LowTh group a two-way RM ANOVA showed significant differences between experimental conditions for the low theta band ($F_{(3,39)}$ = 6.642, p = 0.001) and for the high theta band ($F_{(3,39)}$ = 3.790, p = 0.0177). *Post hoc* Sidak's multiple comparison tests showed that power was significantly different between resting and locomotion for both bands of theta at speeds of 15 m/min and 20 m/min, and between 10 m/min and 20 m/min (**Figures 6B,C**). There were no significant differences between the different behavioral states in the HighTh group. Moreover, the difference between LowTh and HighTh groups for locomotion at 20 m/min was significant (**Figure 6C**).

For the power of the beta band, the differences between various behavioral states (i.e., resting and locomotion at different speeds) were significant ($F_{(3,39)}$ = 3.071, p = 0.0389) only in the LowTh group (**Figure 6D**). The power observed at rest was significantly different from that observed during locomotion at 20 m/min (Sidak's test, p = 0.0026).

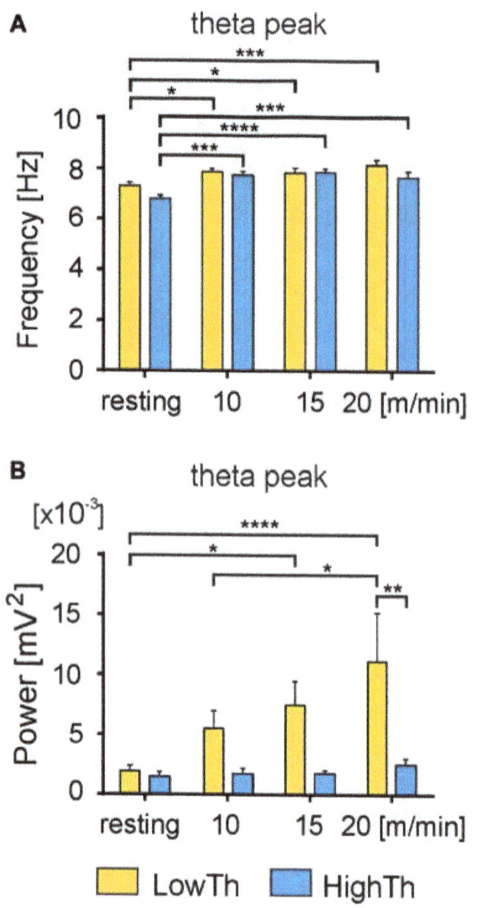

FIGURE 5 | Changes in frequency and power of the theta peak with the transition from resting state to locomotion. A significant increase in the frequency of theta peak was observed with the transition from resting to locomotion in both LowTh and HighTh animals **(A)**. Note significant increase in power of the theta peak in the LowTh group between resting and locomotion at 15 m/min and 20 m/min, and between 10 m/min and 20 m/min **(B)**. The power of the theta peak was significantly different when comparing LowTh and HighTh rats during locomotion at the highest speed (20 m/min). *$P < 0.05$, **$P < 0.01$, ***$P < 0.001$, ****$P < 0.0001$.

For the low gamma band we found significant differences between various behavioral states ($F_{(3,39)} = 4.189$, $p = 0.0116$). *Post hoc* analysis showed differences between resting and locomotion at 20 m/min, and locomotion at speeds of 10 m/min and 20 m/min (**Figure 6E**) only in the LowTh group. The same results were obtained for the high gamma band ($F_{(3,39)} = 4.203$, $p = 0.0114$; **Figure 6F**). These results show that there are progressive changes for all frequency bands as locomotion increases in speed.

Results shown in **Figure 6** suggested the possibility of a relationship between the power of frequency bands and the speed. Thus, we performed linear regression analysis which showed that changes in power of delta, theta, beta and gamma bands are related to the speed changes (data not shown). As the relation between speed and the power of delta and theta bands were much stronger (for delta $R^2 = 0.96$, $p = 0.016$; for theta high $R^2 = 0.97$, $p = 0.015$) than for the other bands and as in both bands there is characteristic peak of frequency visible, we decided to analyze their parameters further, i.e., the frequency and power of the peak frequency in relation to the speed of locomotion. **Figure 7** shows the regression lines for LowTh and HighTh groups. For the peak of the power spectra of the theta band the changes of both the frequency (**Figure 7A**) and power (**Figure 7C**) were positively related to the speed in the LowTh group (slopes of both regression lines were significantly different from zero ($p < 0.05$ and $p < 0.02$, respectively). For the peak of the delta band such a relationship was significant only for the power (slope significantly different from zero at $p < 0.05$) but not for the frequency of the delta peak (**Figures 7B,D**). This suggests that the theta rhythm represents a more meaningful biomarker for effective MLR sites.

Because the LFP frequency is a potential means of localizing the most effective sites for DBS for therapeutic purposes, we also determined whether the theta rhythm in LFPs persists after SCI. As **Figure 8** illustrates, in rats after chronic SCI the theta oscillations can be observed in MLR LFP spectrograms and power spectra during locomotion, similar to those we have described for intact rats. These characteristics of LFP that we describe here can therefore be considered reliable indices of the location of potentially effective MLR stimulus sites in injured animals. These LFP characteristics were observed in all of the rats with SCI with low threshold MLR sites ($n = 8$) included in this article. In each of these animals, DBS improved locomotor activity. A full analysis of the effect of MLR stimulation on locomotor activity observed following contusive SCI will be presented elsewhere.

DISCUSSION

LFPs in Functionally Defined MLR in Intact Rats Display a Characteristic Theta Rhythm during Voluntary Locomotor Activity

This is the first observation of LFP activity recorded in freely moving rats from functionally identified locomotion-inducing MLR sites. We found that the onset of voluntary locomotor activity was invariably accompanied by a transition from disorganized activity to a prominent theta rhythm. This is in accordance with previous studies on hypothalamic locomotor sites that were functionally identified (Sławińska and Kasicki, 1995, 1998). This is also the typical LFP frequency band observed in hippocampal CA1 at bipolar recording sites during locomotion (Kramis et al., 1975; Bland, 1986). Our data confirm our hypothesis that the theta rhythm is a characteristic of LFP activity in the MLR during voluntary locomotion, and are consistent with the suggestion that the theta rhythm serves to link different cell groups together in functional ensembles (Tort et al., 2008; Colgin, 2016).

The transition from resting to locomotion was associated with increases in the power spectra. For two bands, delta and theta, the increase was clear. Moreover, in both bands clear

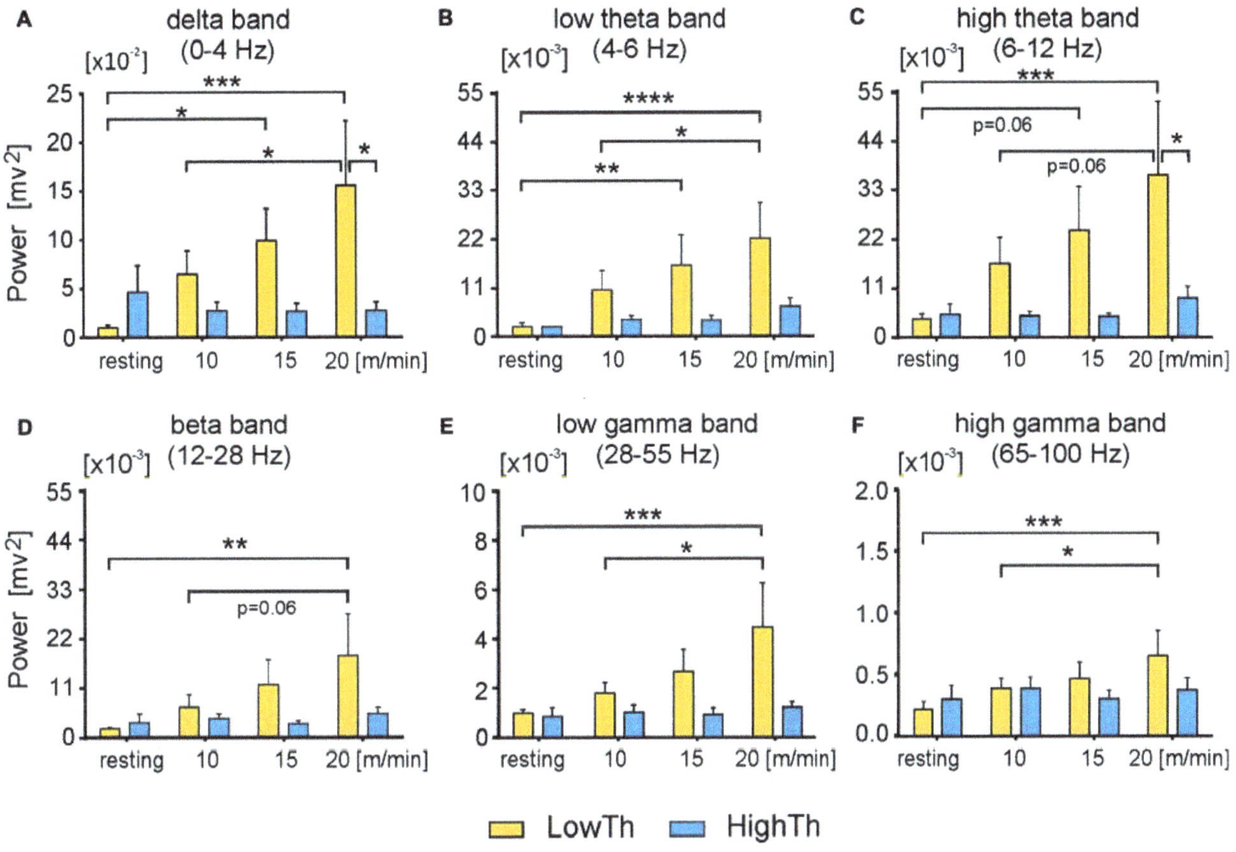

FIGURE 6 | Power of all analyzed frequency bands in LFPs significantly increases in low threshold MLR sites but not high threshold sites as locomotor speed increases. Power of delta **(A)** low and high theta band (**B,C** respectively) and beta band **(D)** significantly increases in LowTh sites, but not HighTh sites as voluntary locomotor speed increases. **(E,F)** Power of low and high gamma band in LowTh sites also shows significant increases as locomotor speed increases. Note, difference in scaling between individual plots for power of different bands. Power of any band is the integral of the power in the specific frequency ranges: delta: 0–4 Hz; theta low: 4–6 Hz; theta high: 6–12 Hz; beta: 12–28 Hz; gamma low: 28–55 Hz; gamma high: 65–100 Hz (n – 8 LowTh; n – 7 HighTh). $^{*}P < 0.05$, $^{**}P < 0.01$, $^{***}P < 0.001$, $^{****}P < 0.0001$).

peaks were visible. Thus, we did a more thorough analysis for those bands. Namely, we analyzed the frequency and power of the peak frequency in both bands. For the delta band, we found that the frequency of the peak was not related to the speed for either the LowTh or the HighTh group. The power of the delta peak frequency was related to the speed for the LowTh group only. Thus, we can conclude that the changes in delta band parameters are not locomotion related. We also analyzed the relationship of the theta rhythm to the speed of locomotion. There are several differences between theta band parameters when comparing the LowTh vs. HighTh groups. The power of the theta band was significantly greater (by up to 5-fold) in the LowTh animals than in the HighTh groups. Furthermore, the power and the frequency of the peak theta frequency was related to the speed of locomotion in the LowTh group of animals, but not in the HighTh group, analogous to our previous finding, where we showed theta recorded from the hippocampus was related to the speed of locomotion (Sławińska and Kasicki, 1998). We consider these facts as further support for the suggestion that locomotion is associated with theta rhythm in structures implicated in the control of locomotion, including the MLR.

Our finding that the peak in the power spectrum is highly correlated with the speed of locomotion in the LowTh cases suggests that the theta oscillations may be a reliable biomarker for electrode placement in an effective MLR site for inducing locomotion. We are aware of the potential for signal contamination due to the use of monopolar recording, but we think this is an unlikely confound. The fact that the power of the theta peak is significantly larger in the LowTh cases than in the HighTh cases that are spatially more remote from the most effective site clearly demonstrates that the LFPs recorded in these cases are generated locally and not due to volume conductance. The placement of our reference electrode also argues against volume conduction from the hippocampus, because it was substantially caudal to the region of the hippocampus, and the hippocampus was not between the reference and the LFP electrodes.

The relationship of our theta LFPs (the peak frequency and power) to speed of locomotion is noteworthy, because

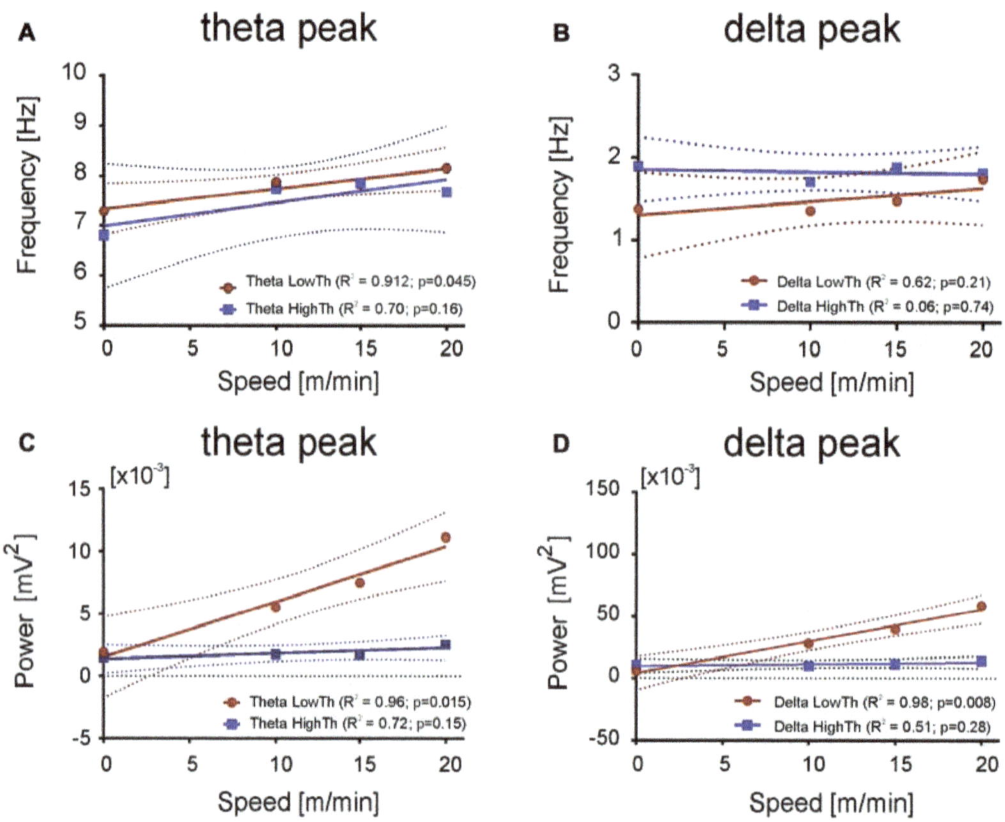

FIGURE 7 | Relationship between the frequency and power of maximum in the delta and theta band and the speed. (A,C) Both frequency and power of theta peak increase with the speed of an animal for LFPs recorded from the LowTh sites, while for the HighTh sites the relationship was not significant. **(B,D)** Opposite to that the frequency of delta peak was not related with the speed of rat both for LowTh and HighTh sites. Note that in contrast to the theta peak, in the delta peak only the power was related to the speed of locomotion of the animals of LowTh group only.

this is typical of other areas in the brain implicated in locomotor control, including the hypothalamus and the hippocampus. Theta oscillations in the hippocampus depend on the activity of the medial septal neurons, and the speed of locomotion is conveyed to the hippocampus via glutamatergic septohippocampal projections (King et al., 1998; Fuhrmann et al., 2015). Optogenetic stimulation at theta frequencies of axons of medial septal GABAergic cells in the hippocampus via an optic fiber implanted above the CA1 area induced theta oscillations but did not initiate locomotion in immobile mice (Bender et al., 2015), while optogenetic activation of the medial septal glutamatergic input to the hippocampus induced locomotion and hippocampal theta rhythm (Fuhrmann et al., 2015). However, both articles described that theta oscillations were correlated with the speed of locomotion. The means whereby the hippocampal activity can modulate or initiate locomotion is not known, but either the hypothalamic or mesencephalic locomotor regions may be involved. This is an issue that needs clarification. It is of particular interest because hippocampal theta oscillations are thought to be involved in encoding the animal's position during spatial navigation (Bender et al., 2015). The presence of a locomotor speed-related theta rhythm in the MLR is consistent with the hypothesis that these areas are coherently bound together during locomotion. Perhaps the purpose of such binding might be to preserve position and speed information throughout the locomotor system.

The presence of similar theta rhythms in multiple sites related to locomotion (MLR, hypothalamic locomotor regions and hippocampus) is consistent with functional coupling of these structures. Although Bland and Vanderwolf (1972) showed electrical stimulation of the hippocampus does not induce locomotion, recent experiments showed chemogenetic or optogenetic activation of hippocampal cells (including CA1 neurons) resulted in enhanced locomotor behavior (Alexander et al., 2009; Fuhrmann et al., 2015). In the chemogenetic study, Alexander et al. (2009) expressed HA-hM3Dq driven by the CaMKIIa promoter in mice and found that the otherwise inert ligand for hM3Dq, clozapine-N-oxide (CNO), markedly increased locomotor activity. These findings are consistent with the well-known coupling between the limbic and motor systems (Mogenson and Nielsen, 1984), and with functional coupling of locomotor regions through a common LFP frequency as previously proposed (Sławińska and Kasicki, 1995).

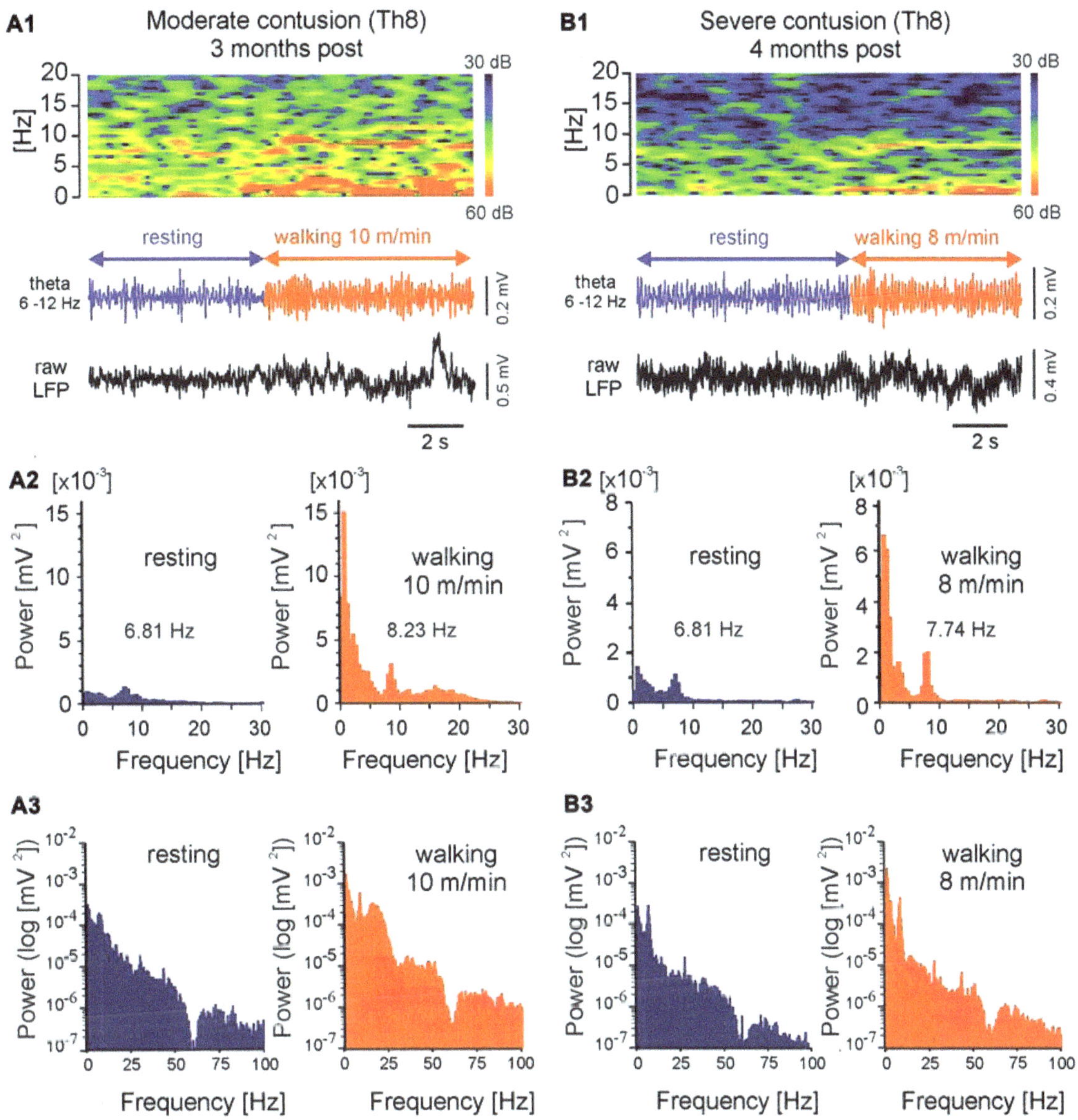

FIGURE 8 | LFPs recorded from LowTh sites in rats with moderate or severe mid-thoracic contusion SCI show similar correlation to locomotor speed as intact animals. Top in **(A1,B1)**: frequency spectrogram plot vs. time; bottom in **(A1,B1)**: LFP, filtered 6–12 Hz and raw; **(A2,B2)**: histograms of power spectra in linear scale; **(A3,B3)**: histograms of power spectra in logarithmic scale. Note increased power within the theta band (<12 Hz) and shift in the dominating theta frequency with the transition to walking.

The persistence of this characteristic theta oscillation at sites that promote locomotor recovery after SCI suggests that it can be used as a biomarker in clinically relevant circumstances, and can guide that placement of DBS electrodes for effective restoration of locomotion in injured subjects. Further studies are needed to determine the impact, if any, of damage or degeneration in cases such as partial SCI on the MLR locomotor system. There is evidence of plasticity in multiple descending pathways after SCI (Ballermann and Fouad, 2006; Filli et al., 2014; Leszczyńska et al., 2015; Fink and Cafferty, 2016; Hansen et al., 2016), and changes in brainstem locomotor circuits are possible. However, our results so far provide a clear indication that the factors producing theta oscillations in the MLR during even impaired locomotion after partial SCI persist to the degree that the potential biomarker role for theta oscillations is maintained.

A predominance of gamma band activity in the MLR might be expected based on the activity of single PPN neurons *in vitro* (Garcia-Rill et al., 2015). However, in contrast to those results, no other peak in higher frequency bands (including gamma) was visible in the power spectra in the rats included in our study. This is consistent with the observation that the firing of single PPN neurons during actual locomotion was less than 6 Hz in normal rats (Geng et al., 2016).These same authors reported LFP results from PPN during locomotion consistent with our findings from effective MLR sites, with the highest percentage of relative LFP power observed in the 0.7–12 Hz range. Their PPN sites were not confirmed to be effective locomotion-inducing sites, however. And their PPN recording sites were anatomically distinct from our MLR sites (more ventral). The much lower power of beta and gamma bands also varied for different experimental conditions (treadmill speed) in the LowTh group but no such variations occurred in the HighTh animals. The frequency of the theta rhythm increased significantly as the animal started to walk. This is consistent with the association of the theta rhythm at these sites with the processes underlying locomotion. These findings have the potential to aid in the identification of brainstem sites that should be the most effective for DBS facilitation of locomotion, providing for the first time a theta rhythm signature for the MLR. Emerging clinical data is consistent with this. According to Tattersall et al. (2014), LFP recordings from the supposed PPN area of the MLR have shown oscillations in both the alpha (6–12 Hz) and beta (12–30 Hz) frequency bands (Weinberger et al., 2008; Shimamoto et al., 2010; Tsang et al., 2010; Thevathasan et al., 2012; Tattersall et al., 2014). Active gait was also accompanied by increased LFP alpha power in this area (Thevathasan et al., 2012; Tattersall et al., 2014). Recordings from DBS electrodes implanted in the PPN area (PD patients) showed an increase of the power in the range 7–11 Hz (the alpha range in human, which overlaps with the high theta; 6–12 Hz in our article) after symptom improvement with levodopa administration (Androulidakis et al., 2008). It was also shown in PD patients after levodopa that LFPs recorded from the PPN area showed "an increase in PPNa alpha (5–12 Hz) oscillatory activity and a decrease in beta (13–35 Hz) and gamma (65–90 Hz) bands activity" (Fraix et al., 2013).

Like most areas of the brain, the MLR region receives input in a range of frequencies. The arrangement of MLR neurons, the orientation of their dendritic fields, and the organization of the synaptic input could create more synchronous LFPs or they could cancel out others in the MLR area. Thus neurons in MLR may be receiving significant gamma frequency input, for example, but because of the microanatomy of local circuits, synchronized extracellular current flow may be minimal in the gamma range. However, we were unable to find evidence for an endogenous rhythm in the gamma range, as suggested for the PPN (Simon et al., 2010; Garcia-Rill et al., 2011).

Effective Stimulus Sites and Parameters for Inducing Locomotion in Freely-Moving Rats

Low threshold MLR sites (below 60 μA, mean 32.8 μA) were found in the CnF and the more rostral DpMe. This is consistent with recent findings from human studies using DBS for treatment of FOG, where it has been suggested that the most effective targets are within the CnF and subcuneiform regions instead of the PPN (Piallat et al., 2009; Alam et al., 2011). This conclusion is in agreement with many previous animal studies (Shik et al., 1966; Ross and Sinnamon, 1984; Steeves and Jordan, 1984; Milner and Mogenson, 1988; Coles et al., 1989; Mori et al., 1989; Jordan, 1998; Takakusaki et al., 2016). A recent trans-synaptic tracing study also implicates the CnF (Xiang et al., 2013). Although there are a number of studies implicating the PPN as the effective site for DBS in humans (reviewed in Collomb-Clerc and Welter, 2015; Hamacher et al., 2015; Nonnekes et al., 2015; Udupa and Chen, 2015), it is widely recognized that the effective sites are difficult to clearly identify (Alam et al., 2011). fMRI of the brainstem in human subjects shows the CnF is activated during imaginary gait (Karachi et al., 2012). Nevertheless, it is common in the clinical literature to equate the PPN with the MLR, and the suggestion has been made that the term MLR can now be "retired" (Garcia-Rill et al., 2015). But Hernández-Chan et al. (2011) and Winn and co-workers (Winn, 2006; Gut and Winn, 2015, 2016) have pointed out weaknesses in the argument that the PPN is an essential component of the MLR, and these arguments along with our data support the notion that a functional definition of the MLR is still valid. Takakusaki et al. (2005, 2016) and Takakusaki (2008, 2013) have directly compared the effects of CnF and PPN stimulation, and they found that the CnF is effective for eliciting locomotion in decerebrate cats, while the PPN controls muscle tone, and stimulation in this region may actually suppress locomotion. Also, they showed the effective MLR sites are not co-extensive with cholinergic neurons that define the location of PPN. Moreover, neurons activated during locomotion (indicated by the presence of the activity-dependent marker Fos) are found in the CnF and other nearby areas, including the DpMe (Jordan, 1998; Vianna et al., 2003; Heise and Mitrofanis, 2006), but not in the PPN. Stimulation in the DpMe area also induces locomotion in the rat (Melnikova, 1975; Milner and Mogenson, 1988; Coles et al., 1989; Cabaj et al., 2017) and does not harbor cholinergic neurons.

PPN cholinergic neurons have been considered essential for MLR initiation of locomotion (Garcia-Rill and Skinner, 1987) in mammals and lamprey (reviewed in Ryczko and Dubuc, 2013). However, recent data does not support a critical role for a cholinergic component of the MLR in the initiation of locomotion. Activation of the cholinergic component of the PPN using a chemogenetic approach induced only subtle effects on locomotion in freely moving, control rats (Pienaar et al., 2015), and optogenetic stimulation of cholinergic neurons in the PPN did not elicit locomotion in stationary mice (Roseberry et al., 2016). Glutamatergic rather than cholinergic neurons of the MLR have been shown to be effective for eliciting locomotion with optogenetic stimulation (Lee et al., 2014; Roseberry et al., 2016). Furthermore, cholinergic antagonists do not impair the initiation of locomotion due to electrical stimulation of the MLR (Jordan et al., 2014). Taken together these data increase the likelihood that components of the MLR other than the PPN should be the target for DBS to restore locomotion.

In clinical DBS studies, the electrode size and methods of detecting electrode placement do not provide sufficient resolution to rule out the possibility that the stimulus activates structures outside of the anatomically defined PPN. As a result the term PPNa, for the area of the brainstem surrounding the PPN, including CnF and precuneiformis, has been introduced (Fraix et al., 2013; Welter et al., 2015). Further research in animal models is required using modern methods of activating and silencing genetically defined putative MLR constituents to clarify this issue, but the continued use of the term PPN instead of MLR to describe effective sites for locomotion induction is misleading.

We determined the most effective stimulation parameters for inducing controllable locomotion (pulses of 1.0 ms duration at 20 Hz). These are relevant to the selection of stimulation parameters for the treatment of gait defects using DBS, but are in contrast to the previous claim, based upon results from PPN stimulation in decerebrate rats and recordings from PPN neurons *in vitro*, that stimuli in the 40–60 Hz range should be required (Garcia-Rill et al., 2015). Our results show that the effective frequency for electrical stimulation is not predicted by the peak frequency of LFP recorded during locomotion in the same area, but must be determined empirically. We contend that the definition of "optimal stimulation frequency" should necessarily take into consideration the ability to induce controllable locomotion, i.e., to "dial-in" locomotor speed and maintain it. According to this definition and in these targeted sites, stimulation frequencies lower than gamma are optimal. In keeping with this, DBS experience for gait improvement in PD has led to the conclusion that the effective frequency of stimulation is often in the range of 10–25 Hz instead of higher frequencies (Androulidakis et al., 2008; Ferraye et al., 2010, 2011; Nosko et al., 2015). Others have also shown that stimulation in the MLR at the lower frequency ranges (5–30 Hz) was suitable for inducing locomotion in adult rats (Melnikova, 1975; MacDonell et al., 2015) and cats (Douglas et al., 1993; Guertin et al., 1995; Noga et al., 2003).

Concluding Remarks

Our results are consistent with earlier observations that the onset of locomotion is characterized by theta frequency oscillations of the LFPs in hippocampus and in locomotion-inducing sites in the subthalamic locomotor region and posterior hypothalamus (Sławińska and Kasicki, 1995, 1998). We suggest that theta oscillatory LFPs may coherently bind cooperating neuronal ensembles during locomotor activity in order to encode the animal's position during spatial navigation. It is clear from our results that after injury the theta rhythm can also be used as a signature for effective sites for DBS, especially as DBS in the MLR dramatically improved locomotion in animals with a SCI.

AUTHOR CONTRIBUTIONS

LMJ, US and BRN: conceptualization; BRN, LMJ, US and SK: methodology; BRN, FJS, CO, LMV, US, MO, AMC and HM: investigation; BRN, US and SK: formal analysis; BRN and US: visualization; BRN, LMJ, US and SK: writing—original draft; BRN, LMJ, US and SK: writing—review and editing; BRN and US: supervision; BRN, US, SK and LMJ: funding acquisition.

ACKNOWLEDGMENTS

This study was supported by The Christopher and Dana Reeve Foundation (Grant no. NA1-1001-2), the Craig H. Neilsen Foundation (Grant no. 190550) and National Institute of Neurological Disorders and Stroke (NINDS) Grant 2 R56NS-46404-061A to BRN, the Nencki Institute to US and SK and Canadian Institutes of Health Research (CIHR; FRN 115147) to LMJ. We would like to thank Sławomir Stasieńko for his contribution to LFP analysis and Ioan Opris for his constructive recommendations on the manuscript and figures.

REFERENCES

Alam, M., Schwabe, K., and Krauss, J. K. (2011). The pedunculopontine nucleus area: critical evaluation of interspecies differences relevant for its use as a target for deep brain stimulation. *Brain* 134, 11–23. doi: 10.1093/brain/awq322

Alexander, G. M., Rogan, S. C., Abbas, A. I., Armbruster, B. N., Pei, Y., Allen, J. A., et al. (2009). Remote control of neuronal activity in transgenic mice expressing evolved G protein-coupled receptors. *Neuron* 63, 27–39. doi: 10.1016/j.neuron.2009.06.014

Androulidakis, A. G., Mazzone, P., Litvak, V., Penny, W., Dileone, M., Gaynor, L. M., et al. (2008). Oscillatory activity in the pedunculopontine area of patients with Parkinson's disease. *Exp. Neurol.* 211, 59–66. doi: 10.1016/j.expneurol.2008.01.002

Ballermann, M., and Fouad, K. (2006). Spontaneous locomotor recovery in spinal cord injured rats is accompanied by anatomical plasticity of reticulospinal fibers. *Eur. J. Neurosci.* 23, 1988–1996. doi: 10.1111/j.1460-9568.2006.04726.x

Basso, D. M., Beattie, M. S., and Bresnahan, J. C. (1996). Graded histological and locomotor outcomes after spinal cord contusion using the NYU weight-drop device versus transection. *Exp. Neurol.* 139, 244–256. doi: 10.1006/exnr.1996.0098

Bender, F., Gorbati, M., Cadavieco, M. C., Denisova, N., Gao, X., Holman, C., et al. (2015). Theta oscillations regulate the speed of locomotion via a hippocampus to lateral septum pathway. *Nat. Commun.* 6:8521. doi: 10.1038/ncomms9521

Bland, B. H. (1986). The physiology and pharmacology of hippocampal formation theta rhythms. *Prog. Neurobiol.* 26, 1–54. doi: 10.1016/0301-0082(86)90019-5

Bland, B. H., and Oddie, S. D. (2001). Theta band oscillation and synchrony in the hippocampal formation and associated structures: the case for its role in sensorimotor integration. *Behav. Brain Res.* 127, 119–136. doi: 10.1016/s0166-4328(01)00358-8

Bland, B. H., and Vanderwolf, C. H. (1972). Electrical stimulation of the hippocampal formation: behavioral and bioelectrical effects. *Brain Res.* 43, 89–106. doi: 10.1016/0006-8993(72)90276-4

Cabaj, A. M., Majczyński, H., Couto, E., Gardiner, P. F., Stecina, K., Sławińska, U., et al. (2017). Serotonin controls initiation of locomotion and afferent modulation of coordination via 5-HT$_7$ receptors in adult rats. *J. Physiol.* 595, 301–320. doi: 10.1113/JP272271

Coles, S. K., Iles, J. F., and Nicolopoulos-Stournaras, S. (1989). The mesencephalic centre controlling locomotion in the rat. *Neuroscience* 28, 149–157. doi: 10.1016/0306-4522(89)90239-x

Colgin, L. L. (2016). Rhythms of the hippocampal network. *Nat. Rev. Neurosci.* 17, 239–249. doi: 10.1038/nrn.2016.21

Collomb-Clerc, A., and Welter, M. L. (2015). Effects of deep brain stimulation on balance and gait in patients with Parkinson's disease: a systematic neurophysiological review. *Neurophysiol. Clin.* 45, 371–388. doi: 10.1016/j.neucli.2015.07.001

Douglas, J. R., Noga, B. R., Dai, X., and Jordan, L. M. (1993). The effects of intrathecal administration of excitatory amino acid agonists and antagonists on the initiation of locomotion in the adult cat. *J. Neurosci.* 13, 990–1000.

Ferraye, M. U., Debû, B., Fraix, V., Goetz, L., Ardouin, C., Yelnik, J., et al. (2010). Effects of pedunculopontine nucleus area stimulation on gait disorders in Parkinson's disease. *Brain* 133, 205–214. doi: 10.1093/brain/awp229

Ferraye, M. U., Debû, B., Fraix, V., Krack, P., Charbardès, S., Seigneuret, E., et al. (2011). Subthalamic nucleus versus pedunculopontine nucleus stimulation in Parkinson disease: synergy or antagonism? *J. Neural Transm. (Vienna)* 118, 1469–1475. doi: 10.1007/s00702-011-0673-y

Filli, L., Engmann, A. K., Zörner, B., Weinmann, O., Moraitis, T., Gullo, M., et al. (2014). Bridging the gap: a reticulo-propriospinal detour bypassing an incomplete spinal cord injury. *J. Neurosci.* 34, 13399–13410. doi: 10.1523/JNEUROSCI.0701-14.2014

Fink, K. L., and Cafferty, W. B. (2016). Reorganization of intact descending motor circuits to replace lost connections after injury. *Neurotherapeutics* 13, 370–381. doi: 10.1007/s13311-016-0422-x

Fraix, V., Bastin, J., David, O., Goetz, L., Ferraye, M., Benabid, A. L., et al. (2013). Pedunculopontine nucleus area oscillations during stance, stepping and freezing in Parkinson's disease. *PLoS One* 8:e83919. doi: 10.1371/journal.pone.0083919

Fuhrmann, F., Justus, D., Sosulina, L., Kaneko, H., Beutel, T., Friedrichs, D., et al. (2015). Locomotion, theta oscillations, and the speed-correlated firing of hippocampal neurons are controlled by a medial septal glutamatergic circuit. *Neuron* 86, 1253–1264. doi: 10.1016/j.neuron.2015.05.001

Garcia-Rill, E., Houser, C. R., Skinner, R. D., Smith, W., and Woodward, D. J. (1987). Locomotion-inducing sites in the vicinity of the pedunculopontine nucleus. *Brain Res. Bull.* 18, 731–738. doi: 10.1016/0361-9230(87)90208-5

Garcia-Rill, E., Hyde, J., Kezunovic, N., Urbano, F. J., and Petersen, E. (2015). The physiology of the pedunculopontine nucleus: implications for deep brain stimulation. *J. Neural Transm. (Vienna)* 122, 225–235. doi: 10.1007/s00702-014-1243-x

Garcia-Rill, E., Simon, C., Smith, K., Kezunovic, N., and Hyde, J. (2011). The pedunculopontine tegmental nucleus: from basic neuroscience to neurosurgical applications: arousal from slices to humans: implications for DBS. *J. Neural Transm. (Vienna)* 118, 1397–1407. doi: 10.1007/s00702-010-0500-x

Garcia-Rill, E., and Skinner, R. D. (1987). The mesencephalic locomotor region. I. Activation of a medullary projection site. *Brain Res.* 411, 1–12. doi: 10.1016/0006-8993(87)90675-5

Garcia-Rill, E., Skinner, R. D., Conrad, C., Mosley, D., and Campbell, C. (1986). Projections of the mesencephalic locomotor region in the rat. *Brain Res. Bull.* 17, 33–40. doi: 10.1016/0361-9230(86)90158-9

Geng, X., Xie, J., Wang, X., Wang, X., Zhang, X., Hou, Y., et al. (2016). Altered neuronal activity in the pedunculopontine nucleus: an electrophysiological study in a rat model of Parkinson's disease. *Behav. Brain Res.* 305, 57–64. doi: 10.1016/j.bbr.2016.02.026

Gillis, G. B., and Biewener, A. A. (2001). Hindlimb muscle function in relation to speed and gait: *in vivo* patterns of strain and activation in a hip and knee extensor of the rat (*Rattus norvegicus*). *J. Exp. Biol.* 204, 2717–2731.

Grillner, S., Georgopoulos, A. P., and Jordan, L. M. (1997). "Selection and initiation of motor behavior," in *Neurons, Network and Motor Behavior*, eds P. S. G. Stein, A. I. Selverston and D. G. Stuart (Cambridge, MA: MIT Press), 3–19.

Gruner, J. A. (1992). A monitored contusion model of spinal cord injury in the rat. *J. Neurotrauma* 9, 123–126; discussion 126–128. doi: 10.1089/neu.1992.9.123

Guertin, P., Angel, M. J., Perreault, M. C., and McCrea, D. A. (1995). Ankle extensor group I afferents excite extensors throughout the hindlimb during fictive locomotion in the cat. *J. Physiol.* 487, 197–209. doi: 10.1113/jphysiol.1995.sp020871

Gut, N. K., and Winn, P. (2015). Deep brain stimulation of different pedunculopontine targets in a novel rodent model of parkinsonism. *J. Neurosci.* 35, 4792–4803. doi: 10.1523/JNEUROSCI.3646-14.2015

Gut, N. K., and Winn, P. (2016). The pedunculopontine tegmental nucleus-A functional hypothesis from the comparative literature. *Mov. Disord.* 31, 615–624. doi: 10.1002/mds.26556

Hamacher, D., Herold, F., Wiegel, P., Hamacher, D., and Schega, L. (2015). Brain activity during walking: a systematic review. *Neurosci. Biobehav. Rev.* 57, 310–327. doi: 10.1016/j.neubiorev.2015.08.002

Hamani, C., Moro, E., and Lozano, A. M. (2011). The pedunculopontine nucleus as a target for deep brain stimulation. *J. Neural Transm. (Vienna)* 118, 1461–1468. doi: 10.1007/s00702-010-0547-8

Hansen, C. N., Faw, T. D., White, S., Buford, J. A., Grau, J. W., and Basso, D. M. (2016). Sparing of descending axons rescues interneuron plasticity in the lumbar cord to allow adaptive learning after thoracic spinal cord injury. *Front. Neural Circuits* 10:11. doi: 10.3389/fncir.2016.00011

He, W., and Bellamkonda, R. V. (2008). "A molecular perspective on understanding and modulating the performance of chronic central nervous system (CNS) recording electrodes," in *Indwelling Neural Implants: Strategies for Contending with the in vivo Environment*, ed. W. M. Reichert (Boca Raton, FL: CRC Press), 151–175.

Heise, C. E., and Mitrofanis, J. (2006). Fos immunoreactivity in some locomotor neural centres of 6OHDA-lesioned rats. *Anat. Embryol. (Berl)* 211, 659–671. doi: 10.1007/s00429-006-0130-0

Hernández-Chan, N. G., Góngora-Alfaro, J. L., Álvarez-Cervera, F. J., Solís-Rodríguez, F. A., Heredia-López, F. J., and Arankowsky-Sandoval, G. (2011). Quinolinic acid lesions of the pedunculopontine nucleus impair sleep architecture, but not locomotion, exploration, emotionality or working memory in the rat. *Behav. Brain Res.* 225, 482–490. doi: 10.1016/j.bbr.2011.08.007

Jordan, L. M. (1998). Initiation of locomotion in mammals. *Ann. N Y Acad. Sci.* 860, 83–93. doi: 10.1111/j.1749-6632.1998.tb09040.x

Jordan, L. M., McVagh, J. R., Noga, B. R., Cabaj, A. M., Majczyński, H., Slawińska, U., et al. (2014). Cholinergic mechanisms in spinal locomotion-potential target for rehabilitation approaches. *Front. Neural Circuits* 8:132. doi: 10.3389/fncir.2014.00132

Jordan, L. M. J., and Sławińska, U. (2014). "The brain and spinal cord networks controlling locomotion," in *Neuronal Networks in Brain Function, CNS Disorders and Therapeutics*, eds C. L. Faingold and H. Blumenfeld (Amsterdam: Academic Press), 215–233.

Karachi, C., André, A., Bertasi, E., Bardinet, E., Lehéricy, S., and Bernard, F. A. (2012). Functional parcellation of the lateral mesencephalus. *J. Neurosci.* 32, 9396–9401. doi: 10.1523/JNEUROSCI.0509-12.2012

Kiehn, O. (2016). Decoding the organization of spinal circuits that control locomotion. *Nat. Rev. Neurosci.* 17, 224–238. doi: 10.1038/nrn.2016.9

King, C., Recce, M., and O'Keefe, J. (1998). The rhythmicity of cells of the medial septum/diagonal band of Broca in the awake freely moving rat: relationships with behaviour and hippocampal theta. *Eur. J. Neurosci.* 10, 464–477. doi: 10.1046/j.1460-9568.1998.00026.x

Kramis, R., Vanderwolf, C. H., and Bland, B. H. (1975). Two types of hippocampal rhythmical slow activity in both the rabbit and the rat: relations to behavior and effects of atropine, diethyl ether, urethane, and pentobarbital. *Exp. Neurol.* 49, 58–85. doi: 10.1016/0014-4886(75)90195-8

Lee, A. M., Hoy, J. L., Bonci, A., Wilbrecht, L., Stryker, M. P., and Niell, C. M. (2014). Identification of a brainstem circuit regulating visual cortical state in parallel with locomotion. *Neuron* 83, 455–466. doi: 10.1016/j.neuron.2014.06.031

Leszczyńska, A. N., Majczynski, H., Wilczynski, G. M., Sławińska, U., and Cabaj, A. M. (2015). Thoracic hemisection in rats results in initial recovery followed by a late decrement in locomotor movements, with changes in coordination correlated with serotonergic innervation of the ventral horn. *PLoS One* 10:e0143602. doi: 10.1371/journal.pone.0143602

MacDonell, C. W., Power, K. E., Chopek, J. W., Gardiner, K. R., and Gardiner, P. F. (2015). Extensor motoneurone properties are altered immediately before and during fictive locomotion in the adult decerebrate rat. *J. Physiol.* 593, 2327–2342. doi: 10.1113/JP270239

MacLaren, D. A., Santini, J. A., Russell, A. L., Markovic, T., and Clark, S. D. (2014). Deficits in motor performance after pedunculopontine lesions in rats—impairment depends on demands of task. *Eur. J. Neurosci.* 40, 3224–3236. doi: 10.1111/ejn.12666

Mazzone, P., Lozano, A., Stanzione, P., Galati, S., Scarnati, E., Peppe, A., et al. (2005). Implantation of human pedunculopontine nucleus: a safe and clinically relevant target in Parkinson's disease. *Neuroreport* 16, 1877–1881. doi: 10.1097/01.wnr.0000187629.38010.12

Melnikova, Z. L. (1975). The locomotion of the rat evoked by stimulation of the midbrain. *Vestn. Moscow. Univ.* 2, 45–51.

Milner, K. L., and Mogenson, G. J. (1988). Electrical and chemical activation of the mesencephalic and subthalamic locomotor regions in freely moving rats. *Brain Res.* 452, 273–285. doi: 10.1016/0006-8993(88)90031-5

Mogenson, G. J., and Nielsen, M. (1984). A study of the contribution of hippocampal-accumbens-subpallidal projections to locomotor activity. *Behav. Neural Biol.* 42, 38–51. doi: 10.1016/s0163-1047(84)90412-6

Mori, S., Matsuyama, K., Kohyama, J., Kobayashi, Y., and Takakusaki, K. (1992). Neuronal constituents of postural and locomotor control systems and their interactions in cats. *Brain Dev.* 14, S109–S120.

Mori, S., Sakamoto, T., Ohta, Y., Takakusaki, K., and Matsuyama, K. (1989). Site-specific postural and locomotor changes evoked in awake, freely moving intact cats by stimulating the brainstem. *Brain Res.* 505, 66–74. doi: 10.1016/0006-8993(89)90116-9

Noga, B. R., Kriellaars, D. J., Brownstone, R. M., and Jordan, L. M. (2003). Mechanism for activation of locomotor centers in the spinal cord by stimulation of the mesencephalic locomotor region. *J. Neurophysiol.* 90, 1464–1478. doi: 10.1152/jn.00034.2003

Nonnekes, J., Snijders, A. H., Nutt, J. G., Deuschl, G., Giladi, N., and Bloem, B. R. (2015). Freezing of gait: a practical approach to management. *Lancet Neurol.* 14, 768–778. doi: 10.1016/S1474-4422(15)00041-1

Nosko, D., Ferraye, M. U., Fraix, V., Goetz, L., Chabardes, S., Pollak, P., et al. (2015). Low-frequency versus high-frequency stimulation of the pedunculopontine nucleus area in Parkinson's disease: a randomised controlled trial. *J. Neurol. Neurosurg. Psychiatry* 86, 674–679. doi: 10.1136/jnnp-2013-307511

Paxinos, G., and Watson, C. (1998). *The Rat Brain in Stereotaxic Coordinates.* New York, NY: Academic Press.

Piallat, B., Chabardès, S., Torres, N., Fraix, V., Goetz, L., Seigneuret, E., et al. (2009). Gait is associated with an increase in tonic firing of the sub-cuneiform nucleus neurons. *Neuroscience* 158, 1201–1205. doi: 10.1016/j.neuroscience.2008.10.046

Pienaar, I. S., Gartside, S. E., Sharma, P., De Paola, V., Gretenkord, S., Withers, D., et al. (2015). Pharmacogenetic stimulation of cholinergic pedunculopontine neurons reverses motor deficits in a rat model of Parkinson's disease. *Mol. Neurodegener.* 10:47. doi: 10.1186/s13024-015-0044-5

Roseberry, T. K., Lee, A. M., Lalive, A. L., Wilbrecht, L., Bonci, A., and Kreitzer, A. C. (2016). Cell-type-specific control of brainstem locomotor circuits by Basal Ganglia. *Cell* 164, 526 537. doi: 10.1016/j.cell.2015.12.037

Ross, G. S., and Sinnamon, H. M. (1984). Forelimb and hindlimb stepping by the anesthetized rat elicited by electrical stimulation of the pons and medulla. *Physiol. Behav.* 33, 201–208. doi: 10.1016/0031-9384(84)90100-8

Ryczko, D., and Dubuc, R. (2013). The multifunctional mesencephalic locomotor region. *Curr. Pharm. Des.* 19, 4448–4470. doi: 10.2174/1381612811319240011

Shik, M. L., Severin, F. V., and Orlovskii, G. N. (1966). Control of walking and running by means of electric stimulation of the midbrain. *Biofizika* 11, 659–666.

Shimamoto, S. A., Larson, P. S., Ostrem, J. L., Glass, G. A., Turner, R. S., and Starr, P. A. (2010). Physiological identification of the human pedunculopontine nucleus. *J. Neurol. Neurosurg. Psychiatry* 81, 80–86. doi: 10.1136/jnnp.2009.179069

Simon, C., Kezunovic, N., Ye, M., Hyde, J., Hayar, A., Williams, D. K., et al. (2010). Gamma band unit activity and population responses in the pedunculopontine nucleus. *J. Neurophysiol.* 104, 463–474. doi: 10.1152/jn.00242.2010

Sławińska, U., and Kasicki, S. (1995).Theta-like rhythm in depth EEG activity of hypothalamic areas during spontaneous or electrically induced locomotion in the rat. *Brain Res.* 678, 117–126. doi: 10.1016/0006-8993(95)00174-o

Sławińska, U., and Kasicki, S. (1998). The frequency of rat's hippocampal theta rhythm is related to the speed of locomotion. *Brain Res.* 796, 327–331. doi: 10.1016/s0006-8993(98)00390-4

Sławińska, U., Majczyński, H., and Djavadian, R. (2000). Recovery of hindlimb notor functions after spinal cord transection is enhanced by grafts of the embryonic raphe nuclei. *Exp. Brain Res.* 132, 27–38. doi: 10.1007/s002219900323

Steeves, J. D., and Jordan, L. M. (1984). Autoradiographic demonstration of the projections from the mesencephalic locomotor region. *Brain Res.* 307, 263–276. doi: 10.1016/0006-8993(84)90480-3

Stefani, A., Lozano, A. M., Peppe, A., Stanzione, P., Galati, S., Tropepi, D., et al. (2007). Bilateral deep brain stimulation of the pedunculopontine and subthalamic nuclei in severe Parkinson's disease. *Brain* 130, 1596–1607. doi: 10.1093/brain/awl346

Takakusaki, K. (2008). Forebrain control of locomotor behaviors. *Brain Res. Rev.* 57, 192–198. doi: 10.1016/j.brainresrev.2007.06.024

Takakusaki, K. (2013). Neurophysiology of gait: from the spinal cord to the frontal lobe. *Mov. Disord.* 28, 1483–1491. doi: 10.1002/mds.25669

Takakusaki, K., Chiba, R., Nozu, T., and Okumura, T. (2016). Brainstem control of locomotion and muscle tone with special reference to the role of the mesopontine tegmentum and medullary reticulospinal systems. *J. Neural Transm. (Vienna)* 123, 695–729. doi: 10.1007/s00702-015-1475-4

Takakusaki, K., Takahashi, K., Saitoh, K., Harada, H., Okumura, T., Kayama, Y., et al. (2005). Orexinergic projections to the cat midbrain mediate alternation of emotional behavioural states from locomotion to cataplexy. *J. Physiol.* 568, 1003–1020. doi: 10.1113/jphysiol.2005.085829

Tattersall, T. L., Stratton, P. G., Coyne, T. J., Cook, R., Silberstein, P., Silburn, P. A., et al. (2014). Imagined gait modulates neuronal network dynamics in the human pedunculopontine nucleus. *Nat. Neurosci.* 17, 449–454. doi: 10.1038/nn.3642

Thevathasan, W., Pogosyan, A., Hyam, J. A., Jenkinson, N., Foltynie, T., Limousin, P., et al. (2012). Alpha oscillations in the pedunculopontine nucleus correlate with gait performance in parkinsonism. *Brain* 135, 148–160. doi: 10.1093/brain/awr315

Thompson, J. A., Lanctin, D., Ince, N. F., and Abosch, A. (2014). Clinical implications of local field potentials for understanding and treating movement disorders. *Stereotact. Funct. Neurosurg.* 92, 251–263. doi: 10.1159/000364913

Tort, A. B., Kramer, M. A., Thorn, C., Gibson, D. J., Kubota, Y., Graybiel, A. M., et al. (2008). Dynamic cross-frequency couplings of local field potential oscillations in rat striatum and hippocampus during performance of a T-maze task. *Proc. Natl. Acad. Sci. U S A* 105, 20517–20522. doi: 10.1073/pnas.0810524105

Tsang, E. W., Hamani, C., Moro, E., Mazzella, F., Poon, Y. Y., Lozano, A. M., et al. (2010). Involvement of the human pedunculopontine nucleus region in voluntary movements. *Neurology* 75, 950–959. doi: 10.1212/wnl.0b013e3181f25b35

Udupa, K., and Chen, R. (2015). The mechanisms of action of deep brain stimulation and ideas for the future development. *Prog. Neurobiol.* 133, 27–49. doi: 10.1016/j.pneurobio.2015.08.001

Vianna, D. M., Borelli, K. G., Ferreira-Netto, C., Macedo, C. E., and Brandao, M. L. (2003). Fos-like immunoreactive neurons following electrical stimulation of the dorsal periaqueductal gray at freezing and escape thresholds. *Brain Res. Bull.* 62, 179–189. doi: 10.1016/j.brainresbull.2003.09.010

Weinberger, M., Hamani, C., Hutchison, W. D., Moro, E., Lozano, A. M., and Dostrovsky, J. O. (2008). Pedunculopontine nucleus microelectrode recordings in movement disorder patients. *Exp. Brain Res.* 188, 165–174. doi: 10.1007/s00221-008-1349-1

Welter, M. L., Demain, A., Ewenczyk, C., Czernecki, V., Lau, B., El Helou, A., et al. (2015). PPNa-DBS for gait and balance disorders in Parkinson's disease: a double-blind, randomised study. *J. Neurol.* 262, 1515–1525. doi: 10.1007/s00415-015-7744-1

Whelan, P. J. (1996). Control of locomotion in the decerebrate cat. *Prog. Neurobiol.* 49, 481–515. doi: 10.1016/0301-0082(96)00028-7

Winn, P. (2006). How best to consider the structure and function of the pedunculopontine tegmental nucleus: evidence from animal studies. *J. Neurol. Sci.* 248, 234–250. doi: 10.1016/j.jns.2006.05.036

Xiang, H. B., Zhu, W. Z., Guan, X. H., and Ye, D. W. (2013). The cuneiform nucleus may be involved in the regulation of skeletal muscle tone by motor pathway: a virally mediated trans-synaptic tracing study in surgically sympathectomized mice. *Brain* 136:e251. doi: 10.1093/brain/awt123

16

Rapid Alleviation of Parkinson's Disease Symptoms via Electrostimulation of Intrinsic Auricular Muscle Zones

Yusuf O. Cakmak[1], Hülya Apaydin[2], Güneş Kiziltan[2], Ayşegül Gündüz[2], Burak Ozsoy[3], Selim Olcer[4], Hakan Urey[4], Ozgur O. Cakmak[5], Yasemin G. Ozdemir[5] and Sibel Ertan[2]*

[1] Department of Anatomy, School of Medical Sciences, Otago University, Dunedin, New Zealand, [2] Department of Neurology, Cerrahpasa School of Medicine, Istanbul University, Istanbul, Turkey, [3] Global Dynamic Systems (GDS) ARGE, Teknopark Istanbul, Istanbul, Turkey, [4] Department of Electrical Engineering, College of Engineering, Koç University, Istanbul, Turkey, [5] Department of Neurology, School of Medicine, Koç University, Istanbul, Turkey

***Correspondence:**
Yusuf O. Cakmak
yusuf.cakmak@otago.ac.nz

Background: Deep brain stimulation of the subthalamic nucleus (STN-DBS) and the pedunculopontine nucleus (PPN) significantly improve cardinal motor symptoms and postural instability and gait difficulty, respectively, in Parkinson's disease (PD).

Objective and Hypothesis: Intrinsic auricular muscle zones (IAMZs) allow the potential to simultaneously stimulate the C2 spinal nerve, the trigeminal nerve, the facial nerve, and sympathetic and parasympathetic nerves in addition to providing muscle feedback and control areas including the STN, the PPN and mesencephalic locomotor regions. Our aim was to observe the clinical responses to IAMZ stimulation in PD patients.

Method: Unilateral stimulation of an IAMZ, which includes muscle fibers for proprioception, the facial nerve, and C2, trigeminal and autonomic nerve fibers, at 130 Hz was performed in a placebo- and sham-controlled, double-blinded, within design, two-armed study of 24 PD patients.

Results: The results of the first arm (10 patients) of the present study demonstrated a substantial improvement in Unified Parkinson's Disease Ratings Scale (UPDRS) motor scores due to 10 min of IAMZ electrostimulation ($p = 0.0003$, power: 0.99) compared to the placebo control ($p = 0.130$). A moderate to large clinical difference in the improvement in UPDRS motor scores was observed in the IAMZ electrostimulation group. The results of the second arm (14 patients) demonstrated significant improvements with dry needling ($p = 0.011$) and electrostimulation of the IAMZ ($p < 0.001$) but not with sham electrostimulation ($p = 0.748$). In addition, there was a significantly greater improvement in UPDRS motor scores in the IAMZ electrostimulation group compared to the IAMZ dry needling group ($p < 0.001$) and the sham electrostimulation ($p < 0.001$) groups. The improvement in UPDRS motor scores of the IAMZ electrostimulation group (ΔUPDRS = 5.29) reached moderate to high clinical significance, which was not the case for the dry needling group (ΔUPDRS = 1.54). In addition, both arms of the study demonstrated bilateral improvements in motor symptoms in response to unilateral IAMZ electrostimulation.

Conclusion: The present study is the first demonstration of a potential role of IAMZ electrical stimulation in improving the clinical motor symptoms of PD patients in the short term.

Keywords: Parkinson's disease, electrostimulation, auricular muscles, PPN, STN, mesencephalon, locomotor, neuromodulation

INTRODUCTION

Bilateral high-frequency stimulation of the subthalamic nucleus (STN), commonly known as deep brain stimulation of the STN (STN-DBS), provides a significant improvement in cardinal motor symptoms and in the control of drug-induced complications of Parkinson's disease (PD). To be clinically effective, stimulation of the STN must be applied at frequencies greater than 100 Hz (Limousin et al., 1995; Limousin et al., 1997), and electrostimulation is usually delivered at 130 Hz (Little and Brown, 2012). Effective stimulation was shown to be associated with a significant decrease in the activity of the ipsilateral primary sensorimotor cortex at rest and a significant increase in premotor, anterior cingulate, pre-supplementary motor areas (pre-SMAs) and dorsolateral prefrontal cortices during movement (Payoux et al., 2004). On the other hand, axial symptoms, such postural instability and gait difficulty (PIGD), freezing of gait, and impaired speech, have been reported to be resistant to STN-DBS and levodopa treatments (Hamani et al., 2007; Tattersall et al., 2014). Recent clinical results have indicated the potential effectiveness of deep brain stimulation of the pedunculopontine nucleus (PPN-DBS) on PGID (Hamani et al., 2007; Tattersall et al., 2014). It has been demonstrated that lesions of the PPN induce gait deficits (Karachi et al., 2010; Tattersall et al., 2014). Moreover, cholinergic cell loss in the caudal PPN is accompanied by PIGD (Hirsch et al., 1987; Zweig et al., 1989; Karachi et al., 2010; Tattersall et al., 2014). Therefore, PIGD is thought to be related to the mesencephalic locomotor region rather than dopaminergic motor centers such as the STN (Garcia-Rill, 1991). The major components of the mesencephalic locomotor region are the PPN and the cuneiform nucleus (Garcia-Rill, 1991). In the context of different outcomes of STN-DBS and PPN-DBS, PPN dysfunction likely contributes to PIGD in PD (Tykocki et al., 2011). The PPN receives direct inputs from the pre-SMA and the basal ganglion to modulate muscle tone by directly exciting pontine reticular formation (Burn, 2013). Central pattern generators in the spinal cord can also be modulated directly and indirectly by the PPN (**Figure 1B**). Notably, sensory proprioceptive afferents have also been demonstrated to modify these patterns (Jankowska et al., 1983; Takakusaki et al., 2008; Burn, 2013).

Although altered proprioception is not a prominent symptom of PD, proprioception deficits have been reported in PD patients (Lee et al., 2013), and improvements in proprioception have been reported with STN stimulation (Lee et al., 2013). Selective muscle afferent nerve stimulation has been reported to cause significant activation in motor-related areas compared with cutaneous stimuli (Wardman et al., 2014). Muscle afferent stimulation evokes more widespread cortical, subcortical, and cerebellar activations than cutaneous afferents (Wardman et al., 2014). Separate precentral and post-central excitation foci were observed with muscle afferent stimulation, emphasizing the importance of muscle afferent nerve stimulation in the modulation of cortical motor areas (Wardman et al., 2014). Therefore, peripheral nerve stimulation may also hold the potential as an alternative and minimally invasive approach to modulate the activity in the premotor, anterior cingulate, pre-SMA and dorsolateral prefrontal cortices and basal ganglia such as the STN and the PPN and should be investigated in PD. Median nerve stimulation has been shown to result in the activation of STN neurons, which form a motor homunculus (Nambu et al., 1996, 1997, 2000; Hanajima et al., 2004). In theory, stimulation of other peripheral motor nerves may also activate motor homunculus of the STN.

Upper facial muscles around the orbital region are controlled bilaterally by the motor cortex through the facial nerve (Mima et al., 1999). In addition, unilateral STN-DBS has been demonstrated to induce strictly contralateral motor-evoked potentials in the trapezius, deltoid, biceps, and thenar muscles; however, the same stimulus reportedly always induces bilateral motor-evoked potentials in the orbicularis oculi, orbicularis oris, masseter, and sternocleidomastoid in Parkinson's patients (Costa et al., 2007). The intrinsic auricular muscles of the tragicus and antitragicus muscles have also been shown to simultaneously contract with the orbicularis oculi muscles (Matsuo and Hirose, 1987). The latter demonstration is also indirect proof of bilateral cortical connections of intrinsic auricular muscles, such as in the orbicularis oculi.

In the context of these anatomical relationships, unilateral stimulation of the intrinsic auricular muscle zones (IAMZs) may hold potential for bilateral feedback stimulation of muscle feedback and motor driver cortical areas. In addition to the possible proprioceptive outcomes of IAMZ stimulation, contributions of the facial nerve branches stimulating the intrinsic auricular muscles (Fujita, 1934; Matsuo and Hirose, 1987), the vagus nerve via the Arnold branch as a parasympathetic contribution (Alvord and Farmer, 1997; Peuker and Filler, 2002), the trigeminal nerve via the auriculotemporal nerve branch (Alvord and Farmer, 1997; Peuker and Filler, 2002) and the C2 spinal nerve within the great auricular nerve (Alvord and Farmer, 1997; Peuker and Filler, 2002) to IAMZ have been demonstrated in the literature (**Figure 1A**). In addition, cervical sympathetic nerves are distributed to the auricula within the ear arteries (Daniel and Paton, 1975; Lambru et al., 2013) (**Figure 1A**). Therefore, stimulation of the IAMZ has the potential for synchronous stimulation of the C2 spinal nerve, the trigeminal nerve, and sympathetic and parasympathetic nerves (**Figure 1A**), each of which may contribute to motor regulation.

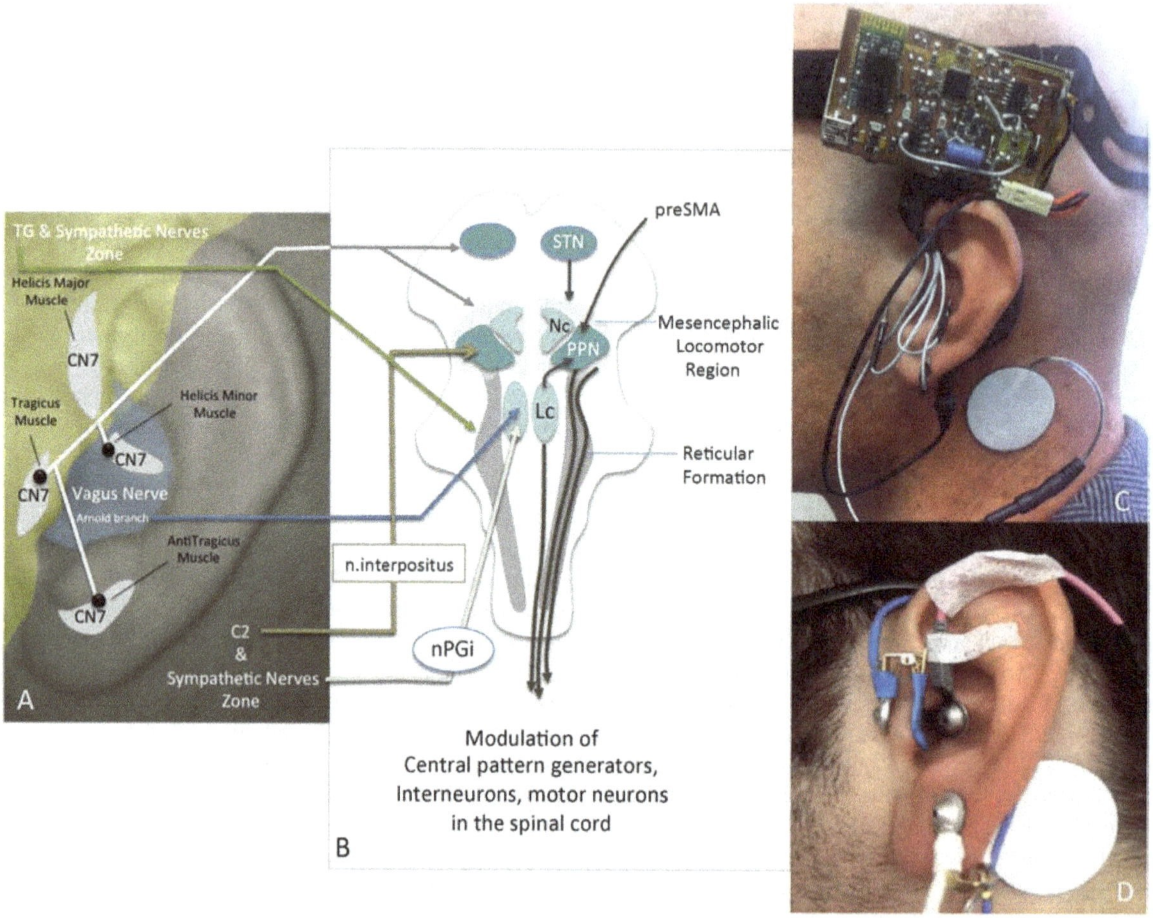

FIGURE 1 | (A) Innervation of the ear, the IAMZs and IAMZ electrode locations (black dots); **(B)** relevant anatomical pathways of IAMZs via auricular nerves for motion regulation and mesencephalic locomotor regions (modified from Burn, 2013); **(C)** active stimulation with needle electrodes of the IAMZ and with TENS electrode of the SCM; **(D)** placebo group TENS electrode placements in the IAMZ and SCM; CN7, facial nerve; C2, C2 spinal nerve; TG, trigeminal nerve; Nc, nucleus cuneatus; Lc, locus coerulei; nPGi, nucleus paragigantocellularis; STN, subthalamic nucleus; PPN, pedunculopontine nucleus. *Yellow zone*: trigeminal nerve + sympathetic nerve zone; *Gray zone*: C2 + sympathetic nerve zone; *White areas*: intrinsic auricular muscles zones. *Blue area*: Arnold branch of the vagus nerve, C2, CN7, and sympathetic nerves overlapping zone.

It has been demonstrated that the C2 spinal nerve forms anatomical connections with the deep cerebellar nucleus of the interpositus (represented by the nucleus globosus and the emboliformis in humans) in animals (Matsushita and Xiong, 2001). The interpositus has projections to the PPN and from the PPN to the STN (Schell and Strick, 1984; Hazrati and Parent, 1992; Lavoie and Parent, 1994; Harting, 1997; McFarland and Haber, 2000; Muthusamy et al., 2007). In addition, the C2-interpositus nucleus-PPN-reticulospinal axis may play a cardinal role in motion and position regulation: a substantial body of evidence suggests that the reticulospinal system is essential and plays a fundamental role in the integration of commands for whole-body movement and postural adjustment rather than the movement of a single limb (Magni and Willis, 1964; Keizer and Kuypers, 1984, 1989; Drew and Rossignol, 1990; Luccarini et al., 1990; Drew, 1991; Massion, 1992; Mori et al., 1992; Kably and Drew, 1998; Schepens and Drew, 2003) (**Figure 1B**). Of note, the reticulospinal system is also directly excited by the PPN and mediates DBS-PPN to modulate muscle tone in PD patients (Burn, 2013) (**Figure 1B**). In addition to the potential effects of the C2 spinal nerve on the reticulospinal system via the interpositus nucleus-PPN axis, the mesencephalic trigeminal nucleus as the principal nucleus of the facial muscles' proprioceptive center, projects to the reticular formation and to the spinal cord via propriospinal neurons (Lawrence and Kuypers, 1968; Gorska and Sybirska, 1980; Alstermark et al., 1981, 1989; Hobbs et al., 1992; Usunoff et al., 1997; Whishaw et al., 1998; Sasaki, 2004; Jankowska and Edgley, 2006) (**Figures 1A,B**). This connection also underlines the potential role of intrinsic auricular muscle proprioception feedback on reticular formation and the possible influences on movement and posture, in addition to C2-related pathways, on reticular formation and propriospinal neurons. The C2 spinal nerve projects to the lower ear lobe and the corresponding skin that overlays the intrinsic muscles of the antitragicus muscle by the greater auricular nerve and the trigeminal nerve; its auriculotemporal branch innervates the skin areas over the tragicus and helicis major muscles (Matsuo and Hirose, 1987; Alvord and Farmer, 1997; Peuker and Filler, 2002; Lambru et al., 2013; Drake et al., 2015) (**Figure 1A**).

In addition to the possible indirect autonomic effects of IAMZ stimulation via the C2 nerve, autonomic fibers of the auricula also directly contribute to these zones. While the sympathetic nerves overlay the IAMZ within the arterial walls, the Arnold branch of the vagus nerve is distributed only over the helicis minor muscle zone (Matsuo and Hirose, 1987; Alvord and Farmer, 1997; Peuker and Filler, 2002; Lambru et al., 2013; Drake et al., 2015) (**Figure 1A**). Thus far, no neuromodulation studies of the Arnold branch or neurotraces of the efferent connections of the Arnold branch have considered the existence of the helicis minor muscle in the concha area where the Arnold branch is distributed.

The earliest accumulation of α-synuclein and Lewy bodies have been shown to occur in the dorsal motor nucleus of the vagus nerve in PD (Braak et al., 2003). A recent study also showed that chronic impairment of vagus nerve function leads to inhibition of dopamine and that low frequency stimulation of the vagus nerve significantly inhibited the dopamine system in rat brain structures (Ziomber et al., 2012). It is worth noting that low- and high-frequency electrostimulation induce opposite outcomes on the autonomic nerve system and neurotransmitters (Cakmak et al., 2008, 2016; Zhao, 2008), so that high frequency of stimulation may result with the stimulation of the dopaminergic system.

In the context of the demonstrated structural and functional anatomical connections of the IAMZ and the underlined mechanisms of deep brain stimulation studies in PD, the IAMZ is the only potential auricular zone to synchronously stimulate the C2 spinal nerve, the trigeminal nerve, autonomic nerve fibers and proprioceptive centers to modulate motor modulatory centers including mesencephalic locomotor region. We hypothesized that the stimulation of IAMZ would be beneficial to alleviate the PD motor symptoms. A clinical trial is designed to investigate the potential clinical outcomes (motor symptoms) of the IAMZ stimulation in PD patients. We stimulated the IAMZ (which includes the helicis minor, tragicus, and antitragicus muscles) unilaterally (ipsilateral to the dominant PD symptoms) at a high frequency and analyzed the efficacy of this technique on 24 PD patients via a double-blind, placebo- and sham controlled within-subject design, two-armed study.

MATERIALS AND METHODS

All subjects provided written informed consent to undergo the procedure. The study was approved by the Ethics Committee of the Koç University, Turkey, and it was carried out in accordance with the Ethical Principles for Medical Research Involving Human (Declaration of Helsinki).

Koç University Clinical Trials Ethics Committee Approval Number: 2015.091.IRB1.018,
ClinicalTrials.gov Identifier: NCT02722824,
Turkey Ministry of Health: Follow up number - 133235.

Research Participants

Ten volunteer patients with idiopathic PD who had been followed in our movement disorders outpatient clinic were enrolled for the first arm of the study. Another 14 volunteer patients with idiopathic PD with the same criteria were enrolled for the second arm of the study. PD diagnoses were made by a neurologist who was an expert in movement disorders using the UK Parkinson's Disease Society Brain Bank clinical diagnostic criteria (Hughes et al., 1992).

All patients underwent a detailed neurological examination, and parkinsonian features were rated according to the Unified Parkinson's Disease Rating Scale (UPDRS) Part III. Patients with a disease duration longer than 2 years and Hoehn and Yahr stage $\geq$ 2 were included. Patients with cognitive impairment that might prevent cooperation during tests and patients with any other neurological or systemic disease in which electrostimulation was contraindicated were excluded.

Electrostimulation and Analysis of Symptoms

Arm 1 [10 patients – 10 min of electrostimulation of the IAMZ with needle electrodes and 10 min of placebo using transcutaneous electrodes (TENS) for IAMZ]: two movement disorder specialists blind to the nature of stimulation rated all patients twice according to the motor section of the UPDRS just before the stimulation (baseline evaluation) and 10 min after the onset of stimulation or placebo application. The patients and two movement disorder specialists were informed that there would be two modes of stimulation, sub-threshold stimulation with TENS of the IAMZ (placebo group, **Figure 1D**) and above the sensory threshold with needle electrodes of the IAMZ (active group, **Figure 1C**). In the placebo-control application in which there was no stimulation and the device was in off mode, the patients and two movement disorder specialists were informed that a new device would be placed on the ear to improve their motor symptoms and that they would not sense the stimulation of the device because of the sub-threshold stimulation of the IAMZ via the TENS. In the active group, the patients and two movement disorder specialists were informed that the stimulation would be above the sensory threshold and applied via the needle electrodes to the IAMZ. In both groups, there was a TENS electrode on the sternocleidomastoid muscle (SCM) (**Figures 1C,D**). The consort flow chart (**Figure 2**) demonstrates the study design in the first arm.

Arm 2 [14 patients – 20 min of stimulation in three sessions: electrostimulation of the IAMZ with needles, needling of the IAMZ without electrostimulation (dry needling) and sham region electrostimulation with needles]: the main aims of the second arm of the study were to assess the following:

- a potential effect of dry needling on the IAMZ without electrostimulation (dry needling of the IAMZ zones without electrostimulation but keeping the needle electrodes connected with to the electrostimulator),
- the potential effect of stimulation of only the C2/sympathetic nerve by ensuring no or minimal

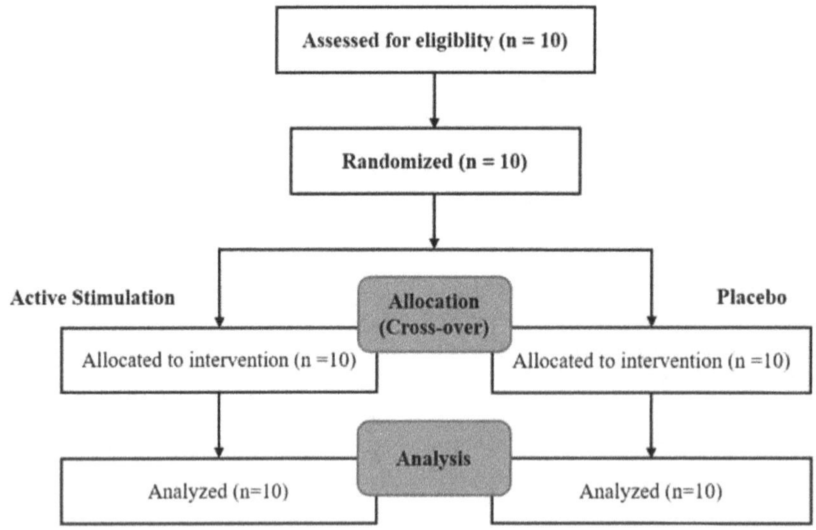

FIGURE 2 | The consort flow chart of the first arm of the study.

stimulation of the SCM, the vagus facial nerve and the trigeminal nerve (sham stimulation),
- the specificity of the IAMZ zone electrostimulation (active group-IAMZ electrostimulation),
- the sole specificity of 130 Hz stimulation (sham stimulation zone),
- a potential long-term effect of the stimulation (50th-minute).

In the second arm of the study, the stimulation duration proceeded to the 20th-minute, and patients were assessed at the 50th-minute (30 min after the termination of 20-min stimulation). The two movement disorder specialists who participated in the first arm and who were blind to the nature of stimulation rated all ($n = 24$) patients twice according to the motor section of the UPDRS.

The two movement disorder specialists were blinded to the type of stimulation by covering the entire auricula with cotton pads, including the needle electrodes (**Figure 3A**). Patients were also informed that there would be three modes of stimulation: sub-threshold stimulation with needles (dry needling of the IAMZ without electrostimulation but with the needles connected to stimulator as in the needle electrostimulation group, **Figure 1C**) and electrostimulation with needle electrodes above the sensory threshold at two different auricular zones (electrostimulation with needle electrodes on the IAMZ **Figure 1C** and a sham region **Figure 3B**). These groups ensured that the patients were blind to the active stimulation group. A part of the upper helix that is innervated by C2/sympathetic nerves but free or with minimal contributions of the SCM, vagal, facial, and trigeminal nerves was selected as the sham electrostimulation region (**Figure 3B**). The consort flow chart in **Figure 4** demonstrates the study flow in the second arm.

Stimulation Procedure

All examinations and electrostimulations were performed during "off" periods of the patients (when the effect of the dopaminergic drug was minimal). We designed and built an electrical signal generator with a changeable voltage output (0–5 V), frequency (2–300 Hz) and pulse length (50–200 μs) with external electrodes able to be connected to press needles (KINGLI, China) placed on the three intrinsic auricular muscles (tragicus, antitragicus, and helicis minor muscles). While the needle electrodes were placed on the IAMZ (**Figure 1C**) in the active stimulation and dry needling groups and over the upper helix in the sham stimulation group (**Figure 3B**), the transcutaneous electrode was placed on the SCM 1-2 cm to its mastoid origin (**Figure 1C**) near the electrical stimulation circuit. In the sham group, the transcutaneous electrode was placed but remained inactive to keep the electrical field of stimulation in the selected helix region for C2/sympathetic nerve stimulation. It was also placed and kept inactive in the dry needling group to maintain observer blindness.

The SCM was chosen for surface electrode placement for three reasons:

(1) STN contribution: bilateral SCM activation has been reported during unilateral STN stimulation, which underlines the bilateral STN connections to each SCM (Costa et al., 2007).
(2) Nucleus cuneatus contribution: the mesencephalic locomotor region has two major components: the PPN and the nucleus cuneatus. SCM proprioception projects to the nucleus cuneatus as the neck muscle proprioception center [6] and as a mesencephalic locomotor component (Garcia-Rill, 1991) (**Figure 1B**).
(3) C2 spinal nerve contribution: the skin over the SCM (1–2 cm to its mastoid origin) is also innervated by the C2 spinal nerve (Matsuo and Hirose, 1987; Alvord and Farmer, 1997;

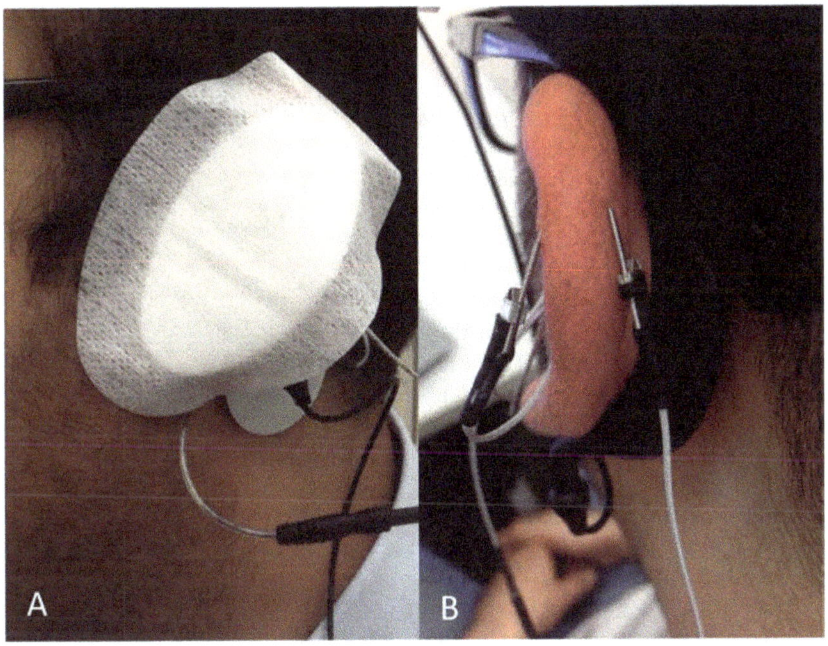

FIGURE 3 | (A) A pad covered the ear to ensure observer blindness in the groups of the second arm of the study. **(B)** Sham stimulation zone needle electrode placement.

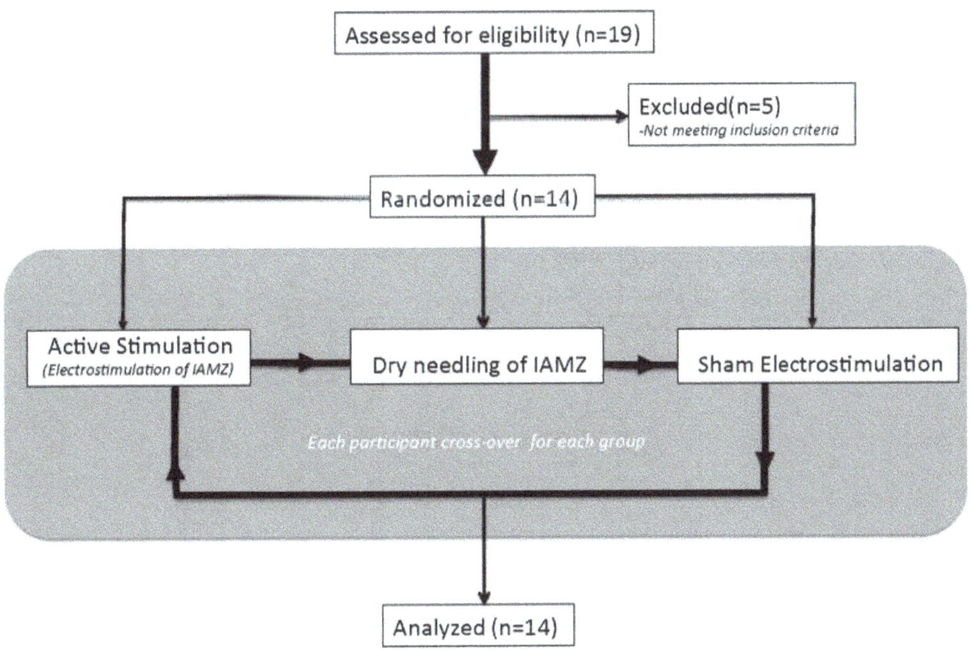

FIGURE 4 | The consort flow chart of the second arm of the study.

Peuker and Filler, 2002; Lambru et al., 2013; Drake et al., 2015) (**Figure 1A**).

In the present study, we used a biphasic wave-form and a stimulation style that alternated the anode and cathode for each stimulus during the stimulation period such that the needle electrodes on the intrinsic auricular muscles and the surface electrode on the SCM served as both the anode and cathode in an alternating manner. Given the much larger contact surface of the transcutaneous electrode compared with the needle electrodes and taking into account the difference in the skin conductance between the needle electrode and the transcutaneous electrode in addition to the low power of the stimulus, the transcutaneous electrode on the SCM would have a minimal impact on the stimulation-related outcomes.

Auricular electrical stimulation was applied with the following STN-DBS parameters: 130 Hz with a wavelength of 100 μs and an intensity just under the pain threshold (1-4 V). The stimulation was administered unilaterally (ipsilateral to the side of prominent symptoms). We did not set a power (V) for the stimulation because such an approach does not eliminate the probability of current differences due to skin conductance differences in different subjects or within subjects during different sessions. To overcome this possible problem, the electrostimulator contained a built-in current-control feature so that the current was stabilized in the range of 100–130 μÅ during the stimulation period by modulating the power and ensuring that the tingling sensation was under the pain threshold. This approach overcomes the interindividual and intraindividual (in active and control sessions) differences in skin conductance.

In addition to the traditional approach of taking into account the dominant symptom side scores of lateralized subitems (items 20–26) for the UPDRS Part-III motor scale scoring, the scores of lateralized subitems on both sides (ipsilateral and contralateral to the dominant symptoms and to the stimulator) were also documented to reveal any potential effects of unilateral stimulation over the bilateral motor symptoms. Moreover, subscores of the UPDRS Part-III were also classified and analyzed as Tremor (items 20–21), Rigidity (item 22), Bradykinesia (items 23–26,31), Gait and Postural Stability (items 27–30) and Bulbar Anomalies (items 18–19), as in previous studies (Postuma et al., 2008). All statistical analyses were performed using Student's paired *t*-tests (Prism 7 demo version, GraphPad Software, Inc., La Jolla, CA, United States, 2016). In addition, the Bonferroni correction was also applied as a conservative approach for the subscore group analysis [$n = 2$ (active and placebo), $p < 0.025$ in Arm 1, and $n = 3$ (active, dry needling, and sham), $p < 0.016$ in Arm 2]. The second arm of the study, which included three groups, also analyzed via analysis of variance (ANOVA) for group comparisons.

RESULTS

Arm 1

The mean age of the patients was 55.7 ±SD 7.8 years, and only one patient was female. The mean disease duration was 8.3 ±SD 4.4 years. Detailed clinical features of the patients are presented in **Table 1**.

There were no statistically significant differences between the baseline UPDRS motor scores of the patients in the active and placebo groups ($p = 0.735$). The UPDRS motor scores showed a statistically significant improvement 10 min after auricular stimulation compared with baseline UPDRS scores ($p = 0.0003$, power: 0.99). The placebo group did not show statistically significant differences in UPDRS motor scores compared with baseline ($p = 0.130$). At the 10th-minute, the mean improvement rates were 35% (ΔUPDRS = 5.9) in the active group [mean UPDRS motor scores: 17.0 at baseline, 11.1

TABLE 1 | Detailed clinical features of the patients in the first arm of the study.

	Patient 1	Patient 2	Patient 3	Patient 4	Patient 5	Patient 6	Patient 7	Patient 8	Patient 9	Patient 10
Age (years)	61	46	55	48	54	48	61	71	52	61
Gender	F	M	M	M	M	M	M	M	M	M
Dominant hand	R	R	R	R	R	R	R	R	R	R
Affected side at onset	Right	Left	Right	Right	Right	Left	Left	Right	Right	Right
Symptoms at onset	UE BK, R > Tr	UE BK, R	UE BK > Tr	UE and LE BK	UE BK, R > Tr	LE BK	UE and LE Tr	UE Tr	UE BK	UE Tr
PD type	Akinetic rigidity	Akinetic rigidity	Akinetic rigidity	Akinetic rigidity	Akinetic rigidity	Akinetic rigidity	Tremor dominant	Tremor dominant	Akinetic rigidity	Tremor dominant
PD duration (years)	12	4	8	12	6	8	6	17	2	8
Wearing off	+	+	+	+	+	+	+	+	−	+
Dyskinesia	+	+	+	+	−	+	−	+	−	+
Medication	LDED: 1100 mg/day, Amantadine	LDED: 500 mg/day, Amantadine	LDED: 700 mg/day, Amantadine	LDED: 600 mg/day, Amantadine	LDED: 650 mg/day, Amantadine, Rasagiline	LDED: 800 mg/day, Rasagiline	LDED: 1025 mg/day	LDED: 950 mg/day, Amantadine	LDED: 450 mg/day, Rasagiline	LDED: 1100 mg/day, Amantadine
H&Y stage	3	3	2	2	2	2	2	2	2	3

F, female; M, male; R, right; L, left; UE, upper extremity; LE, lower extremity; BK, bradykinesia; R, rigidity; Tr, tremor; PD, Parkinson's disease; LDED, levodopa equivalent dose; H&Y, Hoehn and Yahr.

at the 10th-minute, standard deviation (SD): 3.6 at baseline and 4.6 at the 10th-minute, ΔUPDRS range = 1.5–12] and 5% (ΔUPDRS = 1) in the placebo-control group (mean UPDRS motor scores: 17.4 at baseline, 16.4 at the 10th-minute, *SD*: 4.6 at baseline and 4.5 at the 10th-minute, ΔUPDRS range = −1.5–4.5).

Figure 5 shows the UPDRS Part-III scores and the group comparison for each case and an overall summary of the first arm. **Figure 6** summarizes the classified UPDRS subscore differences for the group comparisons with *t*-tests, **Figure 7** gives these differences for the group comparisons after the Bonferroni correction. **Table 2** summarizes the *p*-values for the *t*-tests and after the Bonferroni correction of the classified UPDRS subscores for the 10th-minute compared with baseline.

The bilateral assessments of the symptomatic improvements of PD patients before and after electrical stimulation revealed that unilateral stimulation of the intrinsic auricular muscles can relieve PD symptoms on both sides at the 10th-minute. The 10th-minute mean improvements in the lateralized (UPDRS Part III subscore 20–26) UPDRS motor subscores were 3.0 on the contralateral side and 3.2 on the ipsilateral side in the active

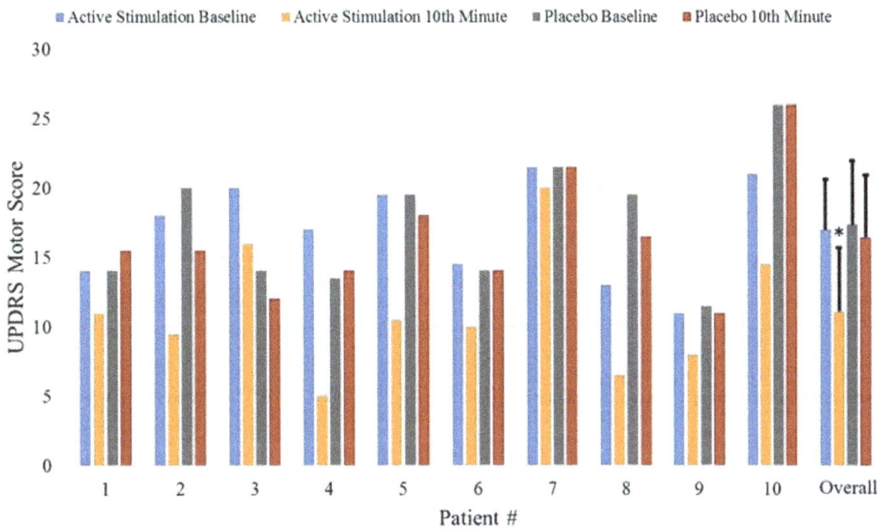

FIGURE 5 | The UPDRS part III scores at baseline and at the 10th-minute for the placebo and active groups and overall comparisons of the first arm. *Statistically significant.

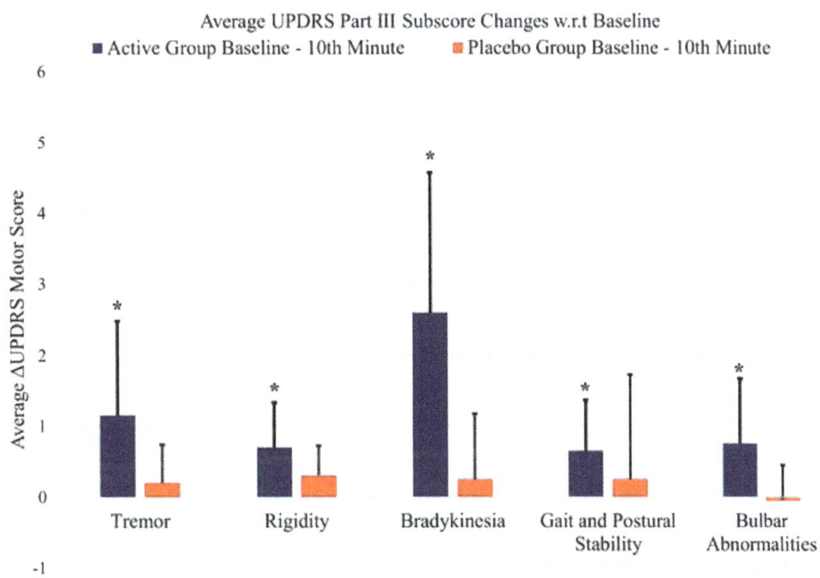

FIGURE 6 | The classified UPDRS subscore differences for group comparisons of the first arm ($p < 0.05$, *t*-test). *Statistically significant.

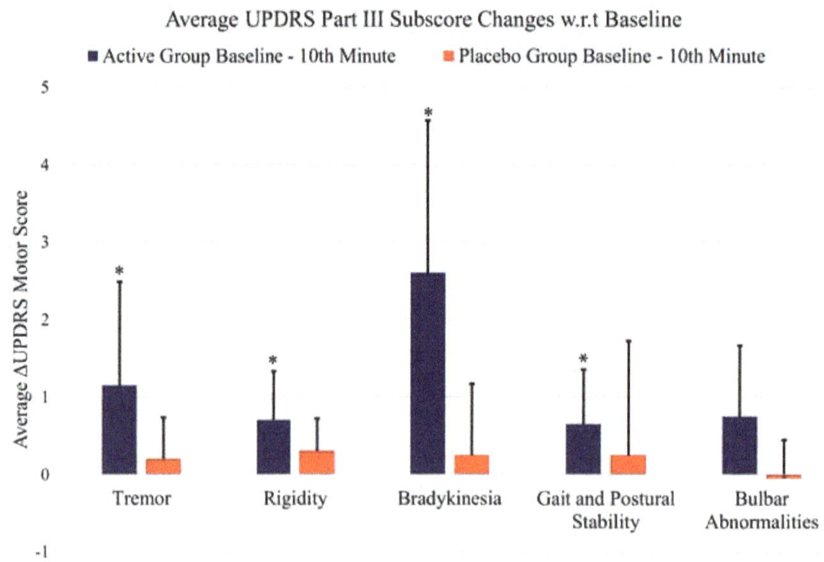

FIGURE 7 | The classified UPDRS subscore differences for group comparisons with Bonferroni correction. *Statistically significant.

TABLE 2 | The p-values after Bonferroni correction of the classified UPDRS subscores for the 10th-minute compared with baseline of the first arm study groups.

Subgroup	p-Value active group	p-Value placebo group
Tremor	***0.023***	0.398
Rigidity	***0.007***	0.051
Bradykinesia	***0.002***	0.413
Gait and postural instability	***0.018***	0.605
Bulbar abnormalities	*0.030*	0.758

t-test; $p < 0.05$, Bonferroni correction $p < 0.025$, Italic: significant in t-test, bold: significant after Bonferroni correction, bold and italic: significant in t-test and Bonferroni.

group. The 10th-minute difference in the lateralized UPDRS motor subscores in the placebo-control group were 0.5 on the contralateral side and 0.8 on the ipsilateral side.

Arm 2

The mean age of the patients was 58.1 ±SD 9.8 years, and 6 of the patients were female. The mean disease duration was 7.9 ±SD 3.7 years. Detailed clinical features of the patients are presented in **Table 3**. Baseline UPDRS motor scores of the three groups were compared via one-way repeated measures ANOVA. There were no statistically significant differences between the baseline UPDRS motor scores of the patients in the active (IAMZ electrostimulation), IAMZ dry needling and sham electrostimulation groups prior to the interventions (pairwise comparison p-values: active vs. dry needling: 0.286, active vs. sham: 0.052, sham vs. dry needling: 1.0).

In the active group, the UPDRS motor scores were significantly improved at the 50th-minute after the initiation of IAMZ electrostimulation (i.e., 30 min after the termination of the 20-min stimulation) compared with baseline UPDRS scores ($p < 0.001$, power: 0.99). The IAMZ dry needling group also showed statistically significant differences in UPDRS motor scores after the dry needling procedure compared with baseline ($p = 0.011$). However, the improvement in UPDRS motor scores of dry needling stimulation of the IAMZ (ΔUPDRS = 1.54) did not reach clinical significance (Shulman et al., 2010) as electrostimulation of the IAMZ (ΔUPDRS = 5.29). The improvement in the UPDRS score observed in the active group (electrostimulation of the IAMZ) was in the range of moderate to high clinical significance (Shulman et al., 2010). There was no significant difference in UPDRS motor scores in the sham electrostimulation group ($p = 0.748$).

The mean improvement rates at the 50th-minute were 31% (ΔUPDRS = 5.29) in the active group (mean UPDRS motor scores: 17.71 at baseline, 12.42 at the 50th-minute, *SD*: 4.27 at baseline and 4.61 at the 50th-minute, ΔUPDRS range = 0.50–9.50), 9% (ΔUPDRS = 1.54) in the dry needling group (mean UPDRS motor scores: 16.04 at baseline, 14.50 at the 50th-minute, *SD*: 3.1 at baseline and 3.3 at the 50th-minute, ΔUPDRS range = 0.50–7.0) and 0% (ΔUPDRS = 0.20) in the sham stimulation group (mean UPDRS motor scores: 15.25 at baseline, 15.05 at the 50th-minute, *SD*: 5.09 at baseline and 5.15 at the 50th-minute, ΔUPDRS range = −3.5 to 4.0).

One-way repeated measures ANOVA was also performed for the difference in each group's baseline and post-stimulation UPDRS scores (ΔUPDRS comparison). The ΔUPDRS comparison for the active vs. dry needling groups and the active vs. sham groups were significant ($p < 0.001$ for both comparisons); however, the comparison of ΔUPDRS for the sham vs. dry needling groups was not statistically significant ($p = 0.319$).

Figure 8 gives the UPDRS Part-III scores and the group comparison for each case and the overall summary of the second arm. **Figure 9** summarizes the classified UPDRS subscore

TABLE 3 | Detailed clinical features of the patients in the second arm of the study.

	Patient 1	Patient 2	Patient 3	Patient 4	Patient 5	Patient 6	Patient 7	Patient 8	Patient 9	Patient 10	Patient 11	Patient 12	Patient 13	Patient 14
Age (years)	56	47	63	58	54	70	64	45	71	45	63	72	45	60
Gender	M	F	M	F	M	F	M	F	M	F	F	M	M	M
Dominant hand	R	R	R	R	R	R	R	R	R	R	R	R	L	R
Affected side at onset	Right	Right	Right	Right	Right	Right	Left	Left	Right	Left	Right	Left	Right	Right
Symptoms at onset	UE BK	UE TR > BK	UE TR	UE TR > BK	UE TR	UE BK	UE BK	UE TR	UE BK	LE TR	LE TR	BK	TR	BK
PD type	Akinetic rigidity	Akinetic rigidity	Akinetic rigidity	Tremor dominant	Akinetic rigidity	Akinetic rigidity	Akinetic rigidity	Tremor dominant	Akinetic rigidity	Tremor dominant	Tremor dominant	Akinetic rigidity	Akinetic rigidity	Akinetic rigidity
PD duration (years)	7	10	8	15	9	8	1	4	5	8	4	13	8	10
Wearing off	+	+	−	+	+	+	−	−	−	−	−	−	+	−
Dyskinesia	−	+	+	−	+	+	−	−	−	−	+	+	−	+
Medication	LDED: 950 mg/day, Amantadine	LDED: 1200 mg/day, Amantadine	LDED: 300 mg/day, Amantadine	LDED: 1400 mg/day, Amantadine, Rasagiline	LDED: 1316.2 mg/day	LDED: 1000 mg/day	LDED: 500 mg/day	LDED: 940 mg/day, Rasagline	LDED: 660 mg/day	LDED: 840 mg/day	LDED: 800 mg/day	LDED: 850 mg/day, Amantadine	LDED:600 mg/day, Rasagline	LDED: 1162.5 mg/day
H&Y stage	2	2	2	2	3	3	2	2	2	2	2	2	2	2

F, female; M, male; R, right; L, left; UE, upper extremity; LE, lower extremity; BK, bradykinesia; R, rigidity; Tr, tremor; PD, Parkinson's disease; LDED, levodopa equivalent dose; H&Y, Hoehn and Yahr.

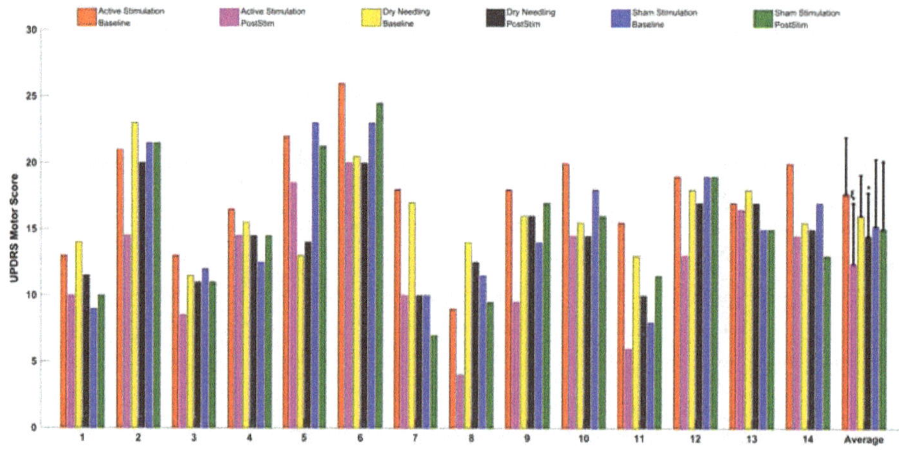

FIGURE 8 | The UPDRS part III scores at baseline and at the 50th-minute for the active group (electrostimulation of the IAMZ), IAMZ dry needling group, and sham stimulation group and overall comparisons of the second arm. *Statistically significant, ξstatistically and clinically significant.

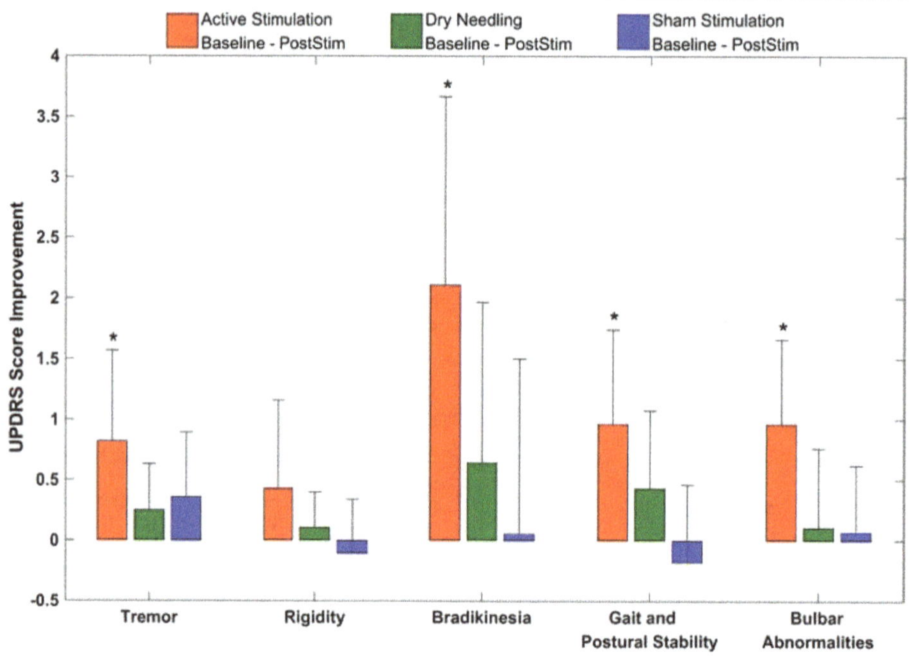

FIGURE 9 | The classified UPDRS subscore differences for group comparisons with Bonferroni correction of the second arm of the study. *Statistically significant.

differences in the group comparisons with Bonferroni correction. **Table 4** summarizes the *p*-values for *t*-tests and after Bonferroni correction of the classified UPDRS subscores for the 50th-minute compared with baseline.

Bilateral assessments of the symptomatic improvements of PD patients before and after electrical stimulation of the IAMZ revealed that unilateral stimulation of the intrinsic auricular muscles can relieve PD symptoms on both sides at the 50th-minute. The 50th-minute mean improvements in the lateralized (UPDRS Part III subscore 20–26) UPDRS motor subscores were 2.39 on the contralateral side and 1.89 on the ipsilateral side in the active group. The 50th-minute differences in the contralateral and ipsilateral UPDRS motor subscores were 0.79 and 0.61 in the dry needling group and 0.48 and 0.0 in the sham group, respectively.

DISCUSSION

The results of the present study demonstrated a substantial improvement in UPDRS motor scores after electrostimulation of the IAMZ but not after placebo or sham stimulation. The UPDRS score improvements in the electrostimulation of IAMZ groups were statistically and clinically significant. Comparison of the ΔUPDRS (5.9 in the first arm and 5.29 in the second arm) of

TABLE 4 | The *p*-values after Bonferroni correction of the classified UPDRS subscores for the 50th-minute compared with baseline of the second arm study groups.

	p-Values - Baseline vs. Post-stim		
Subgroup	**Active**	**Dry needling**	**Sham**
Tremor	***0.001***	*0.029*	*0.027*
Rigidity	*0.047*	0.189	0.385
Bradykinesia	***<0.001***	0.092	0.892
Gait and postural instability	***<0.001***	*0.028*	0.315
Bulbar abnormalities	***<0.001***	0.551	0.635

t-test; $p < 0.05$, Bonferroni correction $p < 0.016$. Italic: significant in t-test, bold: significant after Bonferroni correction, bold and italic: significant in t-test and Bonferroni.

the active groups considering the clinically important difference (CID) values described by Shulman et al. (ΔUPDRS 2.5, 5.2, and 10.8 for minimal, moderate, and large CIDs, respectively) indicated that the improvement in UPDRS scores obtained with electrostimulation of the IAMZ in the present study falls between a moderate and large CID (Shulman et al., 2010). In addition, dry needling of IAMZ group reached to a statistically significant improvement (but not a CID) in UPDRS scores which was not the case for the sham or placebo groups. The dry needling group results also underlined the significance of the IAMZ. Invasive deep brain stimulation modalities of neuromodulation utilize bilateral approaches to document UPDRS improvement rates. It must be noted that the results of the present study were obtained using only unilateral stimulation, and bilateral stimulation needs to be investigated.

In addition to UPDRS score improvements, the classified UPDRS subitem paired *t*-test analysis also demonstrated that symptomatic suppression for all subitem groups in both arms of the study, including tremor, rigidity, bradykinesia, gait and postural stability and bulbar abnormalities, were statistically significant for only the electrostimulation of IAMZ group. All of the other study groups were not statistically significant after *t*-test analysis for all of the subitem analysis.

The Bonferroni correction is a conservative approach that has advantages and disadvantages, especially for pilot studies. To clarify the outcomes of the conservative Bonferroni correction, we also performed analyses of the subscore groups. The suppression of tremor, rigidity, gait and postural stability and bradykinesia symptoms were still statistically significant after Bonferroni correction in the first arm of the study, and all subgroups (except rigidity) exhibited statistically significant reductions after bonferroni correction in the second arm of the study. In addition, although the improvements in bulbar abnormalities of the first arm and rigidity in the second arm were not statistically significant after the Bonferroni correction, there was a trend toward significance in both groups (p-crit: 0.025, *p*: 0.030 for bulbar abnormalities in arm 1; and p-crit: 0.016, *p*: 0.047 for rigidity in arm 2). Axial symptoms, including speech, have also been reported to worsen with DBS-STN (Tornqvist et al., 2005; Hammer et al., 2010; Moreau et al., 2011; Sidiropoulos et al., 2013). None of the subitems worsened in the active stimulation group in the present study, in contrast to other DBS-STN applications (Tornqvist et al., 2005; Hammer et al., 2010; Moreau et al., 2011; Sidiropoulos et al., 2013). On the other hand, DBS-PPN has been reported to induce greater improvements in PIGD (Hamani et al., 2007; Tykocki et al., 2011). In the context of the different outcomes of DBS-STN and DBS-PPN on motor symptoms and the outcomes in the present study, we suggest that the underlying mechanism of IAMZ stimulation may be related to PPN-associated pathways rather than STN-associated pathways or that both the STN and the PPN may be responsible for the observed effect; however, a sole contribution of the STN is not suggested.

The results of the bilateral assessments of the symptomatic improvements of PD patients before and after electrical stimulation of the IAMZ revealed that unilateral stimulation (ipsilateral to dominant, lateralized motor symptoms) of the IAMZ relieved PD symptoms on both sides of patients in both arms of this study. These improved contralateral motor symptoms may suggest a bihemispheric contribution of the intrinsic auricular muscles. Whether the stimulation of facial nerve branches over the intrinsic auricular muscles is solely responsible for all of the bilateral symptomatic improvements observed in this study or whether other nerves in the IAMZ also contribute remains unclear. The C2 spinal nerve may also play a role in bilateral symptomatic improvement. Although the C2-related role of the propriospinal tracts is more active on the ipsilateral side, animal studies demonstrated that C2 spinal nerves have ipsilateral and contralateral connections with the interpositus nucleus of the cerebellum (Matsushita and Xiong, 2001). As such, C2 spinal nerve stimulation may act on the bilateral PPN through bilateral cerebellar nuclei, and bilateral PPN stimulation may act on the bilateral reticulospinal tract to modulate bilateral motor symptoms. However, C2 zone stimulation in the sham group of the second arm was ineffective.

Autonomic nerve modulation may also contribute to the bilateral symptomatic relief observed in the present study. Low-frequency vagal nerve stimulation leads to impaired vagus nerve function and inhibition of the dopamine system in brain structures (Ziomber et al., 2012). Considering that low- and high-frequency electrostimulation have different outcomes on the autonomic nerve system and on neurotransmitters (Cakmak et al., 2008, 2016; Zhao, 2008), high-frequency stimulation of the Arnold branch of the vagus nerve may in fact have the opposite effect. The present study used 130 Hz stimulation, which is very high compared with the frequency (0.5 Hz) that inhibits the dopaminergic system via vagus nerve stimulation (Ziomber et al., 2012). Therefore, the beneficial bilateral effects obtained in the present study may also be derived from improved dopamine levels. Although there was not a formal feedback survey, the patients in the active group also reported that they felt like they had their levodopa pills. The underlying neurotransmitter related mechanism of action will be the focus of animal studies in addition to levodopa integrated clinical trials for the IAMZ stimulation.

A recent study reported bilateral c-fos activation in the nucleus tractus solitarius (NTS) and the locus coerulei (LC) after stimulation of the left cavum concha area, which is located in the bed of the Arnold branch of the vagus nerve in rats (Ay et al., 2015) (**Figures 1A,B**). On the other hand, transganglionic neurotracing studies with horseradish peroxidase (HRP) injections to the central cut end of the Arnold branch did not result in LC labeling (Nomura and Mizuno, 1984). Interestingly, the same study investigated left cavum concha stimulation and reported c-fos activation in the facial nerve nucleus in one of the experimental animals. The cavum concha is located next to the helicis minor muscle, and facial nerve fibers to the helicis minor may also be distributed in this area. Therefore, it is always possible that some facial nerve fibers will be stimulated along with the Arnold branch of the vagus nerve within the cavum concha. The authors attributed the c-fos labeling in the bilateral LC to projections from the NTS and as a result of stimulation of the Arnold branch of the vagus nerve. The Arnold branch of the vagus-NTS-LC axis may not be the only option for bilateral LC c-fos labeling after cavum concha stimulation, as sympathetic nerves also contribute to the cavum concha area within the arterial walls, and the cervical sympathetic ganglia were not investigated for possible labeling in that particular study. A major input to the LC originates from the nucleus paragigantocellularis (nPGi) in the reticular formation (Ennis and Aston-Jones, 1988; Kessel et al., 2008) (**Figure 1B**). The nPGi directly innervates sympathetic neurons and receives inputs (Ennis and Aston-Jones, 1988; Aston-Jones et al., 1996; Berntson et al., 1998) (**Figures 1A,B**). This pathway is involved in transmitting information of sympathetic control and state between the nPGi and the LC (Garcia-Rill, 1991; Limousin et al., 1997) (**Figures 1A,B**). In addition, the nPGi has been shown to be antidromically activated by electrostimulation of the LC, which may also be the case for sympathetic afferents. The major efferent pathways of the LC, the major wakefulness-promoting nucleus, project to the PPN (Samuels and Szabadi, 2008) (**Figure 1B**). Therefore, the possible role of the auricular sympathetic nerves in LC activation and, as a consequence, their possible effects on motor regulation via the LC-PPN axis, cannot be excluded. In contrast, the sham stimulation zone, which included the C2 and sympathetic nerves in the second arm of the study, did not affect the UPDRS motor scores, which may suggest that the sympathetic nerves had a minimal role in the UPDRS improvements observed in the present study. On the other hand, the distribution of the sympathetic nerves may have less contribution to sham zone stimulation area in comparison to the IAMZ electrostimulation zones so that sympathetic nerves may still have a potential role in the observed clinical improvement.

Although there are different possible anatomical pathways from the IAMZ to the LC-PPN axis that need to be investigated, the demonstration of bilateral LC activation through unilateral stimulation of the cavum concha area (Ay et al., 2015) may also explain the bilateral motor improvements observed in our study.

Proprioception nerve fibers of the intrinsic auricular muscles may project to the mesencephalic trigeminal nucleus, to the cuneate nucleus, or both. The mesencephalic trigeminal nucleus projects to the reticular formation and to the spinal cord (Usunoff et al., 1997) (**Figures 1A,B**). This connection indicates the presence of potential intrinsic auricular muscle proprioception feedback over reticular formation, which is the PPN's gateway for influencing movement and posture. On the other hand, imaging studies have revealed that the cortical representation of the ear is distributed not as a single zone over the cortical face-head representation area but as numerous different zones over the face, head and neck representation areas (Nihashi et al., 2001). If this unique auricular sensory representation finding is extrapolated to intrinsic auricular muscle representations, then the proprioceptive feedback of the intrinsic auricular muscles may also contribute to the neck proprioceptive center, the nucleus cuneatus. A recent study also supported such a connection: in an fMRI study, stimulation of the antitragicus muscle zone as a control demonstrated activation of the nucleus cuneatus, whereas there was no activation in the nucleus cuneatus when a non-muscular area of the ear was stimulated (Frangos et al., 2015) (**Figures 1A,B**). The nucleus cuneatus and the PPN are the two major components of the mesencephalic locomotor region that modulates PGID (Garcia-Rill, 1991). The SCM, where the transcutaneous electrode was placed, may also play a role in nucleus cuneatus modulation because of the alternating anode-cathode stimulation method that we used in the present study. On the other hand, the effect would be relatively small compared with the effect that occurs by IAMZ stimulation because of the transcutaneous electrode usage and the very low power of the stimulus. We did not observe any contractions of the SCM during stimulation. In addition, the patients also reported a distinct tingling sensation over the IAMZ but not of the SCM where the transcutaneous electrode was placed. The different surface size of the needle electrodes placed on the IAMZ compared with the transcutaneous electrodes on the SCM may be the reason behind this difference, in addition to the skin conductance factor between the needle electrodes and the transcutaneous electrodes. In conclusion, the contribution of the SCM electrode to the symptomatic improvements observed in the present study, if any, would be minimal. The sham region in the present study is selected to eliminate the potential effect of stimulation of only the C2/sympathetic nerve by ensuring no or minimal stimulation of the SCM, the vagus facial nerve and the trigeminal nerve, on the other hand the character of the sham design has limitations for surface SCM stimulation contributions (if any). Different sham group designs are needed to eliminate the SCM only stimulation effects.

The upper face muscles, such as the orbicularis oculi and frontalis muscles, have similar bilateral hemispheric connections; however, reports of the muscle spindle content of the orbicularis oculi highlight the lack of muscle spindles in this muscle group (Urban et al., 2004). In addition, these muscles are actively used to as mimics and as sphincters, and the contraction of these muscles with external electrostimulation may induce visible contractions that counteract their functions. In conclusion, these muscles are not the ideal targets, not only because they lack muscle spindles but also because they are actively used in daily life, and therefore, the contraction of these muscles may be annoying to patients. Subthreshold stimulation that does not induce visible contractions of these muscles may be another option for an alternative non-invasive electrostimulation modality for modulating similar networks related to IAMZ, but the lack of muscle spindles is still a major concern. On the other hand, intrinsic auricular muscles have active roles in shaping the external ear surface features during the prenatal period and become functionally regressed but anatomically intact in adult humans, such that stimulation of intrinsic muscles does not induce the visible contractions observed in the frontalis and orbicularis oculi (Zerin et al., 1982; Yotsuyanagi et al., 1999). Finally, although no studies on the muscle spindle content of human intrinsic auricular muscles have been published thus far, muscle spindles have been examined in peri-auricular muscles in non-human primates, including, rhesus monkeys (Lovell et al., 1977). The statistically significant (but clinically not significant) effect that was observed in the IAMZ dry needling group in the second arm of the study also underlines the significance of the IAMZ zone during minimal stimulation. In addition, it is worth noting that electrostimulation with the same parameters of a muscle-free area of the auricula in the sham group had no effect on UPDRS scores.

The current study was a pilot study performed on a small group of patients that investigated the immediate effects of IAMZ stimulation on PD motor symptoms. Although the study includes numerous groups including sham, placebo, dry needling and active, the SCM contribution (if any), and the potential perception differences of the sham and real IAMZ stimulations were the limitations. The results require further validation in subsequent studies with more participants. Further investigations of bilateral stimulation applications and different stimulation frequencies are also needed to clarify the efficacy of the technique, as in DBS, for patient-specific frequency effects on tremor. In addition, although postural tremor and tremor at rest significantly improved after active stimulation, we observed that tremor developed more erratically and was modulated by the emotional states of patients. In addition, the patients also well-tolerated the device without any side effect or discomfort with short term (20 min) stimulation. The usability of the device for longer terms will be the focus of future trials. Responsiveness regarding the stage of the disease, different stimulation frequencies and long-term effects should also be investigated. Moreover, we only observed the short-term effects of stimulation, and the second arm of the study indicates that the effect may persist up to the 30th-minute after termination of stimulation, which corresponded to the 50th-minute after the initiation of the stimulation. Prolonged efficacy will also be the focus of the next phase of clinical trials. Responsiveness regarding the stage of the disease must also be investigated in future studies.

CONCLUSION

We provide the first demonstration of a potential role of IAMZ electrical stimulation in improving (moderate to large clinical improvement) the clinical motor symptoms of PD patients in the short term. The underlying neuronal pathways and mechanisms need to be investigated in future studies.

AUTHOR CONTRIBUTIONS

Developed the concept: YC; experiment design: YC, YO, SE; performed stimulation experiments: YC, BO; performed patient enrollments and/or clinical assessments: HA, GK, SE, AG, OC; development of hardware: HU, SO, YC; development of software and code writing: HU, SO, BO, YC; development of analytical tools: HU, SO, BO, YC; data collection: BO, YC, OC, SO; analyzed data: YC, SE, AG, BO, YO, SE; wrote the draft: YC; wrote the main paper: YC, HA, GK, SE, AG, BO, OC, YO, HU, BO.

FUNDING

This project was supported by Koç University, School of Medicine.

REFERENCES

Alstermark, B., Isa, T., Lundberg, A., Pettersson, L. G., and Tantisira, B. (1989). The effect of low pyramidal lesions on forelimb movements in the cat. *Neurosci. Res.* 7, 71–75. doi: 10.1016/0168-0102(89)90038-2

Alstermark, B., Lundberg, A., Norrsell, U., and Sybirska, E. (1981). Integration in descending motor pathways controlling the forelimb in the cat. 9. Differential behavioural defects after spinal cord lesions interrupting defined pathways from higher centres to motoneurones. *Exp. Brain Res.* 42, 299–318. doi: 10.1007/BF00237496

Alvord, L. S., and Farmer, L. B. (1997). Anatomy and orientation of the human external ear. *J. Am. Acad. Audiol.* 8, 383–390.

Aston-Jones, G., Rajkowski, J., Kubiak, P., Valentino, R. J., and Shipley, M. T. (1996). Role of the locus coeruleus in emotional activation. *Prog. Brain Res.* 107, 379–402. doi: 10.1016/S0079-6123(08)61877-4

Ay, I., Napadow, V., and Ay, H. (2015). Electrical stimulation of the vagus nerve dermatome in the external ear is protective in rat cerebral ischemia. *Brain Stimul.* 8, 7–12. doi: 10.1016/j.brs.2014.09.009

Berntson, G. G., Sarter, M., and Cacioppo, J. T. (1998). Anxiety and cardiovascular reactivity: the basal forebrain cholinergic link. *Behav. Brain Res.* 94, 225–248. doi: 10.1016/S0166-4328(98)00041-2

Braak, H., del Tredici, K., Rub, U., de Vos, R. A., Jansen Steur, E. N., and Braak, E. (2003). Staging of brain pathology related to sporadic Parkinson's disease. *Neurobiol. Aging* 24, 197–211. doi: 10.1016/S0197-4580(02)00065-9

Burn, D. (2013). *Oxford Textbook of Movement Disorders.* Oxford: Oxford University Press, 16–22. doi: 10.1093/med/9780199609536.001.0001

Cakmak, Y. O., Akpinar, I. N., Ekinci, G., and Bekiroglu, N. (2008). Point- and frequency-specific response of the testicular artery to abdominal electroacupuncture in humans. *Fertil. Steril.* 90, 1732–1738. doi: 10.1016/j.fertnstert.2007.08.013

Cakmak, Y. O., Akpinar, I. N., and Yoldemir, T. (2016). Decreasing the uterine blood flow with electroacupuncture: bidermatomal and monodermatomal applications. *Gynecol. Obstet. Invest.* 82, 151–156. doi: 10.1159/000446947

Costa, J., Valls-Sole, J., Valldeoriola, F., Rumia, J., and Tolosa, E. (2007). Motor responses of muscles supplied by cranial nerves to subthalamic nucleus deep brain stimuli. *Brain* 130, 245–255. doi: 10.1093/brain/awl336

Daniel, E. E., and Paton, D. M. (1975). *Methods in Pharmacology, Smooth Muscle,* Vol. 3. New York, NY: Plenum Press, 442. doi: 10.1007/978-1-4684-2751-6

Drake, R. L., Vogl, W., and Mitchell, A. W. M. (2015). *Gray's Anatomy for Students.* Philadelphia, PA: Churchill Livingstone, 954.

Drew, T. (1991). Functional organization within the medullary reticular formation of the intact unanesthetized cat. III. Microstimulation during locomotion. *J. Neurophysiol.* 66, 919–938.

Drew, T., and Rossignol, S. (1990). Functional organization within the medullary reticular formation of intact unanesthetized cat. I. movements evoked by microstimulation. *J. Neurophysiol.* 64, 767–781.

Ennis, M., and Aston-Jones, G. (1988). Activation of locus coeruleus from nucleus paragigantocellularis: a new excitatory amino acid pathway in brain. *J. Neurosci.* 8, 3644–3657.

Frangos, E., Ellrich, J., and Komisaruk, B. R. (2015). Non-invasive access to the vagus nerve central projections via electrostimulation of the external ear: fMRI evidence in humans. *Brain Stimul.* 8, 624–636. doi: 10.1016/j.brs.2014.11.018

Fujita, T. (1934). Die motorische innervation der genuinen aurikularmuskeln beim menschen, nebst bemerkungen zu ihrer phylogenetischen herkunft. *Anat. Anz.* 78, 321.

Garcia-Rill, E. (1991). The pedunculopontine nucleus. *Prog. Neurobiol.* 36, 363–389. doi: 10.1016/0301-0082(91)90016-T

Gorska, T., and Sybirska, E. (1980). Effects of pyramidal lesions on forelimb movements in the cat. *Acta Neurobiol. Exp.* 40, 843–859.

Hamani, C., Stone, S., Laxton, A., and Lozano, A. M. (2007). The pedunculopontine nucleus and movement disorders: anatomy and the role for deep brain stimulation. *Parkinsonism Relat. Disord.* 13, S276–S280. doi: 10.1016/S1353-8020(08)70016-6

Hammer, M. J., Barlow, S. M., Lyons, K. E., and Pahwa, R. (2010). Subthalamic nucleus deep brain stimulation changes speech respiratory and laryngeal control in Parkinson's disease. *J. Neurol.* 257, 1692–1702. doi: 10.1007/s00415-010-5605-5

Hanajima, R., Chen, R., Ashby, P., Lozano, A. M., Hutchison, W. D., Davis, K. D., et al. (2004). Very fast oscillations evoked by median nerve stimulation in the human thalamus and subthalamic nucleus. *J. Neurophysiol.* 92, 3171–3182. doi: 10.1152/jn.00363.2004

Harting, J. K. (1997). *The Global Cerebellum '97.* Ph.D. thesis, University of Wisconsin Medical School, Madison, WI.

Hazrati, L. N., and Parent, A. (1992). Projection from the deep cerebellar nuclei to the pedunculopontine nucleus in the squirrel monkey. *Brain Res.* 585, 267–271. doi: 10.1016/0006-8993(92)91216-2

Hirsch, E. C., Graybiel, A. M., Duyckaerts, C., and Javoy-Agid, F. (1987). Neuronal loss in the pedunculopontine tegmental nucleus in Parkinson's disease and in progressive supranuclear palsy. *Proc. Natl. Acad. Sci. U.S.A.* 84, 5976–5980. doi: 10.1073/pnas.84.16.5976

Hobbs, S. F., Oh, U. T., Chandler, M. J., Fu, Q. G., Bolser, D. C., and Foreman, R. D. (1992). Evidence that C1 and C2 propriospinal neurons mediate the inhibitory effects of viscerosomatic spinal afferent input on primate spinothalamic tract neurons. *J. Neurophysiol.* 67, 852–860.

Hughes, A. J., Daniel, S. E., Kilford, L., and Lees, A. J. (1992). Accuracy of clinical diagnosis of idiopathic Parkinson's disease: a clinico-pathological study of 100 cases. *J. Neurol. Neurosurg. Psychiatry* 55, 181–184. doi: 10.1136/jnnp.55.3.181

Jankowska, E., and Edgley, S. A. (2006). How can corticospinal tract neurons contribute to ipsilateral movements? A question with implications for recovery of motor functions. *Neuroscientist* 12, 67–79. doi: 10.1177/107385840528 3392

Jankowska, E., Lundberg, A., and Stuart, D. (1983). Propriospinal control of interneurons in spinal reflex pathways from tendon organs in the cat. *Brain Res.* 261, 317–320. doi: 10.1016/0006-8993(83)90636-4

Kably, B., and Drew, T. (1998). Corticoreticular pathways in the cat. I. Projection patterns and collaterization. *J. Neurophysiol.* 80, 389–405.

Karachi, C., Grabli, D., Bernard, F. A., Tande, D., Wattiez, N., Belaid, H., et al. (2010). Cholinergic mesencephalic neurons are involved in gait and postural disorders in Parkinson's disease. *J. Clin. Invest.* 120, 2745–2754. doi: 10.1172/JCI42642

Keizer, K., and Kuypers, H. G. (1984). Distribution of corticospinal neurons with collaterals to lower brain stem reticular formation in cat. *Exp. Brain Res.* 54, 107–120. doi: 10.1007/BF00235823

Keizer, K., and Kuypers, H. G. (1989). Distribution of corticospinal neurons with collaterals to the lower brain stem reticular formation in monkey (*Macaca fascicularis*). *Exp. Brain Res.* 74, 311–318. doi: 10.1007/BF00248864

Kessel, F., Rosenfield, P., and Anderson, N. (2008). *Expanding the Boundaries of Health and Social Science: Case Studies in Interdisciplinary Innovation.* New York, NY: Oxford University Press, 27.

Lambru, G., Miller, S., and Matharu, M. S. (2013). The red ear syndrome. *J. Headache Pain* 2:83. doi: 10.1186/1129-2377-14-83

Lavoie, B., and Parent, A. (1994). Pedunculopontine nucleus in the squirrel monkey: projections to the basal ganglia as revealed by anterograde tract-tracing methods. *J. Comp. Neurol.* 344, 210–231. doi: 10.1002/cne.903440204

Lawrence, D. G., and Kuypers, H. G. (1968). The functional organization of the motor system in the monkey: I. The effects of bilateral pyramidal lesions. *Brain* 91, 1–14. doi: 10.1093/brain/91.1.1

Lee, D., Henriques, D. Y., Snider, J., Song, D., and Poizner, H. (2013). Reaching to proprioceptively defined targets in Parkinson's disease: effects of deep brain stimulation therapy. *Neuroscience* 244, 99–112. doi: 10.1016/j.neuroscience.2013.04.009

Limousin, P., Greene, J., Pollak, P., Rothwell, J., Benabid, A. L., and Frackowiak, R. (1997). Changes in cerebral activity pattern due to subthalamic nucleus or internal pallidum stimulation in Parkinson's disease. *Ann. Neurol.* 42, 283–291. doi: 10.1002/ana.410420303

Limousin, P., Pollak, P., Benazzouz, A., Hoffmann, D., Le Bas, J. F., Broussolle, E., et al. (1995). Effect of parkinsonian signs and symptoms of bilateral subthalamic nucleus stimulation. *Lancet* 345, 91–95. doi: 10.1016/S0140-6736(95)90062-4

Little, S., and Brown, P. (2012). What brain signals are suitable for feedback control of deep brain stimulation in Parkinson's disease? *Ann. N. Y. Acad. Sci.* 1265, 9–24. doi: 10.1111/j.1749-6632.2012.06650.x

Lovell, M., Sutton, D., and Lindeman, R. C. (1977). Muscle spindles in nonhuman primate extrinsic auricular muscles. *Anat. Rec.* 189, 519–523. doi: 10.1002/ar.1091890310

Luccarini, P., Gahery, Y., and Pompeiano, O. (1990). Cholinoceptive pontine reticular structures modify the postural adjustments during the limb movements induced by cortical stimulation. *Arch. Ital. Biol.* 128, 19–45.

Magni, F., and Willis, W. D. (1964). Cortical control of brain stem reticular neurons. *Arch. Ital. Biol.* 102, 418–433.

Massion, J. (1992). Movement, posture and equilibrium: interaction and coordination. *Prog. Neurobiol.* 38, 35–56. doi: 10.1016/0301-0082(92)90034-C

Matsuo, K., and Hirose, T. (1987). Tragicus and antitragicus muscles as constrictors of the external auditory meatus. *Eur. J. Plastic Surg.* 10, 82–83. doi: 10.1007/BF00578381

Matsushita, M., and Xiong, G. (2001). Uncrossed and crossed projections from the upper cervical spinal cord to the cerebellar nuclei in the rat, studied by anterograde axonal tracing. *J. Comp. Neurol.* 432, 101–118. doi: 10.1002/cne.1091

McFarland, N. R., and Haber, S. N. (2000). Convergent inputs from thalamic motor nuclei and frontal cortical areas to the dorsal striatum in the primate. *J. Neurosci.* 20, 3798–3813.

Mima, T., Sadato, N., Yazawa, S., Hanakawa, T., Fukuyama, H., Yonekura, Y., et al. (1999). Brain structures related to active and passive finger movements in man. *Brain* 122, 1989–1997. doi: 10.1093/brain/122.10.1989

Moreau, C., Pennel-Ployart, O., Pinto, S., Plachez, A., Annic, A., Viallet, F., et al. (2011). Modulation of dysarthropneumophonia by low-frequency STN DBS in advanced Parkinson's disease. *Mov. Disord.* 26, 659–663. doi: 10.1002/mds.23538

Mori, S., Matsuyama, K., Kohyama, J., Kobayashi, Y., and Takakusaki, K. (1992). Neuronal constituents of postural and locomotor control systems and their interactions in cats. *Brain Dev.* 14, S109–S120.

Muthusamy, K. A., Aravamuthan, B. R., Kringelbach, M. L., Jenkinson, N., Voets, N. L., Johansen-Berg, H., et al. (2007). Connectivity of the human pedunculopontine nucleus region and diffusion tensor imaging in surgical targeting. *J. Neurosurg.* 107, 814–820. doi: 10.3171/JNS-07/10/0814

Nambu, A., Takada, M., Inase, M., and Tokuno, H. (1996). Dual somatotopical representations in the primate subthalamic nucleus: evidence for ordered but reversed body-map transformations from the primary motor cortex and the supplementary motor area. *J. Neurosci.* 16, 2671–2683.

Nambu, A., Tokuno, H., Hamada, I., Kita, H., Imanishi, M., Akazawa, T., et al. (2000). Excitatory cortical inputs to pallidal neurons via the subthalamic nucleus in the monkey. *J. Neurophysiol.* 84, 289–300.

Nambu, A., Tokuno, H., Inase, M., and Takada, M. (1997). Corticosubthalamic input zones from forelimb representations of the dorsal and ventral divisions of the premotor cortex in the macaque monkey: comparison with the input zones from the primary motor cortex and the supplementary motor area. *Neurosci. Lett.* 239, 13–16. doi: 10.1016/S0304-3940(97)00877-X

Nihashi, T., Kakigi, R., Kawakami, O., Hoshiyama, M., Itomi, K., Nakanishi, H., et al. (2001). Representation of the ear in human primary somatosensory cortex. *Neuroimage* 13, 295–304. doi: 10.1006/nimg.2000.0695

Nomura, S., and Mizuno, N. (1984). Central distribution of primary afferent fibers in the Arnold's nerve (the auricular branch of the vagus nerve): a transganglionic HRP study in the cat. *Brain Res.* 292, 199–205. doi: 10.1016/0006-8993(84)90756-X

Payoux, P., Remy, P., Damier, P., Miloudi, M., Loubinoux, I., Pidoux, B., et al. (2004). Subthalamic nucleus stimulation reduces abnormal motor cortical overactivity in Parkinson disease. *Arch. Neurol.* 61, 1307–1313. doi: 10.1001/archneur.61.8.1307

Peuker, T. E., and Filler, T. J. (2002). The nerve supply of the human auricle. *Clin. Anat.* 15, 35–37. doi: 10.1002/ca.1089

Postuma, R. B., Gagnon, J. F., Vendette, M., Charland, K., and Montplaisir, J. (2008). Research paper REM sleep behaviour disorder in Parkinson's disease is associated with specific motor features. *J. Neurol. Neurosurg. Psychiatry* 79, 1117–1121. doi: 10.1136/jnnp.2008.149195

Samuels, E. R., and Szabadi, E. (2008). Functional neuroanatomy of the noradrenergic locus coeruleus: its roles in the regulation of arousal and autonomic function part I: principles of functional organisation. *Curr. Neuropharmacol.* 6, 235–253. doi: 10.2174/157015908785777229

Sasaki, S. (2004). Dexterous finger movements in primate without monosynaptic corticomotoneuronal excitation. *J. Neurophysiol.* 92, 3142–3147. doi: 10.1152/jn.00342.2004

Schell, G. R., and Strick, P. L. (1984). The origin of thalamic inputs to the arcuate premotor and supplementary motor areas. *J. Neurosci.* 4, 539–560.

Schepens, B., and Drew, T. (2003). Strategies for the integration of posture and movement during reaching in the cat. *J. Neurophysiol.* 90, 3066–3086. doi: 10.1152/jn.00339.2003

Shulman, L. M., Gruber-Baldini, A. L., Anderson, K. E., Fishman, P. S., Reich, S. G., and Weiner, W. J. (2010). The clinically important difference on the unified Parkinson's disease rating scale. *Arch. Neurol.* 67, 64–70. doi: 10.1001/archneurol.2009.295

Sidiropoulos, C., Walsh, R., Meaney, C., Poon, Y. Y., Fallis, M., and Moro, E. (2013). Low-frequency subthalamic nucleus deep brain stimulation for axial symptoms in advanced Parkinson's disease. *J. Neurol.* 260, 2306–2311. doi: 10.1007/s00415-013-6983-2

Takakusaki, K., Tomita, N., and Yano, M. (2008). Substrates for normal gait and pathophysiology of gait disturbances with respect to the basal ganglia dysfunction. *J. Neurol.* 255, 19–29. doi: 10.1007/s00415-008-4004-7

Tattersall, T. L., Stratton, P. G., Coyne, T. J., Cook, R., Silberstein, P., Silburn, P. A., et al. (2014). Imagined gait modulates neuronal network dynamics in the human pedunculopontine nucleus. *Nat. Neurosci.* 17, 449–454. doi: 10.1038/nn.3642

Tornqvist, A. L., Schalen, L., and Rehncrona, S. (2005). Effects of different electrical parameter settings on the intelligibility of speech in patients with Parkinson's disease treated with subthalamic deep brain stimulation. *Mov. Disord.* 20, 416–423. doi: 10.1002/mds.20348

Tykocki, T., Mandat, T., and Nauman, P. (2011). Pedunculopontine nucleus deep brain stimulation in Parkinson's disease. *Arch. Med. Sci.* 7, 555–564. doi: 10.5114/aoms.2011.24119

Urban, P., Bohl, J., Abrao, L., and Stofft, E. (2004). Absence of muscle spindles in human facial muscles. *Klin. Neurophysiol.* 35, 297.

Usunoff, K. G., Marani, E., and Schoen, J. H. R. (1997). *The Trigeminal System in Man: Advances in Anatomy, Embryology and Cell Biology*, Vol. 136. Berlin: Springer, 1–126. doi: 10.1007/978-3-642-60779-0

Wardman, D. L., Gandevia, S. C., and Colebatch, J. G. (2014). Cerebral, subcortical, and cerebellar activation evoked by selective stimulation of muscle and cutaneous afferents: an fMRI study. *Physiol. Rep.* 2:e00270. doi: 10.1002/phy2.270

Whishaw, I. Q., Gorny, B., and Sarna, J. (1998). Paw and limb use in skilled and spontaneous reaching after pyramidal tract, red nucleus and combined lesions in the rat: behavioral and anatomical dissociations. *Behav. Brain Res.* 93, 167–183. doi: 10.1016/S0166-4328(97)00152-6

Yotsuyanagi, T., Nihei, Y., Shinmyo, Y., and Sawada, Y. (1999). Stahl's ear caused by an abnormal intrinsic auricular muscle. *Plast. Reconstr. Surg.* 103, 171–174. doi: 10.1097/00006534-199901000-00027

Zerin, M., Van Allen, M. I., and Smith, D. W. (1982). Intrinsic auricular muscles and auricular form. *Pediatrics* 69, 91–93.

Zhao, Z. Q. (2008). Neural mechanism underlying acupuncture analgesia. *Prog. Neurobiol.* 85, 355–375. doi: 10.1016/j.pneurobio.2008.05.004

Ziomber, A., Thor, P., Krygowska-Wajs, A., Zalecki, T., Moskala, M., Romanska, I., et al. (2012). Chronic impairment of the vagus nerve function leads to inhibition of dopamine but not serotonin neurons in rat brain structures. *Pharmacol. Rep.* 64, 1359–1367. doi: 10.1016/S1734-1140(12)70933-7

Zweig, R. M., Jankel, W. R., Hedreen, J. C., Mayeux, R., and Price, D. L. (1989). The pedunculopontine nucleus in Parkinson's disease. *Ann. Neurol.* 26, 41–46. doi: 10.1002/ana.410260106

17

Evaluation of the Cortical Silent Period of the Laryngeal Motor Cortex in Healthy Individuals

Mo Chen[1]*, Rebekah L. S. Summers*[1]*, George S. Goding*[2]*, Sharyl Samargia*[3]*, Christy L. Ludlow*[4]*, Cecília N. Prudente*[1] *and Teresa J. Kimberley*[1*]

[1] *Divisions of Physical Therapy and Rehabilitation Science, Department of Rehabilitation Medicine, School of Medicine, University of Minnesota, Minneapolis, MN, USA,* [2] *Department of Otolaryngology-Head and Neck Surgery, University of Minnesota, Minneapolis, MN, USA,* [3] *Department of Communication Sciences and Disorders, University of Wisconsin River Falls Campus, River Falls, WI, USA,* [4] *Department of Communication Sciences and Disorders, James Madison University, Harrisonburg, VA, USA*

Correspondence:
Teresa J. Kimberley
tjk@umn.edu

Objective: This work aimed to evaluate the cortical silent period (cSP) of the laryngeal motor cortex (LMC) using the bilateral thyroarytenoid (TA) muscles with transcranial magnetic stimulation (TMS).

Methods: In 11 healthy participants, fine-wire electromyography (EMG) was used to record bilateral TA muscle responses to single pulse TMS delivered to the LMC in both hemispheres. Peripheral responses to stimulation over the mastoid, where the vagus nerve exits the skull, were collected to verify the central origin of the cortical stimulation responses by comparing the latencies.

Results: The cSP duration ranged from 41.7 to 66.4 ms. The peripherally evoked motor-evoked potential (MEP) peak occurred 5–9 ms earlier than the cortical responses (for both sides of TAs: $p < 0.0001$) with no silent period. The right TA MEP latencies were earlier than the left TA responses for both peripheral and cortical measures ($p \leq 0.0001$).

Conclusion: These findings demonstrate the feasibility of measuring cSP of LMC based on intrinsic laryngeal muscles responses during vocalization in healthy volunteers.

Significance: The technique could be used to study the pathophysiology of neurological disorders that affect TA muscles, such as spasmodic dysphonia. Further, the methodology has application to other muscles of the head and neck not accessible using surface electrodes.

Keywords: Transcranial magnetic stimulation, TMS, larynx, motor cortex excitability, fine wire electrode, cortical silent period, cSP

INTRODUCTION

The laryngeal motor cortex (LMC) plays a significant role in human voice and speech production (Henriquez et al., 2007; Simonyan et al., 2009; Ludlow, 2015). However, its functional organization and interactions with other brain regions in both healthy humans and patients with neurological voice and speech disorders warrants further investigation (Simonyan and Horwitz, 2011). Specifically, for example, it is unknown how neurotransmitters, such as dopamine and gamma-aminobutyric acid (GABA) influence and modulate the human LMC network during voice and speech production and how these neurotransmitters are altered in people with neurological voice and speech disorders. This information is crucial in identifying the target brain regions for the development of new neuropharmacological options to modulate the LMC activity in patients with neurological voice problems, such as spasmodic dysphonia (Ludlow et al., 2008).

Transcranial magnetic stimulation (TMS) provides an important non-invasive way to evaluate the corticospinal excitability in a wide range of healthy and disease populations (for review: Eldaief et al., 2013). If the TMS stimulus is delivered to the motor cortex, a response in the peripheral muscles can be measured using electromyography (EMG). The response is defined as a motor-evoked potential (MEP). By assessing the MEPs induced by single or paired pulse techniques, TMS can be used to evaluate different aspects of cortical excitability, e.g., motor threshold, MEP latency and amplitude, and the cortical silent period (cSP) (Hallett, 2007).

Among these excitability measures, cSP is a widely adopted and highly reliable way to evaluate motor cortex excitability and its responses to neuromodulation (Wolters et al., 2008; Chen et al., 2015). Since the first reported cSP evoked by TMS (Calancie et al., 1987), cSP has been studied extensively in physiological and pathological conditions. Currently, it is thought that the cSP reflects intracortical inhibitory process mediated by $GABA_A$ (Paulus et al., 2008) and $GABA_B$ receptors (Wolters et al., 2008). This unique feature makes the cSP a powerful tool to non-invasively probe the GABA receptor mediated intracortical inhibitory process, especially in people with pathological conditions, such as dystonia (Siebner et al., 1998). Significantly shorter cSP has been reported in hand muscles in people with focal hand dystonia (Tinazzi et al., 2005; Kimberley et al., 2009), facial muscles in people with cranial dystonia (Currà et al., 2000) and hand muscles in people with spasmodic dysphonia (Samargia et al., 2014). Thus, cSP has the potential to reveal the abnormal inhibition in neurological disorders and may serve as a biomarker to help with diagnosis and early intervention.

Testing of the cSP can be performed by applying a single suprathreshold TMS pulse to the motor cortical representation of a tonically preactivated target muscle, producing a period of EMG silence in contralateral target muscles (Wolters et al., 2008). The hand region of the motor cortex has been the primary location of cSP testing due to the ease of accessing the corresponding muscles, such as first dorsal interosseous (FDI) or abductor pollicis brevis. The EMG signal from these peripheral muscles is large in amplitude with sufficient latency from the TMS pulse to make it easily identifiable and unaffected by TMS artifact. Furthermore, these muscles are easily accessible with surface electrodes which summate MEPs from a large number of motor units, making the EMG signal less sensitive to noise or the firing of individual motor unit. However, in order to evaluate the cSP from the deep muscles (i.e., the intrinsic laryngeal muscles in people with spasmodic dysphonia), intramuscular electrodes, i.e., fine-wire or needle electrodes, must be used. Signals from intramuscular electrodes are more difficult to assess than surface electrodes (Konrad, 2005). Reasons for the difficulties are as follows: (1) Electrode placement is technically difficult. (2) The position of the two fine-wire electrodes cannot be altered once inserted. If the initial insertion is not accurate another insertion is required; and (3) Fine-wire or needle electrodes summate evoked potentials from fewer motor units than surface electrodes, reducing the MEP amplitude and making it difficult to differentiate the MEP from spontaneous firing of intrinsic motor units. A challenge specific to measurements from the LMC is that the EMG electrode location is close to the stimulation site, which results in a large stimulus artifact. When the stimulation artifact is lengthened due to amplifier saturation, it is difficult to identify MEPs with early latencies. Finally, the LMC brain representation is relatively small compared to regions, such as the hand and, therefore, stimulation location may be challenging to locate.

Overcoming these difficulties, several groups have studied the MEP responses to TMS over the LMC. MEP latency and amplitude values from the cricopharyngeal sphincter muscles during cortical stimulation have been reported (Ertekin et al., 2001); single pulse responses from the cricothyroid muscles were also reported (Espadaler et al., 2012; Rogić Vidaković et al., 2015). Another laryngeal intrinsic muscle, the thyroarytenoid (TA), which directly controls the vocal folds by modulating vocal-fold tension when opposed by other intrinsic muscles, is highly relevant for the pathophysiology of speech related neurological disorders, i.e., spasmodic dysphonia and voice tremor (Ludlow, 2005; Simonyan et al., 2009; Simonyan and Horwitz, 2011). However, the TA muscle has only been used to evaluate the latency of MEPs during cortical stimulation to LMC (Khedr and Aref, 2002; Rödel et al., 2004). These latencies were relatively early ($\leq$10 ms) and some were close to TA latencies found with peripheral stimulation over the mastoid (Sims et al., 1996). Moreover, the excitability of the LMC as measured by cSP in TA muscles has not been investigated. Considering that investigation of the excitability of corticobulbar projections to the TA would be relevant for understanding the neural controls of voice production in both healthy and pathological conditions, the purpose of the current study was to assess the excitability of the LMC by measuring the cSP in the TA muscles. The use of TMS with fine-wire electrodes to measure the cSP of the LMC will provide a tool to evaluate the GABA receptor mediated inhibition process. This will further lead to a better understanding of the pathophysiology of disorders of the larynx i.e., spasmodic dysphonia and voice tremor.

METHODS

Participants

Data from eleven healthy participants (mean age, 54 $\pm$ 7.4 years; 3 females) were collected. Participants gave written, informed consent prior to participation according to the Declaration of Helsinki (World Medical Association, 2013). The study was approved by the Clinical and Translational Science Institute and the Institutional Review Board of the University of Minnesota.

Devices

Transcranial magnetic stimulation (TMS) pulses were delivered using a 70 mm figure-of-eight coil connected to the Bistim^2 and 200^2 stimulator set (The Magstim Company Ltd, UK). Two pairs of fine-wire electrodes were connected to two bi-polar active pre-amps (Y03-002, Motion Lab Systems, Inc., Baton Rouge, LA) powered by two 9-volt batteries. EMG signals were amplified with a gain of x300, passed through a band-pass filter (15–2000 Hz), and digitized by a 24-bit analog-to-digital converter (NI9234, National Instruments Co., Austin, TX) in AC coupling mode (0.5 Hz) with the sampling rate of 6.4 k Hz. All data were collected and stored using a custom data acquisition program written with LabVIEW (V2012, National Instruments, Austin, TX) on a laptop computer (Latitude, Dell Co., Ltd, Round Rock, TX) which was also used to monitor real-time EMG activity.

Experiment Procedures

Participants were seated comfortably in a reclined armchair with the subject tracker band of a frameless stereotactic neuronavigation system (BrainSight, Rogue Research Inc., Canada) attached to their forehead. The hand region was assessed prior to the laryngeal area.

Hand Region Assessment

Hand region excitability was evaluated by using surface electrodes (6030-TP, Nicolet, CA, USA) attached to right hand FDI muscle. The experiment procedure was the same as previously published protocols (Chen et al., 2015; Rossini et al., 2015). Briefly, the resting motor threshold was determined as the lowest intensity that generated MEPs with the peak-to-peak amplitude >50 μV in 5 out of 10 consecutive trials. The hotspot was the location of the coil where the resting motor threshold was determined. The 1-mV threshold was determined by using a similar protocol with the MEP amplitude response ≥ 1 mV. The 1-mV threshold intensity was used as the initial stimulation intensity for the LMC assessment.

Laryngeal Region Assessment

Skin preparation

Skin around the area of the laryngeal prominence was cleaned using alcohol wipes. A topical anesthetic cream (LMX 4% Lidocaine, Ferndale Laboratories, Inc., Ferndale, MI) was applied to the cleaned area. After approximately 15 min, a numbing agent (Xylocaine, 2% lidocaine HCL and epinephrine, 1:100,000, Professional Veterinary Laboratories, NB, Canada) was injected into the skin of the numbed region.

Electrodes placement

A 30 mm, 27 gauge needle loaded with a pair of fine-wire hooked electrodes (#019-772800, Nicolet Co., Middleton, WI) was inserted into left and right TA muscle by an experienced otolaryngologist following standard procedures for laryngeal EMG (Hirano and Ohala, 1969). Using a percutaneous approach, the needle was passed through the cricothyroid membrane at an angle off midline but medial to the ipsilateral inferior tubercle, to directly enter the TA muscle while avoiding the airway. During insertion, the electrodes were connected to an audio monitor (Grass AM10, Natus Medical Incorporated Co., San Carlos, CA) to allow monitoring of muscle activity in real-time. After the location was confirmed, the needle was removed leaving the fine-wires in the TA muscles (**Figure 1A**). A silver-silver chloride strap with a Velcro fastener (TD-431, Discount Disposables, St. Albans, VT) was attached to the participant's forehead serving as a ground (**Figure 1B**).

Peripheral stimulation

Peripheral stimulation was delivered over the mastoid to: (1) confirm electrode placement in the TA muscles, (2) determine peripheral stimulation response latency, and (3) contrast with the cortical stimulation responses to ensure that there was not stimulus spread to the vagus nerve during cortical stimulation. Ten peripheral stimulation trials were collected; 5 at rest and 5 during a production of sustained /i/. The TMS coil was placed over the mastoid bone to activate the vagus nerve. Placement was tangential to the tip of mastoid bone in a posterior-anterior direction (**Figure 2B**). The center of the coil was located above the mastoid (the exit of vagus nerve from the skull through the jugular foramen) behind the ear. This placement is consistent with previous studies (Sims et al., 1996; Khedr and Aref, 2002). The stimulation intensity was set to 40% of maximum TMS output. Preliminary work determined that 40% was the lowest intensity that consistently generated peripheral evoked potentials in all participants with very little variation. Higher stimulation intensities induced facial muscle contractions during the experiment and caused the magnetic field spread to the electrode area, resulting in amplifier saturation.

Cortical stimulation

An anatomical T1 magnetic resonance image (MRI) with high-resolution ($1 \times 1 \times 1$ mm^3) was acquired on a separate day prior to the TMS experiment visit. The image was imported into the neuronavigation system to guide the localization of the LMC in the primary motor cortex (M1). The location of the LMC, as determined by Simonyan et al. (2009), was used to help direct neuronavigation of initial coil placement on each participant's skull. This location is reported as approximately 0.5–1 cm anterior and 2–4 cm lateral to the hotspot determined in the afore-determined hand region assessment (Simonyan et al., 2009). This LMC location is similar to the 2 cm anterior and 4–8 cm lateral to the Cz EEG electrode position in the 10–20 system reported by Ertekin et al. (2001). The coil was held tangential to the skull over the targeted area in a posterior-anterior direction parallel to the midline (**Figure 2A**) and was systematically moved in an approximate 1 cm grid. The procedure was monitored by the neuronavigation system in real time. Initially, the intensity used for single TMS pulses was the 1-mV threshold for the FDI muscle as determined in the aforementioned hand region assessment; however, in most cases, the intensity was increased to induce an MEP in TA muscles. Conventional motor threshold determination protocol was attempted with the observation that the MEP amplitude was not modulated with TMS intensity within participant's acceptable/comfortable range (80% of the maximum stimulator output). However, a silent period was clearly observed following the superimposed MEP when a given TMS intensity was reached. Thus, cSP threshold was defined as the lowest TMS intensity that elicits a cSP in 5 out of 10 consecutive trials. The location that corresponded to the lowest

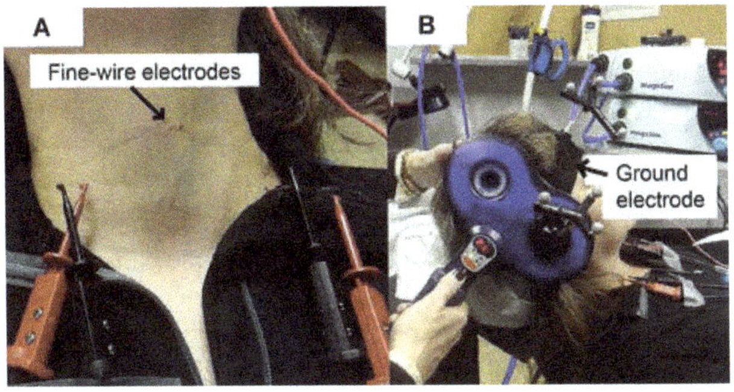

FIGURE 1 | Experimental Set up. (A) Fine-wire electrodes. There were two channels (pairs of fine-wires) inserted into bilateral thyroarytenoid muscles; **(B)** Ground electrode. The strap ground electrode was placed under the BrainSight subject tracker band.

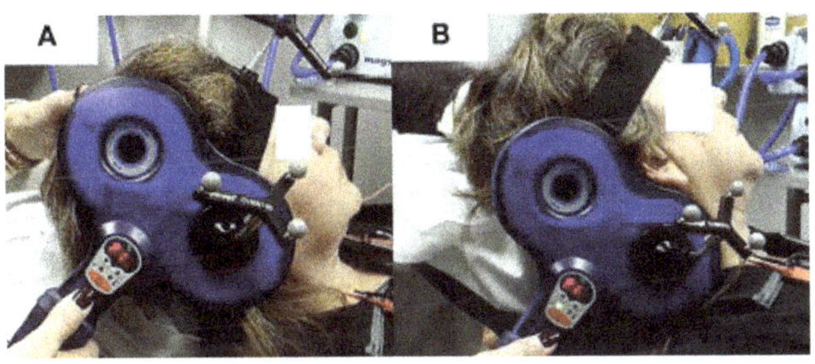

FIGURE 2 | TMS coil placement for laryngeal motor cortex (LMC) and peripheral stimulation. (A) Coil position and angle for LMC stimulation (cSP test), **(B)** coil position and angle for peripheral stimulation.

stimulation intensity (cSP threshold) was used as the LMC "hotspot" in the following experiment procedures. The hotspot coordinates were recorded by the neuronavigation system in MNI standard space using template ICBM152 with 1 mm^3 resolution (Mazziotta et al., 2001).

Outcome measure

cSP was the outcome measure for LMC excitability. The cSP threshold was used as the stimulation intensity. Single pulse cortical stimulations were performed during vocalization of sustained /i/. Participants were instructed to produce a comfortable pitch and volume of vocalization that was kept similar throughout the trials. The single pulse was applied approximately 1 s after initiation of the sustained vocalization. Participants were instructed to relax approximately 2 s after the pulse was delivered. In all participants, cSP threshold and cSP responses were first collected in the left hemisphere followed by the right hemisphere. Fifty trials of bilateral cSP responses in left and right TA muscles were collected in response to stimulation in both hemispheres. Given the low signal-to-noise ratio (SNR) with the fine wire responses, 50 trials were collected and traces were averaged to cancel out noise and increase the SNR. Average MEP amplitude was also calculated.

Data Processing

The cSP data were first averaged and rectified. Then, a 10-ms moving standard deviation (SD) window was applied to generate an SD curve of the signal. The average value of the SD curve during baseline (100–5 ms before stimulus) was calculated as the baseline contraction level. This value was used to define the offset of the cSP when the signal returned to pre-stimulus level. The onset of the cSP was defined as the time point of the stimulus. cSP duration was calculated by subtracting the onset from the offset of the cSP (Wolters et al., 2008; Chen et al., 2015). The MEP peak latency for both cortical and peripheral stimulation was defined as the duration between the stimulation artifact and the first peak of the MEP. The latency of the MEP to peripheral stimulation was calculated from each trial of stimulation; the latency of the MEP from cortical stimulation was identified from the average of 50 trials. The advantage of using the average of 50 trials was that it overcame any obscured response secondary to the active contraction of the TA muscle. MEP amplitude was calculated by the following procedures: in the averaged cSP trace, MEP was first identified within the range of 10–30 ms after the stimulus artifact. Then the peak-to-peak amplitude was extracted to represent the corresponding participant's MEP amplitude.

Data Analysis

Motor-evoked potential (MEP) latencies for peripheral stimulation under both active and resting conditions, and cortical stimulation for each hemisphere were compared. All data were normally distributed as determined by the Shapiro-Wilk W test. Multi-factor ANOVAs were used to examine the following three hypotheses to confirm the cortical nature of the evoked responses. (1) Cortical latencies are longer than peripheral latencies for the TA muscle on the same side. (2) MEP latencies from the left TA are longer than the right TA within the same type of stimulation (due to the longer length of the left recurrent laryngeal nerve Atkins, 1973). (3) There are no differences in latency for TA muscle on the same side when tested under different conditions. This hypothesis was tested with two sub-hypotheses: (3a) There are no differences in TA latency between resting and active with peripheral stimulation; (3b) there are no differences in TA latency between the cortical stimulation on the left and right hemispheres. These three hypotheses have to be tested separately because the cortical and peripheral data are not balanced. That is, all cortical data were collected during active contraction and peripheral data were collected under active and resting. Therefore, a three-step approach was used: for hypotheses 1 and 2 (cortical comparison), cortical and active peripheral data were tested by a two-way ANOVA with "stimulation type" (cortical vs. peripheral) and "TA side" (left vs. right) as interaction factors. For hypotheses 2 (peripheral comparison) and 3a, peripheral data were tested by a two-way ANOVA with "TA state" (rest vs. active) and "TA side" (left vs. right) as interaction factors. For hypothesis 3b, cortical data were tested by a two-way ANOVA with "stimulation side" (left vs. right) and "TA side" (left vs. right) as interaction factors. The significance level was set as $p < 0.05$ for all tests.

TABLE 1 | Participant information.

Participant	Sex	Age (years)	Stimulation intensity (% MSO)	
			L-cortical	R-cortical
1	F	42	60	60
2	F	56	63	63
3	F	49	63	63
4	M	62	57	61
5	M	58	64	65
6	M	67	52	52
7	M	60	67	58
8	M	56	55	52
9	M	47	60	60
10	M	49	60	60
11	M	46	50	52

MSO, maximum stimulator output; L, left hemisphere cortical stimulation; R, right hemisphere cortical stimulation.

RESULTS

No serious or unexpected adverse effects were reported. All participants tolerated the procedures with expected adverse events including skin soreness ($n = 4$), bruising ($n = 1$), and a tender throat ($n = 2$). Cortical stimulation intensities (percentage of the maximum stimulator output) are listed in **Table 1**. Average coordinates (MNI standard space) of the LMC hotspot were $x = -56$, $y = -3$, $z = 36$ in the left hemisphere and $x = 56$, $y = 3$, $z = 37$ in the right hemisphere. Individual coordinates are listed in Supplementary Table 1.

Peripheral stimulation induced unilateral (ipsilateral) responses of shorter latencies both during rest (left TA: 9.1 ± 2.2 ms; right TA: 6.9 ± 1.4 ms) and active contraction (left TA: 9.3 ± 2.2 ms; right TA: 6.8 ± 1.3 ms). Individual responses are listed in Supplementary Table 2. Importantly, no silent period was observed after active peripheral stimulation. Cortical stimulation evoked bilateral responses with silent periods. Average MEP latencies for left hemisphere cortical stimulation were 15.6 ± 2.3 ms in the left TA and 13.1 ± 2.0 ms in the right TA; average MEP latencies for right hemisphere cortical stimulation were 15.5 ± 2.8 ms in the left TA and 13.1 ± 2.3 ms in the right TA. The cSP duration and MEP peak latency values are listed in **Table 2**. Average cSP duration from left hemisphere cortical stimulation was 53.7 ± 7.8 ms in the left TA and 52.8 ± 7.3 ms in the right TA; average cSP duration from right hemisphere cortical stimulation was 53.4 ± 7.8 ms in the left TA and 54.5 ± 5.9 ms in the right TA. The average MEP amplitude from the left hemisphere cortical stimulation was 89.2 ± 80.0 μV in the left TA and 142.1 ± 142.5 μV in the right TA; the average MEP amplitude from the right hemisphere cortical stimulation was 110.6 ± 106.4 μV in the left TA and 196.3 ± 194.0 μV in the right TA. Individual MEP amplitude details are listed in **Table 2**. Samples of MEP responses are shown in **Figure 3** and cSP responses during right cortical stimulation are shown in **Figure 4**.

The two-way ANOVA tested cortical and active peripheral data with "stimulation type" and "TA side" as interaction factors with significant effects in "stimulation type" [$F_{(1, 59)} = 113.4894$, $p < 0.0001$] and "TA side" [$F_{(1, 59)} = 18.0334$, $p < 0.0001$] factors. No significant effect was found in the interaction of the two factors [$F_{(1, 59)} = 0.0140$, $p = 0.9062$]. This indicates that the cortical MEP latencies were longer than the peripheral MEP latencies regardless of TA side; and the left TA MEP latencies were longer than the right TA MEP latencies regardless of stimulation type. These results support hypotheses 1 and 2 (cortical comparison).

The two-way ANOVA test on peripheral data showed a significant effect with "TA side" [$F_{(1, 38)} = 18.2670$, $p = 0.0001$] as a significant factor. No significant effects were found in either "TA state" [$F_{(1, 38)} = 0.0011$, $p = 0.9734$] or the interaction of the two factors [$F_{(1, 38)} = 0.0213$, $p = 0.8849$]. This indicates that the left TA peripheral MEP latencies were longer than the right TA peripheral MEP latencies regardless of the "TA state" (rest vs. active) and that there was no difference in peripheral MEP latencies between the two TA states (rest and active). These findings support hypotheses 2 (peripheral comparison) and 3a.

The final two-way ANOVA test on cortical data with "stimulation side" and "TA side" as interaction factors showed significant effects in "TA side" [$F_{(1, 38)} = 10.5621$, $p = 0.0024$]. No significant effects were observed in either "stimulation side" [$F_{(1, 38)} = 0.0027$, $p = 0.9592$] or the interaction between the two factors [$F_{(1, 38)} = 0.0048$, $p = 0.9450$]. This indicates that in cortical stimulation, left TA latencies were longer than right TA latencies regardless of stimulation side (hemispheres) and that there was no difference between cortical MEP latencies evoked by stimulation to different hemispheres. These results support hypothesis 3b (**Figure 5**).

DISCUSSION

In this work we evaluated the feasibility and validity of testing cortical excitability of LMC with the cSP measurement using fine-wire electrodes inserted into TA muscles. TMS evoked MEP responses were confirmed as cortical in origin by observation of bilateral responses secondary to cortical stimulation, the occurrence of a silent period, and contrasting the MEP peak latencies of peripheral and cortical responses. These results suggest that the cSP may be used as a measure of cortical excitability for the LMC. To our knowledge, these cSP findings were the first report of cSP as a measure of the cortical excitability of the LMC.

Cortical vs. Peripheral Responses

The significant difference in MEP latencies between the peripheral and cortical stimulation confirmed that the cSP and MEP were generated cortically. No early response in the cortical data was observed at a similar latency as the peripheral stimulation, confirming that there was no current spread to the peripheral vagus nerve during cortical stimulation.

TABLE 2 | Cortical stimulation MEP latency, MEP amplitude and CSP duration.

Participant	MEP latency (ms)				MEP amplitude (μV)				CSP duration (ms)			
	Left hemisphere		Right hemisphere		Left hemisphere		Right hemisphere		Left hemisphere		Right hemisphere	
	L-TA	R-TA	L-TA	R-TA	L-TA	R-TA	L-TA	R-TA	L-TA	R-TA	L-TA	R-TA
1	12.3	8.9	11.9	8.6	32.7	296.2	33.5	34.1	51.4	44.8	50.3	46.4
2	12.5	11.4	13.0	11.1	81.0	26.5	95.5	34.3	43.3	44.2	42.5	49.2
3	16.1	13.4	14.2	12.7	26.3	105.1	40.9	100.0	53.6	53.4	53.0	53.0
4	16.3	13.9	15.9	11.6	58.1	23.3	12.6	92.1	50.2	47.7	53.8	55.3
5	16.6	13.6	16.3	12.7	10.0	10.3	7.4	3.9	65.3	62.8	64.7	60.9
6	17.8	13.8	15.2	13.8	26.1	10.7	71.2	16.7	48.4	46.1	48.4	49.2
7	13.9	13.0	13.8	11.7	59.1	398.6	128.8	467.3	41.7	46.7	43.9	46.9
8	N/A	15.5	N/A	15.5	N/A	383.1	N/A	322.6	N/A	55.9	N/A	56.4
9	13.4	10.3	15.3	13.9	246.8	101.0	270.3	314.5	60.0	59.2	63.6	63.1
10	19.7	15.5	22.5	17.0	128.0	165.7	344.0	606.2	63.6	66.4	64.4	63.8
11	17.3	14.5	17.0	15.5	224.5	42.4	101.8	167.3	59.5	53.6	53.4	55.6

Values are calculated from averaged trace. MEP amplitude, peak to peak amplitude; MEP, motor evoked potential; cSP, cortical silent period; TA, thyroarytenoid; L-TA, left TA; R-TA, right TA; N/A, no signal was observed from the corresponding channel.

Cortical Silent Period

The cSP duration for the TA muscles reported in this work were much shorter than previously reported values collected from the hand muscles (Chen et al., 2015). Previous studies have reported that the cSP duration is longest in small hand muscles (up to 300 ms), shorter in leg muscles (up to 100 ms), proximal arm muscles (Roick et al., 1993), axial muscles (Ferbert et al., 1992; Lefaucheur and Lofaso, 2002; Lefaucheur, 2005), facial muscles (the triangularis, range 69–169 ms, and orbicularis oculi, range 68–111 ms) (Werhahn et al., 1995; Paradiso et al., 2005) and the tongue (64.2 ± 4.5 ms at 50% maximum stimulator output) (Katayama et al., 2001). Our reported values are in line with other cranial muscles. Of note, as the brain volume decreases with age, the cSP duration gets shorter (Silbert et al., 2006). Considering the age range (54 ± 7.4 years) of participants in this study, this could also be part of the reason for the early cSP offset observed.

The cSP duration values collected from the left and right TA regardless of hemisphere stimulation were similar, the differences were within 2 ms. This symmetry is consistent with previously reported results of the low interhemispheric difference of cSP duration (usually <10 ms) in healthy subjects (Wolters et al., 2008). Although the motor cortical representation of the cSP is lateralized to the contralateral motor cortex for distal limb muscles, for axial muscles the cSP shows a more bilateral distribution (Wolters et al., 2008) which is consistent with our findings here.

Of note, MEP amplitude was not observed to modulate with changes in TMS intensity. This may be due to the small summation area of fine-wire electrodes, in contrast to surface electrodes on larger muscles, which do demonstrate changes in MEP size with different TMS stimulation intensities. This lack of modulation likely has little effect on cSP values (Rossini et al., 1994), but may render paired pulse responses or stimulus response curve measures unreliable. Also, given that the TA muscles are always active during breathing (Kuna et al., 1988), this makes resting measures difficult to reliably execute. Furthermore, it has been reported that the cSP induced by TMS can be elicited at lower stimulation intensities in the absence of a preceding MEP (Davey et al., 1994; Classen and Benecke, 1995). This low stimulation intensity advantage helps with the suppression of the stimulus artifact due to saturation of the amplifier, especially when the two inputs of the differential amplifier are not balanced, which is very likely with fine-wire electrodes, and the ground impedance is not low enough. Altogether, these inherent limitations of the laryngeal measurements suggest that cSP may be the ideal cortical excitability measure.

Latency of Motor Evoked Potential

The MEP latencies for peripheral and cortical stimulation measured in the current study were longer than those previously reported (Thumfart et al., 1992; Khedr and Aref, 2002). In those investigations, the cortical latency was reported as 9.6 ms in the left TA and 11.1 ms in the right TA contralateral to stimulation; and 9.3 and 9.5 ms in the TA ipsilateral to cortical stimulation. They also reported shorter peripheral latencies (between 2.7 and 6 ms), 1–7 ms shorter than the 3.2–13.2 ms range as we report here. These differences may be due to different definitions of the MEP latency. Khedr and Aref (2002) defined MEP latency as the interval between the stimulation artifact and the *onset* of the MEP. In this study, we measured the interval between the stimulation artifact and the first *peak* of the MEP. We chose this definition because the peak is more easily identified and less ambiguous than the MEP onset due to background EMG activity caused by breathing or voice activation. When compared with the studies using the same definition for MEP latency, our results are in agreement with others' reported values (Atkins, 1973; Rödel et al., 2004). Although it has been reported that the age can be a factor to cause a later onset of MEP (Eisen and Shtybel, 1990), in our findings no such a trend was observed.

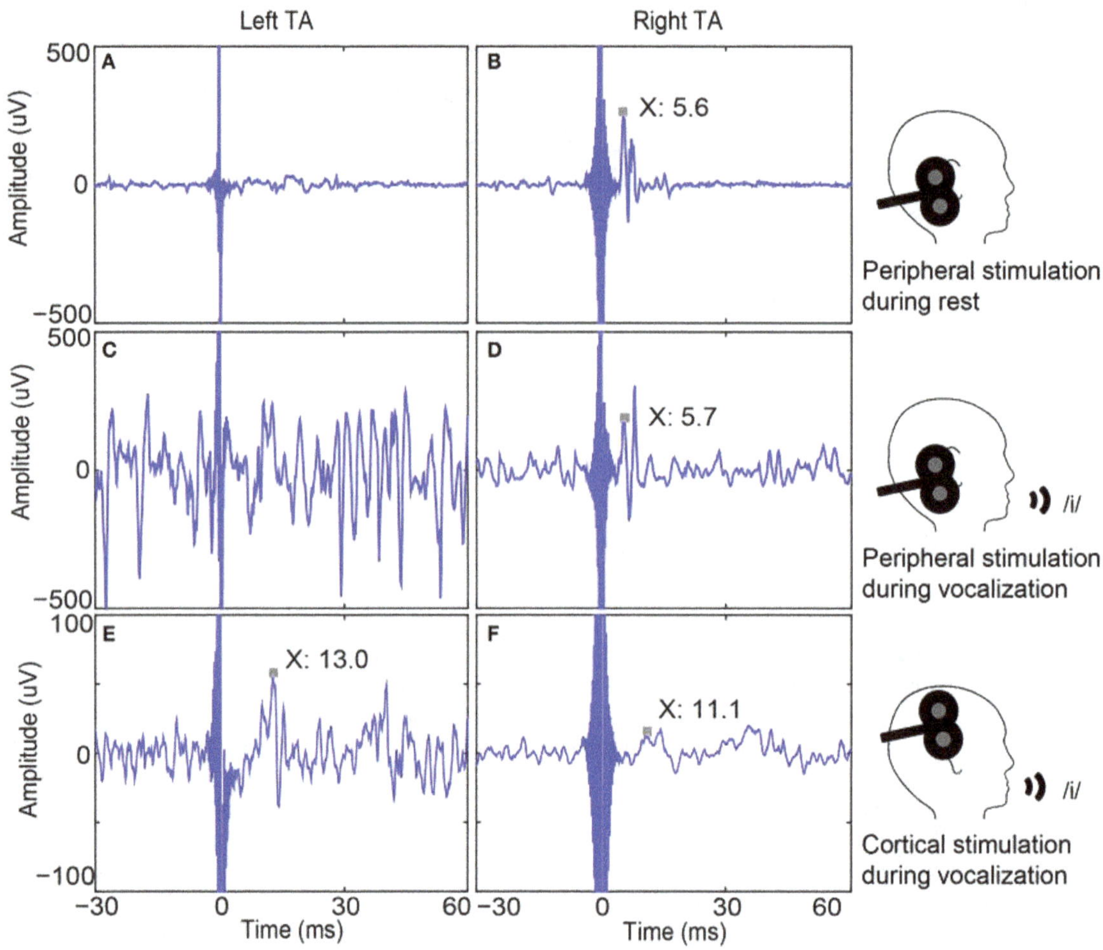

FIGURE 3 | Bilateral thyroarytenoid (TA) muscle responses to right peripheral and cortical stimulation in one participant. (A) Left TA recording without a response to right peripheral stimulation during rest (sample trace); **(B)** Right TA response to right peripheral stimulation during rest (MEP latency is 5.6 ms.); **(C)** Left TA recording without a response to right peripheral stimulation during vocalization (sample trace); **(D)** Right TA response to right peripheral stimulation (MEP peak latency is 5.7 ms.); **(E)** Average of 50 left TA responses to right cortical stimulation (MEP peak latency is 13.0 ms); **(F)** Average of 50 right TA responses to right cortical stimulation (MEP peak latency is 11.1 ms). Note the unilateral (ipsilateral) responses to peripheral stimulation and bilateral responses to cortical stimulation, which demonstrates the validity of cortical responses. MEP: motor evoked potential.

Furthermore, the differences in latency between the left and right TA muscles (2–4 ms) are consistent with the previous reported values (Atkins, 1973; Thumfart et al., 1992; Sims et al., 1996; Khedr and Aref, 2002; Rödel et al., 2004), as are the latency differences between peripheral and cortical responses (4–6 ms) (Thumfart et al., 1992; Khedr and Aref, 2002). The consistency of our results with others supports the validity of this method.

Methodological Considerations

Stimulation Artifact Suppression

Key considerations regarding stimulation artifact suppression were applied for improved signal quality as follows: *First*, a large contact area of the ground electrode suppressed the stimulation artifact, which was essential when the stimulation intensity was high (>80% of the maximum output). We determined that this procedure significantly reduced amplifier saturation as illustrated in **Figure 3**. *Second*, the ground electrode should be located between the stimulation site and the acquisition site and as close to the acquisition site as possible. For the TA or other intrinsic larynx muscles, the forehead or chin were ideal areas to attach the ground electrode. Our testing revealed that participants preferred the head strap due to comfort. Additional ground electrodes can be attached to achieve even greater suppression of the stimulation artifact. *Also*, a relatively low gain (such as x300 or x100) along with a large dynamic range of the amplifier (e.g., using a power supply generated by 9-V batteries or greater) decreased the chances of amplifier saturation. However, the low gain was compensated for by a high quantification resolution analog-to-digital convertor, such as the 24-bit used here. This high quantification resolution helped to improve the signal-noise ratio and increased the quantification accuracy that could have been diminished by the low gain. *Last*, the battery power to the amplifier also had the benefit of reducing

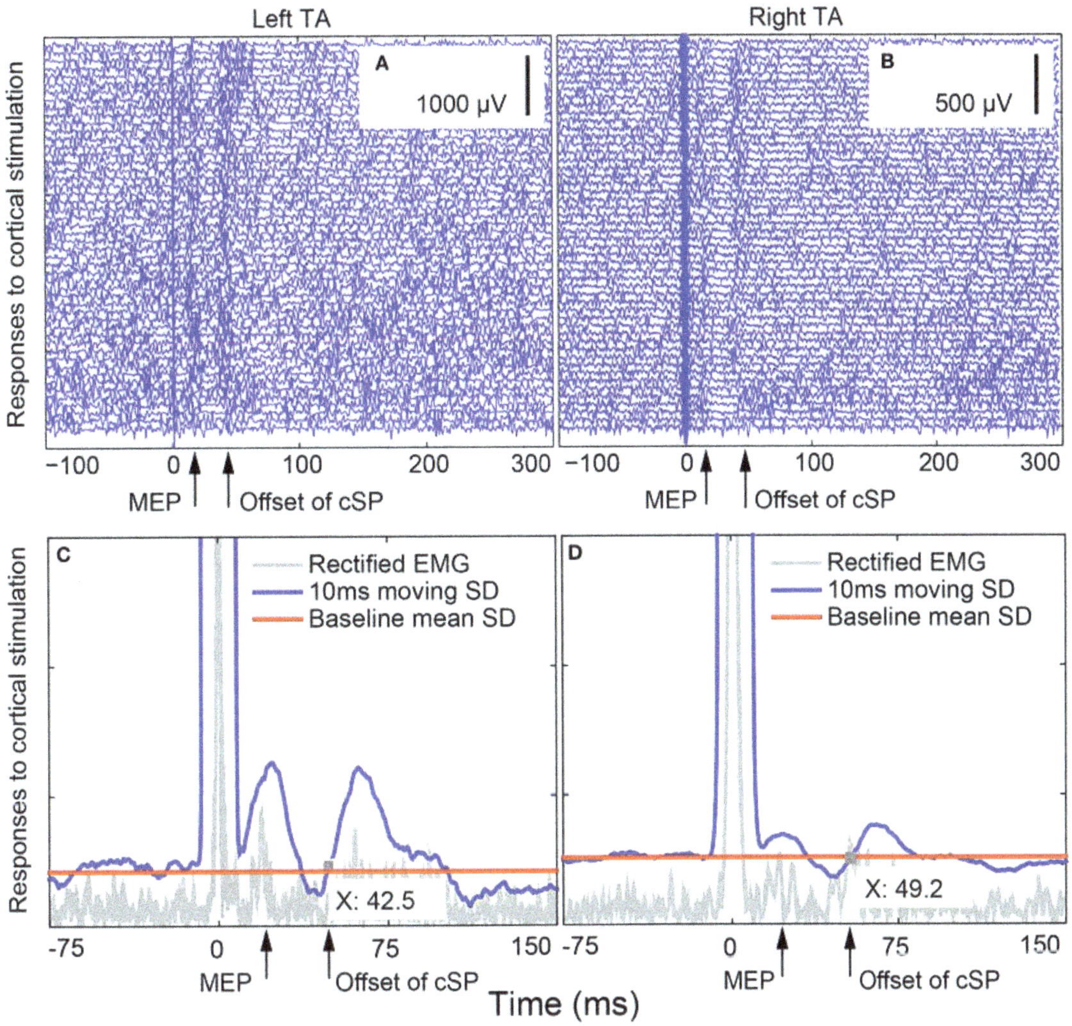

FIGURE 4 | Bilateral thyroarytenoid (TA) motor evoked potential (MEP) responses to right cortical stimulation during voice production in Subject 02. **(A)** 50 individual traces of left TA responses to right cortical stimulation; **(B)** 50 individual traces of right TA responses to right cortical stimulation; **(C)** cSP from the left TA during right cortical stimulation (offset X at 42.5 ms); **(D)** cSP from the right TA during right cortical stimulation (offset X at 49.2 ms). The cSP moving average was calculated based on the average of the 50 trials. The stimuli were delivered at 0 ms. cSP: cortical silent period.

susceptibility to main noise (e.g., 50 or 60 Hz) without requiring a notch filter which should be avoided during EMG/MEP data acquisition because a notch filter would also filter out the informative components of the EMG/MEP within the 50–60 Hz range (Konrad, 2005).

Insertion of Fine-Wire Electrodes

Fine-wire electrodes were chosen instead of needle electrodes because they adapt to the muscle movement. During our experiment, the participants were asked to vocalize "/i/" which contracts the muscles in the vocal folds. Rigid needle electrodes resist muscle contraction causing pain during vocalization and dry swallows. However, insertion accuracy of bi-polar fine-wire pair electrodes is critical to data quality. An experienced otolaryngologist inserted the electrodes in this experiment. In some participants, however, re-insertion was necessary after an insertion did not yield an EMG signal.

In some participants, the two TA muscles had different EMG signal amplitudes, as shown in **Figure 3** (e.g., left > right). This occurred frequently likely due to differences in the insertion angle and depth of the fine-wire electrodes. With different placement in the muscles, the number and size of the motor units between the two poles of the fine-wire electrodes will vary, resulting in differences in the signal amplitude. For this reason, the traditional peak-to-peak motor evoked potentials may not be a valid measure for assessing cortical excitability. The use of cSP, however, diminishes the impact of this issue because the cSP is a temporal/duration measure, not an amplitude measure. Thus, the shape of the MEP has less effect on cSP duration than that of the MEP amplitude. This makes the cSP a useful method for quantifying cortical excitability when using fine-wire electrodes.

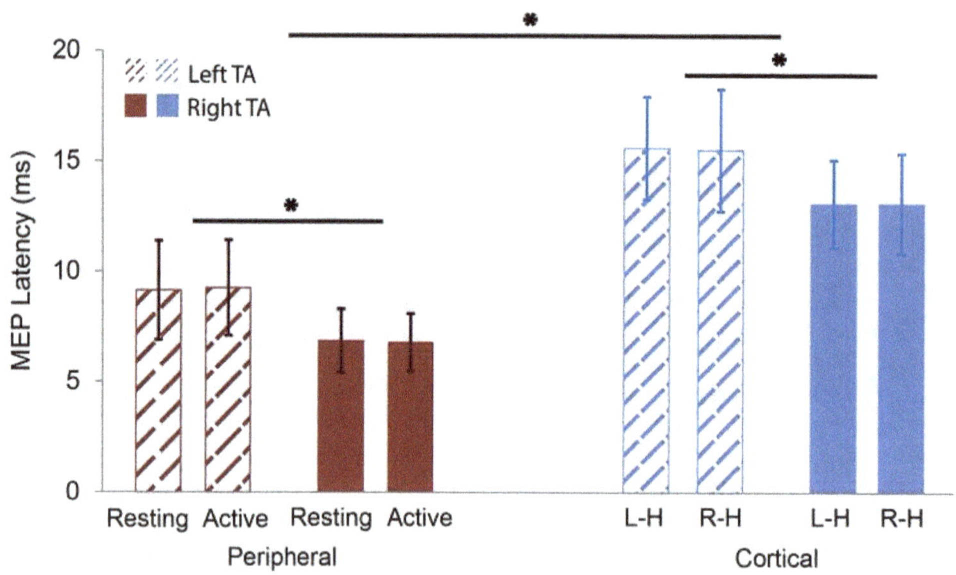

FIGURE 5 | MEP latency comparisons. Red color represents peripheral stimulation responses (left). Blue color represents cortical stimulation responses **(right)**. Thatched represents left TA responses. Solid represents right TA responses. The MEP latencies of left TA were significantly longer than the right TA in both peripheral and cortical stimulation. The MEP latencies of the cortical stimulation were significantly longer than the peripheral one in both left and right TAs. L-H: cortical Left Hemisphere; R-H: cortical Right Hemisphere. $^{*}p < 0.05$.

LIMITATIONS

During data collection, we did not attempt to control TA muscle contraction level as a percent of maximum voluntary contraction (MVC), as is typically performed for hand muscles. The rationale for this decision was that to control the contraction level of TA muscles, both the pitch and the amplitude of vocalization need to be standardized. For the standardization of voice pitch, it is required that the full range of vocal pitch of each participant is measured (similar to the MVC measurement in the conventional TMS test) and, that all participants generate a normalized relative pitch (similar to the 20% of MVC in the conventional hand TMS test) during the experiment. The same procedures apply to the standardization of the amplitude. To control the two factors (pitch and amplitude) synchronously may be difficult for participants to follow, especially when there are fine-wires inserted into their larynx. Thus, in this work we used a compromised but practical method to standardize the TA muscle contraction: participants were instructed to vocalize with their comfortable and natural pitch and volume consistently in each trial. This methodology will allow for future comparisons with populations that have difficulty in controlling their voice, such as people with spasmodic dysphonia. Although the cSP values were likely unaffected by this limitation, as contraction strength of the target muscle does not significantly influence cSP duration (Haug et al., 1992; Inghilleri et al., 1993; Roick et al., 1993; Taylor et al., 1997; Wu et al., 2002; Säisänen et al., 2008). Of note, these previously reported studies were done in large peripheral muscles, i.e., FDI. It is possible that this characteristic is different when measured in intrinsic laryngeal muscles. Thus, it is worth further investigation and may be a useful addition in future experiments.

In the current study, the cSP threshold was used instead of the conventionally adopted 120–130% of resting motor threshold in previous cSP studies (Wolters et al., 2008). This was because that it was difficult to determine a resting motor threshold from the constantly-firing TA muscles. However, it has been reported that the MEP threshold and cSP threshold are usually related (Kimiskidis et al., 2005), suggesting that the stimulation intensity used (cSP threshold) was valid.

Cortical silent period (cSP) threshold and responses were collected first in the left hemisphere followed by the right hemisphere in all participants. Given that the fine-wire electrodes may change position due to swallowing or head rotation during the experiment, we collected data from the hemisphere with higher priority first. The left LMC has been reported to have a more dominant role than the right LMC in vocalization (Simonyan et al., 2009) thus, it was tested first.

Considering the invasive procedure of the fine-wire insertion during the experiment, there was no reliability re-tests attempted in the study design. Although according to previous studies, the intersession variability of cSP is typically <10% (Kukowski and Haug, 1991; Orth and Rothwell, 2004), but this is unknown for laryngeal data.

The MEP amplitudes reported were calculated based on the averaged trace of the 50 cSP trials. Conventionally, the MEP amplitude is calculated based on individual traces and then the average values are reported. However, given the noisy nature of the TA EMG and the relatively low amplitude of the MEP, it is difficult to determine MEP amplitude based on each individual trace. Using the averaged trace provides a clear background to distinguish the MEP from noise or random firing spikes.

CONCLUSION

We assessed the excitability of LMC using the TMS evoked cSP in the TA muscles. The cSP duration was in line with other healthy cranial muscles, such as the tongue (Katayama et al., 2001). The responses were confirmed by contrasting the difference in the MEP peak latencies that were generated by cortical and peripheral stimulation, respectively. Given there are reports of the low intersession variability of the cSP duration in a given subject, typically $<10\%$ (Kukowski and Haug, 1991; Orth and Rothwell, 2004), measurement of cSP may be exceptionally suitable for longitudinal studies in patients, or before and after experimental manipulation. We conclude that the TMS evoked cortical excitability cSP measure can be safely tested in intrinsic laryngeal muscles in healthy volunteers. The use of fine-wire electrodes to measure the cSP of the LMC as validated in this work provides a tool to evaluate GABA receptor mediated inhibition process in the LMC. This will enable the direct comparison of inhibitory responses in healthy individuals and people with neurological voice disorders, such as spasmodic dysphonia and voice tremor which in turn will lead to a better understanding of the pathophysiology of these conditions

AUTHOR CONTRIBUTORS

MC, experimental system design, methodology, data collection, data processing, data analysis, data interpretation, drafting the work, final approval of the version to be published; RS, conception of the study, data collection, data interpretation, drafting the work, final approval of the version to be published; GG, conception of the study, methodology, data collection, final approval of the version to be published; SS, methodology assistance, data interpretation, final approval of the version to be published; CL, methodology, data interpretation, final approval of the version to be published; CP, data collection, drafting the work, final approval of the version to be published; TK, conception of the study, methodology, data collection, data analysis, data interpretation, drafting the work, final approval of the version to be published.

FUNDING

This work was partly supported by the National Institute of Communication Disorders and Deafness, National Institutes of Health (grant number R21DC012344), the University of Minnesota's MnDRIVE (Minnesota's Discovery, Research and Innovation Economy) initiative, the National Center for Advancing Translational Sciences of the National Institutes of Health (award number UL1TR000114) and, National Institute of Biomedical Imaging and Bioengineering (grant number P41 EB015894).

ACKNOWLEDGMENTS

This work was partly supported by the University of Minnesota Clinical and Translational Science Institute and Center for Magnetic Resonance Research at University of Minnesota.

REFERENCES

Atkins, J. P. (1973). An electromyographic study of recurrent laryngeal nerve conduction and its clinical applications. *Laryngoscope* 83, 796–807. doi: 10.1288/00005537-197305000-00015

Calancie, B., Nordin, M., Wallin, U., and Hagbarth, K. E. (1987). Motor-unit responses in human wrist flexor and extensor muscles to transcranial cortical stimuli. *J. Neurophysiol.* 58, 1168–1185.

Chen, M., Deng, H., Schmidt, R. L., and Kimberley, T. J. (2015). Low-Frequency repetitive transcranial magnetic stimulation targeted to premotor cortex followed by primary motor cortex modulates excitability differently than premotor cortex or primary motor cortex stimulation alone. *Neuromodulation* 18, 678–685. doi: 10.1111/ner.12337

Classen, J., and Benecke, R. (1995). Inhibitory phenomena in individual motor units induced by transcranial magnetic stimulation. *Electroencephalogr. Clin. Neurophysiol.* 97, 264–274. doi: 10.1016/0924-980X(95)00099-2

Currà, A., Romaniello, A., Berardelli, A., Cruccu, G., and Manfredi, M. (2000). Shortened cortical silent period in facial muscles of patients with cranial dystonia. *Neurology* 54, 130–135. doi: 10.1212/WNL.54.1.130

Davey, N. J., Romaiguère, P., Maskill, D. W., and Ellaway, P. H. (1994). Suppression of voluntary motor activity revealed using transcranial magnetic stimulation of the motor cortex in man. *J. Physiol.* 477(Pt 2), 223–235.

Eldaief, M. C., Press, D. Z., and Pascual-Leone, A. (2013). Transcranial magnetic stimulation in neurology: a review of established and prospective applications. *Neurol. Clin. Pract.* 3, 519–526. doi: 10.1212/01.CPJ.0000436213.11132.8e

Ertekin, C., Turman, B., Tarlaci, S., Celik, M., Aydogdu, I., Secil, Y., et al. (2001). Cricopharyngeal sphincter muscle responses to transcranial magnetic stimulation in normal subjects and in patients with dysphagia. *Clin. Neurophysiol.* 112, 86–94. doi: 10.1016/S1388-2457(00)00504-6

Eisen, A. A., and Shtybel, W. (1990). AAEM minimonograph #35: clinical experience with transcranial magnetic stimulation. *Muscle Nerve* 13, 995–1011. doi: 10.1002/mus.880131102

Espadaler, J., Rogić, M., Deletis, V., Leon, A., Quijada, C., and Conesa, G. (2012). Representation of cricothyroid muscles at the primary motor cortex (M1) in healthy subjects, mapped by navigated transcranial magnetic stimulation (nTMS). *Clin. Neurophysiol.* 123, 2205–2211. doi: 10.1016/j.clinph.2012.04.008

Ferbert, A., Caramia, D., Priori, A., Bertolasi, L., and Rothwell, J. C. (1992). Cortical projection to erector spinae muscles in man as assessed by focal transcranial magnetic stimulation. *Electroencephalogr. Clin. Neurophysiol.* 85, 382–387. doi: 10.1016/0168-5597(92)90051-C

Hallett, M. (2007). Transcranial magnetic stimulation: a primer. *Neuron* 55, 187–199. doi: 10.1016/j.neuron.2007.06.026

Haug, B. A., Schönle, P. W., Knobloch, C., and Köhne, M. (1992). Silent period measurement revives as a valuable diagnostic tool with transcranial magnetic stimulation. *Electroencephalogr. Clin. Neurophysiol.* 85, 158–160. doi: 10.1016/0168-5597(92)90081-L

Henriquez, V. M., Schulz, G. M., Bielamowicz, S., and Ludlow, C. L. (2007). Laryngeal reflex responses are not modulated during human voice and respiratory tasks. *J. Physiol.* 585(Pt 3), 779–789. doi: 10.1113/jphysiol.2007.143438

Hirano, M., and Ohala, J. (1969). Use of hooked-wire electrodes for electromyography of the intrinsic laryngeal muscles. *J. Speech Hear. Res.* 12:362. doi: 10.1044/jshr.1202.362

Inghilleri, M., Berardelli, A., Cruccu, G., and Manfredi, M. (1993). Silent period evoked by transcranial stimulation of the human cortex and cervicomedullary junction. *J. Physiol.* 466, 521–534.

Katayama, T., Aizawa, H., Kuroda, K., Suzuki, Y., Kikuchi, K., Kimura, T., et al. (2001). Cortical silent period in the tongue induced by transcranial magnetic stimulation. *J. Neurol. Sci.* 193, 37–41. doi: 10.1016/S0022-510X(01)00647-5

Khedr, E. M., and Aref, E.-E. M. (2002). Electrophysiological study of vocal-fold mobility disorders using a magnetic stimulator. *Eur. J. Neurol.* 9, 259–267. doi: 10.1046/j.1468-1331.2002.00394.x

Kimberley, T. J., Borich, M. R., Prochaska, K. D., Mundfrom, S. L., Perkins, A. E., and Poepping, J. M. (2009). Establishing the definition and inter-rater reliability of cortical silent period calculation in subjects with focal hand dystonia and healthy controls. *Neurosci. Lett.* 464, 84–87. doi: 10.1016/j.neulet.2009.08.029

Kimiskidis, V. K., Papagiannopoulos, S., Sotirakoglou, K., Kazis, D. A., Kazis, A., and Mills, K. R. (2005). Silent period to transcranial magnetic stimulation: construction and properties of stimulus–response curves in healthy volunteers. *Exp. Brain Res.* 163, 21–31. doi: 10.1007/s00221-004-2134-4

Konrad, P. (2005). *The ABC of EMG: A Practical Introduction to Kinesiological Electromyography*. Scottsdale, AZ: Noraxon INC.

Kukowski, B., and Haug, B. (1991). Quantitative evaluation of the silent period, evoked by transcranial magnetic stimulation during sustained muscle contraction, in normal man and in patients with stroke. *Electromyogr. Clin. Neurophysiol.* 32, 373–378.

Kuna, S. T., Insalaco, G., and Woodson, G. E. (1988). Thyroarytenoid muscle activity during wakefulness and sleep in normal adults. *J. Appl. Physiol.* 65, 1332–1339.

Lefaucheur, J.-P. (2005). Excitability of the motor cortical representation of the external anal sphincter. *Exp. Brain Res.* 160, 268–272. doi: 10.1007/s00221-004-2170-0

Lefaucheur, J.-P., and Lofaso, F. (2002). Diaphragmatic silent period to transcranial magnetic cortical stimulation for assessing cortical motor control of the diaphragm. *Exp. Brain Res.* 146, 404–409. doi: 10.1007/s00221-002-1197-3

Ludlow, C. L. (2005). Central nervous system control of the laryngeal muscles in humans. *Respir. Physiol. Neurobiol.* 147, 205–222. doi: 10.1016/j.resp.2005.04.015

Ludlow, C. L. (2015). Central nervous system control of voice and swallowing. *J. Clin. Neurophysiol.* 32, 294–303. doi: 10.1097/WNP.0000000000000186

Ludlow, C. L., Adler, C. H., Berke, G. S., Bielamowicz, S. A., Blitzer, A., Bressman, S. B., et al. (2008). Research priorities in spasmodic dysphonia. *Otolaryngol. Head Neck Surg.* 139, 495–505. doi: 10.1016/j.otohns.2008.05.624

Mazziotta, J., Toga, A., Evans, A., Fox, P., Lancaster, J., Zilles, K., et al. (2001). A four-dimensional probabilistic atlas of the human brain. *J. Am. Med. Inform. Assoc.* 8, 401–430. doi: 10.1136/jamia.2001.0080401

Orth, M., and Rothwell, J. (2004). The cortical silent period: intrinsic variability and relation to the waveform of the transcranial magnetic stimulation pulse. *Clin. Neurophysiol.* 115, 1076–1082. doi: 10.1016/j.clinph.2003.12.025

Paradiso, G. O., Cunic, D. I., Gunraj, C. A., and Chen, R. (2005). Representation of facial muscles in human motor cortex. *J. Physiol.* 567, 323–336. doi: 10.1113/jphysiol.2005.088542

Paulus, W., Classen, J., Cohen, L. G., Large, C. H., Di Lazzaro, V., Nitsche, M., et al. (2008). State of the art: pharmacologic effects on cortical excitability measures tested by transcranial magnetic stimulation. *Brain Stimul.* 1, 151–163. doi: 10.1016/j.brs.2008.06.002

Rödel, R. M. W., Olthoff, A., Tergau, F., Simonyan, K., Kraemer, D., Markus, H., et al. (2004). Human cortical motor representation of the larynx as assessed by Transcranial Magnetic Stimulation (TMS). *Laryngoscope* 114, 918–922. doi: 10.1097/00005537-200405000-00026

Rogić Vidaković, M., Schönwald, M. Z., Rotim, K., Jurić, T., Vulević, Z., Tafra, R., et al. (2015). Excitability of contralateral and ipsilateral projections of corticobulbar pathways recorded as corticobulbar motor evoked potentials of the cricothyroid muscles. *Clin. Neurophysiol.* 126, 1570–1577. doi: 10.1016/j.clinph.2014.11.001

Roick, H., von Giesen, H. J., and Benecke, R. (1993). On the origin of the postexcitatory inhibition seen after transcranial magnetic brain stimulation in awake human subjects. *Exp. Brain Res.* 94, 489–498. doi: 10.1007/BF00230207

Rossini, P. M., Barker, A. T., Berardelli, A., Caramia, M. D., Caruso, G., Cracco, R. Q., et al. (1994). Non-invasive electrical and magnetic stimulation of the brain, spinal cord and roots: basic principles and procedures for routine clinical application. Report of an IFCN committee. *Electroencephalogr. Clin. Neurophysiol.* 91, 79–92. doi: 10.1016/0013-4694(94)90029-9

Rossini, P. M., Burke, D., Chen, R., Cohen, L. G., Daskalakis, Z., Di Iorio, R., et al. (2015). Non-invasive electrical and magnetic stimulation of the brain, spinal cord, roots and peripheral nerves: basic principles and procedures for routine clinical and research application. An updated report from an I.F.C.N. Committee. *Clin. Neurophysiol.* 126, 1071–1107. doi: 10.1016/j.clinph.2015.02.001

Säisänen, L., Pirinen, E., Teitti, S., Könönen, M., Julkunen, P., Määttä, S., et al. (2008). Factors influencing cortical silent period: optimized stimulus location, intensity and muscle contraction. *J. Neurosci. Methods* 169, 231–238. doi: 10.1016/j.jneumeth.2007.12.005

Samargia, S., Schmidt, R., and Kimberley, T. J. (2014). Shortened cortical silent period in adductor spasmodic dysphonia: evidence for widespread cortical excitability. *Neurosci. Lett.* 560, 12–15. doi: 10.1016/j.neulet.2013.12.007

Siebner, H. R., Dressnandt, J., Auer, C., and Conrad, B. (1998). Continuous intrathecal baclofen infusions induced a marked increase of the transcranially evoked silent period in a patient with generalized dystonia. *Muscle Nerve* 21, 1209–1212. doi: 10.1002/(SICI)1097-4598(199809)21:9<1209::AID-MUS15>3.0.CO;2-M

Silbert, L. C., Nelson, C., Holman, S., Eaton, R., Oken, B. S., Lou, J. S., et al. (2006). Cortical excitability and age-related volumetric MRI changes. *Clin. Neurophysiol.* 117, 1029–1036. doi: 10.1016/j.clinph.2006.02.003

Simonyan, K., and Horwitz, B. (2011). Laryngeal motor cortex and control of speech in humans. *Neuroscientist* 17, 197–208. doi: 10.1177/1073858410386727

Simonyan, K., Ostuni, J., Ludlow, C. L., and Horwitz, B. (2009). Functional but not structural networks of the human laryngeal motor cortex show left hemispheric lateralization during syllable but not breathing production. *J. Neurosci.* 29, 14912–14923. doi: 10.1523/JNEUROSCI.4897-09.2009

Sims, H. S., Yamashita, T., Rhew, K., and Ludlow, C. L. (1996). Assessing the clinical utility of the magnetic stimulator for measuring response latencies in the laryngeal muscles. *Otolaryngol. Head Neck Surg.* 114, 761–767. doi: 10.1016/S0194-5998(96)70099-2

Taylor, J. L., Allen, G. M., Butler, J. E., and Gandevia, S. C. (1997). Effect of contraction strength on responses in biceps brachii and adductor pollicis to transcranial magnetic stimulation. *Exp. Brain Res.* 117, 472–478. doi: 10.1007/s002210050243

Thumfart, W. F., Zorowka, P., Pototschnig, C., and Eckel, H. E. (1992). Electrophysiologic investigation of lower cranial nerve diseases by means of magnetically stimulated neuromyography of the larynx. *Ann. Otol. Rhinol. Laryngol.* 101, 629–634. doi: 10.1177/000348949210100801

Tinazzi, M., Farina, S., Edwards, M., Moretto, G., Restivo, D., Fiaschi, A., et al. (2005). Task-specific impairment of motor cortical excitation and inhibition in patients with writer's cramp. *Neurosci. Lett.* 378, 55–58. doi: 10.1016/j.neulet.2004.12.015

Werhahn, K. J., Classen, J., and Benecke, R. (1995). The silent period induced by transcranial magnetic stimulation in muscles supplied by cranial nerves: normal data and changes in patients. *J. Neurol. Neurosurg. Psychiatr.* 59, 586–596. doi: 10.1136/JNNP.59.6.586

Wolters, A., Ziemann, U., and Benecke, R. (2008). "The cortical silent period," in *Oxford Handbook of Transcranial Stimulation*, eds C. M. Epstein, E. M. Wassermann, and U. Ziemann (New York, NY: Oxford University Press), 1–23.

World Medical Association (2013). World Medical Association Declaration of Helsinki: ethical principles for medical research involving human subjects. *JAMA.* 310, 2191–2194. doi: 10.1001/jama.2013.281053

Wu, L., Goto, Y., Taniwaki, T., Kinukawa, N., and Tobimatsu, S. (2002). Different patterns of excitation and inhibition of the small hand and forearm muscles from magnetic brain stimulation in humans. *Clin. Neurophysiol.* 113, 1286–1294. doi: 10.1016/S1388-2457(02)00160-8

18

Integration of Descending Command Systems for the Generation of Context-Specific Locomotor Behaviors

Linda H. Kim [1,2†], *Sandeep Sharma* [1,3†], *Simon A. Sharples* [1,2], *Kyle A. Mayr* [1,2], *Charlie H. T. Kwok* [1,3] *and Patrick J. Whelan* [1,2,3*]

[1] Hotchkiss Brain Institute, University of Calgary, Calgary, AB, Canada, [2] Department of Neuroscience, University of Calgary, Calgary, AB, Canada, [3] Department of Comparative Biology and Experimental Medicine, University of Calgary, Calgary, AB, Canada

***Correspondence:**
Patrick J. Whelan
whelan@ucalgary.ca

[†] *These authors have contributed equally to this work.*

Over the past decade there has been a renaissance in our understanding of spinal cord circuits; new technologies are beginning to provide key insights into descending circuits which project onto spinal cord central pattern generators. By integrating work from both the locomotor and animal behavioral fields, we can now examine context-specific control of locomotion, with an emphasis on descending modulation arising from various regions of the brainstem. Here we examine approach and avoidance behaviors and the circuits that lead to the production and arrest of locomotion.

Keywords: locomotor behavior, supraspinal, descending, goal-directed, approach, aversion

INTRODUCTION

Animals produce a wide array of locomotor behaviors in response to internal and external cues. Normally, animals survey the environment in search of appropriate olfaction, audition, visual, or tactile sensory inputs. Internally motivated cues may be due to appetitive drive such as food and reproduction, and other physiological needs like safety, shelter, or adaptation to a new environment. These cues inform ongoing movement sequences by converging onto locomotor

Abbreviations: A10, Dopaminergic cell group A10; A11, Dopaminergic cell group A11; A13, Dopaminergic cell group A13; ABA, Accessory basal amygdala; AMG, Amygdala; BG, Basal ganglia; BLA, Basolateral amygdala complex; CeA, Central nucleus of the amygdala; CeM, Medial central nucleus of the amygdala; ChR2, Channelrhodopsin 2; Chx10, Transcription factor Chx10; CnF, Cuneiform nucleus; D1, Dopamine receptor subtype 1; D2, Dopamine receptor subtype 2; DDS, Diencephalospinal dopamine system (in zebrafish); dlPAG, Dorsolateral periaqueductal gray; DLR, Diencephalic locomotor region; dMSNs, Direct pathway medium spiny neurons; dPAG, Dorsal periaqueductal gray; GABA, gamma-Aminobutyric acid; GAD65, glutamic acid decarboxylase; Gi, Gigantocellular reticular nucleus; GiA, Gigantocellular reticular nucleus alpha part; GiV, Gigantocellular reticular nucleus ventral part; GP, Globus pallidus; GPe, Globus pallidus external; GPi, Globus pallidus internal; iMSNs, Indirect pathway medium spiny neurons; LH, Lateral hypothalamus; Lhx3, Transcription factor Lhx3; lPAG, Lateral periaqueductal gray; LPGi, Lateral paragigantocellular nucleus; MdV, Ventral part of medullary reticular formation; MLR, Mesencephalic locomotor region; MRF, Medullary reticular formation; NAc, Nucleus accumbens; PAG, Periaqueductal gray; PMH, Premammillary nucleus of the hypothalamus; PnC, Pontine reticular nucleus caudal; PnO, Pontine reticular nucleus oral; PPN, Pedunculopontine nuclei; PPTg, Pedunculopontine tegmental nucleus; SC, Superior colliculus; SLR, Subthalamic locomotor region; SN, Substantia nigra; SNc, Substantia nigra pars compacta; SNr, Substantia nigra pars reticulata; STh/ STN, Subthalamic nucleus; V1, Primary visual cortex; V1 L5, Layer 5 of the primary visual cortex; Vglut2, Vesicular glutamate 2; vlPAG, Ventrolateral periaqueductal gray; VMH, Ventromedial hypothalamus; VP, Ventral pallidum; VTA, Ventral tegmental area; ZI, Zona incerta.

control centers in the brainstem and spinal cord, thus facilitating the generation of context-appropriate locomotor behaviors.

In the first part of this review, we focus on key supraspinal regions for locomotor control, with emphasis placed on how technological advances are beginning to reveal cell types and the underlying functional connectome. In the second part of this review, we will explore the afferent projections to these locomotor regions and discuss how internal and external triggers can drive appetitive (approach) or aversive (avoidance) locomotor responses.

DESCENDING COMMAND SYSTEMS FOR LOCOMOTION

Over the past 75 years, studies on the descending control of locomotion have been directed toward three regions (Whelan, 1996; Jordan et al., 2008); the Subthalamic Locomotor Region (SLR), the Mesencephalic Locomotor Region (MLR: **Figure 1**), and the Medullary Reticular Formation (MRF: **Figure 1**). These regions were initially identified based on their ability to elicit various forms of locomotor behaviors in response to direct electrical stimulation of these regions. The term "locomotor region" was used since electrical stimulation cannot be confined to anatomically-defined nuclei. These regions are conserved across vertebrate species studied (reviews Rossignol et al., 2006; Fetcho et al., 2008; Grillner et al., 2008; Jordan et al., 2008; Ryczko and Dubuc, 2013) with initial experiments being performed in cats (Shik et al., 1969—English translation of their 1966 publication; reviews Armstrong, 1986; Whelan, 1996), later in rats (Mel'nikova, 1975, 1977 as cited by Ross and Sinnamon, 1984; Sinnamon et al., 1984; Skinner and Garcia-Rill, 1984), and recently in mice (Bouvier et al., 2015; Roseberry et al., 2016).

Investigations into the underlying cellular and system mechanisms for the generation of locomotor behaviors begun in tandem with the identification of locomotor regions. Earlier work was performed in relatively simple organisms (Gillette et al., 1978; Olson and Krasne, 1981; Edwards et al., 1999; Esch and Kristan, 2002) and primitive vertebrates (Grillner et al., 2008). Work on the leech, lamprey and xenopus have provided fascinating similarities between swim behaviors and circuit organization of organisms separated by up to 560 million years of evolution (Mullins et al., 2011). Recent advances in molecular biology and genetic tools have enabled the functional connectivity of locomotor circuit elements in mammalian systems to be explored (Bouvier et al., 2015; Roseberry et al., 2016).

THE MEDULLARY RETICULAR FORMATION: A CENTRE FOR LOCOMOTOR STOP AND GO

The MRF contains groups of diffusely located nuclei that form an important integration center for the control of locomotion, with descending projections onto interneurons and motoneurons of the cervical and lumbar spinal cord (Grillner et al., 1968; Peterson et al., 1979; Bouvier et al., 2015). Shik et al. (1969) were the first to show the existence of a pathway from the MLR to the MRF. Although, activity in the MRF is known to correspond to locomotor activity, recordings from the MRF in freely walking cats showed that activity patterns were complex, as only some units corresponded to the rhythmic electromyographic activity of muscles while others did not (Drew et al., 1986; Perreault et al., 1993). Both electrical and direct drug-based stimulation of the MRF can elicit locomotion (Garcia-Rill and Skinner, 1987a,b; Noga et al., 1988; Jordan, 1998). Similarly, rhythmic patterns or locomotor-like rhythmicity in the isolated *in vitro* brainstem-spinal cord preparation can be evoked (Liu and Jordan, 2005; Hägglund et al., 2010; Kiehn, 2016). Additionally, stimulation of ventrolateral funiculi, containing the reticulospinal projections, can produce bouts of rhythmic motor activity (Magnuson et al., 1995). Acute lesions of this tract eliminate locomotion elicited by stimulation of the MLR in decerebrate cats (Steeves and Jordan, 1980) and result in changes of gait in freely moving animals (Brustein and Rossignol, 1998).

Classically, the MRF has been subdivided into four key nuclei distributed across the medulla and the pons and is also

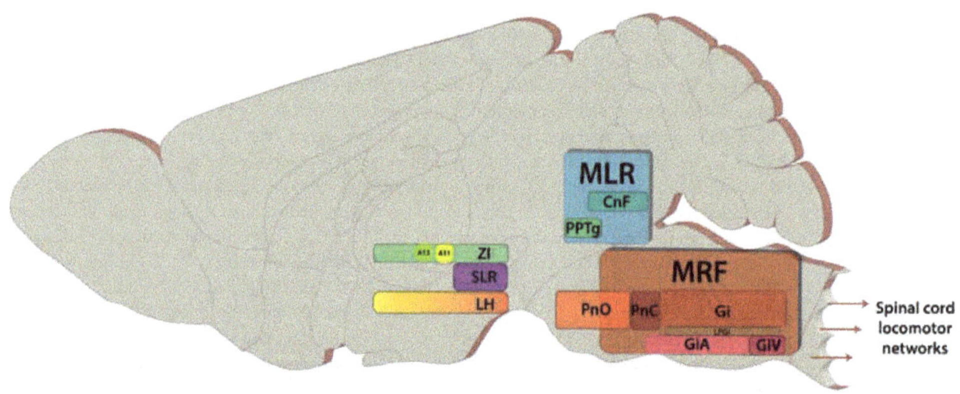

FIGURE 1 | Key areas of the brain discussed in the review. The brain areas are included here have diverse functions in addition to modulating locomotion. Sagittal view of representative locations of locomotor centers.

known as ponto-medullary reticular formation (review Drew et al., 2004). In rodents, these regions correspond with pontine reticular nucleus oral (PnO) and caudal (PnC), gigantocellular reticular nucleus (Gi), and magnocellular nucleus of medulla which encompasses lateral paragigantocellular nucleus (LPGi), gigantocellular reticular nucleus alpha (GiA), and ventral section (GiV), respectively (Paxinos and Franklin, 2008; Esposito et al., 2014). Recent work has focused on the Gi, LPGi, GiA, and GiV. These nuclei form the reticulospinal pathway, and contain cells that descend ipsilaterally via the ventrolateral and ventromedial funiculi (Petras, 1967; Peterson et al., 1979). Contralateral projections also exist (Jankowska et al., 2003; Krutki et al., 2003; Szokol et al., 2011). Recent work using genetic and intersectional viral tracing has revealed that reticulospinal pathways are more diverse than previously thought, and cells can be organized into clusters based on their projections either in the cervical or lumbar spinal cord (Esposito et al., 2014). The ventral part of the MRF (MdV) was highlighted as a region with functional connectivity to forelimb motor neurons suggesting that MRF regions may be organized somatotopically. Interestingly in cat MRF cells were observed to project over long distances to multiple segments (Matsuyama et al., 1999). These differences may represent the different demands of grasping for rodents compared to cats (Whishaw et al., 2008). However, projections to multiple segments have also been observed in the monkey (Kneisley et al., 1978; Coulter et al., 1979).

Most descending MRF cells are glutamatergic and were traditionally thought to form the excitatory command signal for locomotion. Photostimulation of vesicular glutamate 2 (Vglut2)-expressing cells in the brainstem with channelrhodopsin 2 (ChR2) can elicit spinal rhythmicity *in vitro* (Hägglund et al., 2010). Subsequent investigations explored a subpopulation of glutamatergic cells in the brainstem that can be identified by the Chx10 and Lhx3 transcription factors. These cells express c-fos (a marker of neuronal activation) following bouts of locomotor activity, receive input from the MLR, and project to the cervical spinal cord (Bretzner and Brownstone, 2013). Manipulation of activity of these cells *in vivo* did not alter locomotor behavior in mice (Bretzner and Brownstone, 2013), however, activation of these cells in zebrafish is sufficient to drive locomotor activity (Kimura et al., 2013). Surprisingly, recent work on the Chx10 population in mice found that activation of this cell-type at the junction between the rostral medulla (rostral Gi) and caudal pons (PnC) disrupted spinally-generated rhythmicity *in vitro*, and caused the animal to stop when activated *in vivo* (Bouvier et al., 2015). Recruitment of spinally-located premotor inhibitory interneurons by the Chx10 MRF neurons was implicated (Bouvier et al., 2015). Conversely, stop commands in fish (Wannier et al., 1995) and tadpoles (Boothby and Roberts, 1992; Perrins et al., 2002; Li et al., 2003) are reported to be mediated by descending inhibitory cells of the MRF, which project mono-synaptically to motoneurons and are triggered by sensory afferents in the head. This poses an interesting possibility for a parallel stopping mechanism in mammals that remains to be discovered (review Klemm, 2001). Indeed, a GABAergic/glycinergic projection from the MRF to the spinal cord exists in rodents but its function in locomotor control remains unknown (Holstege, 1991).

In addition to the glutamatergic and GABAergic/glycinergic descending pathways within the brainstem are several monoaminergic neuromodulatory pathways that can modulate locomotor activity. The major descending brainstem modulatory pathways are the serotonergic raphespinal pathway and the noradrenergic coeruleospinal pathways. These systems have been reviewed elsewhere (Jordan et al., 2008). Recent work suggests that monoamines (5-HT and noradrenaline) increase in concentration many seconds before locomotion and decrease gradually to baseline once locomotion is terminated. These long timeframes suggest that monoamines are not involved in moment-to-moment modulation of spinal cord circuits and may possibly be released extrasynaptically (Noga B. R. et al., 2017).

THE MESENCEPHALIC LOCOMOTOR REGION: AN INTEGRATIVE HUB FOR LOCOMOTOR SPEED AND GAIT

The MLR is located on the mesopontine border and comprises of the cuneiform (CnF) and the pedunculopontine nuclei (PPN) (**Figure 1**). In basal vertebrates, the MLR comprises the laterodorsal tegmental nucleus and the PPN. In mammals, it comprises the PPN, but also the CnF (Ryczko and Dubuc, 2013, 2017). It can be described as a classical region for locomotor control. Electrical stimulation of the mesopontine border with increasing intensity led to a serial progression from walking to running to galloping (Shik et al., 1969). Initially it was thought that the MLR projects serially to the MRF and acts as a "volume-control" for locomotion, as ablation of the MRF abolished MLR-evoked responses in the spinal cord (Noga et al., 2003). Since the original finding the location of the nuclei comprising the MLR and its projections have been steadily refined.

The PPN, referred to as the pedunculopontine tegmental nucleus (PPTg) in rodents (Paxinos and Franklin, 2008) and sometimes the nucleus tegmenti pedulculopontinus in humans (Schaltenbrand and Wahren, 1977), is located in the ventrolateral portion of the MLR (Olszewski and Baxter, 1954). It is composed of cells with heterogeneous neurotransmitter phenotypes including but not limited to: GABA, glutamate, acetylcholine, and calcium-binding proteins and neuropeptides (Clements and Grant, 1990; Lavoie and Parent, 1994; Fortin and Parent, 1999; Vincent, 2000; Mena-Segovia et al., 2008, 2009). There is no doubt that the use of different terms has led to confusion in the field. In this review we will refer to the PPTg when discussing rodent relevant papers and PPN when referring to cat, monkey, or human work. In terms of projections, the PPN and CnF connect to sensorimotor, associative, and limbic areas of the basal ganglia and the thalamus in monkeys and humans (Sébille et al., 2017). Analysis of these projections suggests that the PPN may integrate sensorimotor, cognitive, and emotional information. The anterior part of the PPN may be related to motor control in the monkey. In contrast, the CnF connectome is more restricted involving predominantly limbic brain regions (Sébille et al., 2017). Some reports have identified the PPTg as an effective site for evoking locomotion, and direct efferent projections to the lumbar spinal cord have been reported (Skinner et al., 1990). Of the two regions, stimulation of the CnF appears to be more robust in driving locomotion in the cat (Shik and Orlovsky, 1976—original article in Russian: Sirota and Shik, 1973). The CnF lies dorsal to PPTg and borders the inferior colliculi ventrally (Allen Brain Atlas: https://tinyurl.com/k8g98tl). Like the PPTg, the CnF is composed of heterogenous cell types including GABAergic (Ford et al., 1995), glutamatergic (Heise and Mitrofanis, 2006), peptidergic (Sar et al., 1978; Beitz, 1982a,b) cells with some cholinergic neurons (Ford et al., 1995).

Recent work examined MLR cell types for their roles in locomotor behaviors (Roseberry et al., 2016; Kroeger et al., 2017; Mena-Segovia and Bolam, 2017). Activity of the glutamatergic MLR cells correlate with spontaneous locomotor episodes and their activation is sufficient to produce locomotor bouts. Conversely, activity of the GABAergic population is associated with stationary states and their activation stops locomotion, partly through suppression of the local MLR glutamatergic population (Roseberry et al., 2016). This suggests that GABAergic and glutamatergic MLR cells collectively control decelerating and accelerating locomotor behaviors. Work in cats shows that the substantia nigra pars reticulata (SNr) projects to the PPN and suppresses muscle tone while another projection from the lateral SNr to the CnF promotes locomotor activity (Takakusaki et al., 2003). It is thought that the cholinergic MLR population modulates locomotion, but activation of these cells is not sufficient to elicit a locomotor bout. Instead, stimulation of cholinergic MLR cells leads to acceleration of locomotion (Roseberry et al., 2016). However, there are interspecies differences in the density of cholinergic cells. For example, in Parkinsonian patients where the number of cholinergic cells in the PPN are reduced (Hirsch et al., 1987; Jellinger, 1988; Zweig et al., 1989), gait disturbances are often observed (reviews Pahapill and Lozano, 2000; Alam et al., 2011). In addition, basal ganglia afferent connectivity onto the PPN, and from the PPN onto the basal ganglia differ between species. This may help explain the uncertainty in the efficacy of deep brain stimulation stimulation in Parkinson's patients (Alam et al., 2011). Some studies have reported beneficial effects but other studies are less supportive. There is a debate about whether stimulation is targeting the PPN, with the most effective site being slightly posterior to the PPN, in the CnF and the subCnF (Ferraye et al., 2010). Notably the location of the nuclei encompassing the MLR is still a matter of debate, and there appears to be interspecies differences (for details refer to Alam et al., 2011, 2013; Liang et al., 2011, 2012; Thankachan et al., 2012; Ryczko and Dubuc, 2013; Xiang et al., 2013; Sherman et al., 2015). The CnF is an important part of MLR in higher mammals such as cats and monkeys, whereas the precuneiform nucleus (PrCnF) is the mouse analog of CnF. In mice the PrCnF projects directly to the spinal cord (Liang et al., 2011, 2012). This is not the case in the cat where the CnF was found to project to the first cervical segment. Likewise, in monkeys, the CnF projects ipsilaterally within segments of the spinal cord. An additional complexity in interpreting the literature is that the size of the PrCnF in cats (Satoda et al., 2002) and possibly monkeys (Castiglioi et al., 1978) is likely underestimated as the boundaries between the PrCnF and CnF in cats are not as distinct (Liang et al., 2011).

To summarize, the MLR is well-studied, but comparing and contrasting studies, especially between species can be difficult. Generally speaking, in rodents, the data suggest that the PPTg (PPN) is better associated with reward-based motor behaviors, place preference, and sensorimotor gating, than locomotion (Koch et al., 1993; Inglis et al., 1994; Olmstead and Franklin, 1994; Alam et al., 2011). On the other hand, the CnF and PrCnF seem to be better associated with locomotion (Garcia-Rill and Skinner, 1987a; Milner and Mogenson, 1988; Noga B. et al., 2017).

THE DIENCEPHALON: A HUB FOR GOAL-DIRECTED LOCOMOTION

The diencephalon is home to several regions that can elicit locomotion. Although, diencephalic sites have been described in several species, they have been named differently based on the differences in anatomy and effective sites for stimulation. A region of the diencephalon that was pro-locomotory was first described in the cat in the 1930's (Ectors et al., 1938; Masserman, 1938), and electrical stimulation of the subthalamic region was conducted by Waller (1940). Additional work in the 1980s from Orlovsky, Sinnamon, and Mori amongst others provided new insight into areas within the posterior hypothalamus, lateral hypothalamus, and zona incerta that could elicit locomotor activity. While differences were observed, a general finding was in freely moving animals, it was found that an initial scan of the area was performed before exploratory activity was initiated (Mori et al., 1989). These behaviors are often indistinguishable from spontaneous locomotor behavior (Grossen and Kelley, 1972; Leppänen et al., 2006; Lamprea et al., 2008).

Initial reports suggested the site for eliciting locomotion in the cat was the subthalamic nucleus (STN) (abbreviated as STh in rodents); and thus, it was named the subthalamic locomotor region (SLR) (Grossman, 1958; Kaelber and Smith, 1979). Work conducted later in the rat found that the zona incerta (or "zone of uncertainty" dorsal to STh) and medial lateral hypothalamus (LH) had lower thresholds for electrical stimulation (**Figure 1**; Sinnamon and Stopford, 1987; Milner and Mogenson, 1988; Sinnamon, 1993). In the lamprey, this region is known as the diencephalic locomotor region (DLR) (Manira et al., 1997; Ménard and Grillner, 2008), and is located ventral to the thalamus—a region analogous to the lateral hypothalamus in mammals (Ménard and Grillner, 2008). Unfortunately, like the MLR, the terminology used over the years has been confusing. Here we will use the historic SLR term but, where possible, we'll specify the anatomical region.

The SLR is necessary for goal-directed locomotion as bilateral ablation of the SLR abolishes spontaneous locomotion for several weeks following surgery (Shik and Orlovsky, 1976—original article in Russian: Sirota and Shik, 1973). Although, the SLR is connected to the MLR, the MLR is not necessary for SLR-evoked locomotor behavior (Shik et al., 1969). It appears from these findings that the SLR serves as a parallel command system for locomotor control. What remains unclear is if the MRF is a necessary integration center to spinal cord to produce locomotion. In the lamprey, the DLR, an analog of the SLR in fish, projects to reticulospinal cells (Manira et al., 1997). However, in mammals, direct descending projections from the SLR and DLR to the spinal cord have been reported (Skagerberg and Lindvall, 1985; Sakurai, 2005; Stoyanova et al., 2010; Koblinger et al., 2014). Therefore, it is possible that an MRF-relay may not be necessary for all locomotor behaviors. A more likely scenario is that parallel pathways converge on spinal circuits to coordinate most behaviors.

Local infusion of glutamate agonists and GABA antagonists into the zona incerta (ZI) or the LH are sufficient to drive locomotor behaviors, suggesting that both inhibitory and excitatory afferents regulate SLR output (Di Scala et al., 1984; Milner and Mogenson, 1988; Sinnamon, 1993). The cell types of the ZI and LH have been well-characterized, and like other locomotor command centers are composed of heterogeneous cell types. These include fast-transmitting GABA, glutamatergic cells, and various peptidergic and neuromodulatory subtypes (review Mitrofanis, 2005; Stuber and Wise, 2016). Two modulatory systems that robustly drive locomotion are orexin (Valenstein et al., 1970; Valenstein, 1971; Ida et al., 1999; Thakkar et al., 2001; Sakurai, 2005; Siegel and Boehmer, 2006) and dopamine (Wagner et al., 1995; Kolmac and Mitrofanis, 1999).

The orexin cells in the brain originate mainly in the LH and activity of orexinergic cells is tightly coupled to the regulation of arousal, sleep, appetite, attention, and sensory modulation (Valenstein et al., 1970; Valenstein, 1971; Ida et al., 1999; Thakkar et al., 2001; Sakurai, 2005; Siegel and Boehmer, 2006). These cells have extensive projections throughout the brain including, but not limited to, the SNr, MLR, MRF, and spinal cord (Peyron et al., 1998; Sakurai, 2005; Stoyanova et al., 2010). Mice exhibit enhanced locomotor activity following intracerebroventricular administration of orexin (Hagan et al., 1999; Ida et al., 1999), and blocking orexin-1 receptors attenuates movement (Duxon et al., 2001). A recent study showed presence of orexin receptors on the reticulospinal MLR cells (Sherman et al., 2015). Moreover, focal injection of orexin into the MLR in decerebrate cats either reduced the intensity to evoke locomotion or elicited locomotion without stimulation, whereas an injection of orexin in either PPTg or SNr increased the intensity required to induce muscle atonia (Takakusaki et al., 2005). Recent work has reported that orexin cells may drive locomotor activity by increasing the activity of glutamic acid decarboxylase (GAD65)—expressing inhibitory neurons located in the LH. This population of inhibitory cells was found to be able to drive locomotor behavior when activated, and suppress locomotion when inhibited. These GAD65-expressing cells send projections to ZI, raphe magnus as well as superior colliculus and periaqueductal gray (Kosse et al., 2017; see section Interactions between Appetitive, Defensive, and Exploratory Behavior); however, the underlying circuitry responsible for orexinergic locomotor control requires further characterization.

The A13 and A11 dopaminergic nuclei are in the ZI and the rostral portion of the posterior hypothalamus, respectively. The contribution of the A11 to locomotor control is well characterized in zebrafish and is known as the diencephalospinal dopamine system (DDS; Tay et al., 2011; Lambert et al., 2012). The most recent work on the DDS demonstrates that these cells are rhythmically active during swimming and are both sufficient and necessary for swimming episodes (Jay et al., 2015). Currently, little is known about the locomotor functions of the A13 and A11 in mammals. However, the A11 projects to the spinal cord (Commissiong and Sedgwick, 1975; Skagerberg and Lindvall, 1985; Holstege et al., 1996; Koblinger et al., 2014; review Sharples et al., 2014) and has known roles in pain modulation (Charbit et al., 2009) and motor control (Ondo et al., 2000; Clemens et al., 2006; Qu et al., 2007). It has also been shown that dopamine modulates mammalian spinal CPG networks (Barrière et al., 2004; Humphreys and Whelan, 2012; Sharples et al., 2015; Picton et al., 2017; Sharples, 2017; Sharples and Whelan, 2017). These data support a possibility for a descending dopamine system in mammalian locomotor control. Nonetheless, the role of A11 and A13 cell populations in locomotor behaviors remains to be tested.

FACTORS MEDIATING DECISION MAKING AND MOTOR SELECTION TO APPROACH OR TO AVOID

So far, we have discussed locomotor regions by illustrating the nuclei and cell types involved in each pathway. These regions must interact with other brain areas to produce behaviorally relevant locomotion. Broadly speaking, there are two basic forms of locomotor responses observed in vertebrate species—approach or avoid—and a balance between these is necessary for survival (Glickman and Schiff, 1967). Here we will describe how internal (affective state, cognitive, reward, motivation, homeostatic, etc.) and external (sensory) cues are integrated to decide on approach or aversion (**Figure 2A**). We will describe the functional role of different types of locomotion based on their behavioral correlates, with emphasis on: (1) the role of the superior colliculus (SC) in deciding the appropriate locomotor response based on external sensory cues; (2) key limbic structures mediating locomotor responses based on internal cognitive and affective information; and (3) subsequent motor selection via the basal ganglia circuitry.

EXTERNAL SENSORY CUES CAN FACILITATE APPROPRIATE MOTOR SELECTION

External sensory cues are broadly classified as olfactory, visual, auditory, and tactile stimuli. When animals encounter such cues they must react appropriately to meet survival needs (**Figure 2B**).

The SC is an integral player in triggering appropriate locomotor responses based on novel visual stimuli in the environment. The superficial layers of the SC make use of retinotopic information relayed via the lateral geniculate nucleus of the thalamus (Nagata and Hayashi, 1984; Born and Schmidt, 2008) and primary visual cortex to orient the eyes, head, and body movement toward objects of interest (reviews Sparks, 1986; Grillner et al., 2008; Gandhi and Katnani, 2011). This permits the SC to trigger approach or avoidance responses based on visuospatial input. The location of visual information

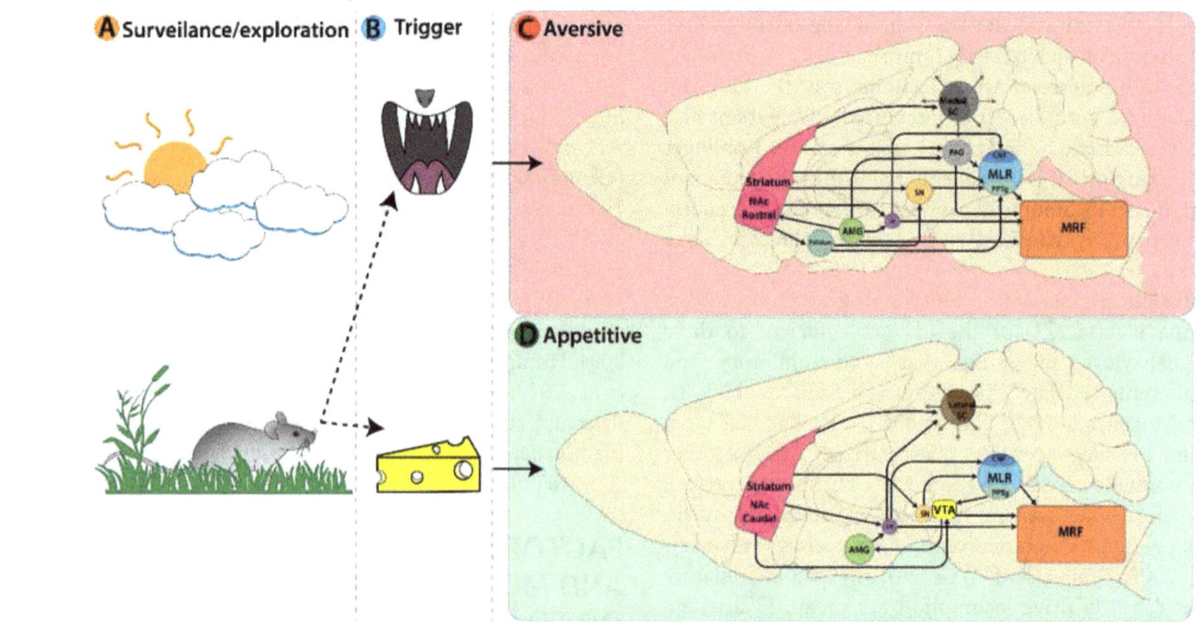

FIGURE 2 | Active nuclei in the mouse brain following a decision or trigger from a surveillance state. **(A)** Representation of an animal's decision process during a surveillance state. In this example a mouse encounters an aversive trigger (**B** top, predatory threat) activating nuclei associated with avoidance behaviors **(C)**. Main nuclei active here are: Striatum, Amygdala, Superior colliculi, etc. On the bottom **(B)** the mouse encounters an appetitive trigger of food/cheese activating nuclei associated with approach behaviors **(D)**.

within the visual field is key for identifying visual cues as food or a threat. Presenting an approaching visual stimulus in the upper visual field can evoke defensive responses such as escape and freezing in mice (Yilmaz and Meister, 2013). In rodents, predatory visual input is in the upper visual field and mapped in the medial SC (**Figure 2C**), whereas appetitive stimuli are detected in the lower visual field and mapped in the lateral SC (Comoli et al., 2012; **Figure 2D**). This functional organization is reflected by increased c-Fos protein expression (sign of recent neural activity) in the lateral SC following a hunting session for roaches on the floor (Favaro et al., 2011). In addition, unilateral electrical stimulation of lateral SC elicits contralateral orienting and approach-like responses, while stimulation of medial SC induces ipsilateral cringe-like defensive movement that develops into locomotion, running, and jumping with increasing stimulation intensity (Sahibzada et al., 1986). Such orienting responses involve contralateral MRF pathways, whereas movement away from the stimulus is mediated exclusively by an ipsilateral MRF pathways originating from the ventral and lateral SC (Sparks, 1986).

The SC projects ipsilaterally to the CnF and contralaterally to PPTg (Dean et al., 1989) with a major projection onto GABAergic MLR cells (Roseberry et al., 2016). The progression of locomotion elicited by stimulation of the medial SC is like that observed following stimulation at the MLR (Shik et al., 1969; Roseberry et al., 2016). One possibility is that this projection is inhibitory in nature, allowing for locomotion to occur via disinhibition of the MLR. Alternatively, if this circuit is glutamatergic, activation of GABAergic MLR neurons could suppress glutamatergic MLR output, producing motor arrest (see section Reflexive Startle Response Driven by Sudden External Sensory Stimuli).

DECISIONS TO APPROACH OR AVOID ARE GUIDED BY INTERNALIZED CONTEXTUAL INFORMATION

Generally, animals approach rewarding stimuli and avoid aversive stimuli. Aside from the positive and negative values associated with external stimuli, the coordination of approach- or aversive-like behaviors depend on the animal's internal affective and motivational states (Loewenstein et al., 2015). In early studies, Denny-Brown (1962) showed that bilateral lesions of the striatum caused animals to follow anything that moved. Since then the limbic system is understood to contribute to context-specific locomotion that drive decisions to approach or avoid.

Within the limbic system, the nucleus accumbens (NAc) of ventral striatum is an important limbic-motor interface underlying reward and motivation states (Mogenson et al., 1980; Roitman et al., 2005; Carlezon and Thomas, 2009; Levita et al., 2009; Humphries and Prescott, 2010; Richard and Berridge, 2011; McCutcheon et al., 2012; Salgado and Kaplitt, 2015). For example, amphetamine injected in the NAc results in hyper-locomotion demonstrating the key role of dopamine in both locomotion and reward. The NAc is divided into two subregions:

the shell and the core. Traditionally, the shell of the NAc orchestrates the response to unconditioned, innate reward and indeed lesions of the shell produce hypolocomotion (Ito et al., 2004; Aragona et al., 2008; Ito and Hayen, 2011). On the other hand, the core mediates approach behaviors associated with Pavlovian reward-associated cues (Parkinson et al., 2000; Ito et al., 2004; Stefanik et al., 2013, 2016; Hamel et al., 2017). The NAc has diverse outputs that enable recruitment of locomotor circuits. The NAc recruits locomotor circuitry via projections to: globus pallidus (GP), substantia nigra pars compacta (SNc), SNr, LH, ventral tegmental area (VTA), periaqueductal gray (PAG), PPTg, and ventral pallidum (VP) (Mogenson et al., 1983; review Nicola, 2007). It may be noted here that in some of these experiments PPTg also included overlapping brain regions including the CnF. Together these outputs explain the strong locomotory effect of stimulation of the NAc [sections Locomotor Response in Anticipation of Reward and Defensive Locomotor Responses (Escape and Freeze) Associated with Aversive Cues].

The amygdala is implicated in decisions regarding approach and avoidance locomotor behaviors (Petrovich, 2011). Learned food cues are relayed to the LH from the basolateral amygdala complex (BLA) to facilitate feeding, and aversive cues can suppress feeding by direct and indirect projections from the central nucleus of the amygdala (CeA) to LH (Petrovich et al., 1996; Petrovich, 2011). Differential modulation by the CeA and BLA onto striatal projection neurons is known and thus can bias approach and avoid behavior selection (Wall et al., 2013). Discrete nuclei within the amygdala have direct and indirect projections to the PAG, which are involved in defensive locomotion (Gross and Canteras, 2012). Although, the amygdala is involved in both approach and avoidance, its role in driving the corresponding locomotor response to associated triggers requires interactions with various brain regions. The role of the amygdala in both appetitive and aversive locomotor behavior will be revisited separately in the following sections (sections from Motivation to Approach: Execution of Forward Locomotion and Reflexive Startle Response Driven by Sudden External Sensory Stimuli).

MOTOR SELECTION DERIVED FROM THE DECISION TO APPROACH OR AVOID

Both external and internal cues interact with basal ganglia (BG) circuits for precise execution and selection of appropriate locomotor behavior. One widely accepted hypothesis is that the direct dopamine pathway facilitates reward-oriented motor behavior (reviews Everitt and Robbins, 2013; Kim and Hikosaka, 2015; Grillner and Robertson, 2016; Averbeck and Costa, 2017) while the indirect pathway suppresses unrewarded movements. Hence, these two pathways may regulate most associative learning and reward-oriented motor actions (Frank, 2006; Kravitz et al., 2010; Hong and Hikosaka, 2011). The two pathways originate from GABAergic striatal projection neurons that are known as the direct and indirect pathway medium spiny neurons, dMSNs, and iMSNs, respectively (review Utter and Basso, 2008). The dMSNs which express dopamine D1 receptors are excited by dopamine and project directly to the output nuclei of the basal ganglia, the SNr and GPi. Tonically active GABAergic projection neurons comprise these output nuclei and are responsible for tonic inhibition of the thalamus, SC, and PPTg. Thus, inhibition of GPi/SNr neurons by GABAergic dMSNs leads to disinhibition of brainstem motor centers and allow movement initiation. In contrast, iMSNs express dopamine D2 receptors and are inhibited by dopamine. These send GABAergic projections to the globus pallidus external (GPe) which in turn projects inhibitory output to the GPi. Sequentially, the GPe sends inhibitory output to excitatory STh that targets the SNr. Therefore, the net effect of the indirect pathway is an enhancement of inhibitory input from GPi and SNr to the descending motor centers. The GPi/SNr projects to the PPTg providing tonic inhibition affecting locomotor behavior. The anatomical tracing studies provide evidence for SNc projections to the PPN in rat (Beckstead et al., 1979; Semba and Fibiger, 1992; Steininger et al., 1992; Ichinohe et al., 2000) and in cat (Edley and Graybiel, 1983). The presence of such descending input was also supported by recordings of short latency antidromic activation of SNc neurons following PPN stimulation in rat (Scarnati et al., 1984, 1987). This is important as it suggests that dopamine has exclusive projections to brainstem nuclei distinct from the BG circuitry (Ryczko and Dubuc, 2013; Ryczko et al., 2016), which adds an extra degree of monoaminergic control over movement initiation.

PRIMARY APPETITIVE LOCOMOTOR SYSTEM: APPROACH-LIKE RESPONSES TO REWARDING & APPETITIVE CUES

Internalized contextual information such as reward and motivation combine to form approach-like behaviors across species. For example, place preference and self-stimulation paradigms often require association with rewarding cues, such as food to facilitate subsequent approach responses toward stimuli. Here we will examine work focused on how locomotion toward a rewarding stimulus is achieved. We will describe the functional connectivity between the limbic circuitry and descending locomotor centers, relevant for mediating forward locomotion in the context of appetitive behaviors (**Figure 3**).

FROM MOTIVATION TO APPROACH: EXECUTION OF FORWARD LOCOMOTION

The motivation to approach a stimulus in the environment stems from associations between the stimulus and its value as a physiological need or reward. Limbic structures such as the amygdala are key in mediating an approach locomotor response toward a rewarding stimulus such as food. As mentioned in section Decisions to Approach or Avoid are Guided by Internalized Contextual Information, the amygdala (BLA) directly projects to the LH which is a key hub for appetitive behaviors. The LH is an

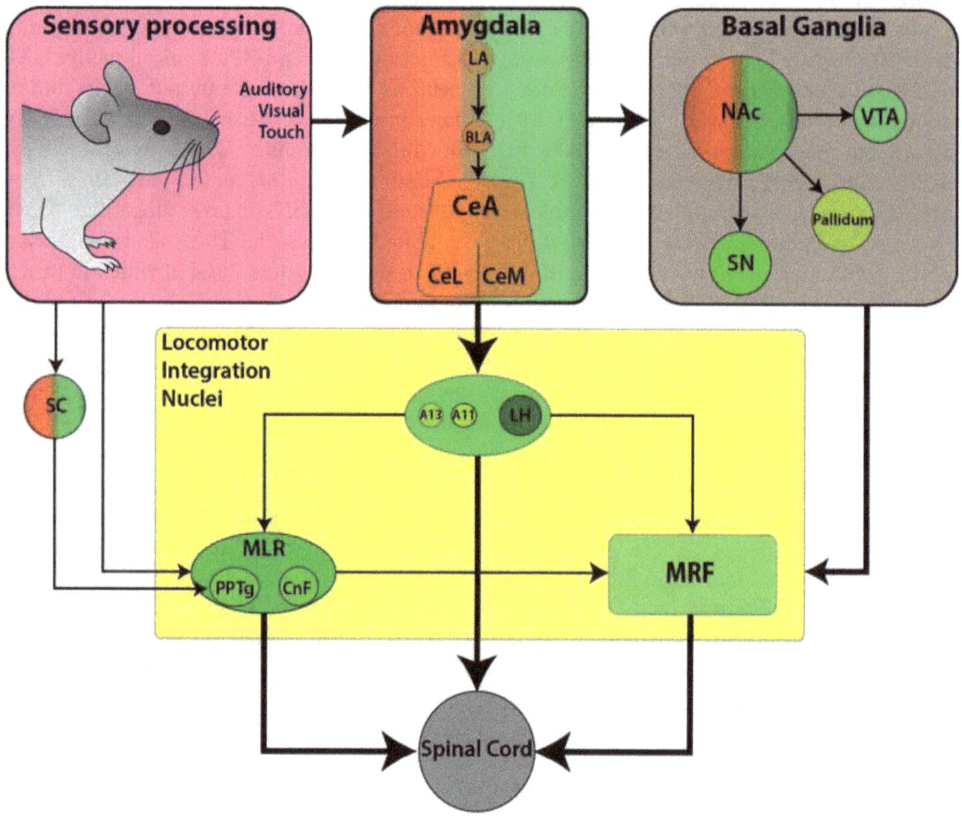

FIGURE 3 | Schematic diagram of the currently known descending connectivity of appetitive (approach) locomotor control. (Complementary to **Figure 2D**. Some connections omitted for lack of data or complexity of connectivity). Weighted arrows represent complex connectivity between regions described in further detail in text. Ascending connectivity has been omitted for clarity.

excellent candidate for investigating how reward-related information integrates with descending locomotor centers to facilitate forward locomotion toward reward-associated stimuli.

The LH is a large structure and has multiple functions. In the locomotor field, the initial descriptions of the LH were studied in the context of appetitive locomotor control (Sinnamon, 1993). However, most recent work has been directed toward the role of the LH in modulating homeostatic demands. Electrical stimulation of the LH elicits diverse responses beyond locomotion, such as feeding, drinking, gnawing and predatory attack that often vary from animal to animal but are linked to the current external stimuli (Coons et al., 1965; Roberts and Carey, 1965; Mogenson and Stevenson, 1967; review Stuber and Wise, 2016). Several LH cell populations have been shown to play a key role in feeding and appetite regulation including orexin, GABAergic, and glutamatergic cells. Projections onto the LH are predictably diverse and include olfactory and pyriform cortex, NAc, dorsal striatum, GP, ZI, perifornical region, most hypothalamic areas including magnocellular and medial preoptic, supraoptic, paraventricular and periventricular nuclei, posterior hypothalamus, arcuate and mammillary nuclei, bed nucleus of stria terminalis, ventral thalamic nuclei, VTA, SN, MRF, PAG, locus coeruleus, and parabrachial region (Barone et al., 1981).

The LH orexinergic transmission plays a key role in mediating locomotor responses via SN and brainstem locomotor regions (section The Diencephalon: A Hub for Goal-Directed Locomotion) and are active during feeding behavior (de Lecea et al., 1998; Sakurai et al., 1998), reward and arousal (Peyron et al., 1998; Baldo et al., 2003; Harris et al., 2005; Swanson et al., 2005; Aston-Jones et al., 2010). Indeed, the orexinergic neuronal population shows the highest level of spiking activity when animals are moving toward a food source. Orexinergic neurons are not the only LH neurons involved in locomotion; recently GABAergic LH cells have been reported to contribute to modulate locomotor activity. Chemogenetic silencing of LH GABAergic cells depresses voluntary locomotion, while stimulation leads to hyper-locomotion (Kosse et al., 2017). Anterograde tracing of these GABAergic cells uncovered substantial projections onto the ZI. The downstream projections are unknown. These ZI cells could also be modulated by orexin since photostimulation of orexinergic cells rapidly recruits GABAergic LH cells, and spiking of these GABAergic LH cells precedes spontaneous running bouts (Kosse et al., 2017).

LOCOMOTOR RESPONSE IN ANTICIPATION OF REWARD

While motivation contributes to an animal's approach behavior toward rewarding stimuli (Mogenson et al., 1980), anticipation of reward can also drive forward locomotion. Such anticipatory reward signals are integrated to locomotor centers via corticolimbic structures including the cortex, striatum and pallidum, which have descending projections to the locomotor regions (Swanson, 2000).

As well as participating in motor selection (section Motor Selection Derived from the Decision to Approach or Avoid), dopamine circuits including mesolimbic, mesocortical, and nigrostriatal pathways govern reward-related behaviors. Dopamine release within the NAc is an important determinant of reward processing. Furthermore, NAc is known to have reciprocal projections to dopaminergic neurons in VTA and the SN which projects to the dorsal striatum (Haber et al., 2000; Ikemoto, 2007). The dorsal striatum and its dopaminergic inputs serve key roles in the regulation of locomotor control (Faure et al., 2005; Belin and Everitt, 2008; Palmiter, 2008). Striatal pathway projections are differentially modulated by dopamine, and are either excitatory via the direct pathway (D1 receptor) or inhibitory via the indirect pathway (D2 receptor) (Surmeier et al., 2007). The locomotor modulation observed within BG circuitry could occur via glutamatergic and cholinergic MLR neurons that mediate initiation and acceleration of locomotion while GABAergic populations could facilitate deceleration, respectively (Roseberry et al., 2016). Dopaminergic fibers have been reported around cholinergic cells in MLR of lamprey (Ryczko et al., 2013), salamander (Ryczko et al., 2016), rat (Ryczko et al., 2016), monkeys (Rolland et al., 2009), and human (Ryczko et al., 2016) indicating that the innervation of the MLR is conserved in vertebrates (Ryczko and Dubuc, 2017). In lamprey and salamander, the origin of this dopaminergic innervation to cholinergic cells in MLR was found to be a diencephalic dopaminergic region termed as posterior tuberculum which sends ascending projections to the striatum and is considered homologous to mammalian SNc and/or VTA (Yamamoto and Vernier, 2011; Wullimann, 2014; Ryczko et al., 2016; Ryczko and Dubuc, 2017). While only a few dopamine neurons sent collaterals to the striatum and the MLR in lampreys and salamanders, numerous SNc dopamine neurons have both ascending and descending collaterals in rats (Ryczko et al., 2016). The number of ascending dopaminergic collaterals may be related to evolutionary expansion of the basal ganglia (Grillner and Robertson, 2016; Ryczko and Dubuc, 2017). These findings suggest that the role of dopaminergic activity in reward-related behavior is bidirectional and could occur in anticipation of obtaining a reward.

Following a similar theme, neurons within the PPTg are important for modulating speed and gait during locomotion (section The Mesencephalic Locomotor Region: An Integrative Hub for Locomotor Speed and Gait), but also respond in anticipation of reward signals. PPTg neurons respond phasically to auditory and visual sensory stimuli that predict reward with a shorter latency (5–10 ms) than dopaminergic VTA/SNc cells (Pan and Hyland, 2005). Furthermore, Norton et al. (2011) examined PPTg neural activity as rats solved a spatial working memory task that involved retrieving rewards of different magnitudes from known locations. Interestingly, they reported separate populations of PPTg neurons independently code for reward or movement. Thus, the reward anticipatory response within PPTg is part of a feedforward mechanism to trigger a fast locomotor response triggered by a reward-associated cue. In support of this idea, photoactivation of cholinergic PPTg terminals at SNc has been shown to increase locomotion (Xiao et al., 2016). Electrical stimulation of PPTg induces a burst firing of midbrain dopaminergic neurons (Lokwan et al., 1999; Floresco et al., 2003) with concomitant release of dopamine in striatum (Chapman et al., 1996; Miller and Blaha, 2004). This suggests that the PPTg may facilitate feedforward and feedback loops with SNc via reciprocal projections. Calcium transients within dopaminergic terminals in dorsal striatum precede (100–150 ms) bouts of locomotion independent of reward expectation (Howe and Dombeck, 2016). Photoactivation of these dopaminergic axons leads to initiation of locomotion bouts. Thus, rapid sub-second phasic signaling contributes to locomotion bout initiation associated with ongoing accelerations. Since glutamatergic MLR cells can facilitate acceleration (Roseberry et al., 2016), the role of these populations in potentiating locomotion in anticipation of reward is of interest.

PRIMARY DEFENSIVE LOCOMOTOR SYSTEM: AVOIDANCE RESPONSES TO AVERSIVE ASSOCIATED CUES

Locomotion is a critical element in the primary defensive system since it serves to increase the distance away from threatening or painful stimuli (Sinnamon, 1993). In general, aversive behaviors are characterized by three types of responses: (1) a reflexive startle response, (2) escape behavior to flee from an aversive stimulus, and (3) a freezing response. Of these three defensive responses, the circuitry for startle response has been best described. On the other hand, escape and freezing responses have often been used as behavioral outcomes in pain and fear related studies, but the associated locomotor components have received less attention (reviews Klemm, 2001; Roseberry and Kreitzer, 2017; **Figure 4**).

REFLEXIVE STARTLE RESPONSE DRIVEN BY SUDDEN EXTERNAL SENSORY STIMULI

The mammalian startle response is characterized by fast twitch of facial and body muscles as well as an arrest of ongoing movement in response to a sudden and intense sensory stimulus (Koch, 1999). It protects the animal from predation by preparing for a flight or fight response, or by freezing so the animal can't be easily seen (Landis and Hunt, 1939). A startle response can be elicited by different sensory modalities which act via separate pathways. These include: (1) trigeminal for sudden tactile stimuli, (2) auditory

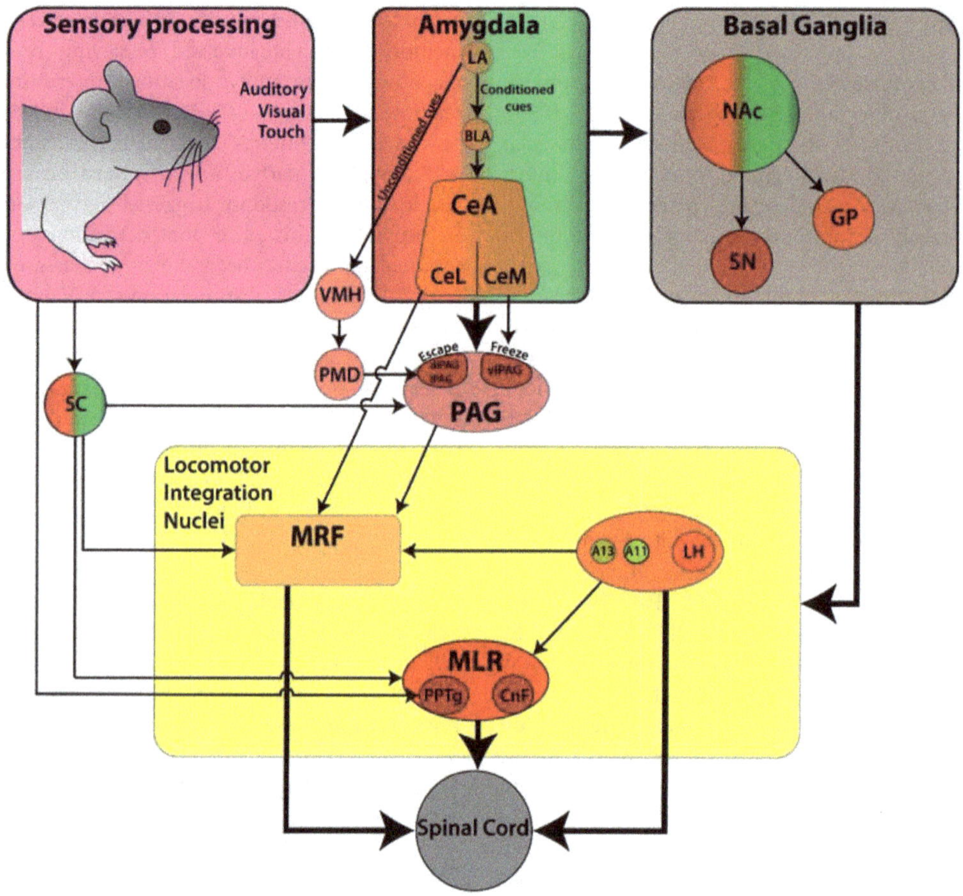

FIGURE 4 | Schematic diagram of the currently known descending connectivity of defensive (avoidance) locomotor control. (Complementary to **Figure 2C**. Some connections omitted for lack of data or complexity of connectivity). Ascending connectivity has been omitted for clarity.

for sudden acoustic stimuli, and (3) vestibular for sudden head movements. Though these startle pathways originate from different second-order afferents (nucleus V for tactile, cochlear root nucleus for auditory, and vestibular nucleus for balance), they converge onto giant neurons in the PnC projecting directly to motoneurons and interneurons of the spinal cord (reviews Koch, 1999; Yeomans et al., 2002). Less well understood is the light-induced startle response characterized by temporary locomotor arrest following brief flashes of light (Liang et al., 2015). This phenomenon can be partly driven by input to the SC from layer 5 of the primary visual cortex (V1 L5). Photoactivation of V1 L5 neurons projecting to SC directly triggers locomotor arrest in running mice (Liang et al., 2015). Inactivating the SC with muscimol reduces the arrest behavior by 76%, whereas silencing V1 by optical activation of parvalbumin-positive inhibitory neurons reduces arrest by 33% (Liang et al., 2015). Overall, these startle pathways are fine-tuned to detect specific triggers from the environment during the default exploration state of the animal, allowing an animal to quickly transition into a defensive state (Yeomans and Frankland, 1995).

DEFENSIVE LOCOMOTOR RESPONSES (ESCAPE AND FREEZE) ASSOCIATED WITH AVERSIVE CUES

In comparison to the startle response, which is reflexive in nature, the choice between escaping a stimulus and freezing is highly dependent on contextual cues. Behavioral outcomes that measure fear and pain such as conditioned place preference/aversion and dynamic weight bearing analysis rely on quantification of locomotor behavior. The descending control of locomotor circuits in response to aversive stimuli has not been fully explored. Nonetheless, aversive responses rely heavily on locomotor circuit interactions between the amygdala and PAG (LeDoux, 2012; Koutsikou et al., 2015, 2017).

Aversive stimuli can be thought of as either unconditioned and innate, or learned and associated with pain and fear. The association between the unconditioned stimulus and the conditioned stimulus required may involve memory processing related to fear. This is mediated in part by both the CeA and BLA of the amygdala (LeDoux, 2000; Medina et al., 2002; Wilensky et al., 2006; Ciocchi et al., 2010; Duvarci et al., 2011;

Li et al., 2013; Han et al., 2015; Sato et al., 2015). The CeA is an important neural substrate for the expression of the freeze response (Davis and Whalen, 2001; Phelps and LeDoux, 2005). It projects to the hypothalamus, dorsal and ventral striatum, PAG, and MRF, and could also modulate cognition in a broader sense, via its outputs to ascending monoaminergic and cholinergic systems such as: noradrenergic LC, dopaminergic SNc and VTA, serotonergic raphe, and the cholinergic nucleus basalis (Davis and Whalen, 2001; Sara, 2009). Recent cell-type-specific viral tracing studies have also revealed a strong projection from the CeA to glutamatergic MLR neurons, which can initiate locomotion from rest when activated (Roseberry et al., 2016). Similarly, chemical or electrical stimulation of CeA can elicit freezing or fleeing behavior (Brandão et al., 1999, 2015; Vianna et al., 2001; Muthuraju et al., 2016). Thus, the CeA is important for orchestrating defensive freeze and escape responses (Sah et al., 2003; Oka et al., 2008).

The PAG also plays a central role in regulating defensive locomotor behaviors. Bandler was the first to show the PAG's direct role in defensive reactions in cats by pharmacological activation with microinjections of glutamate (Bandler, 1982) and excitatory amino acids (Bandler and Carrive, 1988). Subsequent studies identified five subregions that can be differentiated based on anatomy, physiology, and behavioral outcomes when activated (Carrive, 1993). The dorsolateral/lateral (dl/l) and ventrolateral (vl) columns of the PAG appear to be the most relevant in the context of defensive locomotor behaviors. Activation of the lPAG can elicit a variety of responses such as: strong hindlimb movements for flight reaction, reactive immobility accompanied by heightened responsiveness to surrounding stimuli, backward locomotion, and forward escape locomotion with occasional jumps (Bandler and Depaulis, 1988; Depaulis et al., 1989, 1992; Carrive, 1993). Meanwhile, activation of the vlPAG can induce hyporeactive immobility characterized by reduced spontaneous activity and/or responsiveness to surrounding stimuli (Bandler and Depaulis, 1988; Depaulis et al., 1992; Carrive, 1993). In line with this, electrolytic lesions of vlPAG in rats decrease freezing induced by unconditioned and conditioned stimuli, whereas lesions of dlPAG enhanced freezing (Fanselow et al., 1995; De Oca et al., 1998). Photoactivation of glutamatergic cells of the dorsal PAG (dPAG) can evoke both freeze and escape behavior in a gradual manner via firing rate and temporal coding mechanism (Chen et al., 2015). Increasing either frequency or intensity of photoactivation progressed defensive phenotype from freeze to escape and then to jump. Given the lack of a clear boundary between observed phenotypes, it is possible that these cells may perform this function through differing neurotransmitter release and/or its afferent and efferent connections.

Sensory cues that trigger aversive behaviors are either unconditioned or conditioned, and are processed through different pathways. Unconditioned odor cues are conveyed via the medial amygdala, whereas auditory and visual cues are conveyed via the accessory basal amygdala. These signals are further processed through the circuitry of the ventromedial hypothalamus (VMH)-premammillary nucleus of the hypothalamus (PMH) and the dPAG. On the other hand, conditioned cues are processed via the LA and intra-amygdala connections onto CeA, and then project onto vlPAG from medial CeA (CeM) (Motta et al., 2009). The CeA also projects directly onto PnC (Davis and Whalen, 2001) where Chx10 stop neurons could be found (Bouvier et al., 2015) and glutamatergic MLR neurons which are associated with acceleration of ongoing movement (Roseberry et al., 2016). Therefore, defensive responses may be mediated through these projections as well. Furthermore, glutamatergic cells within PAG innervate the GiA, GiV, and LPGi (Tovote et al., 2016). Most work has focused primarily on fear induced freezing; however, the neural circuitry of PAG-mediated defensive locomotor control remains undefined. Considering this, Tovote et al. (2016) selectively manipulated inhibitory projections from the CeA to local inhibitory interneurons within the vlPAG. Glutamatergic neurons of the vlPAG are under local inhibition, and upon disinhibition by the CeA, they induce freezing via GiA, GiV, and LPGi targets. In contrast to activation of glutamatergic vlPAG neurons, photostimulation of glutamatergic dl/lPAG neurons evoke bouts of escape locomotor behavior intermingled with short freezing periods (Tovote et al., 2016). It seems that the PAG could play an important role in translating locomotor behaviors related to freezing or escape and may interact with locomotor command centers. A few studies suggest that an interaction between PAG and locomotor command centers (e.g., CnF) may be relevant for locomotor behaviors in freezing and/or escape (Ferreira-Netto et al., 2007). Connectivity between PAG and Chx10 neurons within caudal PnC and rostral Gi which can evoke stop has not yet been explored. With these multiple possible points of integration between the pain, limbic, and motor systems that have been found through tracing techniques, we can begin to create testable models of functional circuitry within specific contexts that modulate locomotion.

INTERACTIONS BETWEEN APPETITIVE, DEFENSIVE, AND EXPLORATORY BEHAVIOR

Appetitive, defensive and exploratory locomotor behavior are all necessary for survival. This is reflected at the neural systems level, where processes for these behaviors are closely intertwined along with circuits involved in maintenance of food and resources, defense, fluid balance, thermoregulation, and reproduction (Saper, 2006). Eating must often co-exist with the threat of predation for many species. The risks need to be weighed with the rewards and clearly, they are weighed differently in satiated compared to hungry animals. In the above sections, we have provided examples of nuclei that contribute to this complex predation calculus such as SC, NAc, and amygdala.

Since the locomotor responses are driven by the animal's interaction with the environment, there are multiple overlapping cognitive or associative and emotional processing structures modulating locomotor responses. Nevertheless, differential signaling processes for various contexts can facilitate approach while suppressing avoidance responses and vice versa. For example, GABA cells in the LH are excited by orexin and activity of these cells drives locomotion (section The Diencephalon: A Hub for Goal-Directed Locomotion). These inhibitory cells project to the SC and the PAG; both of which drive aversive locomotor behaviors. These inhibitory circuits are strong candidates for the suppression of aversive locomotor behaviors in situations where motivation to seek food is high.

In summary, innervation onto NAc could disinhibit the MLR via VP and the SNr to initiate, modulate or terminate locomotion. In addition, BLA and CeA send efferents to dMSNs preferentially (Roseberry et al., 2016) and the LH area (Petrovich et al., 1996; Petrovich, 2011), which could facilitate approach locomotion for cues associated with food and reward, or mediate suppression of appetitive behavior during defensive response and unrewarded movement, respectively. For example, in a behavioral conflict between aversion and reward, cholinergic and glutamatergic PPTg projections onto the dopaminergic VTA neurons may mediate a bias toward reward-oriented locomotion. Furthermore, PPTg projections to dopaminergic SNc neurons may facilitate suppression of unrewarded movements via the indirect pathway, or reinforce reward oriented motor action via direct pathway (Frank, 2006; Kravitz et al., 2010; Hong and Hikosaka, 2011). In addition, A11 and A13 (DLR) could provide a parallel dopaminergic modulation to mediate a balance between approach and avoidance behaviors.

FUTURE DIRECTIONS

This review has examined how locomotion is integrated into contextual demands. Recent advances in functional connectomics will enable us to decipher the circuits that underlie different approach and avoid motor behaviors. Specifically, optogenetics and chemogenetics coupled with viral-vector based approaches provide the tool kits necessary to advance our understanding. These methods can overcome limitations of electrical stimulation, and lesion approaches. That said direct comparisons with electrical stimulation remain useful since translational approaches using deep brain stimulation rely on this technology. In some cases, electrical stimulation may be advantageous since it's lack of selectivity may be required to adequately activate a network. Electrical stimulation will recruit more neurons due to failures in transfection. While optogenetics and chemogenetics are an excellent choice for understanding the connectome we need to carefully evaluate if these are the tool of choice for clinical use.

It is sobering to consider that establishing the connectome from an anatomical point of view is only half the story; the dynamic recruitment of multiple parallel pathways also needs to be considered. No matter which nuclei one focuses on there are multiple projections to other members within the overall circuit. We need to consider sampling key areas of the circuit simultaneously when designing studies so that we can begin to understand the dynamic recruitment of several centers during approach and avoidance tasks. These centers will include the PPTg, CnF, and MRF since they form key integrative centers in the brain. Depending on the type of study recordings need to be captured from the striatum, hypothalamic nuclei, and the LC.

CHALLENGES FACED IN DRIVING CONTEXTUAL BEHAVIORAL RESPONSE

Meanwhile, as more sophisticated technologies and experimental tools became readily available, thus enabling the study of underlying mechanisms and circuitries associated with motor functions with much higher precision, there are several caveats. It is important to consider that the study of motor behaviors using experimental animal models generally require extensive training or conditioning, which rely on memory and learning processes. The impact of this training on the motor behavior being tested needs to be understood.

Learning and memory formation were initially thought to be driven by dynamic changes in synaptic strengths, which can be experimentally induced by high frequency stimulation (Bliss and Lomo, 1973). A few key regions of the brain were implicated, including the hippocampus, the neocortex, cerebellar, and brainstem nuclei (Medina et al., 2002). This is known as the synaptic plasticity and memory hypothesis, within this there are assumptions that synaptic inputs converge, or there are specific "relay centres" for information processing. This hypothesis has been reappraised because the mechanisms underlying the initial encoding and subsequent learning are likely to be different (Medina et al., 2002). This can be demonstrated by the observations that: (1) habituation occurs over relatively short periods of time for certain behaviors (e.g., forced swim, open field induced anxiety); and (2) neuronal plasticity often persists even when the conditioned behavior has fully extinguished (Hansel et al., 2001). The key point here is that whilst neuronal plasticity in specific regions contributes to the initiation of behavior, the maintenance may involve activity of other neuronal populations or pathways.

Similarly, the extinction of behaviors (e.g., fear extinction), indicate that learning is a state-dependent process. It was established that the amygdala, a brain region important for the regulation of emotion, receives input from the hippocampus and provides "context" (i.e., based on the animal's affective states) during conditioning (Phelps and LeDoux, 2005). In line with this review, modulation of locomotor behaviors is also context-dependent and are driven by the animal's need and/or adaptation to the ever-changing environments. At present, many studies investigating changes in cellular mechanisms or functional circuitry associated with motor behaviors are relatively short-term compared to behavior studies from other fields, such as sensory and cognitive neuroscience. Future studies must consider appropriate experiment paradigms to account for the changes in behaviors over time, and that there may be multiple changes at both cellular and systems levels in context-driven motor learning.

CONCLUSION

To navigate through the environment, animals need to make on-the-fly adjustments to gait. Consider a baseball player running to catch a ball. The person will need to be motivated to run quickly to catch the ball, and this motivation may be higher at the World Series compared to a regular training day. Catching the ball requires visual input which is integrated through the dorsal stream to the motor cortex, which is then relayed back to diencephalic circuits including the BG and hypothalamic circuits. Modifications to gait need to be accomplished to execute accelerations, jumps, and slides. This is presumably integrated at the level of the MRF and MLR and integrated into ongoing activity within rhythm centers of the spinal cord. We are at a critical juncture in our understanding of how emotional and contextual cues affect locomotor performance. Many tools exist to tease apart circuit function in awake behaving animals and show how they affect downstream brainstem and spinal cord function. This of course dramatically increases the complexity of experiments directed at understanding motor control, but it will serve to highlight the interplay between regions of the brain involved in movement decisions that evolved to maximize survival of the organism.

AUTHOR CONTRIBUTIONS

All authors (LK, SS, SAS, KM, CC, and PW) contributed to the conception, drafting, and critical revision of the review.

FUNDING

We would like to acknowledge funding awarded to PW from the Canadian Institute for Health Research (CIHR MOP-130528; PJT-148682), Natural Sciences and Engineering Research Council of Canada (NSERC RGPIN/356153-2013), Wings for Life (WFL-CA011/15), the Hotchkiss Brain Institute (HBI) and Faculty for Veterinary Medicine. LK was supported by the Alberta Parkinson's Society and the Cumming School of Medicine, KM was supported by the Branch Out Foundation and HBI and SAS supported by Alberta Innovates and HBI.

ACKNOWLEDGMENTS

We would like to acknowledge support from members of the Whelan Lab.

REFERENCES

Alam, M., Schwabe, K., and Krauss, J. K. (2011). The pedunculopontine nucleus area: critical evaluation of interspecies differences relevant for its use as a target for deep brain stimulation. *Brain* 134, 11–23. doi: 10.1093/brain/awq322

Alam, M., Schwabe, K., and Krauss, J. (2013). Reply: the cuneiform nucleus may be involved in the regulation of skeletal muscle tone by motor pathway: a virally mediated trans-synaptic tracing study in surgically sympathectomized mice. *Brain* 136, e252. doi: 10.1093/brain/awt125

Aragona, B. J., Cleaveland, N. A., Stuber, G. D., Day, J. J., Carelli, R. M., Wightman, R. M. (2008). Preferential enhancement of dopamine transmission within the nucleus accumbens shell by cocaine is attributable to a direct increase in phasic dopamine release events. *J Neurosci.* 28, 8821–8831. doi: 10.1523/JNEUROSCI.2225-08.2008

Armstrong, D. M. (1986). Supraspinal contributions to the initiation and control of locomotion in the cat. *Prog. Neurobiol.* 26, 273–361. doi: 10.1016/0301-0082(86)90021-3

Aston-Jones, G., Smith, R., Sartor, G., Moorman, D., Massi, L., Tahsili-Fahadan, P., et al. (2010). Lateral hypothalamic orexin/hypocretin neurons: a role in reward-seeking and addiction. *Brain Res.* 1314, 74–90. doi: 10.1016/j.brainres.2009.09.106

Averbeck, B. B., and Costa, V. D. (2017). Motivational neural circuits underlying reinforcement learning. *Nat. Neurosci.* 20, 505–512. doi: 10.1038/nn.4506

Baldo, B. A., Daniel, R. A., Berridge, C. W., and Kelley, A. E. (2003). Overlapping distributions of orexin/hypocretin- and dopamine-β-hydroxylase immunoreactive fibers in rat brain regions mediating arousal, motivation, and stress. *J. Comp. Neurol.* 464, 220–237. doi: 10.1002/cne.10783

Bandler, R. (1982). Induction of "page" following microinjections of glutamate into midbrain but not hypothalamus of cats. *Neurosci. Lett.* 30, 183–188. doi: 10.1016/0304-3940(82)90294-4

Bandler, R., and Carrive, P. (1988). Integrated defence reaction elicited by excitatory amino acid microinjection in the midbrain periaqueductal grey region of the unrestrained cat. *Brain Res.* 439, 95–106. doi: 10.1016/0006-8993(88)91465-5

Bandler, R., and Depaulis, A. (1988). Elicitation of intraspecific defence reactions in the rat from midbrain periaqueductal grey by microinjection of kainic acid, without neurotoxic effects. *Neurosci. Lett.* 88, 291–296. doi: 10.1016/0304-3940(88)90226-1

Barone, F. C., Wayner, M. J., Scharoun, S. L., Guevara-Aguilar, R., and Aguilar-Baturoni, H. U. (1981). Afferent connections to the lateral hypothalamus: a horseradish peroxidase study in the rat. *Brain Res. Bull.* 7, 75–88. doi: 10.1016/0361-9230(81)90101-5

Barrière, G., Mellen, N., and Cazalets, J. (2004). Neuromodulation of the locomotor network by dopamine in the isolated spinal cord of newborn rat. *Eur. J. Neurosci.* 19, 1325–1335. doi: 10.1111/j.1460-9568.2004.03210.x

Beckstead, R. M., Domesick, V. B., and Nauta, W. J. (1979). Efferent connections of the substantia nigra and ventral tegmental area in the rat. *Brain Res.* 175, 191–217. doi: 10.1016/0006-8993(79)91001-1

Beitz, A. J. (1982a). The sites of origin brain stem neurotensin and serotonin projections to the rodent nucleus raphe magnus. *J. Neurosc.* 2, 829–842.

Beitz, A. J. (1982b). The nuclei of origin of brain stem enkephalin and substance pprojections to the rodent nucleus raphe magnus. *Neuroscience* 7, 2753–2768. doi: 10.1016/0306-4522(82)90098-7

Belin, D., and Everitt, B. (2008). Cocaine seeking habits depend upon dopamine-dependent serial connectivity linking the ventral with the dorsal Striatum. *Neuron* 57, 432–441. doi: 10.1016/j.neuron.2007.12.019

Bliss, T. V., and Lomo, T. (1973). Long-lasting potentiation of synaptic transmission in the dentate area of the anaesthetized rabbit following stimulation of the perforant path. *J. Physiol.* 232, 331–356. doi: 10.1113/jphysiol.1973.sp010273

Boothby, K. M., and Roberts, A. (1992). The stopping response of *Xenopus laevis* embryos: behaviour, development and physiology. *J. Comp. Physiol. A* 170, 171–180. doi: 10.1007/BF00196899

Born, G., and Schmidt, M. (2008). A reciprocal connection between the ventral lateral geniculate nucleus and the pretectal nuclear complex and the superior colliculus: an *in vitro* characterization in the rat. *Vis. Neurosci.* 25, 39–51. doi: 10.1017/S0952523808080048

Bouvier, J., Caggiano, V., Leiras, R., Caldeira, V., Bellardita, C., Balueva, K., et al. (2015). Descending command neurons in the brainstem that halt locomotion. *Cell* 163, 1191–1203. doi: 10.1016/j.cell.2015.10.074

Brandão, M. L., Anseloni, V. Z., Pandóssio, J. E., Araújo, J. E., and Castilho, V. M. (1999). Neurochemical mechanisms of the defensive behavior in the dorsal midbrain. *Neurosci. Biobehav. Rev.* 23, 863–875. doi: 10.1016/S0149-7634(99)00038-X

Brandão, M., de Oliveira, A., Muthuraju, S., Colombo, A., Saito, V., and Talbot, T. (2015). Dual role of dopamine D_2-like receptors in the mediation of conditioned and unconditioned fear. *FEBS Lett.* 589, 3433–3437. doi: 10.1016/j.febslet.2015.02.036

Bretzner, F., and Brownstone, R. (2013). Lhx3-Chx10 reticulospinal neurons in locomotor circuits. *J. Neurosci.* 33, 14681–14692. doi: 10.1523/JNEUROSCI.5231-12.2013

Brustein, E., and Rossignol, S. (1998). Recovery of locomotion after ventral and ventrolateral spinal lesions in the cat. I. Deficits and adaptive mechanisms. *J. Neurophysiol.* 80, 1245–1267.

Carlezon, W. A., and Thomas, M. J. (2009). Biological substrates of reward and aversion: a nucleus accumbens activity hypothesis. *Neuropharmacology* 56, 122–132. doi: 10.1016/j.neuropharm.2008.06.075

Carrive, P. (1993). The periaqueductal gray and defensive behavior: functional representation and neuronal organization. *Behav. Brain Res.* 58, 27–47. doi: 10.1016/0166-4328(93)90088-8

Castiglioi, A. J., Gallaway, M. C., and Coulter, J. D. (1978). Spinal projections from the midbrain in monkey. *J. Comp. Neurol.* 178, 329–345. doi: 10.1002/cne.901780208

Chapman, C., Yeomans, J., Blaha, C., and Blackburn, J. (1996). Increased striatal dopamine efflux follows scopolamine administered systemically or to the tegmental pedunculopontine nucleus. *Neuroscience* 76, 177–186. doi: 10.1016/S0306-4522(96)00358-2

Charbit, A. R., Akerman, S., Holland, P. R., and Goadsby, P. J. (2009). Neurons of the dopaminergic/calcitonin gene-related peptide A11 cell group modulate neuronal firing in the trigeminocervical complex: an electrophysiological and immunohistochemical study. *J. Neurosci.* 29, 12532–12541. doi: 10.1523/JNEUROSCI.2887-09.2009

Chen, S., Zhou, H., Guo, S., Zhang, J., Qu, Y., Feng, Z., et al. (2015). Optogenetics based rat–robot control: optical stimulation encodes "stop" and "escape" commands. *Ann. Biomed. Eng.* 43, 1851–1864. doi: 10.1007/s10439-014-1235-x

Ciocchi, S., Herry, C., Grenier, F., Wolff, S. B., Letzkus, J., Vlachos, I., Ehrlich, I., et al. (2010). Encoding of conditioned fear in central amygdala inhibitory circuits. *Nature* 468, 277–282. doi: 10.1038/nature09559

Clemens, S., Rye, D., and Hochman, S. (2006). Restless legs syndrome: revisiting the dopamine hypothesis from the spinal cord perspective. *Neurology* 67, 125–130. doi: 10.1212/01.wnl.0000223316.53428.c9

Clements, J. R., and Grant, S. (1990). Glutamate-like immunoreactivity in neurons of the laterodorsal tegmental and pedunculopontine nuclei in the rat. *Neurosci. Lett.* 120, 70–73. doi: 10.1016/0304-3940(90)90170-E

Commissiong, J. W., and Sedgwick, E. M. (1975). Letter: dopamine and noradrenaline in human spinal cord. *Lancet* 1, 347. doi: 10.1016/S0140-6736(75)91269-6

Comoli, E., Favaro, P., Vautrelle, N., Leriche, M., Overton, P. G., and Redgrave, P. (2012). Segregated anatomical input to sub-regions of the rodent superior colliculus associated with approach and defense. *Front. Neuroanat.* 6:9. doi: 10.3389/fnana.2012.00009

Coons, E. E., Levak, M., and Miller, N. E. (1965). Lateral hypothalamus: learning of food-seeking response motivated by electrical stimulation. *Science* 150, 1320–1321. doi: 10.1126/science.150.3701.1320

Coulter, J. D., Bowker, R. M., Wise, S. P., Murray, E. A., Castiglioni, A. J., and Westlund, K. N. (1979). Cortical, tectal and medullary descending pathways to the cervical spinal cord. *Prog. Brain Res.* 50, 263–274. doi: 10.1016/S0079-6123(08)60827-4

Davis, M., and Whalen, P. (2001). The amygdala: vigilance and emotion. *Mol. Psychiatry* 6, 13–34. doi: 10.1038/sj.mp.4000812

de Lecea, L., Kilduff, T. S., Peyron, C., Gao, X.-B., Foye, P. E., Danielson, P. E., et al. (1998). The hypocretins: hypothalamus-specific peptides with neuroexcitatory activity. *Proc. Natl. Acad. Sci. U.S.A.* 95, 322–327. doi: 10.1073/pnas.95.1.322

De Oca, B. M., DeCola, J. P., Maren, S., and Fanselow, M. S. (1998). Distinct regions of the periaqueductal gray are involved in the acquisition and expression of defensive responses. *J. Neurosci.* 18, 3426–3432.

Dean, P., Redgrave, P., and Westby, G. W. M. (1989). Event or emergency? Two response systems in the mammalian superior colliculus. *Trends Neurosci.* 12, 137–147. doi: 10.1016/0166-2236(89)90052-0

Denny-Brown, D. (1962). *The Basal Ganglia and Their Relation to Disorder of Movement.* New York, NY: Oxford University Press Inc.

Depaulis, A., Bandler, R., and Vergnes, M. (1989). Characterization of pretentorial periaqueductal gray matter neurons mediating intraspecific defensive behaviors in the rat by microinjections of kainic acid. *Brain Res.* 486, 121–132. doi: 10.1016/0006-8993(89)91284-5

Depaulis, A., Keay, K. A., and Bandler, R. (1992). Longitudinal neuronal organization of defensive reactions in the midbrain periaqueductal gray region of the rat. *Exp. Brain Res.* 90, 307–318. doi: 10.1007/BF00227243

Di Scala, G., Schmitt, P., and Karli, P. (1984). Flight induced by infusion of bicuculline methiodide into periventricular structures. *Brain Res.* 309, 205–209. doi: 10.1016/0006-8993(84)90585-7

Drew, T., Dubuc, R., and Rossignol, S. (1986). Discharge patterns of reticulospinal and other reticular neurons in chronic, unrestrained cats walking on a treadmill. *J. Neurophysiol.* 55, 375–401.

Drew, T., Prentice, S., and Schepens, B. (2004). Cortical and brainstem control of locomotion. *Prog. Brain Res.* 143, 251–261. doi: 10.1016/S0079-6123(03)43025-2

Duvarci, S., Popa, D., and Paré, D. (2011). Central amygdala activity during fear conditioning. *J. Neurosci.* 31, 289–294. doi: 10.1523/JNEUROSCI.4985-10.2011

Duxon, M., Stretton, J., Starr, K., Jones, D., Holland, V., Riley, G., et al. (2001). Evidence that orexin-A-evoked grooming in the rat is mediated by orexin-1 (OX_1) receptors, with downstream 5-HT_{2C} receptor involvement. *Psychopharmacology* 153, 203–209. doi: 10.1007/s002130000550

Ectors, L., Brookens, N. L., and Gerard, R. W. (1938). Autonomic and motor localization in the hypothalamus. *Arch. Neurol. Psychiatry* 39, 789–798. doi: 10.1001/archneurpsyc.1938.02270040145009

Edley, S. M., and Graybiel, A. M. (1983). The afferent and efferent connections of the feline nucleus tegmenti pedunculopontinus, pars compacta. *J. Comp. Neurol.* 217, 187–215. doi: 10.1002/cne.902170207

Edwards, D. H., Heitler, W. J., and Krasne, F. B. (1999). Fifty years of a command neuron: the neurobiology of escape behavior in the crayfish. *Trends Neurosci.* 22, 153–161. doi: 10.1016/S0166-2236(98)01340-X

Esch, T., and Kristan, W. (2002). Decision-making in the leech nervous system. *Integr. Comp. Biol.* 42, 716–724. doi: 10.1093/icb/42.4.716

Esposito, M. S., Capelli, P., and Arber, S. (2014). Brainstem nucleus MdV mediates skilled forelimb motor tasks. *Nature* 508, 351–356. doi: 10.1038/nature13023

Everitt, B. J., and Robbins, T. W. (2013). From the ventral to the dorsal striatum: devolving views of their roles in drug addiction. *Neurosci. Biobehav. Rev.* 37, 1946–1954. doi: 10.1016/j.neubiorev.2013.02.010

Fanselow, M., Decola, J., Oca, B., and Landeira-Fernandez, J. (1995). Ventral and dorsolateral regions of the midbrain periaqueductal gray (PAG) control different stages of defensive behavior: dorsolateral PAG lesions enhance the defensive freezing produced by massed and immediate shock. *Aggress. Behav.* 21, 63–77. doi: 10.1002/1098-2337(1995)21:1<63::AID-AB2480210109>3.0.CO;2-F

Faure, A., Haberland, U., Condé, F., and Massioui, N. (2005). Lesion to the nigrostriatal dopamine system disrupts stimulus-response habit formation. *J. Neurosci.* 25, 2771–2780. doi: 10.1523/JNEUROSCI.3894-04.2005

Favaro, P. D. N., Gouvêa, T. S., de Oliveira, S. R., Vautrelle, N., Redgrave, P., and Comoli, E. (2011). The influence of vibrissal somatosensory processing in rat superior colliculus on prey capture. *Neuroscience* 176, 318–327. doi: 10.1016/j.neuroscience.2010.12.009

Ferraye, M. U., Debû, B., Fraix, V., Goetz, L., Ardouin, C., Yelnik, J., et al. (2010). Effects of pedunculopontine nucleus area stimulation on gait disorders in Parkinson's disease. *Brain* 133, 205–214. doi: 10.1093/brain/awp229

Ferreira-Netto, C., Borelli, K. G., and Brandão, M. L. (2007). Distinct Fos expression in the brain following freezing behavior elicited by stimulation with NMDA of the ventral or dorsal inferior colliculus. *Exp. Neurol.* 204, 693–704. doi: 10.1016/j.expneurol.2006.12.023

Fetcho, J. R., Higashijima, S., and McLean, D. L. (2008). Zebrafish and motor control over the last decade. *Brain Res. Rev.* 57, 86–93. doi: 10.1016/j.brainresrev.2007.06.018

Floresco, S. B., West, A. R., Ash, B., Moore, H., and Grace, A. A. (2003). Afferent modulation of dopamine neuron firing differentially regulates tonic and phasic dopamine transmission. *Nat. Neurosci.* 6, 968–973. doi: 10.1038/nn1103

Ford, B., Holmes, C. J., Mainville, L., and Jones, B. E. (1995). GABAergic neurons in the rat pontomesencephalic tegmentum: codistribution with cholinergic and other tegmental neurons projecting to the posterior lateral hypothalamus. *J. Comp. Neurol.* 363, 177–196. doi: 10.1002/cne.903630203

Fortin, M., and Parent, A. (1999). Calretinin-immunoreactive neurons in primate pedunculopontine and laterodorsal tegmental nuclei. *Neuroscience* 88, 535–547. doi: 10.1016/S0306-4522(98)00214-0

Frank, M., J. (2006). Dynamic dopamine modulation in the basal ganglia: a neurocomputational account of cognitive deficits in medicated and nonmedicated Parkinsonism. *J. Cogn. Neurosci.* 17, 51–72. doi: 10.1162/0898929052880093

Gandhi, N. J., and Katnani, H. A. (2011). Motor functions of the superior colliculus. *Annu. Rev. Neurosci.* 34, 205–231. doi: 10.1146/annurev-neuro-061010-113728

Garcia-Rill, E., and Skinner, R. D. (1987a). The mesencephalic locomotor region. I. Activation of a medullary projection site. *Brain Res.* 411, 1–12. doi: 10.1016/0006-8993(87)90675-5

Garcia-Rill, E., and Skinner, R. D. (1987b). The mesencephalic locomotor region. II. Projections to reticulospinal neurons. *Brain Res.* 411, 13–20. doi: 10.1016/0006-8993(87)90676-7

Gillette, R., Kovac, M. P., and Davis, W. J. (1978). Command neurons in Pleurobranchaea receive synaptic feedback from the motor network they excite. *Science* 199, 798–801. doi: 10.1126/science.622571

Glickman, S. E., and Schiff, B. B. (1967). A biological theory of reinforcement. *Psychol. Rev.* 74, 81–109. doi: 10.1037/h0024290

Grillner, S., and Robertson, B. (2016). The basal ganglia over 500 million years. *Curr. Biol.* 26, R1088–R1100. doi: 10.1016/j.cub.2016.06.041

Grillner, S., Hongo, T., and Lund, S. (1968). The origin of descending fibres monosynaptically activating spinoreticular neurones. *Brain Res.* 10, 259–262. doi: 10.1016/0006-8993(68)90130-3

Grillner, S., Wallén, P., Saitoh, K., Kozlov, A., and Robertson, B. (2008). Neural bases of goal-directed locomotion in vertebrates—An overview. *Brain Res. Rev.* 57, 2–12. doi: 10.1016/j.brainresrev.2007.06.027

Gross, C. T., and Canteras, N. S. (2012). The many paths to fear. *Nat. Rev. Neurosci.* 13, 651–658. doi: 10.1038/nrn3301

Grossen, N. E., and Kelley, M. J. (1972). Species-specific behavior and acquisition of avoidance behavior in rats. *J. Comp. Physiol. Psychol.* 81, 307. doi: 10.1037/h0033536

Grossman, R. (1958). Effects of stimulation of non-specific thalamic system on locomotor movements in cat. *J. Neurophysiol.* 21, 85–93.

Haber, S. N., Fudge, J. L., and McFarland, N. R. (2000). Striatonigrostriatal pathways in primates form an ascending spiral from the shell to the dorsolateral striatum. *J. Neurosci.* 20, 2369–2382. Available online at: http://www.jneurosci.org/content/20/6/2369

Hagan, J. J., Leslie, R. A., and Patel, S. (1999). Orexin A activates locus coeruleus cell firing and increases arousal in the rat. *Proc. Natl. Acad. Sci. U.S.A.* 96, 10911–10916. doi: 10.1073/pnas.96.19.10911

Hägglund, M., Borgius, L., Dougherty, K. J., and Kiehn, O. (2010). Activation of groups of excitatory neurons in the mammalian spinal cord or hindbrain evokes locomotion. *Nat. Neurosci.* 13, 246–252. doi: 10.1038/nn.2482

Hamel, L., Thangarasa, T., Samadi, O., and Ito, R. (2017). Caudal nucleus accumbens core is critical in the regulation of cue-elicited approach-avoidance decisions. *eNeuro* 4:ENEURO.0330-16.2017. doi: 10.1523/ENEURO.0330-16.2017

Han, S., Soleiman, M. T., Soden, M. E., Zweifel, L. S., and Palmiter, R. D. (2015). Elucidating an affective pain circuit that creates a threat memory. *Cell* 162, 363–374. doi: 10.1016/j.cell.2015.05.057

Hansel, C. E., Linden, D. J., and D'Angelo, E. (2001). Beyond parallel fiber LTD: the diversity of synaptic and non-synaptic plasticity in the cerebellum. *Nat. Neurosci.* 4, 467–475. doi: 10.1038/87419

Harris, G., Wimmer, M., and Aston-Jones, G. (2005). A role for lateral hypothalamic orexin neurons in reward seeking. *Nature* 437, 556–559. doi: 10.1038/nature04071

Heise, C., and Mitrofanis, J. (2006). Fos immunoreactivity in some locomotor neural centres of 6OHDA-lesioned rats. *Anat. Embryol.* 211, 659–671. doi: 10.1007/s00429-006-0130-0

Hirsch, E. C., Graybiel, A. M., Duyckaerts, C., and Javoy-Agid, F. (1987). Neuronal loss in the pedunculopontine tegmental nucleus in Parkinson disease and in progressive supranuclear palsy. *Proc. Natl. Acad. Sci. U.S.A.* 84, 5976–5980. doi: 10.1073/pnas.84.16.5976

Holstege, J. C. (1991). Ultrastructural evidence for GABAergic brain stem projections to spinal motoneurons in the rat. *J. Neurosci.* 11, 159–167.

Holstege, J. C., Van Dijken, H., Buijs, R. M., Goedknegt, H., Gosens, T., and Bongers, C. M. (1996). Distribution of dopamine immunoreactivity in the rat, cat, and monkey spinal cord. *J. Comp. Neurol.* 376, 631–652. doi: 10.1002/(SICI)1096-9861(19961223)376:4<631::AID-CNE10>3.0.CO;2-P

Hong, S., and Hikosaka, O. (2011). Dopamine-mediated learning and switching in cortico-striatal circuit explain behavioral changes in reinforcement learning. *Front. Behav. Neurosci.* 5:15. doi: 10.3389/fnbeh.2011.00015

Howe, M. W., and Dombeck, D. A. (2016). Rapid signalling in distinct dopaminergic axons during locomotion and reward. *Nature* 535, 505–510. doi: 10.1038/nature18942

Humphreys, J. M., and Whelan, P. J. (2012). Dopamine exerts activation-dependent modulation of spinal locomotor circuits in the neonatal mouse. *J. Neurophysiol.* 108, 3370–3381. doi: 10.1152/jn.00482.2012

Humphries, M. D., and Prescott, T. J. (2010). The ventral basal ganglia, a selection mechanism at the crossroads of space, strategy, and reward. *Prog. Neurobiol.* 90, 385–417. doi: 10.1016/j.pneurobio.2009.11.003

Ichinohe, N., Teng, B., and Kitai, S. T. (2000). Morphological study of the tegmental pedunculopontine nucleus, substantia nigra and subthalamic nucleus, and their interconnections in rat organotypic culture. *Anat. Embryol.* 201, 435–453. doi: 10.1007/s004290050331

Ida, T., Nakahara, K., Katayama, T., and Murakami, N. (1999). Effect of lateral cerebroventricular injection of the appetite-stimulating neuropeptide, orexin and neuropeptide Y, on the various behavioral activities of rats. *Brain Res.* 821, 526–529. doi: 10.1016/S0006-8993(99)01131-2

Ikemoto, S. (2007). Dopamine reward circuitry: two projection systems from the ventral midbrain to the nucleus accumbens–olfactory tubercle complex. *Brain Res. Rev.* 56, 27–78. doi: 10.1016/j.brainresrev.2007.05.004

Inglis, W. L., Dunbar, J. S., and Winn, P. (1994). Outflow from the nucleus accumbens to the pedunculopontine tegmental nucleus: a dissociation between locomotor activity and the acquisition of responding for conditioned reinforcement stimulated by d-amphetamine. *Neuroscience* 62, 51–64. doi: 10.1016/0306-4522(94)90314-X

Ito, R., and Hayen, A. (2011). Opposing roles of nucleus accumbens core and shell dopamine in the modulation of limbic information processing. *J. Neurosci.* 31, 6001–6007. doi: 10.1523/JNEUROSCI.6588-10.2011

Ito, R., Robbins, T. W., and Everitt, B. (2004). Differential control over cocaine-seeking behavior by nucleus accumbens core and shell. *Nat. Neurosci.* 7, 389–397. doi: 10.1038/nn1217

Jankowska, E., Hammar, I., Slawinska, U., Maleszak, K., and Edgley, S. A. (2003). Neuronal basis of crossed actions from the reticular formation on feline hindlimb motoneurons. *J. Neurosci.* 23, 1867–1878. Available online at: http://www.jneurosci.org/content/23/5/1867.long

Jay, M., De Faveri, F., and McDearmid, J. (2015). Firing dynamics and modulatory actions of supraspinal dopaminergic neurons during zebrafish locomotor behavior. *Curr. Biol.* 25, 435–444. doi: 10.1016/j.cub.2014.12.033

Jellinger, K. (1988). The pedunculopontine nucleus in Parkinson's disease, progressive supranuclear palsy and Alzheimer's disease. *J. Neurol. Neurosurg. Psychiatry* 51, 540–543. doi: 10.1136/jnnp.51.4.540

Jordan, L. M. (1998). Initiation of locomotion in mammals. *Ann. N.Y. Acad. Sci.* 860, 83–93. doi: 10.1111/j.1749-6632.1998.tb09040.x

Jordan, L. M., Liu, J., Hedlund, P. B., Akay, T., and Pearson, K. G. (2008). Descending command systems for the initiation of locomotion in mammals. *Brain Res. Rev.* 57, 183–191. doi: 10.1016/j.brainresrev.2007.07.019

Kaelber, W. W., and Smith, T. B. (1979). Projections of the zona incerta in the cat, with stimulation controls. *Exp. Neurol.* 63, 177–200. doi: 10.1016/0014-4886(79)90192-4

Kiehn, O. (2016). Decoding the organization of spinal circuits that control locomotion. *Nat. Rev. Neurosci.* 17, 224–238. doi: 10.1038/nrn.2016.9

Kim, H. F., and Hikosaka, O. (2015). Parallel basal ganglia circuits for voluntary and automatic behaviour to reach rewards. *Brain* 138, 1776–1800. doi: 10.1093/brain/awv134

Kimura, Y., Satou, C., Fujioka, S., Shoji, W., Umeda, K., Ishizuka, T., et al. (2013). Hindbrain V2a neurons in the excitation of spinal locomotor circuits during zebrafish swimming. *Curr. Biol.* 23, 843–849. doi: 10.1016/j.cub.2013.03.066

Klemm, W. R. (2001). Behavioral arrest: in search of the neural control system. *Prog. Neurobiol.* 65, 453–471. doi: 10.1016/S0301-0082(01)00016-8

Kneisley, L. W., Biber, M. P., and LaVail, J. H. (1978). A study of the origin of brainstem projections to monkey spinal cord using the retrograde transport method. *Exp. Neurol.* 60, 116–139. doi: 10.1016/0014-4886(78)90172-3

Koblinger, K., Füzesi, T., Ejdrygiewicz, J., Krajacic, A., Bains, J., and Whelan, P. (2014). Characterization of A11 neurons projecting to the spinal cord of mice. *PLoS ONE* 9:e109636. doi: 10.1371/journal.pone.0109636

Koch, M. (1999). The neurobiology of startle. *Prog. Neurobiol.* 59, 107–128. doi: 10.1016/S0301-0082(98)00098-7

Koch, M., Kungel, M., and Herbert, H. (1993). Cholinergic neurons in the pedunculopontine tegmental nucleus are involved in the mediation of prepulse inhibition of the acoustic startle response in the rat. *Exp. Brain Res.* 97, 71–82. doi: 10.1007/BF00228818

Kolmac, C., and Mitrofanis, J. (1999). Distribution of various neurochemicals within the zona incerta: an immunocytochemical and histochemical study. *Anat. Embryol.* 199, 265–280. doi: 10.1007/s004290050227

Kosse, C., Schöne, C., Bracey, E., and Burdakov, D. (2017). Orexin-driven GAD65 network of the lateral hypothalamus sets physical activity in mice. *Proc. Natl. Acad. Sci. U.S.A.* 114, 4525–4530. doi: 10.1073/pnas.1619700114

Koutsikou, S., Apps, R., and Lumb, B. (2017). Top down control of spinal sensorimotor circuits essential for survival. *J. Physiol.* 595, 4151–4158. doi: 10.1113/JP273360

Koutsikou, S., Watson, T. C., Crook, J. J., Leith, J. L., Lawrenson, C. L., Apps, R., et al. (2015). The periaqueductal gray orchestrates sensory and motor circuits at multiple levels of the neuraxis. *J. Neurosci.* 35, 14132–14147. doi: 10.1523/JNEUROSCI.0261-15.2015

Kravitz, A., Freeze, B., Parker, P., Kay, K., Thwin, M., Deisseroth, K., et al. (2010). Regulation of parkinsonian motor behaviours by optogenetic control of basal ganglia circuitry. *Nature* 466, 622–626. doi: 10.1038/nature09159

Kroeger, D., Ferrari, L., Petit, G., Mahoney, C., Fuller, P., Arrigoni, E., et al. (2017). Cholinergic, glutamatergic, and GABAergic neurons of the pedunculopontine tegmental nucleus have distinct effects on sleep/wake behavior in mice. *J. Neurosci.* 37, 1352–1366. doi: 10.1523/JNEUROSCI.1405-16.2016

Krutki, P., Jankowska, E., and Edgley, S. A. (2003). Are crossed actions of reticulospinal and vestibulospinal neurons on feline motoneurons mediated by the same or separate commissural neurons? *J. Neurosci.* 23, 8041–8050.

Lambert, A. M., Bonkowsky, J. L., Masino, M. A. (2012). The conserved dopaminergic diencephalospinal tract mediates vertebrate locomotor development in zebrafish larvae. *J. Neuroscience.* 32, 13488–13500. doi: 10.1523/JNEUROSCI.1638-12.2012

Lamprea, M. R., Cardenas, F. P., Setem, J., and Morato, S. (2008). Thigmotactic responses in an open-field. *Braz. J. Med. Biol. Res.* 41, 135–140. doi: 10.1590/S0100-879X2008000200010

Landis, C., and Hunt, W. (1939). *The Startle Pattern.* Oxford: Farrar & Rinehart.

Lavoie, B., and Parent, A. (1994). Pedunculopontine nucleus in the squirrel monkey: cholinergic and glutamatergic projections to the substantia nigra. *J. Comp. Neurol.* 344, 232–241. doi: 10.1002/cne.903440205

LeDoux, J. (2000). Emotion circuits in the brain. *Annu. Rev. Neurosci.* 23, 155–184. doi: 10.1146/annurev.neuro.23.1.155

LeDoux, J. (2012). Rethinking the emotional brain. *Neuron* 73, 653–676. doi: 10.1016/j.neuron.2012.02.004

Leppänen, P., Ravaja, N., and Ewalds-Kvist, S. B. M. (2006). Twenty-three generations of mice bidirectionally selected for open-field thigmotaxis: selection response and repeated exposure to the open field. *Behav. Process.* 72, 23–31. doi: 10.1016/j.beproc.2005.11.010

Levita, L., Hare, T. A., Voss, H., Glover, G., Ballon, D. J., and Casey, B. J. (2009). The bivalent side of the nucleus accumbens. *Neuroimage* 44, 1178–1187. doi: 10.1016/j.neuroimage.2008.09.039

Li, H., Penzo, M. A., Taniguchi, H., Kopec, C. D., Huang, Z. J., and Li, B. (2013). Experience-dependent modification of a central amygdala fear circuit. *Nat. Neurosci.* 16, 332–339. doi: 10.1038/nn.3322

Li, W.-C. C., Perrins, R., Walford, A., and Roberts, A. (2003). The neuronal targets for GABAergic reticulospinal inhibition that stops swimming in hatchling frog tadpoles. *J. Comp. Physiol. A* 189, 29–37. doi: 10.1007/s00359-002-0372-0

Liang, F., Xiong, X., Zingg, B., Ji, X., Zhang, L., and Tao, H. (2015). Sensory cortical control of a visually induced arrest behavior via corticotectal projections. *Neuron* 86, 755–767. doi: 10.1016/j.neuron.2015.03.048

Liang, H., Paxinos, G., and Watson, C. (2011). Projections from the brain to the spinal cord in the mouse. *Brain Struct. Funct.* 215, 159–186. doi: 10.1007/s00429-010-0281-x

Liang, H., Paxinos, G., and Watson, C. (2012). Spinal projections from the presumptive midbrain locomotor region in the mouse. *Brain Struct. Funct.* 217, 211–219. doi: 10.1007/s00429-011-0337-6

Liu, J., and Jordan, L. M. (2005). Stimulation of the parapyramidal region of the neonatal rat brain stem produces locomotor-like activity involving spinal 5-HT7 and 5-HT2A receptors. *J. Neurophysiol.* 94, 1392–1404. doi: 10.1152/jn.00136.2005

Loewenstein, G., O'donoghue, T., and Bhatia, S. (2015). Modeling the interplay between affect and deliberation. *Decision* 2, 55–81. doi: 10.1037/dec0000029

Lokwan, S. J., Overton, P. G., Berry, M. S., and Clark, D. (1999). Stimulation of the pedunculopontine tegmental nucleus in the rat produces burst firing in A9 dopaminergic neurons. *Neuroscience* 92, 245–254. doi: 10.1016/S0306-4522(98)00748-9

Magnuson, D., Schramm, M., and MacLean, J. (1995). Long-duration, frequency-dependent motor responses evoked by ventrolateral funiculus stimulation in the neonatal rat spinal cord. *Neurosci. Lett.* 192, 97–100. doi: 10.1016/0304-3940(95)99208-M

Manira, E., Pombal, M. A., and Grillner, S. (1997). Diencephalic projection to reticulospinal neurons involved in the initiation of locomotion in adult lampreys *Lampetra fluviatilis*. *J. Comp. Neurol.* 389, 603–616. doi: 10.1002/(SICI)1096-9861(19971229)389:4<603::AID-CNE5>3.0.CO;2-4

Masserman, J. H. (1938). Destruction of the hypothalamus in cats: effects of activity of the central nervous system and its reaction to sodium amytal. *Arch. Neurol. Psychiatry* 39, 1250–1271. doi: 10.1001/archneurpsyc.1938.02270060140007

Matsuyama, K., Mori, F., Kuze, B., and Mori, S. (1999). Morphology of single pontine reticulospinal axons in the lumbar enlargement of the cat: a study using the anterograde tracer PHA-L. *J. Comp. Neurol.* 410, 413–430. doi: 10.1002/(SICI)1096-9861(19990802)410:3<413::AID-CNE5>3.0.CO;2-Q

McCutcheon, J., Ebner, S., Loriaux, A., and Roitman, M. (2012). Encoding of aversion by dopamine and the nucleus accumbens. *Front. Neurosci.* 6:137. doi: 10.3389/fnins.2012.00137

Medina, J., Repa, C., Mauk, M., and LeDoux, J. (2002). Parallels between cerebellum- and amygdala-dependent conditioning. *Nat. Rev. Neurosci.* 3, 122–131. doi: 10.1038/nrn728

Mel'nikova, Z. L. (1975). Locomotion of rats induced by stimulation of the mesencephalon. *Bull. Moscow Univ.* 30, 45–51.

Mel'nikova, Z. L. (1977). Study of the relationships between the "locomotor regions" of the subthalamus and midbrain in rats. *Neiřofiziol. Neurophysiol.* 9, 275–280.

Ménard, A., and Grillner, S. (2008). Diencephalic locomotor region in the lamprey—Afferents and efferent control. *J. Neurophysiol.* 100, 1343–1353. doi: 10.1152/jn.01128.2007

Mena-Segovia, J., and Bolam, J. P. (2017). Rethinking the pedunculopontine nucleus: from cellular organization to function. *Neuron* 94, 7–18. doi: 10.1016/j.neuron.2017.02.027

Mena-Segovia, J., Micklem, B. R., Nair-Roberts, R. G., Ungless, M. A., and Bolam, J. P. (2009). GABAergic neuron distribution in the pedunculopontine nucleus defines functional subterritories. *J. Comp. Neurol.* 515, 397–408. doi: 10.1002/cne.22065

Mena-Segovia, J., Sims, H. M., Magill, P. J., and Bolam, J. P. (2008). Cholinergic brainstem neurons modulate cortical gamma activity during slow oscillations. *J. Physiol.* 586, 2947–2960. doi: 10.1113/jphysiol.2008.153874

Miller, A., and Blaha, C. (2004). Nigrostriatal dopamine release modulated by mesopontine muscarinic receptors. *Neuroreport* 15:1805. doi: 10.1097/01.wnr.0000135692.81613.85

Milner, K., and Mogenson, G. (1988). Electrical and chemical activation of the mesencephalic and subthalamic locomotor regions in freely moving rats. *Brain Res.* 452, 273–285. doi: 10.1016/0006-8993(88)90031-5

Mitrofanis, J. (2005). Some certainty for the "zone of uncertainty"? Exploring the function of the zona incerta. *Neuroscience* 130, 1–15. doi: 10.1016/j.neuroscience.2004.08.017

Mogenson, G. J., and Stevenson, J. A. F. (1967). Drinking induced by electrical stimulation of the lateral hypothalamus. *Exp. Neurol.* 17, 119–127. doi: 10.1016/0014-4886(67)90139-2

Mogenson, G. J., Jones, D., and Yim, C. (1980). From motivation to action: functional interface between the limbic system and the motor system. *Prog. Neurobiol.* 14, 69–97. doi: 10.1016/0301-0082(80)90018-0

Mogenson, G. J., Swanson, L. W., and Wu, M. (1983). Neural projections from nucleus accumbens to globus pallidus, substantia innominata, and lateral preoptic-lateral hypothalamic area: an anatomical and electrophysiological investigation in the rat. *J. Neurosci.* 3, 189–202.

Mori, S., Sakamoto, T., Ohta, Y., Takakusaki, K., and Matsuyama, K. (1989). Site-specific postural and locomotor changes evoked in awake, freely moving intact cats by stimulating the brainstem. *Brain Res.* 505, 66–74. doi: 10.1016/0006-8993(89)90116-9

Motta, S., Goto, M., Gouveia, F., Baldo, M., Canteras, N., and Swanson, L. (2009). Dissecting the brain's fear system reveals the hypothalamus is critical for responding in subordinate conspecific intruders. *Proc. Natl. Acad. Sci. U.S.A.* 106, 4870–4875. doi: 10.1073/pnas.0900939106

Mullins, O., Hackett, J., Buchanan, J., and Friesen, O. (2011). Neuronal control of swimming behavior: comparison of vertebrate and invertebrate model systems. *Prog. Neurobiol.* 93, 244–269. doi: 10.1016/j.pneurobio.2010.11.001

Muthuraju, S., Talbot, T., and Brandão, M. (2016). Dopamine D_2 receptors regulate unconditioned fear in deep layers of the superior colliculus and dorsal periaqueductal gray. *Behav. Brain Res.* 297, 116–123. doi: 10.1016/j.bbr.2015.10.005

Nagata, T., and Hayashi, Y. (1984). The visual field representation of the rat ventral lateral geniculate nucleus. *J. Comp. Neurol.* 227, 582–588. doi: 10.1002/cne.902270409

Nicola, S. (2007). The nucleus accumbens as part of a basal ganglia action selection circuit. *Psychopharmacology* 191, 521–550. doi: 10.1007/s00213-006-0510-4

Noga, B. R., Kettler, J., and Jordan, L. M. (1988). Locomotion produced in mesencephalic cats by injections of putative transmitter substances and antagonists into the medial reticular formation and the pontomedullary locomotor strip. *J. Neurosci.* 8, 2074–2086.

Noga, B. R., Kriellaars, D. J., Brownstone, R. M., and Jordan, L. M. (2003). Mechanism for activation of locomotor centers in the spinal cord by stimulation of the mesencephalic locomotor region. *J. Neurophysiol.* 90, 1464–1478. doi: 10.1152/jn.00034.2003

Noga, B., Sanchez, F., Villamil, L., O'Toole, C., Kasicki, S., Olszewski, M., et al. (2017). LFP oscillations in the mesencephalic locomotor region during voluntary locomotion. *Front. Neural Circuit* 11:34. doi: 10.3389/fncir.2017.00034

Noga, B. R., Turkson, R. P., Xie, S., Taberner, A., Pinzon, A., and Hentall, I. D. (2017). Monoamine release in the cat lumbar spinal cord during fictive locomotion evoked by the mesencephalic locomotor region. *Front. Neural Circuits* 11:59. doi: 10.3389/fncir.2017.00059

Norton, A., Jo, Y., Clark, E., Taylor, C., and Mizumori, S. (2011). Independent neural coding of reward and movement by pedunculopontine tegmental nucleus neurons in freely navigating rats. *Eur. J. Neurosci.* 33, 1885–1896. doi: 10.1111/j.1460-9568.2011.07649.x

Oka, T., Tsumori, T., Yokota, S., and Yasui, Y. (2008). Neuroanatomical and neurochemical organization of projections from the central amygdaloid nucleus to the nucleus retroambiguus via the periaqueductal gray in the rat. *Neurosci. Res.* 62, 286–298. doi: 10.1016/j.neures.2008.10.004

Olmstead, M. C., and Franklin, K. B. (1994). Lesions of the pedunculopontine tegmental nucleus abolish catalepsy and locomotor depression induced by morphine. *Brain Res.* 662, 134–140. doi: 10.1016/0006-8993(94)90805-2

Olson, G., and Krasne, F. (1981). The crayfish lateral giants as command neurons for escape behavior. *Brain Res.* 214, 89–100. doi: 10.1016/0006-8993(81)90440-6

Olszewski, J., and Baxter, D. (1954). *Cytoarchitecture of the Human Brain Stem.* New York, NY: Basle: S. Karger.

Ondo, W. G., He, Y., Rajasekaran, S., and Le, W. D. (2000). Clinical correlates of 6-hydroxydopamine injections into A11 dopaminergic neurons in rats: a possible model for restless legs syndrome. *Mov. Disord.* 15, 154–158. doi: 10.1002/1531-8257(200001)15:1<154::AID-MDS1025>3.0.CO;2-Q

Pahapill, P., and Lozano, A. (2000). The pedunculopontine nucleus and Parkinson's disease. *Brain* 123, 1767–1783. doi: 10.1093/brain/123.9.1767

Palmiter, R. (2008). Dopamine signaling in the dorsal striatum is essential for motivated behaviors. *Ann. N.Y. Acad. Sci.* 1129, 35–46. doi: 10.1196/annals.1417.003

Pan, W.-X., and Hyland, B. (2005). Pedunculopontine tegmental nucleus controls conditioned responses of midbrain dopamine neurons in behaving rats. *J. Neurosci.* 25, 4725–4732. doi: 10.1523/JNEUROSCI.0277-05.2005

Parkinson, J. A., Cardinal, R. N., and Everitt, B. J. (2000). Limbic cortical-ventral striatal systems underlying appetitive conditioning. *Prog. Brain Res.* 126, 263–285. doi: 10.1016/S0079-6123(00)26019-6

Paxinos, G., and Franklin, K. B. (2008). *The Mouse Brain in Stereotaxic Coordinates, Compact, Third Edition: The Coronal Plates and Diagrams, 3rd Edn.* New York, NY: Elsevier Publishing.

Perreault, M. C., Drew, T., and Rossignol, S. (1993). Activity of medullary reticulospinal neurons during fictive locomotion. *J. Neurophysiol.* 69, 2232–2247.

Perrins, R., Walford, A., and Roberts, A. (2002). Sensory activation and role of inhibitory reticulospinal neurons that stop swimming in hatchling frog tadpoles. *J. Neurosci.* 22, 4229–4240.

Peterson, B. W., Pitts, N. G., and Fukushima (1979). Reticulospinal connections with limb and axial motoneurons. *Exp. Brain Res.* 36, 1–20. doi: 10.1007/BF00238464

Petras, J. M. (1967). Cortical, tectal and tegmental fiber connections in the spinal cord of the cat. *Brain Res.* 6, 275–324. doi: 10.1016/0006-8993(67)90196-5

Petrovich, G. D. (2011). Learning and the motivation to eat: forebrain circuitry. *Physiol. Behav.* 104, 582–589. doi: 10.1016/j.physbeh.2011.04.059

Petrovich, G. D., Risold, P. Y., and Swanson, L. W. (1996). Organization of projections from the basomedial nucleus of the amygdala: a PHAL study in the rat. *J. Comp. Neurol.* 374, 387–420. doi: 10.1002/(SICI)1096-9861(19961021)374:3<387::AID-CNE6>3.0.CO;2-Y

Peyron, C., Tighe, D. K., van den Pol, A. N., de Lecea, L., Heller, H. C., Sutcliffe, J. C., et al. (1998). Neurons containing hypocretin (orexin) project to multiple neuronal systems. *J. Neurosci.* 18, 9996–10015.

Phelps, E., and LeDoux, J. (2005). Contributions of the amygdala to emotion processing: from animal models to human behavior. *Neuron* 48, 175–187. doi: 10.1016/j.neuron.2005.09.025

Picton, L., Nascimento, F., Broadhead, M., Sillar, K., and Miles, G. (2017). Sodium pumps mediate activity-dependent changes in mammalian motor networks. *J. Neurosci.* 37, 906–921. doi: 10.1523/JNEUROSCI.2005-16.2016

Qu, S., Le, W., Zhang, X., Xie, W., Zhang, A., and Ondo, W. (2007). Locomotion is increased in a11-lesioned mice with iron deprivation: a possible animal model for restless legs syndrome. *J. Neuropathol. Exp. Neurol.* 66, 383–388. doi: 10.1097/nen.0b013e3180517b5f

Richard, J., and Berridge, K. (2011). Nucleus accumbens dopamine/glutamate interaction switches modes to generate desire versus dread: D1 alone for appetitive eating but D1 and D2 together for fear. *J. Neurosci.* 31, 12866–12879. doi: 10.1523/JNEUROSCI.1339-11.2011

Roberts, W. W., and Carey, R. J. (1965). Rewarding effect of performance of gnawing aroused by hypothalamic stimulation in the rat. *J. Comp. Physiol. Psychol.* 59, 317–324. doi: 10.1037/h0022030

Roitman, M., Wheeler, R., and Carelli, R. (2005). Nucleus accumbens neurons are innately tuned for rewarding and aversive taste stimuli, encode their predictors, and are linked to motor output. *Neuron* 45, 587–597. doi: 10.1016/j.neuron.2004.12.055

Rolland, A.-S. S., Tandé, D., Herrero, M.-T. T., Luquin, M.-R. R., Vazquez-Claverie, M., Karachi, C., et al. (2009). Evidence for a dopaminergic innervation of the pedunculopontine nucleus in monkeys, and its drastic reduction after MPTP intoxication. *J. Neurochem.* 110, 1321–1329. doi: 10.1111/j.1471-4159.2009.06220.x

Roseberry, T. K., Lee, A. M., Lalive, A. L., Wilbrecht, L., Bonci, A., and Kreitzer, A. C. (2016). Cell-type-specific control of brainstem locomotor circuits by basal ganglia. *Cell* 164, 526–537. doi: 10.1016/j.cell.2015.12.037

Roseberry, T., and Kreitzer, A. (2017). Neural circuitry for behavioural arrest. *Philos. Trans. R. Soc. B* 372:20160197. doi: 10.1098/rstb.2016.0197

Ross, G. S., and Sinnamon, H. M. (1984). Forelimb and hindlimb stepping by the anesthetized rat elicited by electrical stimulation of the pons and medulla. *Physiol. Behav.* 33, 201–208. doi: 10.1016/0031-9384(84)90100-8

Rossignol, S., Dubuc, R., and Gossard, J.-P. (2006). Dynamic sensorimotor interactions in locomotion. *Physiol. Rev.* 86, 89–154. doi: 10.1152/physrev.00028.2005

Ryczko, D., Cone, J., Alpert, M., Goetz, L., Auclair, F., Dubé, C., et al. (2016). A descending dopamine pathway conserved from basal vertebrates to mammals. *Proc. Natl. Acad. Sci. U.S.A.* 113, E2440–E2449. doi: 10.1073/pnas.1600684113

Ryczko, D., and Dubuc, R. (2013). The multifunctional mesencephalic locomotor region. *Curr. Pharm. Des.* 19, 4448–4470. doi: 10.2174/1381612811319240011

Ryczko, D., and Dubuc, R. (2017). Dopamine and the brainstem locomotor networks: from lamprey to human. *Front. Neurosci.* 11:295. doi: 10.3389/fnins.2017.00295

Ryczko, D., Grätsch, S., Auclair, F., Dubé, C., Bergeron, S., Alpert, M. H., et al. (2013). Forebrain dopamine neurons project down to a brainstem region controlling locomotion. *Proc. Natl. Acad. Sci. U.S.A.* 110, E3235–E3242. doi: 10.1073/pnas.1301125110

Sah, P., Faber, E., Armentia, L. M., and Power, J. (2003). The amygdaloid complex: anatomy and physiology. *Physiol. Rev.* 83, 803–834. doi: 10.1152/physrev.00002.2003

Sahibzada, N., Dean, P., and Redgrave, P. (1986). Movements resembling orientation or avoidance elicited by electrical stimulation of the superior colliculus in rats. *J. Neurosci.* 6, 723–733.

Sakurai, T. (2005). *The Orexin/Hypocretin System.* Totowa, NJ: Humana Press.

Sakurai, T., Amemiya, A., Ishii, M., Matsuzaki, I., Chemelli, R. M., Tanaka, H., et al. (1998). Orexins and orexin receptors: a family of hypothalamic neuropeptides and G protein-coupled receptors that regulate feeding behavior. *Cell* 92, 573–585. doi: 10.1016/S0092-8674(00)80949-6

Salgado, S., and Kaplitt, M. G. (2015). The nucleus accumbens: a comprehensive review. *Stereot. Funct. Neuros* 93, 75–93. doi: 10.1159/000368279

Saper, C. B. (2006). Staying awake for dinner: hypothalamic integration of sleep, feeding, and circadian rhythms. *Prog. Brain Res.* 153, 243–252. doi: 10.1016/S0079-6123(06)53014-6

Sar, M., Stumpf, W., Miller, R., Chang, K., and Cuatrecasas, P. (1978). Immunohistochemical localization of enkephalin in rat brain and spinal cord. *J. Comp. Neurol.* 182, 17–37. doi: 10.1002/cne.901820103

Sara, S. (2009). The locus coeruleus and noradrenergic modulation of cognition. *Nat. Rev. Neurosci.* 10, 211–223. doi: 10.1038/nrn2573

Sato, M., Ito, M., Nagase, M., Sugimura, Y., Takahashi, Y., Watabe, A., et al. (2015). The lateral parabrachial nucleus is actively involved in the acquisition of fear memory in mice. *Mol. Brain* 8, 1–15. doi: 10.1186/s13041-015-0108-z

Satoda, T., Matsumoto, H., Zhou, L., Rose, P. K., and Richmond, F. J. (2002). Mesencephalic projections to the first cervical segment in the cat. *Exp. Brain Res.* 144, 397–413. doi: 10.1007/s00221-002-1047-3

Scarnati, E., Campana, E., and Pacitti, C. (1984). Pedunculopontine-evoked excitation of substantia nigra neurons in the rat. *Brain Res.* 304, 351–361. doi: 10.1016/0006-8993(84)90339-1

Scarnati, E., Proia, A., Di Loreto, S., and Pacitti, C. (1987). The reciprocal electrophysiological influence between the nucleus tegmenti pedunculopontinus and the substantia nigra in normal and decorticated rats. *Brain Res.* 423, 116–124. doi: 10.1016/0006-8993(87)90831-6

Schaltenbrand, G., and Wahren, W. (1977). *Atlas for Stereotaxy of the Human Brain.* Stuttgart; New York, NY: Thieme.

Sébille, S. B., Belaid, H., Philippe, A.-C. C., André, A., Lau, B., François, C., et al. (2017). Anatomical evidence for functional diversity in the mesencephalic locomotor region of primates. *Neuroimage* 147, 66–78. doi: 10.1016/j.neuroimage.2016.12.011

Semba, K., and Fibiger, H. C. (1992). Afferent connections of the laterodorsal and the pedunculopontine tegmental nuclei in the rat: a retro- and antero-grade transport and immunohistochemical study. *J. Comp. Neurol.* 323, 387–410. doi: 10.1002/cne.903230307

Sharples, S. A. (2017). Dopamine pumping up spinal locomotor network function. *J. Neurosci.* 37, 3103–3105. doi: 10.1523/JNEUROSCI.0019-17.2017

Sharples, S. A., and Whelan, P. J. (2017). Modulation of rhythmic activity in mammalian spinal networks is dependent on excitability state. *eNeuro* 4:ENEURO.0368-16.2017. doi: 10.1523/ENEURO.0368-16.2017

Sharples, S. A., Humphreys, J. M., Jensen, A. M., Dhoopar, S., Delaloye, N., Clemens, S., et al. (2015). Dopaminergic modulation of locomotor network activity in the neonatal mouse spinal cord. *J. Neurophysiol.* 113, 2500–2010. doi: 10.1152/jn.00849.2014

Sharples, S. A., Koblinger, K., Humphreys, J. M., and Whelan, P. J. (2014). Dopamine: a parallel pathway for the modulation of spinal locomotor networks. *Front. Neural Circuits* 8:55. doi: 10.3389/fncir.2014.00055

Sherman, D., Fuller, P., Marcus, J., Yu, J., Zhang, P., Chamberlin, N., et al. (2015). Anatomical location of the mesencephalic locomotor region and its possible role in locomotion, posture, cataplexy, and parkinsonism. *Front. Neurol.* 6:140. doi: 10.3389/fneur.2015.00140

Shik, M. L., and Orlovsky, G. N. (1976). Neurophysiology of locomotor automatism. *Physiol. Rev.* 56, 465–501.

Shik, M. L., Severin, F. V., and Orlovsky, G. N. (1969). Control of walking and running by means of electrical stimulation of the mesencephalon. *Electr. Clin. Neurol.* 26:549.

Siegel, J., and Boehmer, L. (2006). Narcolepsy and the hypocretin system—where motion meets emotion. *Nat. Clin. Pract. Neurol.* 2, 548–556. doi: 10.1038/ncpneuro0300

Sinnamon, H. (1993). Preoptic and hypothalamic neurons and the initiation of locomotion in the anesthetized rat. *Prog. Neurobiol.* 41, 323–344. doi: 10.1016/0301-0082(93)90003-B

Sinnamon, H. M., Lee, S. H., Adams, D. B., and Stopford, C. K. (1984). Locomotor stepping elicited by electrical stimulation of the lateral hypothalamus requires an ipsilateral descending pathway. *Physiol. Behav.* 33, 209–215. doi: 10.1016/0031-9384(84)90101-X

Sinnamon, H., and Stopford, K. (1987). Locomotion elicited by lateral hypothalamic stimulation in the anesthetized rat does not require the dorsal midbrain. *Brain Res.* 402, 78–86. doi: 10.1016/0006-8993(87)91049-3

Sirota, M. G., and Shik, M. L. (1973). Locomotion of the cat on stimulation of the mesencephalon. *Fiziol. Zhurnal Sssr Imeni M Sechenova* 59, 1314–1321.

Skagerberg, G., and Lindvall, O. (1985). Organization of diencephalic dopamine neurones projecting to the spinal cord in the rat. *Brain Res.* 342, 340–351. doi: 10.1016/0006-8993(85)91134-5

Skinner, R. D., and Garcia-Rill, E. (1984). The mesencephalic locomotor region (MLR) in the rat. *Brain Res.* 323, 385–389.

Skinner, R. D., Kinjo, N., Henderson, V., and Garcia-Rill, E. (1990). Locomotor projections from the pedunculopontine nucleus to the spinai cord. *Neuroreport* 1, 183–186. doi: 10.1097/00001756-199011000-00001

Sparks, D. L. (1986). Translation of sensory signals into commands for control of saccadic eye movements: role of primate superior colliculus. *Physiol. Rev.* 66, 118–171.

Steeves, J., and Jordan, L. (1980). Localization of a descending pathway in the spinal cord which is necessary for controlled treadmill locomotion. *Neurosci. Lett.* 20, 283–288. doi: 10.1016/0304-3940(80)90161-5

Stefanik, M., Kupchik, Y., and Kalivas, P. (2016). Optogenetic inhibition of cortical afferents in the nucleus accumbens simultaneously prevents cue-induced transient synaptic potentiation and cocaine-seeking behavior. *Brain Struct. Funct.* 221, 1681–1689. doi: 10.1007/s00429-015-0997-8

Stefanik, M., Kupchik, Y., Brown, R., and Kalivas, P. (2013). Optogenetic evidence that pallidal projections, not nigral projections, from the nucleus accumbens core are necessary for reinstating cocaine seeking. *J. Neurosci.* 33, 13654–13662. doi: 10.1523/JNEUROSCI.1570-13.2013

Steininger, T. L., Rye, D. B., and Wainer, B. H. (1992). Afferent projections to the cholinergic pedunculopontine tegmental nucleus and adjacent midbrain extrapyramidal area in the albino rat. I. Retrograde tracing studies. *J. Comp. Neurol.* 321, 515–543. doi: 10.1002/cne.903210403

Stoyanova, I. I., Rutten, W. L., and le Feber, J. (2010). Orexin-A and orexin-B during the postnatal development of the rat brain. *Cell. Mol. Neurobiol.* 30, 81–89. doi: 10.1007/s10571-009-9433-z

Stuber, G. D., and Wise, R. A. (2016). Lateral hypothalamic circuits for feeding and reward. *Nat. Neurosci.* 19, 198–205. doi: 10.1038/nn.4220

Surmeier, J., Ding, J., Day, M., Wang, Z., and Shen, W. (2007). D1 and D2 dopamine-receptor modulation of striatal glutamatergic signaling in striatal medium spiny neurons. *Trends Neurosci.* 30, 228–235. doi: 10.1016/j.tins.2007.03.008

Swanson, L. W. (2000). Cerebral hemisphere regulation of motivated behavior. *Brain Res.* 886, 113–164. doi: 10.1016/S0006-8993(00)02905-X

Swanson, L., Sanchez-Watts, G., and Watts, A. (2005). Comparison of melanin-concentrating hormone and hypocretin/orexin mRNA expression patterns in a new parceling scheme of the lateral hypothalamic zone. *Neurosci. Lett.* 387, 80–84. doi: 10.1016/j.neulet.2005.06.066

Szokol, K., Glover, J., and Perreault, M.-C. (2011). Organization of functional synaptic connections between medullary reticulospinal neurons and lumbar descending commissural interneurons in the neonatal mouse. *J. Neurosci.* 31, 4731–4742. doi: 10.1523/JNEUROSCI.5486-10.2011

Takakusaki, K., Habaguchi, T., Ohtinata-Sugimoto, J., Saitoh, K., and Sakamoto, T. (2003). Basal ganglia efferents to the brainstem centers controlling postural muscle tone and locomotion: a new concept for understanding motor disorders in basal ganglia dysfunction. *Neuroscience* 119, 293–308. doi: 10.1016/S0306-4522(03)00095-2

Takakusaki, K., Takahashi, K., Saitoh, K., Harada, H., Okumura, T., Kayama, Y., et al. (2005). Orexinergic projections to the cat midbrain mediate alternation of emotional behavioural states from locomotion to cataplexy. *J. Physiol.* 568, 1003–1020. doi: 10.1113/jphysiol.2005.085829

Tay, T., Ronneberger, O., Ryu, S., Nitschke, R., and Driever, W. (2011). Comprehensive catecholaminergic projectome analysis reveals single-neuron integration of zebrafish ascending and descending dopaminergic systems. *Nat. Commun.* 2:171. doi: 10.1038/ncomms1171

Thakkar, M. M., Ramesh, V., Strecker, R. E., and McCarley, R. W. (2001). Microdialysis perfusion of orexin-A in the basal forebrain increases wakefulness in freely behaving rats. *Arch. Ital. Biol.* 139, 313–328. doi: 10.4449/aib.v139i3.506

Thankachan, S., Fuller, P. M., and Lu, J. (2012). Movement- and behavioral state-dependent activity of pontine reticulospinal neurons. *Neuroscience* 221, 125–139. doi: 10.1016/j.neuroscience.2012.06.069

Tovote, P., Esposito, M., Botta, P., Chaudun, F., Fadok, J., Markovic, M., et al. (2016). Midbrain circuits for defensive behaviour. *Nature* 534, 206–212. doi: 10.1038/nature17996

Utter, A., and Basso, M. (2008). The basal ganglia: an overview of circuits and function. *Neurosci. Biobehav. Rev.* 32, 333–342. doi: 10.1016/j.neubiorev.2006.11.003

Valenstein, E. (1971). Channeling of responses elicited by hypothalamic stimulation. *J. Psychiatr. Res.* 8, 335–344. doi: 10.1016/0022-3956(71)90029-X

Valenstein, E., Cox, V., and Kakolewski, J. (1970). Reexamination of the role of the hypothalamus in motivation. *Psychol. Rev.* 77:16. doi: 10.1037/h0028581

Vianna, D. M. L., Landeira-Fernandez, J., and Brandão, M. L. (2001). Dorsolateral and ventral regions of the periaqueductal gray matter are involved in distinct types of fear. *Neurosci. Biobehav. Rev.* 25, 711–719. doi: 10.1016/S0149-7634(01)00052-5

Vincent, S. R. (2000). The ascending reticular activating system–from aminergic neurons to nitric oxide. *J. Chem. Neuroanat.* 18, 23–30. doi: 10.1016/S0891-0618(99)00048-4

Wagner, C. K., Eaton, M. J., Moore, K. E., and Lookingland, K. J. (1995). Efferent projections from the region of the medial zona incerta containing A13 dopaminergic neurons: a PHA-L anterograde tract-tracing study in the rat. *Brain Res.* 677, 229–237. doi: 10.1016/0006-8993(95)00128-D

Wall, N., De La Parra, M., Callaway, E., and Kreitzer, A. (2013). Differential innervation of direct- and indirect-pathway striatal projection neurons. *Neuron* 79, 347–360. doi: 10.1016/j.neuron.2013.05.014

Waller, W. H. (1940). Progression movements elicited by subthalamic stimulation. *J. Neurophysiol.* 3, 300–307.

Wannier, T., Orlovsky, G., and Grillner, S. (1995). Reticulospinal neurones provide monosynaptic glycinergic inhibition of spinal neurones in lamprey. *Neuroreport* 6, 1597. doi: 10.1097/00001756-199508000-00003

Whelan, P. J. (1996). Control of locomotion in the decerebrate cat. *Prog. Neurobiol.* 49, 481–515. doi: 10.1016/0301-0082(96)00028-7

Whishaw, I., Alaverdashvili, M., and Kolb, B. (2008). The problem of relating plasticity and skilled reaching after motor cortex stroke in the rat. *Behav. Brain Res.* 192, 124–136. doi: 10.1016/j.bbr.2007.12.026

Wilensky, A., Schafe, G., Kristensen, M., and LeDoux, J. (2006). Rethinking the fear circuit: the central nucleus of the amygdala is required for the acquisition, consolidation, and expression of pavlovian fear conditioning. *J. Neurosci.* 26, 12387–12396. doi: 10.1523/JNEUROSCI.4316-06.2006

Wullimann, M. F. (2014). Ancestry of basal ganglia circuits: new evidence in teleosts. *J. Comp. Neurol.* 522, 2013–2018. doi: 10.1002/cne.23525

Xiang, H.-B. B., Zhu, W.-Z. Z., Guan, X.-H. H., and Ye, D.-W. W. (2013). The cuneiform nucleus may be involved in the regulation of skeletal muscle tone by motor pathway: a virally mediated trans-synaptic tracing study in surgically sympathectomized mice. *Brain* 136:e251. doi: 10.1093/brain/awt123

Xiao, C., Cho, J., Zhou, C., Treweek, J., Chan, K., McKinney, S., et al. (2016). Cholinergic mesopontine signals govern locomotion and reward through dissociable midbrain pathways. *Neuron* 90, 333–347. doi: 10.1016/j.neuron.2016.03.028

Yamamoto, K., and Vernier, P. (2011). The evolution of dopamine systems in chordates. *Front. Neuroanat.* 5:21. doi: 10.3389/fnana.2011.00021

Yeomans, J. S., and Frankland, P. W. (1995). The acoustic startle reflex: neurons and connections. *Brain Res. Rev.* 21, 301–314. doi: 10.1016/0165-0173(96)00004-5

Yeomans, J., Li, L., Scott, B., and Frankland, P. (2002). Tactile, acoustic and vestibular systems sum to elicit the startle reflex. *Neurosci. Biobehav. Rev.* 26, 1–11. doi: 10.1016/S0149-7634(01)00057-4

Yilmaz, M., and Meister, M. (2013). Rapid innate defensive responses of mice to looming visual stimuli. *Curr. Biol.* 23, 2011–2015. doi: 10.1016/j.cub.2013.08.015

Zweig, R., Jankel, W., Hedreen, J., Mayeux, R., and Price, D. (1989). The pedunculopontine nucleus in Parkinson's disease. *Ann. Neurol.* 26, 41–46. doi: 10.1002/ana.410260106

Permissions

All chapters in this book were first published by Frontiers; hereby published with permission under the Creative Commons Attribution License or equivalent. Every chapter published in this book has been scrutinized by our experts. Their significance has been extensively debated. The topics covered herein carry significant findings which will fuel the growth of the discipline. They may even be implemented as practical applications or may be referred to as a beginning point for another development.

The contributors of this book come from diverse backgrounds, making this book a truly international effort. This book will bring forth new frontiers with its revolutionizing research information and detailed analysis of the nascent developments around the world.

We would like to thank all the contributing authors for lending their expertise to make the book truly unique. They have played a crucial role in the development of this book. Without their invaluable contributions this book wouldn't have been possible. They have made vital efforts to compile up to date information on the varied aspects of this subject to make this book a valuable addition to the collection of many professionals and students.

This book was conceptualized with the vision of imparting up-to-date information and advanced data in this field. To ensure the same, a matchless editorial board was set up. Every individual on the board went through rigorous rounds of assessment to prove their worth. After which they invested a large part of their time researching and compiling the most relevant data for our readers.

The editorial board has been involved in producing this book since its inception. They have spent rigorous hours researching and exploring the diverse topics which have resulted in the successful publishing of this book. They have passed on their knowledge of decades through this book. To expedite this challenging task, the publisher supported the team at every step. A small team of assistant editors was also appointed to further simplify the editing procedure and attain best results for the readers.

Apart from the editorial board, the designing team has also invested a significant amount of their time in understanding the subject and creating the most relevant covers. They scrutinized every image to scout for the most suitable representation of the subject and create an appropriate cover for the book.

The publishing team has been an ardent support to the editorial, designing and production team. Their endless efforts to recruit the best for this project, has resulted in the accomplishment of this book. They are a veteran in the field of academics and their pool of knowledge is as vast as their experience in printing. Their expertise and guidance has proved useful at every step. Their uncompromising quality standards have made this book an exceptional effort. Their encouragement from time to time has been an inspiration for everyone.

The publisher and the editorial board hope that this book will prove to be a valuable piece of knowledge for researchers, students, practitioners and scholars across the globe.

List of Contributors

Bowen Dempsey, Sheng Le, Anita Turner, Phil Bokiniec, Radhika Ramadas, Ann K. Goodchild and Simon McMullan
Faculty of Medicine and Health Sciences, Neurobiology of Vital Systems, Macquarie University, Sydney, NSW, Australia

Jan G. Bjaalie
Department of Anatomy, Institute of Basic Medical Sciences, University of Oslo, Oslo, Norway

Clement Menuet and Andrew M. Allen
Department of Physiology, University of Melbourne, Melbourne, VIC, Australia

Laura Légat, Sofie Brouwers and Alain G. Dupont
Laboratory of Pharmaceutical Chemistry, Drug Analysis and Drug Information (FASC), Research Group Experimental Pharmacology (EFAR), Center for Neurosciences (C4N), Vrije Universiteit Brussel, Brussels, Belgium Cardiovascular Center, Universitair Ziekenhuis Brussel, Brussels, Belgium Department of Clinical Pharmacology and Clinical Pharmacy, Universitair Ziekenhuis Brussel, Brussels, Belgium

Ilse J. Smolders
Laboratory of Pharmaceutical Chemistry, Drug Analysis and Drug Information (FASC), Research Group Experimental Pharmacology (EFAR), Center for Neurosciences (C4N), Vrije Universiteit Brussel, Brussels, Belgium

Dimitri Ryczko
Groupe de Recherche sur le Système Nerveux Central, Département de Neurosciences, Université de Montréal, Montréal, QC, Canada

Réjean Dubuc
Groupe de Recherche sur le Système Nerveux Central, Département de Neurosciences, Université de Montréal, Montréal, QC, Canada Groupe de Recherche en Activité Physique Adaptée, Département des Sciences de l'Activité Physique, Université du Québec à Montréal, Montréal, QC, Canada

Wen-Wen Wang
The Center of Traditional Chinese Medicine, The Second Affiliated Hospital, Yuying Children's Hospital of Wenzhou Medical University, Wenzhou, China

Man-Man Zhang, Xing-Ru Zhang, Zeng-Rui Zhang, Jie Chen, Liang Feng and Cheng-Long Xie
Department of Neurology, The First Affiliated Hospital of Wenzhou Medical University, Wenzhou, China

Lili Hou
Department of Respiratory and Critical Care Medicine, Shanghai General Hospital, Shanghai Jiao Tong University, Shanghai, China Department of Neurobiology, School of Basic Medical Sciences, Fudan University, Shanghai, China Department of Respiratory Medicine, Zhongshan Hospital, Fudan University, Shanghai, China

Min Zhang, Xingyi Zhang, Zhenwei Liu, Pengyu Zhang and Xin Zhou
Department of Respiratory and Critical Care Medicine, Shanghai General Hospital, Shanghai Jiao Tong University, Shanghai, China

Dongying Qiu
Department of Neurobiology, School of Basic Medical Sciences, Fudan University, Shanghai, China Department of Physiology and Pathophysiology, School of Basic Medical Sciences, Fudan University, Shanghai, China Department of Gerontology, Zhongshan Hospital, Fudan University, Shanghai, China

Lei Zhu
Department of Respiratory Medicine, Zhongshan Hospital, Fudan University, Shanghai, China

Shashwati Geed
Motor Systems Physiology Laboratory, Department of Kinesiology, University of Wisconsin–Madison, Madison, WI, USA Department of Rehabilitation Medicine, Georgetown University Medical Center, Washington, DC, USA

Martha L. McCurdy and Peter L. E. van Kan
Motor Systems Physiology Laboratory, Department of Kinesiology, University of Wisconsin–Madison, Madison, WI, USA

Hui-Zhong Wen, Shi-Hao Gao, Yan-Dong Zhao and Huai-Zhen Ruan
Department of Neurobiology, College of Basic Medical Science, Chongqing Key Laboratory of Neurobiology, Third Military Medical University, Chongqing, China

Wen-Juan He
Department of Pathophysiology and High Altitudepathology, College of High Altitude Military Medicine, Third Military Medical University, Chongqing, China

Xue-Long Tian
Bioengineering College, Chongqing University, Chongqing, China

Kazunori Sasaki
Interdisciplinary Research Center for Catalytic Chemistry, National Institute of Advanced Industrial Science and Technology, Tsukuba, Japan Faculty of Pure and Applied Sciences, University of Tsukuba, Tsukuba, Japan

Mahmoud B. Othman
Alliance for Research on North Africa, University of Tsukuba, Tsukuba, Japan

Mikihide Demura
Algal Biomass and Energy System R&D Center, University of Tsukuba, Tsukuba, Japan

Makoto Watanabe
Algal Biomass and Energy System R&D Center, University of Tsukuba, Tsukuba, Japan Faculty of Life and Environmental Sciences, University of Tsukuba, Tsukuba, Japan

Hiroko Isoda
Alliance for Research on North Africa, University of Tsukuba, Tsukuba, Japan Faculty of Life and Environmental Sciences, University of Tsukuba, Tsukuba, Japan

Kazuo Nakamoto, Fuka Aizawa, Megumi Kinoshita and Shogo Tokuyama
Department of Clinical Pharmacy, School of Pharmaceutical Sciences, Kobe Gakuin University, Kobe, Japan

Yutaka Koyama
Laboratory of Pharmacology, Faculty of Pharmacy, Osaka Ohtani University, Osaka, Japan

Yi Yuan and Zhitao Ma
Institute of Electrical Engineering, Yanshan University, Qinhuangdao, China

Jiaqing Yan
School of Electrical and Control Engineering, North China University of Technology, Beijing, China

Xiaoli Li
State Key Laboratory of Cognitive Neuroscience and Learning and IDG/McGovern Institute for Brain Research, Beijing Normal University, Beijing, China
Center for Collaboration and Innovation in Brain and Learning Sciences, Beijing Normal University, Beijing, China

Walter J. Jermakowicz
The Miami Project to Cure Paralysis, Miller School of Medicine, University of Miami, Miami, FL, USA
Department of Neurological Surgery, Miller School of Medicine, University of Miami, Miami, FL, USA

Ian D. Hentall and Eva Widerström-Noga
The Miami Project to Cure Paralysis, Miller School of Medicine, University of Miami, Miami, FL, USA
Department of Neurological Surgery, Miller School of Medicine, University of Miami, Miami, FL, USA
Research Service, Bruce W. Carter Department of Veterans Affairs Medical Center, Miami, FL, USA

Jonathan R. Jagid and James Adcock
The Miami Project to Cure Paralysis, Miller School of Medicine, University of Miami, Miami, FL, USA
Research Service, Bruce W. Carter Department of Veterans Affairs Medical Center, Miami, FL, USA

Corneliu C. Luca
Research Service, Bruce W. Carter Department of Veterans Affairs Medical Center, Miami, FL, USA
Department of Neurology, Miller School of Medicine, University of Miami, Miami, FL, USA

Alberto Martinez-Arizala
The Miami Project to Cure Paralysis, Miller School of Medicine, University of Miami, Miami, FL, USA
Department of Neurological Surgery, Miller School of Medicine, University of Miami, Miami, FL, USA
Research Service, Bruce W. Carter Department of Veterans Affairs Medical Center, Miami, FL, USA
Department of Neurology, Miller School of Medicine, University of Miami, Miami, FL, USA

Yang Bai, Zhenhu Liang and Yong Wang
Institute of Electrical Engineering, Yanshan University, Qinhuangdao, China

Xiaoyu Xia, Yi Yang and Jianghong He
Department of Neurosurgery, PLA General Hospital, Beijing, China

Céline Jean-Xavier and Marie-Claude Perreault
Department of Physiology, Emory University School of Medicine, Atlanta, GA, United States

Bin Li, Xiao-Yang Zhang, Xiao-Chun Peng, Zhang-Peng Chen, Jia-Yuan Zhou, Jian-Jun Wang and Jing-Ning Zhu
State Key Laboratory of Pharmaceutical Biotechnology and Department of Biological Science and Technology, School of Life Sciences, Nanjing University, Nanjing, China

Ai-Hong Yang
State Key Laboratory of Pharmaceutical Biotechnology and Department of Biological Science and Technology, School of Life Sciences, Nanjing University, Nanjing, ChinaDepartment of Medicine, Huaibei Vocational and Technical College, Huaibei, China

Ying-Shing Chan
Department of Physiology, LKS Faculty of Medicine, The University of Hong Kong, Hong Kong

Brian R. Noga, Francisco J. Sanchez, Luz M. Villamil and Christopher O'Toole
The Miami Project to Cure Paralysis, Department of Neurological Surgery, University of Miami Miller School of Medicine, Miami, FL, United States

Stefan Kasicki, Maciej Olszewski, Anna M. Cabaj, Henryk Majczyński and Urszula Sławińska
Department of Neurophysiology, Nencki Institute of Experimental Biology, Warsaw, Poland

Larry M. Jordan
Department of Physiology, Spinal Cord Research Centre, University of Manitoba, Winnipeg, MB, Canada

Yusuf O. Cakmak
Department of Anatomy, School of Medical Sciences, Otago University, Dunedin, New Zealand

Hülya Apaydin, Güneş Kiziltan, Ayşegül Gündüz and Sibel Ertan
Department of Neurology, Cerrahpasa School of Medicine, Istanbul University, Istanbul, Turkey

Burak Ozsoy
Global Dynamic Systems (GDS) ARGE, Teknopark Istanbul, Istanbul, Turkey

Selim Olcer and Hakan Urey
Department of Electrical Engineering, College of Engineering, Koç University, Istanbul, Turkey

Ozgur O. Cakmak and Yasemin G. Ozdemir
Department of Neurology, School of Medicine, KoçUniversity, Istanbul, Turkey

Mo Chen, Rebekah L. S. Summers, Cecília N. Prudente and Teresa J. Kimberley
Divisions of Physical Therapy and Rehabilitation Science, Department of Rehabilitation Medicine, School of Medicine, University of Minnesota, Minneapolis, MN, USA

George S. Goding
Department of Otolaryngology-Head and Neck Surgery, University of Minnesota, Minneapolis, MN,USA

Sharyl Samargia
Department of Communication Sciences and Disorders University of Wisconsin River Falls Campus, River Falls, WI, USA

Christy L. Ludlow
Department of Communication Sciences and Disorders, James Madison University, Harrisonburg, VA, USA

Linda H. Kim, Simon A. Sharples and Kyle A. Mayr
Hotchkiss Brain Institute, University of Calgary, Calgary, AB, Canada Department of Neuroscience, University of Calgary, Calgary, AB, Canada

Sandeep Sharma and Charlie H. T. Kwok
Hotchkiss Brain Institute, University of Calgary, Calgary, AB, Canada Department of Comparative Biology and Experimental Medicine, University of Calgary, Calgary, AB, Canada

Patrick J. Whelan
Hotchkiss Brain Institute, University of Calgary, Calgary, AB, Canada Department of Neuroscience, University of Calgary, Calgary, AB, Canada Department of Comparative Biology and Experimental Medicine, University of Calgary, Calgary, AB, Canada

Index

www.ingramcontent.com/pod-product-compliance
Lightning Source LLC
LaVergne TN
LVHW082211200926
848484LV00008B/2240

* 9 7 9 8 8 8 7 4 0 3 1 6 8 *